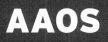

Fourth Edition

First Responder

Your First Response in Emergency Care

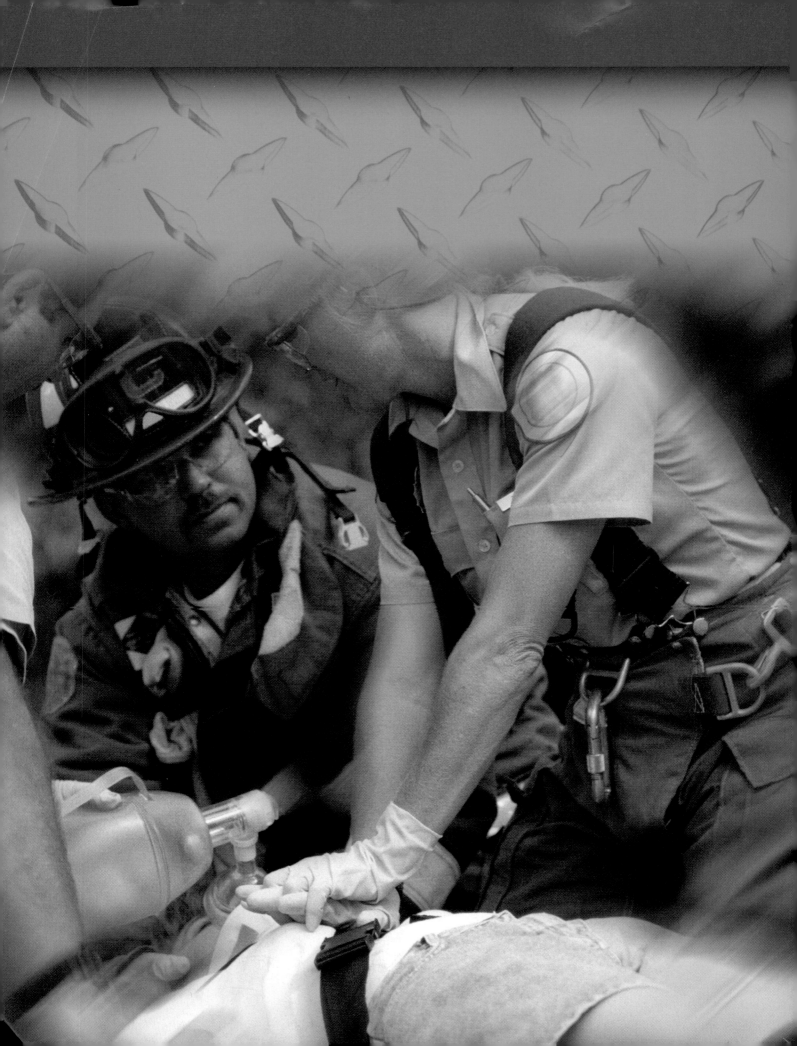

First Responder
Your First Response in Emergency Care

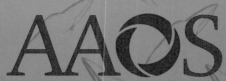

AMERICAN ACADEMY OF ORTHOPAEDIC SURGEONS

Series Editor:
Andrew N. Pollak, MD, FAAOS

Author:
David Schottke, RN, NREMT-P, MPH

JONES AND BARTLETT PUBLISHERS

Sudbury, Massachusetts

BOSTON   TORONTO   LONDON   SINGAPORE

World Headquarters

Jones and Bartlett Publishers
40 Tall Pine Drive
Sudbury, MA 01776
978-443-5000
info@jbpub.com
www.EMSzone.com

Jones and Bartlett Publishers Canada
6339 Ormindale Way
Mississauga, ON L5V 1J2
Canada

Jones and Bartlett Publishers International
Barb House, Barb Mews
London W6 7PA
United Kingdom

Jones and Bartlett's books and products are available through most bookstores and online booksellers. To contact Jones and Bartlett Publishers directly, call 800-832-0034, fax 978-443-8000, or visit our website www.jbpub.com.

Substantial discounts on bulk quantities of Jones and Bartlett's publications are available to corporations, professional associations, and other qualified organizations. For details and specific discount information, contact the special sales department at Jones and Bartlett via the above contact information or send an email to specialsales@jbpub.com.

AAOS
AMERICAN ASSOCIATION OF
ORTHOPAEDIC SURGEONS

Editorial Credits
Chief Education Officer: Mark W. Wieting
Director, Department of Publications: Marilyn L. Fox, PhD
Managing Editor: Barbara A. Scotese

ISBN-13: 978-0-7637-4031-3
ISBN-10: 0-7637-4031-4

Production Credits
Chief Executive Officer: Clayton E. Jones
Chief Operating Officer: Donald W. Jones, Jr.
President, Higher Education and Professional Publishing: Robert W. Holland, Jr.
V.P., Sales and Marketing: William J. Kane
V.P., Production and Design: Anne Spencer
V.P., Manufacturing and Inventory Control: Therese Connell
Publisher, Public Safety Group: Kimberly Brophy
Acquisitions Editor, EMS: Christine Emerton
Production Editor: Susan Schultz

Text Design: Anne Spencer and Kristin Ohlin
Composition: Graphic World
Cover Design: Kristin Ohlin
Photo Research Manager: Kimberly Potvin
Cover Photograph: © Craig Jackson/ InTheDarkPhotography.com
Voices of Experience photo: © Comstock Images/ Alamy Images
Printing and Binding: Courier Corporation

The procedures and protocols in this book are based on the most current recommendations of responsible medical sources. The American Academy of Orthopaedic Surgeons and the Publisher, however, make no guarantee as to, and assume no responsibility for the correctness, sufficiency or completeness of such information or recommendations. Other or additional safety measures may be required under particular circumstances.

This textbook is intended solely as a guide to the appropriate procedures to be employed when rendering emergency care to the sick and injured. It is not intended as a statement of the standards of care required in any particular situation, because circumstances and the patient's physical condition can vary widely from one emergency to another. Nor is it intended that this textbook shall in any way advise emergency personnel concerning legal authority to perform the activities or procedures discussed. Such local determinations should be made only with the aid of legal counsel.

Notice: The patients described in "You are the Provider" and "Assessment in Action" throughout this text are fictitious.

Library of Congress Cataloging-in-Publication Data
Schottke, David.
 First responder : your first response in emergency care / Dave Schottke. — 4th ed.
   p. ; cm.
 ISBN 0-7637-4031-4 (pbk.)
1. Medical emergencies. 2. Emergency medical technicians. 3. First aid in illness and injury. I. American Academy of Orthopaedic Surgeons. II. Title.
 [DNLM: 1. Emergencies—Examination Questions. 2. Emergency Medical Technicians—education—Examination Questions. 3. Emergency Medical Technicians—standards—Examination Questions. 4. Emergency Treatment—Examination Questions. WB 18.2 S375f 2007]
 RC86.7.S35 2007
 616.02'5—dc22
                         2006013535
6048

Additional illustration and photo credits appear on page 536, which constitutes a continuation of this copyright page.
Printed in the United States of America
11 10 09 08 07   10 9 8 7 6 5 4 3

Brief Contents

Contents

SECTION 1
Preparing to Be a First Responder 2

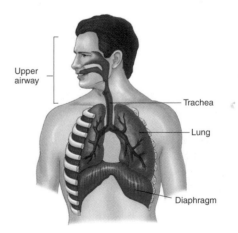

Upper airway

Trachea

Lung

Diaphragm

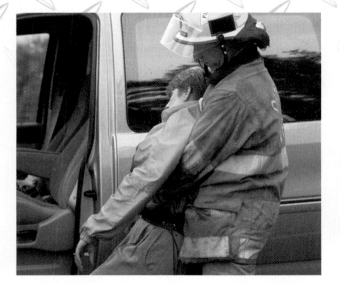

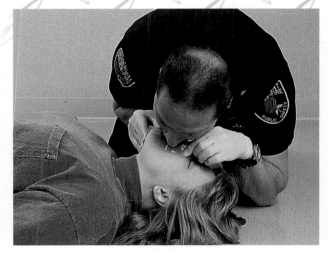

5   Lifting and Moving Patients 66

SECTION 2
Airway   98

6   Airway Management   100

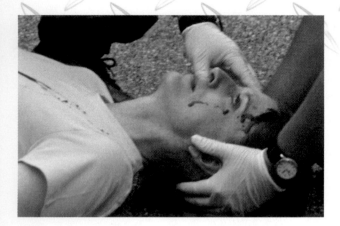

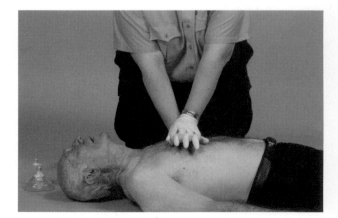

SECTION 5
Illness and Injury   228

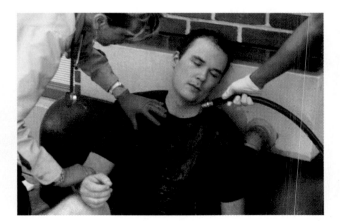

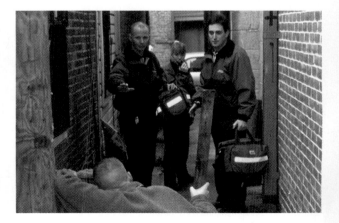

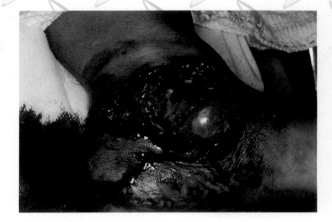

13   Bleeding, Shock, and Soft-Tissue Injuries   288

14   Injuries to Muscles and Bones   326

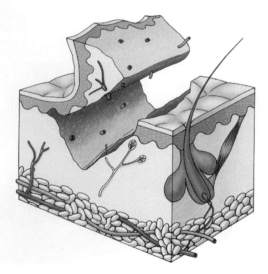

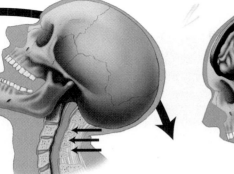
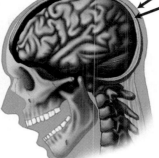

SECTION 6
Childbirth, Pediatrics, and Geriatrics 368

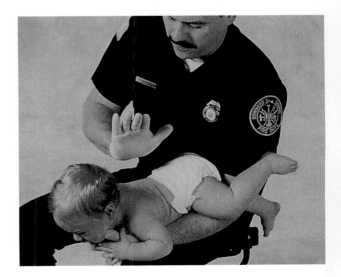

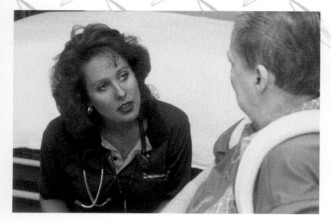

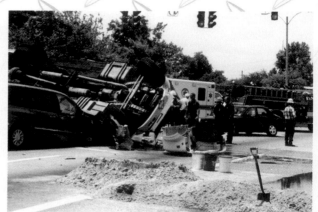

SECTION 7
EMS Operations   **432**

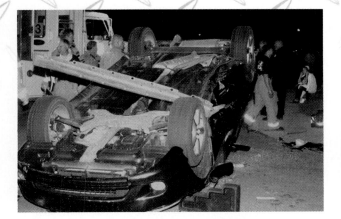

SECTION 8
Enrichment   478

First Responder Skill Drills

Resource Preview

The American Academy of Orthopaedic Surgeons is pleased to bring you *First Responder, Fourth Edition*, a modern integrated teaching and learning system. The Fourth Edition offers an assessment-based approach to first responder training and has been revised to reflect the latest Cardiopulmonary Resuscitation and Emergency Cardiac Care Guidelines.

First Responder fully addresses the objectives in the U.S. Department of Transportation (DOT) First Responder National Standard Curriculum to provide the knowledge and skills needed to work as a first responder. Additionally, some topics are covered in greater depth and are identified as supplemental material by an FYI icon.

Effective first responders need to understand four basic principles. These are:

1. Know what you should not do.
2. Know how to use your first responder life support kit.
3. Know how to improvise.
4. Know how to assist other emergency medical services providers.

This text has been written with these principles in mind. By continuing to remember the four principles, students will be able to better understand the different roles they will have as first responders.

Chapter Resources

The text is the core of the teaching and learning system with features that reinforce and expand on essential information. These features include:

Chapter Objectives Department of Transportation (DOT) First Responder National Standard Curriculum objectives and additional chapter-specific objectives are provided for each chapter, with corresponding page references.

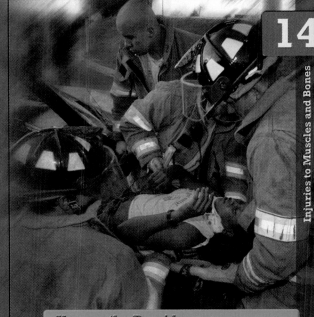

You are the Provider Each chapter contains a case study to help students begin thinking about what they might do if they encountered a similar case in the field. A summary of the case study concludes the chapter. This feature is a valuable learning tool that encourages critical thinking skills.

Technology Toolbar Found at the beginning of each chapter, the technology toolbar guides the student through the resources available for that chapter at **www.FirstResponder.EMSzone.com**.

---

106   Section 2 Airway

Introduction

This chapter introduces the two most important lifesaving skills: airway care and rescue breathing. Patients must have an open airway passage and must maintain adequate breathing to survive. By learning and practicing the simple skills in this chapter, you can often make the difference between life and death for a patient.

A review of the major structures of the respiratory system is needed before you practice airway and rescue breathing skills. Once you learn the functions of these structures, you will be a long way down the road to becoming proficient in performing these skills.

The skills of airway care and rescue breathing are as easy as A and B—the "A" stands for airway, and the "B" stands for breathing. Because you must assess and correct the airway before you turn your attention to the patient's breathing status, it is helpful to remember the AB sequence. In Chapter 9, "C" will be added for the assessment and correction of the patient's circulation. As you learn the skills presented in this chapter and in Chapter 9, remember the ABC sequence. A second mnemonic that will be used throughout both this chapter and Chapter 9 is "check and correct." By using this two-step sequence for each of the ABCs, you will be able to remember the steps needed to check

and correct problems involving the patient's airway, breathing, and circulation.

The "A" or airway section presents airway skills, including how to check the level of consciousness (responsiveness) and manually correct a blocked airway by using the head tilt–chin lift and jaw-thrust techniques. You must check the patient's airway for foreign objects. If you find foreign objects, you must correct the problem and remove the objects by using either a manual technique or a suction device. You will learn when and how to use oral and nasal airways to keep the patient's airway open.

The "B" or breathing section describes how to check patients to determine whether they are breathing adequately. You will learn how to correct breathing problems by using three rescue breathing techniques: mouth-to-mask, mouth-to-barrier device, and mouth-to-mouth.

Finally, you will learn how to check patients to determine if they have an airway obstruction that can cause death in only a few minutes. You will learn how to correct this condition using manual techniques that require no special equipment.

As you study this chapter, remember the check-and-correct process for both airway and breathing skills. Do not forget that the A and B skills presented in this chapter will be followed by C (for circulation) skills in Chapter 9. After you have learned the airway, breathing, and circulation skills (the ABCs), you will be able to perform **cardiopulmonary resuscitation (CPR)**. CPR is used to save the lives of people suffering from cardiac arrest.*

Anatomy and Function of the Respiratory System

To maintain life, all organisms must receive a constant supply of certain substances. In human beings, these basic life-sustaining substances are food, water, and **oxygen (O₂)**. A person can live several weeks without food because the body can

*The material presented in this book concerning CPR is intended to follow the CPR guidelines of the American Heart Association (AHA). Although the information presented here follows AHA guidelines at the time of publication, these guidelines are subject to periodic revision. You should follow the AHA's most current CPR guidelines.

Technology

Interactivities
Vocabulary Explorer
Anatomy Review
Web Links
Online Review Manual

www.FirstResponder.EMSzone.com

Skill Drills Provide written step-by-step explanations and visual summaries of key skills in a format that enhances student comprehension.

Chapter 9 Professional Rescuer CP

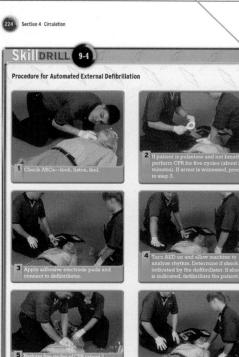

Figure 9-17
An automated external defibrillator.

Performing Automated External Defibrillation

The steps for using an AED are listed in Skill Drill 9-4 ▶.

1. If you arrive on the scene before an AED is available, check the patient for responsiveness, airway, breathing, and circulation Step 1. If the patient is unresponsive, is not breathing, and has no pulse, you should begin CPR Step 2.

2. If you arrive with an AED and have been trained in its use, first check the patient for responsiveness, airway, breathing, and circulation. If the patient's cardiac arrest was not witnessed, perform five cycles of CPR (about 2 minutes) before beginning the AED procedure. If the cardiac arrest was witnessed, apply the AED as soon as possible.

3. Once the AED is brought to the scene, quickly attach the adhesive electrode pads to the patient Step 3. Minimize interruptions in performing CPR.

4. Stop CPR and remove your hands from the patient before you turn on the

defibrillator. No one should touch t
patient once the machine has been
on and is analyzing the heart rhythr

5. Allow the defibrillator to analyze fo
shockable rhythm. If a shockable rh
found, the machine quickly recommends
defibrillation. You should first say, "Clear
the patient" and ensure that no one i
touching the patient before you pres
"shock" button on the defibrillator

6. After one shock is delivered, immed
resume CPR. Perform five cycles of
(about 2 minutes) starting with che
compressions Step 5. Stop CPR and
remove your hands from the patien
Press the defibrillator to analyze the
rhythm. If another shock is recommended, "clear" the patient, and
administer another shock. Continu
sequence of five cycles of CPR, anal
and shock until the defibrillator
recommends no further shocks.

7. Check the patient's pulse. If a pulse
present, check breathing and suppo
ventilations if necessary Step 6.

8. If no pulse, resume five cycles of CP
(about 2 minutes) starting with che
compressions. Check rhythm every
cycles. Continue until ALS provider
over or the patient starts to move.

If, after five cycles (about 2 minu
CPR, the defibrillator advises no shock,
the patient's pulse for at least 5 seconds
more than 10 seconds. If the pulse is a
resume CPR. If the pulse is present, ch
breathing. Support ventilations if nec
When advanced life support personnel
at the scene, they will assume control a
sponsibility for the patient's care.

AEDs vary in their operation so lea
to use your specific AED. You must have th
ing required by your medical director in o
practice this procedure. Practice until y
perform the procedure quickly and safe
cause the recommended guidelines for pe
ing AED change, always follow the most c
Emergency Cardiac Care (ECC) guidelin

---

224   Section 4 Circulation

SkillDRILL   9-4

Procedure for Automated External Defibrillation

1 Check ABCs—look, listen, feel.

2 If patient is pulseless and not breathing, perform CPR for five cycles (about 2 minutes). If arrest is witnessed, proceed to step 3.

3 Apply adhesive electrode pads and connect to defibrillator.

4 Turn AED on and allow machine to analyze rhythm. Determine if shock is indicated by the defibrillator. If shock is indicated, defibrillate the patient.

5 Perform five cycles of CPR (about 2 minutes) starting with chest compressions. Repeat Steps 4 and 5 until defibrillator no longer recommends a shock.

6 When no shock is recommended, check the pulse. If no pulse is present, check and correct breathing.

Vital Vocabulary Key terms are easily identified and explained within the text. A complete list with definitions follows each chapter.

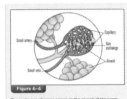

flapper valve that allows air to enter the trachea but helps prevent food or water from doing so. Air passes from the throat to the larynx (voice box), which can be seen externally as the Adam's apple in the neck. Below the trachea, the **airway** divides into the **bronchi** (two large tubes). The bronchi branch into smaller and smaller airways in the **lungs**. The lungs are located on either side of the heart and are protected by the sternum at the front and by the rib cage at the sides and back Figure 6-3.

The airways branch into smaller and smaller passages, which end as tiny air sacs called **alveoli**. The alveoli are surrounded by very small blood vessels, the **capillaries**. The actual exchange of gases takes place across a thin membrane that separates the capillaries of the circulatory system from the alveoli of the lungs Figure 6-4. The incoming oxygen passes from the alveoli into the blood, and the outgoing carbon dioxide passes from the blood into the alveoli.

The lungs consist of soft, spongy tissue with no muscles. Therefore, movement of air into the lungs depends on movement of the rib cage and the diaphragm. As the rib cage expands, air is drawn into the lungs through the trachea. The diaphragm, a muscle that separates the abdominal cavity from the chest, is dome shaped when it is relaxed. When the diaphragm contracts, it flattens and moves downward. This action in-

creases the size of the chest cavity and draws air into the lungs through the trachea. In normal breathing, the combined actions of the diaphragm and the rib cage automatically produce adequate inhalation and exhalation Figure 6-5.

Figure 6-4

The exchange of gases occurs in the alveoli of the lungs.

Special Populations

- The structures of the respiratory systems in children and infants are smaller than they are in adults. Thus the air passages of children and infants may be more easily blocked by secretions or by foreign objects.
- In children and infants, the tongue is proportionally larger than it is in adults. Thus, the tongue of these smaller patients is more likely to block their airway than it would in an adult patient.
- Because the trachea of an infant or child is more flexible than that of an adult, it is more likely to become narrowed or blocked than that of an adult.
- The head of a child or an infant is proportionally larger than the head of an adult. You will have to learn slightly different techniques for opening the airways of children.
- Children and infants have smaller lungs than adults. You need to give them smaller breaths when you perform rescue breathing.
- Most children and infants have healthy hearts. When a child or infant suffers cardiac arrest (stoppage of the heart), it is usually because the patient has a blocked airway or has stopped breathing, not because there is a problem with the heart.

Figure 6-3

Anatomy of the respiratory system.

Epiglottis
Larynx (voicebox)
Trachea (windpipe)
Esophagus
Bronchi
Rib cage
Lung

Special Populations Discuss the specific needs and emergency care of special populations.

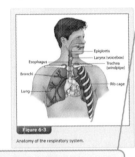

6 Airway Management   117

Voices of Experience

Making a Difference

It was a dark and stormy night—really, it was! My family and I were traveling on Interstate 5 to my parent's house to spend Christmas. It was cold and getting icy on some of the overpasses. As my car crested the top of one of the overpasses, I saw six headlights in my lane pointing in various directions. I may not know much about cars, but I did know that this wasn't right.

I walked up to the three cars that had obviously slid on the ice coming over the overpass. They had struck each other and spun around so that all three were facing the wrong way on the freeway. Two people were getting out of one of the cars; this car looked the worst. The second car looked a little better, but the driver was still inside. I walked up to the door, thinking that if the people in the more damaged car were all right, this driver would be all right also.

> **The patient was breathing, and all I could think was: "Did I do that?"**

Well, math doesn't always work like it should and patients *never* read the textbook. I remember asking if he was OK as I looked up and saw the lights of a fire engine approaching. I thought it was strange that the man didn't answer me, so I looked down and froze; the man didn't talk, he didn't move—he wasn't breathing. The next thing I knew I was yelling for help, but the fire fighters didn't come. They couldn't hear me over the traffic.

Even while I was panicking, I saw my hand reach in and lift the patient's head. Just that fast, he changed from a man to a patient. Without even realizing what I was doing, my hand reached in and lifted his head; my other hand also entered the car and I was doing a jaw thrust on the patient. While I was wondering if I had actually done the airway maneuver or just imagined it, I heard something. It sounded like thunder bursting out of the patient's chest and mouth. It was a breath! The patient was breathing, and all I could think was: "Did I do that?" I must have, although I didn't remember doing anything. Then I looked down at my hands and the patient (my instructors would be proud); I was doing a perfect jaw-thrust maneuver.

I felt a hand on my back. I looked and it was a paramedic telling me he would take over the airway. I let go and watched as the paramedics packaged "my" patient and put him in the ambulance. Later, I was told that I had done a good job and that I had probably saved the patient's life. I think I told that story to everyone I knew—and a few people I didn't know—that Christmas.

The night of that accident, I wasn't a paramedic; I wasn't an EMT. I was a first responder. I was debating whether I wanted to go on to EMT training or do other things. I hadn't even used my skills on a real person, except for my "victim" during my practical exam. That night the training took over; it worked as if it was the most natural thing in the world. I was a first responder and I had helped someone and saved his life. Anyone who tells you that you are "just" a first responder is wrong! If a first responder hadn't been there on that dark and stormy night, that man would have died. As a first responder, you can and will make a difference.

Fifteen years later, I look back and smile. I made a difference that night.

David K. Anderson, BS, EMT-P
Director of Paramedic Education
Northwest Regional Training Center
Vancouver, Washington

Voices of Experience Veteran EMS providers share accounts of memorable incidents and offer advice and encouragement.

FYI FYI sections cover additional information for further study. This material goes beyond the scope of the DOT curriculum and may be incorporated at the instructor's discretion.

Treatment Tips Offer additional treatment information or reinforce treatment information provided in the text.

---

334   Section 5 Illness and Injury

each relevant term. Regardless of the terminology used, the most important part of the first responder's job is to provide the best assessment and treatment for the patient.

Types of Injuries

It is often difficult to distinguish one type of musculoskeletal extremity injury from another. All three types are serious, and all extremity injuries must be identified so they can receive appropriate medical treatment.

Fractures

A *fracture* is a broken bone. Fractures can be caused by a variety of mechanisms, but require a significant force, unless the bone is weakened by a disease such as osteoporosis. Fractures are generally classified as either closed or open **Figure 14-6 ▾**. In the more common **closed fracture**, the bone is broken but there is no break in the skin.

In an **open fracture**, the bone is broken and the overlying skin is lacerated. The open wound can be caused by a penetrating object, such as a bullet, or by the fractured bone end itself protruding through the skin. Open fractures are contaminated by dirt and bacteria that may lead to

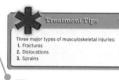

Treatment Tips

Three major types of musculoskeletal injuries:
1. Fractures
2. Dislocations
3. Sprains

infection. Both open and closed fractures injure adjacent soft tissues, resulting in bleeding at the fracture site. Fractures can also injure nearby nerves and blood vessels, causing severe nerve injury and excessive bleeding.

Dislocations

A **dislocation** is a disruption that tears the supporting ligaments of the joint. The bone ends that make up the joint separate completely from each other and can lock in one position. Any attempt to move a dislocated joint is very painful. Because many nerves and blood vessels lie near joints, a dislocation can damage these structures as well.

Sprains and Strains

A **sprain** is a joint injury caused by excessive stretching of the supporting ligaments. It can be

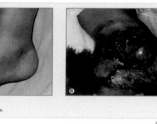

Figure 14-6
A, Closed fracture. B, Open fracture.

Chapter 14 Injuries to Muscles and Bones   335

thought of as a partial dislocation. Strains are caused by stretching or tearing of a muscle.

Body Substance Isolation and Musculoskeletal Injuries

As you examine and treat patients with musculoskeletal injuries, you need to practice BSI. These patients may have open wounds related to the musculoskeletal injury or to a separate, open soft-tissue injury. You should assume that trauma patients have open wounds that pose a threat of infection. Wear approved gloves. When responding to motor vehicle crashes or other situations that may present a hazard from broken glass or other sharp objects, it is wise to wear heavy rescue gloves that provide protection from sharp objects. Some first responders wear latex or vinyl gloves under the heavy rescue gloves for added BSI protection. If the patient has active bleeding that may splatter, you should have protection for your eyes, nose, and mouth as well.

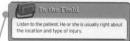

Safety Tips

BSI is for your protection.

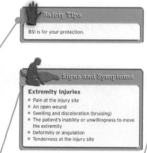

Signs and Symptoms

Extremity Injuries
- Pain at the injury site
- An open wound
- Swelling and discoloration (bruising)
- The patient's inability or unwillingness to move the extremity
- Deformity or angulation
- Tenderness at the injury site

Examination of Musculoskeletal Injuries

There are three essential steps in examining a patient with a limb injury:
1. General assessment of the patient according to the patient assessment sequence
2. Examination of the injured part
3. Evaluation of the circulation and sensation in the injured limb

General Patient Assessment

A general, initial assessment of the injured patient must be carried out before focusing attention on any injured limb. All of the steps in the patient assessment must be followed. Once you have checked and stabilized the patient's airway, breathing, and circulation (ABCs), you can then direct your attention to the injured limb identified during the physical examination.

Limb injuries are not life threatening unless there is excessive bleeding from an open wound. Therefore, it is essential that you stabilize the airway, breathing, and circulation before you focus on the limb injury, regardless of the pain or deformity that may be present at that injury site.

As you examine and treat patients with musculoskeletal injuries remember that this is a scary and painful experience for them. Explain what you are doing as you conduct your examination and stabilize the patient. Treat the patient with the same care and consideration that you would give to a close member of your own family.

Examining the Injured Limb

As a first responder, you should initially inspect the injured limb and compare it to the

In the Field

Listen to the patient. He or she is usually right about the location and type of injury.

Safety Tips Reinforce safety concerns for both the responder and the patient.

In the Field Discuss practical applications of material for use in the field.

Signs and Symptoms List signs and symptoms of the relevant injury/illness.

Prep Kit End-of-chapter materials and activities reinforce important concepts and evaluate students' mastery of the subject.
- **Ready for Review** thoroughly summarizes chapter content.
- **Vital Vocabulary** provides key terms and definitions from the chapter.
- **Assessment in Action** promotes critical thinking through the use of case studies and provides instructors with discussion points for classroom presentation.

Prep Kit

Ready for Review

The Ready for Review thoroughly summarizes the chapter.

- The first responder is the first medically trained person to arrive on the scene. The initial care provided is essential because it is available sooner than more advanced emergency medical care and could mean the difference between life and death.
- The four basic goals of first responder training are to know what not to do, know how to use your first responder life support kit, know how to improvise, and know how to assist other EMS providers.
- First responders should understand their roles in the EMS system. The typical sequence of events of the EMS system is reporting, dispatch, first response, EMS response, and hospital care.
- As a first responder, your primary goal is to provide immediate care for a sick or injured patient. As more highly trained personnel (EMTs or paramedics) arrive on the scene, you will assist them in treating and preparing the patient for transportation.
- Once your role in treating the patient is finished, it is important that you record your observations about the scene, the patient's condition, and the treatment you provided. Documentation should be clear, concise, accurate, and according to the accepted policies of your organization.
- Remember that medical information about a patient is confidential and should be shared only with other medical personnel who are involved in the care of that particular patient.
- The overall leader of the medical care team is the physician or medical director. To ensure that the patient receives appropriate medical treatment, it is important that first responders receive direction from a physician.

Vital Vocabulary

The Vital Vocabulary are the key terms for this chapter.

advanced life support (ALS) The use of specialized equipment such as cardiac monitors, defibrillators, intravenous fluids, drug infusion, and endotracheal intubation to stabilize the patient.

appropriate medical facility A hospital with adequate medical resources to provide continuing care to sick or injured patients who are transported after field treatment by first responders.

basic life support (BLS) Emergency lifesaving procedures performed without advanced emergency procedures to stabilize patients who have experienced sudden illness or injury.

defibrillation Delivery of an electric current through a person's chest wall and heart for the purpose of ending lethal heart rhythms such as ventricular fibrillation.

emergency medical technician-basic (EMT-B) A person who is trained and certified to provide basic life support and certain other noninvasive prehospital medical procedures.

emergency services dispatch center A fire, police, or emergency medical services (EMS) agency; a 9-1-1 center; or a seven-digit telephone number used by one or all of the emergency agencies to receive and dispatch requests for emergency care.

paramedics Emergency medical technicians who have completed an extensive course of 800 or more hours, successfully passed a national or state certification, and who can perform advanced life support skills.

Technology
- Interactivities
- Vocabulary Explorer
- Anatomy Review
- Web Links
- Online Review Manual

Assessment in Action

Assessment in Action presents a fictitious scenario to help you review what you learned in this chapter.

As a first responder, you are often the first step in the process of a patient getting the necessary care needed in an emergency situation. You will work closely with a variety of other emergency and nonemergency personnel. Your role may vary greatly depending upon the scene and the additional resources available.

1. What are some of the responsibilities of a first responder?

2. What is your role in the initial treatment of a patient?
   - A. Perform patient assessment.
   - B. Administer emergency medical care and reassurance.
   - C. Move patients only when necessary.
   - D. All of the above.

3. In what way can you be of assistance to emergency medical providers of a higher level?
   - A. Start an IV.
   - B. Interpret cardiac rhythms.
   - C. Help prepare the patient for transport.
   - D. Give epinephrine.

4. What is your role in the continuing treatment and subsequent transportation of a patient?

5. What are some of the differences in the treatment that a first responder can provide versus that of an EMT-B or paramedic?

6. What are some of the standard components of an EMS system?
   - A. Medical and support facilities
   - B. Communications system
   - C. Public information and education
   - D. Medical direction
   - E. All of the above

7. When documenting a scene, what information should you NOT include in your report?
   - A. Condition of the patient when found
   - B. The patient's description of the injury or illness
   - C. The initial and later vital signs
   - D. Patient's work history

Online Resources

At www.First Responder.EMSzone.com, innovative and interactive activities help students become great first responders.

Chapter Pretests prepare students for training. Each chapter has a pretest and provides instant results, feedback on incorrect answers, and page references for further study.

Interactivities allow your students to experiment with skills and procedures in the safety of a virtual environment.

Anatomy Review provides interactive anatomical figure labeling exercises to reinforce students' knowledge of human anatomy.

Vocabulary Explorer is your virtual dictionary. Here, students can review key terms, test their knowledge of key terms through flashcards, and complete crossword puzzles.

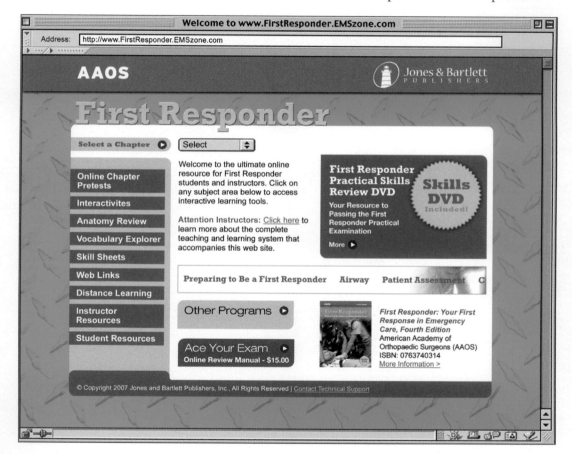

Ace Your Exam!

Online Review Manual

ISBN: 0-7637-4608-8

The **Online Review Manual** is designed to evaluate mastery of material learned in class and covered in *First Responder, Fourth Edition*. Each chapter in the book is supplemented with:

- An exam consisting of multiple-choice questions to test students' knowledge of key concepts and procedures
- A special grading feature for immediate results and answers to all of the questions
- Page references to the *Fourth Edition*

Instructor Resources

First Responder, Fourth Edition is supported by a complete teaching and learning system that was developed by educators with an intimate knowledge of the obstacles you face every day. The supplements provide practical, hands-on, time-saving tools such as PowerPoint™ presentations, customizable test banks, and web-based resources to better support you and your students.

Instructor's ToolKit CD-ROM

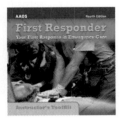

ISBN: 0-7637-4268-6

We have made it easy for you with fully adaptable:

- **Lecture Outlines** Complete, ready-to-use lesson plans from the *Instructor's Resource Manual* outline all the topics covered in the text. Lesson plans can be modified and edited to meet your needs.
- **PowerPoint™ Presentations** Provide you with a powerful way to make presentations that are educational and engaging to your students. The slides can be modified and edited to fit your individual presentation.
- **Image Bank and Table Bank** Provide many of the images and tables found in the text, allowing you to incorporate more images into the PowerPoint presentations, make handouts, or enlarge a specific image for further discussion.
- **Test Bank** A new bank of test questions that corresponds to the chapters in the text and includes both general knowledge and critical thinking questions.
- **Skill Sheets** Ready-to-use sheets that allow you to track students' skills and conduct skill proficiency exams.

The resources found on the Instructor's ToolKit CD-ROM have been formatted so that you can seamlessly integrate them into the most popular course administration tools. Please contact Jones and Bartlett Publishers technical support at any time with questions.

Instructor's Resource Manual on CD-ROM

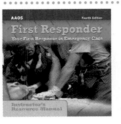

ISBN: 0-7637-4269-4

The **Instructor's Resource Manual** is your guide to the entire teaching and learning system. It has been designed to assist you with creative ideas and tools to incorporate all of the components of the teaching and learning system. For each chapter, this indispensable manual contains:

- Chapter overview and objectives
- Support materials
- Enhancements
- Teaching tips
- Readings and preparations
- Presentation overview
- Lesson plans and corresponding PowerPoint slide text
- Skill Drill evaluation sheets
- Answers to all end-of-chapter student questions found in the text
- Activities and assignments
- National Registry skill sheets

Student Resources

To help students retain the most important information and to assist them in preparing for exams, we have developed the following resources:

Student Workbook

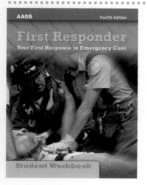

ISBN: 0-7637-4271-6

Designed to encourage critical thinking and aid comprehension of course material, a variety of interesting exercises and scenarios are provided to reinforce the objectives and concepts found in the text. It will help students achieve a fuller understanding of the role of the first responder in emergency care. The workbook offers:

- Case studies and corresponding questions
- Skill drill activities
- Figure labeling exercises
- Crossword puzzles
- Matching, fill-in-the-blank, short answer, and multiple-choice questions

First Responder Practical Skills Review DVD

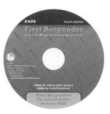

ISBN: 0-7637-4270-8

Packaged with each copy of the *Fourth Edition*, this DVD provides students with a walk-through of the skills that are required to successfully complete the national first responder practical examination process. For each skill, students can visually learn the steps and will find helpful information, tips, and pointers designed to facilitate their progression through the practical examination, specifically:

- Objectives
- Equipment
- Key steps to perform to successfully complete the skill
- Critical errors that result in failure

To the Student

As recently as the mid-1950s there were no commonly used medical techniques that were effective for restarting stopped hearts, and victims often died. Today, simple and advanced techniques can restart a stopped heart. A trained first responder can keep a person alive until advanced techniques can be performed by other medical personnel. Opening a patient's airway, performing rescue breathing, controlling external bleeding, and treating a patient for the signs and symptoms of shock can make a critical difference. Because first responders are often the first medically trained personnel on the scene of an emergency, they supply the first and vital link in a chain of survival. As you study this book, realize that you are about to become a first responder, an emergency care provider who can make a real difference to patients.

Before studying the knowledge and skills needed to become a medical first responder, it is important to understand more about the following topics:

1. Overview of the first responder course
2. Criteria for first responder certification

1. Overview of the First Responder Course

The first responder course presents an exciting opportunity to develop emergency medical skills and knowledge that will enable you to assist people who have sustained an accidental injury or who are suffering from a sudden illness or medical problem. This course follows a national curriculum that was developed by representatives from many federal and state agencies and from professional medical groups. The material you will learn is divided into seven sections, which follow the national standard curriculum. We have added an eighth section, which covers supplemental skills that may be taught to first responders in some communities. The decision about whether to cover this material will be made by course directors. These modules are:

Section 1   Preparing to Be a First Responder
Section 2   Airway
Section 3   Patient Assessment
Section 4   Circulation
Section 5   Illness and Injury
Section 6   Childbirth, Pediatrics, and Geriatrics
Section 7   EMS Operations
Section 8   Enrichment

2. Criteria for First Responder Certification

The process of becoming a first responder begins with your thorough study and mastery of the knowledge and skills presented in this book. To practice these skills you must be certified or registered as a first responder in the state where you will be working. Some states require certification or registration through a state agency such as a department of health. Other states may require you to become registered through the National Registry of Emergency Medical Technicians.

In either case, you will be required to successfully complete this course and then pass a written and practical test. Your certification or registration is good for a limited period of time. To maintain your certification or recertification, you will be required to complete certain course work to refresh your knowledge and skills and probably take a written and/or practical test. It is important to remember that your ability to function as a first responder depends on maintaining your certification or registration. It is your responsibility to do this even though you may receive help from the agency for which you work.

Acknowledgments

The American Academy of Orthopaedic Surgeons acknowledge the contributors and reviewers of *First Responder: Your First Response in Emergency Care, Fourth Edition.*

Contributors

David K. Anderson, BS, EMT-P
NW Regional Training Center
Vancouver, Washington

Sally Becker
President
Becker Training Associates
Webster, New Hampshire

T.J. Bishop, NREMT-P, WASEI
North Country EMS
Yacolt, Washington

Major Raymond W. Burton, retired
Plymouth Regional Police Academy
Plymouth, Massachusetts

Julie Chase, BS, NREMT-P
Emergency Medical Training and Consulting,
  LLC
Austin, Texas

Shaun Froshour, NREMT–P
Managing Partner
Public Safety Management Solutions
Telford, Pennsylvania

Roxann M. Gabany, RN, BSBA, EMT Instructor
New Horizons Regional Education Center
Hampton, Virginia

Samuel A. Getz, Jr., NREMT–P
President and CEO
EMS Systems Consulting Service
Austintown, Ohio

Joseph A. Grafft, MS
Retired EMS Manager, MN State Colleges &
  Universities, Office of the Chancellor
Community Faculty, Metropolitan State University, School
  of Law Enforcement
St. Paul, Minnesota

Guy H. Haskell, PhD, NREMT-P
Fire fighter, Benton Township Volunteer Fire Department,
Unionville, Indiana
Paramedic, Brown Township Fire and Rescue
Mooresville, Indiana
Director, Emergency Medical and Safety Services
  Consultants
Bloomington, Indiana

Michael Hay, MHA, LP, NREMT-P
EMS Specialist
Texas Department of State Health Services
EMS Compliance
San Antonio, Texas

Alan E. Joos, Fire Fighter/EMT-I
Assistant Director—Training
Utah Fire & Rescue Academy
Provo, Utah

Fred P. LaFemina
Battalion Chief, Rescue Operations, and Special
  Operations Command
New York City Fire Department
New York, New York

Sheri Polley, NREMT-B
Linesville Volunteer Fire Department
  Ambulance
Linesville, Pennsylvania

Terry Pool, EMT-P
Galesburg Area EMS System Coordinator
Galesburg, Illinois

Stephen J. Rahm, NREMT–P
EMS Professions Educator
Bulverde—Spring Branch EMS
Spring Branch, Texas

Angela D. Reed, EMT-B, Program Director
Pima Community College
Tucson, Arizona

John Reed, RN, EMT-P
Birmingham Regional Emergency Medical
  Services System
Birmingham, Alabama

Brent Ricks, MS, REMT-P
Hudson Valley Community College
Troy, New York

Jose V. Salazar, MPH, NREMT-P
Captain
Loudoun County Fire-Rescue
Leesburg, Virginia

Tammy Samarripa, AAS, EMT-LP
EMT/Paramedic Course Coordinator
Central Texas College
Killeen, Texas

David M. Schwartz
Director of Public Safety, retired
Forest Lake Police Department
Forest Lake, Minnesota

Robert Shields
Lieutenant, Paramedic
Cumberland Rescue Service
Cumberland, Rhode Island

Michael D. Smith, EMT-P, AS, EMSI
Grant Medical Center Lifelink
City of Grandview Heights Division of Fire
Lancaster, Ohio

Sherm Syverson, BS, NREMT-P
Emergency Medical Education Center at F-M
  Ambulance
Fargo, North Dakota

Matthew S. Zavarella, RN, REMT-P, MS, CCRN,
  CFRN, CEN
St. Vincent's Life Flight
Ypsilanti, Michigan

Reviewers

David K. Anderson, BS, EMT-P
NW Regional Training Center
Vancouver, Washington

T.J. Bishop, NREMT-P, WASEI
North Country EMS
Yacolt, Washington

Ronald R. Bowser
Maryland Fire and Rescue Institute
College Park, Maryland

Sandra Brotzman
Northampton Community College
Northampton County, Pennsylvania

Major Raymond W. Burton, Retired
Plymouth Regional Police Academy
Plymouth, Massachusetts

Catherine Camargo, EMT-B, I/C, MA
Bernalillo High School
Bernalillo, New Mexico

Paul H. Coffey, EMT-I
Massachusetts Department of Public Health,
  Office of EMS
Boston, Massachusetts

Jim Cox, EMT-P
MAST Ambulance
Kansas City, Missouri

Roxann M. Gabany, RN, BSBA, EMT Instructor
New Horizons Regional Education Center
Hampton, Virginia

Linda J Frissora-Gosselin, MS, REMT IC Ed.
Massachusetts Emergency Care Training
  Academy
Millbury, Massachusetts

Lynn Henley, NREMT-P
AAA Ambulance
Hattiesburg, Mississippi

Jan Hershberger
Southeast Community College
Lincoln, Nebraska

Camille C. Klein, RN, CCRN, BS
Hanna West Side High School Extension
Anderson, South Carolina

Shawn Komorn, MA, Licensed Paramedic,
  LVN, Assistant Professor
University of Texas Health Science Center at
  San Antonio
San Antonio, Texas

Louis B. Mallory, MBA, REMT-P
Santa Fe Community College
Gainesville, Florida

Trooper William D. McElhiney
Massachusetts State Police Academy
New Braintree, Massachusetts

Nicholas F. Miller, Jr., CCEMT-P
Barnhart, Missouri

Captain William R. Montrie, EMT-P
Owens Community College
Perrysburg, Ohio

Charles Morris, Director
North Mississippi EMS
Tupelo, Mississippi

Timothy Murphy, EMT-P
Carl Sandburg College
Galesburg, Illinois

Nona Niemeier, MS
South Central College
North Mankato, Minnesota

Cynthia Osborne
New Mexico State University
Alamogordo, New Mexico

Terry Pool, EMT-P
Galesburg Area EMS System Coordinator
Galesburg, Illinois

Angela D. Reed, EMT-B, Program Director
Pima Community College
Tucson, Arizona

John Reed, RN, EMT-P
Birmingham Regional Emergency Medical
  Services System
Birmingham, Alabama

Lisa Robles, NREMT-P, BS, EMS Program Director
Arkansas Tech University, Ozark Campus
Ozark, Arkansas

Robert F. Shields, Jr., NREMT-P, EMS
Instructor/Coordinator
Public Safety Training Associates
Chepachet, Rhode Island

Frank Slaughtner, EMT
Powell County Ambulance
Deer Lodge, Montana

Michael D. Smith, EMT-P, AS, EMSI
Grant Medical Center Lifelink
City of Grandview Heights Division of Fire
Lancaster, Ohio

Stanley M. Striefsky, EMT-P
Emergency Medical Services of N.E. Pennsylvania
Pittston, Pennsylvania

Sherm Syverson, BS, NREMT-P
Emergency Medical Education Center at F-M
  Ambulance
Fargo, North Dakota

Joe Welsh, BS, EMT-B, EMT-Instructor
Life-Savers, Inc.
Louisville, Kentucky

Lauri Wempen, EMT-I
Fremont County Ambulance
Riverton, Wyoming

Antonio A. Zamarron, EMT-P, Instructor/Coordinator
Mid Michigan Medical Center
Midland Emergency Medical Services
  Educational Services and Development
Midland, Michigan

Matthew S. Zavarella, RN, REMT-P, MS, CCRN,
  CFRN, CEN
St. Vincent's Life Flight
Ypsilanti, Michigan

Preparing to Be a First Responder

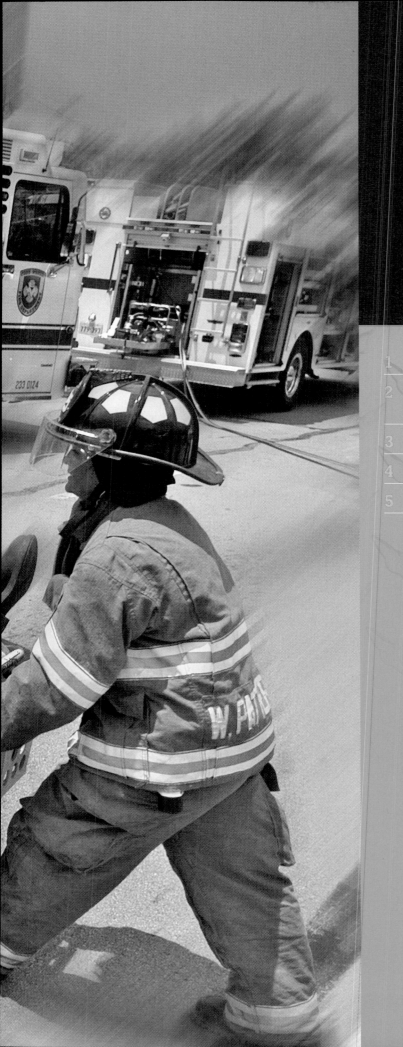

1

Introduction to the EMS System

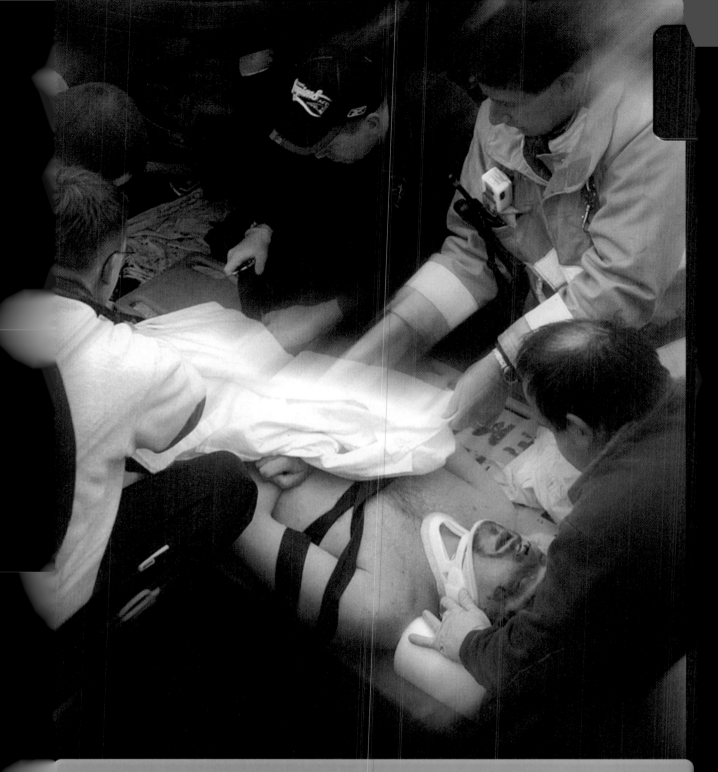

You are the Provider

Now that you have completed your first responder course, you are responsible for providing the first tier of EMS in your community. Basic and advanced life support services complement your initial response, provide additional treatment, and transport the patient to an appropriate medical facility.

1. Why is it important to learn about the components of an EMS system?
2. How does good interaction between different levels of the EMS team improve patient care?
3. Why is your role as a first responder sometimes the most important for the welfare of the patient?

Introduction

The first responder is, by definition, the first medically trained person to arrive on the scene. The initial care you give as the first responder is essential because it is available sooner than more advanced emergency medical care and could mean the difference between life and death. Your initial care is usually followed by more sophisticated care given by emergency medical technicians (EMTs), paramedics, nurses, physicians, and other allied health professionals.

First Responder Training

This book has been written for a first responder training course. Although the book alone can teach you many things, it is best to use it as part of an approved first responder course. A first responder course will teach you the basics of good patient care and the skills you will need to deliver appropriate care to the victim of an accident or sudden illness until more highly trained emergency personnel arrive. The skills and knowledge you will gain from this course provide the foundation for the entire emergency medical services

(EMS) system **Figure 1-1** . Your actions can prevent a minor situation from becoming serious and may even determine whether a patient lives or dies.

In this first responder course, you will learn how to examine patients and how to use basic emergency medical skills. These skills are divided into two main groups: (1) those needed to treat injured trauma patients and (2) those needed to care for patients suffering from illness or serious medical problems.

You will learn the following skills to stabilize and treat persons who have been injured:

- Controlling airway, breathing, and circulation (Chapters 6 and 9)
- Controlling external bleeding (hemorrhage) (Chapter 13)
- Treating shock (Chapter 13)
- Treating wounds (Chapter 13)
- Splinting injuries to stabilize extremities (Chapter 14)

In addition to these trauma skills, you will learn to recognize, stabilize, and provide initial treatment for the following medical conditions:

- Heart attacks (Chapter 10)
- Seizures (Chapter 10)
- Problems associated with excessive heat or cold (Chapter 10)
- Alcohol and drug abuse (Chapter 11)
- Poisonings (Chapter 11)
- Bites and stings (Chapter 11)
- Altered mental status (Chapter 10)
- Behavioral or psychological crises (Chapter 12)
- Emergency childbirth (Chapter 15)

Goals of First Responder Training

It is important for you to understand the basic goals of first responder training. This training aims to teach you how to evaluate, stabilize, and treat patients using a minimum of specialized equipment. As a first responder, you will find yourself in situations where little or no emergency medical equipment is readily available, so you must know how to improvise. Finally, first responder

Technology

- Interactivities
- Vocabulary Explorer
- Anatomy Review
- Web Links
- Online Review Manual

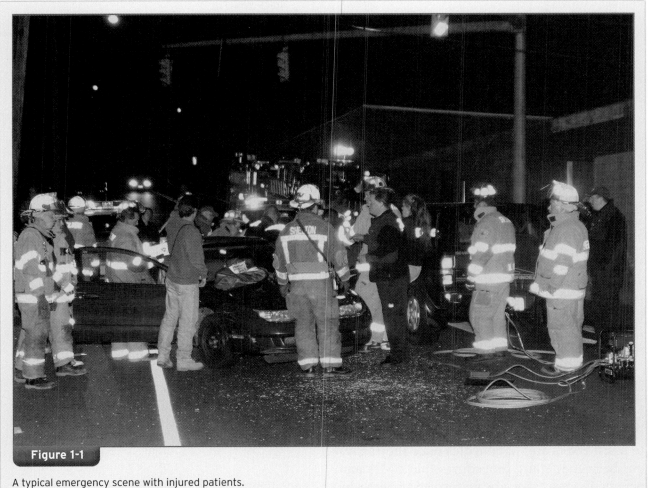

Figure 1-1

A typical emergency scene with injured patients.

training teaches you what you can do to help EMTs and paramedics when they arrive on the scene.

Know What You Should Not Do

The first lesson you must learn as a first responder is what *not* to do! For example, it may be better for you to leave a patient in the position found rather than attempt to move him or her without the proper equipment or an adequate number of trained personnel. It is also critical that you not judge a patient based on his or her cultural background, gender, age, or socioeconomic status; doing so may undermine the quality of care you provide.

Know How to Use Your First Responder Life Support Kit

The second goal of first responder training is to teach you to treat patients using limited emer-

gency medical supplies. A first responder life support kit should be small enough to fit in the trunk of an automobile or on almost any police, fire, or rescue vehicle. Although the contents of the kit are limited, such supplies are all you need to provide immediate care for most patients you will encounter. The suggested contents of a first responder life support kit are shown in **Figure 1-2 ▸** and described in **Table 1-1 ▸**.

Know How to Improvise

The third goal of first responder training is to teach you to improvise. As a trained first responder, you will often be in situations with little or no emergency medical equipment. Therefore, it is important that you know how to improvise. Although no course can teach improvisation, this course provides examples that can be applied to real-life situations. You will learn, for example, how to

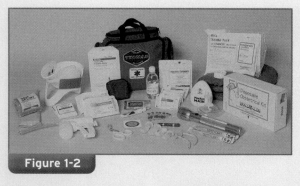

Figure 1-2

Suggested contents of a first responder life support kit.

TABLE 1-1	Suggested Contents of a First Responder Life Support Kit
Patient Examination Equipment	1 flashlight
Personal Safety Equipment	5 pairs of vinyl or latex gloves 5 face masks 1 bottle of hand sanitizer
Resuscitation Equipment	1 mouth-to-mask resuscitation device 1 portable hand-powered suction device 1 set oral airways 1 set nasal airways
Bandaging and Dressing Equipment	10 gauze-adhesive strips 1" 10 gauze pads 4" × 4" 5 gauze pads 5" × 9" 2 universal trauma dressings 10" × 30" 1 occlusive dressing for sealing chest wounds 4 conforming gauze rolls 3" × 15' 4 rolls 4½" × 15' 6 triangular bandages 1 adhesive tape 2" 1 burn sheet
Patient Immobilization Equipment	2 (each) cervical collars: small, medium, large *or* 2 adjustable cervical collars 3 rigid conforming splints (SAM splints) *or* 1 set air splints for arm and leg *or* 2 (each) cardboard splints 18" and 24"
Extrication Equipment	1 spring-loaded center punch 1 pair heavy leather gloves
Miscellaneous Equipment	2 blankets (disposable) 2 cold packs 1 bandage scissors
Other Equipment	1 set personal protective clothing (helmet, eye protection, EMS jacket) 1 reflective vest 1 fire extinguisher (5 lb ABC dry chemical) 1 *Emergency Response Guidebook* 6 fusees 1 set of binoculars

use articles of clothing and handkerchiefs to stop bleeding and how to use wooden boards, magazines, or newspapers to immobilize injured extremities.

Know How to Assist Other EMS Providers

Finally, first responder training teaches you how to assist EMTs and paramedics once they arrive on the scene. Many procedures that EMTs and paramedics use cannot be performed correctly by fewer than three people. Thus you may have to assist with these procedures and you must know what to do.

Additional Skills

First responders operate in a variety of settings. Many problems encountered in urban areas differ sharply from those found in rural settings. In addition, regional variations in climate create conditions that not only affect the situations you encounter but also require you to use different skills and equipment in treating patients. Certain skills and equipment mentioned in this book are beyond the essential, minimum knowledge level that you need to successfully complete a first responder course. However, these supplemental skills and equipment may be required in your local EMS system. Supplemental skills are identified by the following icon: FYI

The Emergency Medical Services System

The EMS system was developed because evidence showed that patients who received appropriate emergency medical care before they reached the hospital had a better chance of surviving a major accident or sudden illness than patients who did not receive such care. It is important that you understand the operation and complexity of an EMS system Figure 1-3 ▼ . Problems that occur in the "prehospital" phase of the EMS operation often focus on control and coordination of resources and personnel. Agencies and personnel need to share a mutual understanding of their roles for an EMS system to operate smoothly in both "routine" and multiple-casualty situations.

This understanding develops through close cooperation, careful planning, communication, and continual effort. You can best understand the EMS system by examining the sequence of events as an injured or ill patient moves through the system.

Reporting

The reporting of the emergency incident activates the EMS system Figure 1-4 ▼ . An **emergency services dispatch center** usually receives the phone call reporting an incident. The dispatch center may be a fire, police, or EMS agency; a 9-1-1 center; or a seven-digit emergency telephone number used by one or all of the emergency agencies. Enhanced 9-1-1 centers can determine the location of the caller by computer as soon as the telephone in the 9-1-1 center is answered.   • E911 - not in all states

Dispatch

Once the emergency services dispatch center is notified of an incident, appropriate equipment and personnel are dispatched to the scene Figure 1-5 ▶ . Dispatch may occur by pager,

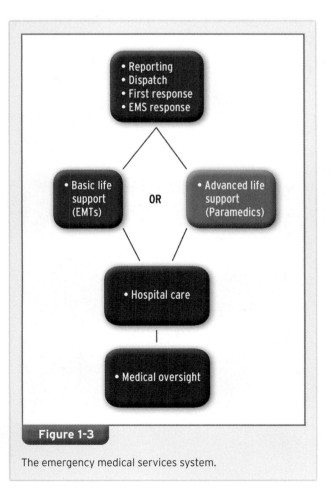

Figure 1-3

The emergency medical services system.

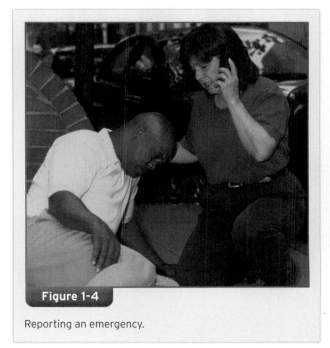

Figure 1-4

Reporting an emergency.

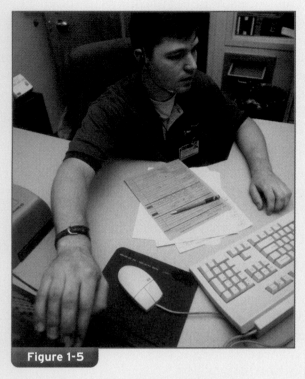

Figure 1-5

A dispatch center receives the call.

radio, telephone, or other means. Agencies, personnel, and equipment that are involved in the first response vary by community.

First Response

Because of their location or speed in responding, fire fighters (paid or volunteer) or law enforcement personnel are likely to be the first responders in most emergencies Figure 1-6 ▼. Most communities have many potential first responders, but few EMTs and even fewer paramedics. A community with four or five fire stations may have only two or three ambulances. In some situations, a first responder's actions can mean the difference between life and death. For example, a key survival factor for people in cardiac arrest is the length of time between when the heartbeat stops and when manual cardiopulmonary resuscitation (CPR) starts. The patient's first and perhaps most crucial contact with the EMS system occurs when the trained first responder arrives. The first responder is a key element in providing emergency care.

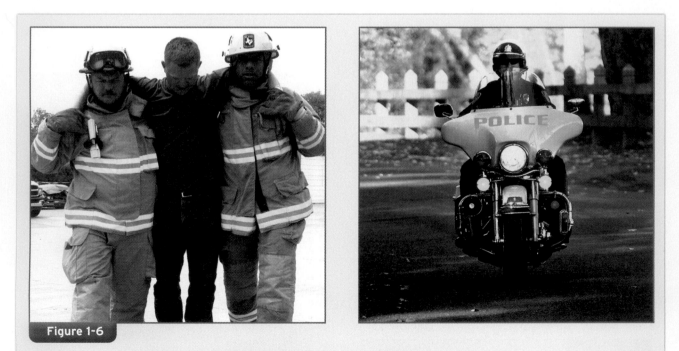

Figure 1-6

Fire fighters and law enforcement personnel are first responders in many emergencies.

EMS Response

The arrival of an emergency medical vehicle (usually an ambulance) Figure 1-7 ▾ staffed by **emergency medical technicians-basic (EMT-Bs)** or paramedics is the patient's second contact with the EMS system. A properly equipped vehicle and the EMTs who staff it make up a **basic life support (BLS)** unit. Each EMT has completed at least 110 hours of training; many may complete even longer training courses.

EMTs continue the care begun by first responders. EMTs stabilize the patient further and prepare the patient for transport to the emergency department of the hospital. Well-trained emergency personnel who can carefully move the patient and provide proper treatment increase the chance that the patient will arrive at the emergency department in the best possible condition.

In addition to BLS services provided by EMTs, patients may receive **advanced life support (ALS)** services from paramedics. **Paramedics** have more than the BLS skills and knowledge of EMTs. They have received additional training so they can ad-

minister intravenous (IV) fluids and certain medications and monitor and treat heart conditions with medications and defibrillation. **Defibrillation** is the administration of an electric shock to the heart of a patient who is suffering from a highly irregular heartbeat, known as ventricular fibrillation. This may also be done by specially trained EMT-Bs and first responders. Paramedics are also trained to place special airway tubes (endotracheal tubes) to keep the patient's airway open.

Emergency medical technicians-intermediate (EMT-Is) are able to perform limited ALS skills. They may work alone or they may work with a paramedic on an ALS unit.

Each level of skill builds on the one that precedes it: The paramedic's skills originate from those of the EMT-B and the techniques used by the EMT-B depend on those of the first responder. All skill levels are based on what is learned in the first responder course: airway maintenance, control of bleeding, and prevention, recognition, and treatment of shock.

The EMS system involves more than emergency medical care. For example, law enforcement personnel are often a crucial part of the system because they may provide protection and control at the scene of an incident. Fire units provide fire protection, specialized rescue, and patient extrication.

Hospital Care

The patient's third contact with the EMS system occurs in the hospital, primarily in the emergency department. After being treated at the scene, the patient is transported to an appropriate hospital, where definitive treatment can be given Figure 1-8 ▸ . It may be necessary for the patient to be transported to the closest appropriate medical facility first, for stabilization, and then to a hospital that provides specialized treatment. Special facilities include trauma centers, stroke centers, burn centers, pediatric centers, poison control centers, and perinatal centers. You must learn and follow your local patient transportation protocols.

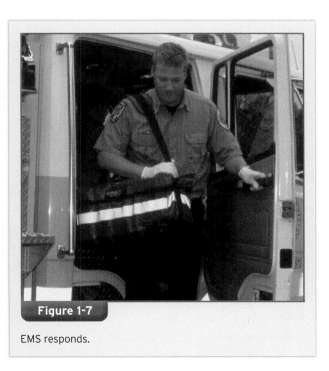

Figure 1-7

EMS responds.

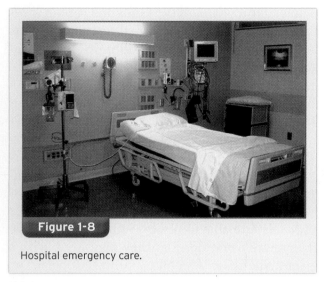

Figure 1-8

Hospital emergency care.

The History of EMS

As an EMS provider, you should have some understanding of the history of EMS. Many advances in civilian EMS have followed progress made first in the military medical system. Ambulances were first used to remove wounded patients from the battlefield during the Civil War. Traction splints were first used in World War I and are credited with greatly reducing the death rate from fractured femurs. During World War II, well-trained corpsmen and field hospitals helped reduce battlefield mortality. In the 1950s, during the Korean Conflict, timely helicopter evacuations to mobile army surgical hospitals (MASH) further reduced battlefield mortality. Additional medical advances were made in the 1960s and 1970s during the Vietnam war.

In the United States during the 1950s and 1960s, funeral homes, hospitals, and volunteer rescue squads provided most ambulance service. The only training available for ambulance attendants was basic first aid. Even interns who staffed hospital-based ambulances had no special training for their prehospital duties. Hearses were commonly used to transport ill and injured patients. The mortality rate from trauma to civilians was much higher than the mortality experienced by military personnel.

Some physicians recognized that civilian prehospital medical care lagged behind military emergency medical care and urged the National

Academy of Sciences to investigate this situation. In 1966, the National Academy of Sciences/National Research Council produced a landmark paper, *Accidental Death and Disability: The Neglected Disease of Modern Society*. This paper described the deficiencies in emergency medical care. It recommended the development of a national course of instruction for prehospital emergency care personnel. It also called for nationally accepted textbooks, ambulance vehicle design guidelines, ambulance equipment guidelines, state regulations for ambulance services, and improvements in hospital emergency departments. As a result of this effort, in the early 1970s, the U.S. Department of Transportation developed a national standard curriculum for training EMTs. This curriculum was the grandfather of the curriculum in use today.

During the 1980s, the use of advanced life support within the EMS services became common. Today paramedics are able to perform many procedures that were limited to physicians in the early days of EMS. Currently, cities, counties, fire departments, third-service EMS departments, rescue squads, and hospitals provide most EMS. Today, EMS providers are trained through standardized courses. Certified personnel use standardized vehicles to transport patients to recognized hospital emergency departments. Hospital emergency departments provide a high level of care for emergency patients.

Ten Standard Components of an EMS System

EMS systems can be categorized in many different ways. Depending on location, the same part of the system may be provided by different agencies. The National Highway Traffic Safety Administration (NHTSA) of the U.S. Department of Transportation evaluates EMS systems based on the following 10 criteria, which are used primarily in the administration of an EMS system:

1. Regulation and policy
2. Resource management
3. Human resources and training
4. Transportation equipment and system
5. Medical and support facilities
6. Communications system

7. Public information and education
8. Medical direction
9. Trauma system and development
10. Evaluation

A Word About Transportation

As a first responder, your primary goal is to provide immediate care for a sick or injured patient. As more highly trained emergency medical service personnel (EMTs or paramedics) arrive on the scene, you will assist them in treating and preparing the patient for transportation. Although other EMS personnel usually provide patient transportation, it is important that you understand when a patient must be transported quickly to a hospital or other medical facility Figure 1-9 ▼.

This book uses three terms to describe proper patient transportation to an appropriate medical facility:

- *Transport.* This means that a patient's condition requires care by medical professionals, but speed in getting the patient to a medical facility is not the most important factor. For example, this might describe the transportation needed by a patient who has sustained an isolated injury to an extremity but whose condition is otherwise stable.

- *Prompt transport.* This phrase is used when a patient's condition is serious enough that the patient needs to be taken to an appropriate medical facility in a fairly short period of time. If the patient is not transported fairly quickly, the condition may get worse and the patient may die.

- *Rapid transport.* This phrase is used for the few cases when EMS personnel are unable to give the patient adequate lifesaving care in the field. This patient may die unless he or she is transported immediately to an appropriate medical facility. This phrase is rarely used in this book.

Each of these three phrases refers to transportation to an **appropriate medical facility**. An appropriate medical facility may be a hospital, trauma center, or medical clinic. It is essential that you be familiar with the services provided by the medical facilities in your community.

EMS personnel must work closely with their medical director to establish transportation protocols that ensure that patients are transported to the closest medical facility capable of providing adequate care. To provide the best possible care for the patient, all members of the EMS team must remember that they are key components in the total system. Smooth operation of the team ensures the best care for the patient.

Roles and Responsibilities of the First Responder

As a first responder, you have several roles and responsibilities. Depending on the emergency situation, you may need to:

- Respond promptly and safely to the scene of an accident or sudden illness.
- Ensure that the scene is safe from hazards.
- Protect yourself.
- Protect the incident scene and patients from further harm.
- Summon appropriate assistance (EMTs, fire department, rescue squad).
- Gain access to the patient.
- Perform patient assessment.

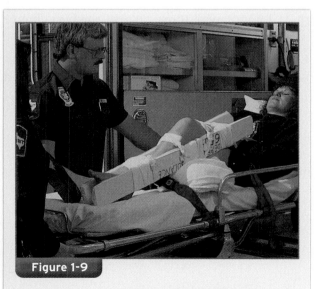

Figure 1-9

Ambulance transport to a hospital or medical facility.

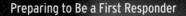

Voices of
Experience

Ready to Respond

It was a cold and rainy April night on a county road, when a car driven by a 16-year-old male with two 14-year-old female passengers crossed the center line and hit another car head on. The second vehicle had a father and son making a pizza run for the family.

> **As you begin your first steps into the EMS system as a first responder, you too will become part of an integrated team, ready and able to respond to those who desperately need you.**

The dispatch center received the call of the crash on County 15, 14 miles from the ACLS base. The local volunteer fire department was paged out with a response time of 5 minutes. The sheriff's office was contacted with a response time of 15 minutes.

The fire department arrived on the scene first. They set up a safety zone, surveyed the scene for hazards, sent fire fighters with lights ahead and behind the scene to warn traffic, and stabilized the vehicles. Other fire fighters checked the vehicles for victims and found the father and son unresponsive. The 16-year-old male was still behind the wheel, but he was not badly injured and was breathing. The smell of alcohol permeated the air. To the fire fighters' collective horror, they discovered that the two 14-year-old girls had been thrown from the vehicle and were in cardiac arrest. The fire fighters decided to do CPR on the two girls in cardiac arrest, but their efforts got no response.

The sheriff's deputy then arrived on the scene and took over the scene safety and possible crime scene. This freed up additional fire fighters to assist at the incident. ACLS arrived a few minutes later and transported the two most seriously injured, the father and son, to a trauma center. The 16-year-old driver was taken to the hospital by a second ACLS unit.

The entire EMS system was stressed by this situation, but because of highly trained dispatchers, first responder fire fighters, and law enforcement officers, all trained in a DOT first responder course, they were ready. This integrated and tiered response with an ACLS unit gave those victims the best chance of survival.

As you begin your first steps into the EMS system as a first responder, you too will become part of an integrated team, ready and able to respond to those who desperately need you. Good luck on your journey.

Joseph A. Grafft, MS
Retired EMS Manager, Minnesota State Colleges & Universities,
Office of the Chancellor Community Faculty,
Metropolitan State University, School of Law Enforcement
St. Paul, Minnesota

- Administer emergency medical care and reassurance.
- Move patients only when necessary.
- Seek and then direct help from bystanders, if necessary.
- Control activities of bystanders.
- Assist EMTs and paramedics, as necessary.
- Document your care.
- Keep your knowledge and skills up to date.

Concern for the patient is primary; you should perform all activities with the patient's well-being in mind. Prompt response to the scene is essential if you are to provide quality care to the patient. It is important that you know your response area well so you can quickly determine the most efficient route to the emergency scene.

When you reach the emergency scene, park your vehicle so that it does not create an additional hazard. The emergency scene should be protected with the least possible disruption of traffic. Do not block the roadway unnecessarily. As first responder, you should assess the scene to determine whether any hazards are present, such as downed electrical wires, gasoline spills, or unstable vehicles. This assessment is necessary to ensure that patients suffer no further injuries and that rescuers, other EMS personnel, and bystanders are not hurt.

If the equipment and personnel already dispatched to the scene cannot cope with the incident, you must immediately summon additional help. It may take some time for additional equipment and personnel to reach the scene, especially in rural areas or communities with systems staffed by volunteers.

Once you have taken the preceding steps, you must gain access to the patient. This may be as simple as opening the door to a car or house or as difficult as squeezing through the back window of a wrecked automobile. Next, examine the patient to determine the extent of the injury or illness. This initial assessment of a patient is called the patient assessment sequence. Once the patient assessment is completed, you must stabilize the patient's condition to prevent it from getting worse. The techniques you use to do this are limited by your training and the equipment available. Correctly applying these techniques can have a positive effect on the patient's condition.

When EMTs or paramedics arrive to assist, it is important to tell them what you have discovered about the patient's condition and what you have done so far to stabilize or treat it. Your next task is to assist the EMTs or paramedics.

In some communities or situations, you may be asked to accompany the patient in the ambulance. If CPR is being performed, you may need to assist or relieve the EMT or paramedic, especially if the hospital is far from the scene. In some EMS systems, you may be asked to drive the ambulance to the hospital so EMS personnel with more advanced training can devote all their efforts to patient care.

The Importance of Documentation

Once your role in treating the patient is finished, it is important that you record your observations about the scene, the patient's condition, and the treatment you provided. Documentation should be clear, concise, accurate, and according to the accepted policies of your organization. This documentation is important because you will not be able to remember the treatment you give to all patients. It also serves as a legal record of your treatment and may be required in the event of a lawsuit. Documentation also provides a basis to evaluate the quality of care given.

Documentation should include:
- Condition of the patient when found
- The patient's description of the injury or illness
- The initial and later vital signs
- The treatment you gave the patient
- The agency and personnel who took over treatment of the patient
- Any other helpful facts

Further information about documentation is included in Chapter 8.

Attitude and Conduct

As a first responder, you will be judged by your attitude and conduct, as well as by the medical care you administer. It is important to understand that professional behavior has a positive impact on your patients. Because you will often be the first medically trained person to arrive on the scene of an emergency, it is important to act in a calm and caring way. You will gain the confidence of both patient and bystanders more easily by using a courteous and caring tone of voice. Show an interest in your patient. Avoid embarrassing your patient and help protect his or her privacy. Talk with your patient and tell him or her what you are doing.

Remember that medical information about a patient is confidential and do not discuss it with your family or friends. This information should be shared only with other medical personnel who are involved in the care of that particular patient.

Your appearance should be neat and professional at all times. You should be well groomed and clean. A uniform helps identify you as a first responder. If you are a volunteer who responds from home, always identify yourself as a first responder. Your professional attitude and neat appearance help provide much needed reassurance to the patient Figure 1-10 ▸.

Medical Oversight

The overall leader of the medical care team is the physician or medical director. To ensure that the patient receives appropriate medical treatment, it is important that first responders receive direction from a physician. Each first responder agency should have a physician who directs training courses, helps set medical policies and procedures, and ensures quality management of the EMS system. This type of medical direction is known as indirect (or off-line) medical control.

A second type of medical control is known as direct (or online) medical control. Online medical control is provided by a physician who is in contact with prehospital EMS providers, usually paramedics or EMTs, by two-way radio or wireless telephone. In cases where large numbers of people are injured, physicians may respond to the scene of the incident to provide on-scene medical control.

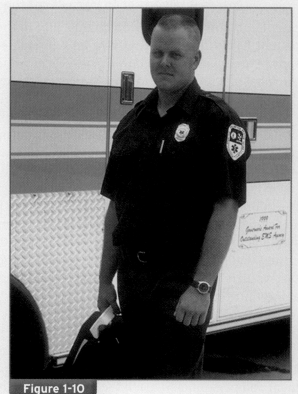

Figure 1-10

A professional attitude and neat appearance provide reassurance to the patient.

You are the Provider

SUMMARY

Review the *You are the Provider* case study provided at the beginning of the chapter.

Now that you have completed your first responder course, you are responsible for providing the first tier of EMS in your community. Basic and advanced life support services complement your initial response, provide additional treatment, and transport the patient to an appropriate medical facility.

1. Why is it important to learn about the components of an EMS system?

It is important to understand the components of the EMS system because you are a part of the system. You provide a vital function in the system and are supported by and interact with people who fulfill other functions within the system.

2. How does good interaction between different levels of the EMS team improve patient care?

Good interactions between different levels of the EMS team improve patient care by relaying vital patient information and by improving the efficiency of patient care.

3. Why is your role as a first responder sometimes the most important for the welfare of the patient?

At times, your actions as a first responder may make a difference in the patient's outcome. Your role is very important because sometimes you will be the only medically trained person at the scene of a medical emergency.

Prep Kit

Ready for Review

The Ready for Review thoroughly summarizes the chapter.

- The first responder is the first medically trained person to arrive on the scene. The initial care provided is essential because it is available sooner than more advanced emergency medical care and could mean the difference between life and death.

- The four basic goals of first responder training are to know what not to do, know how to use your first responder life support kit, know how to improvise, and know how to assist other EMS providers.

- First responders should understand their roles in the EMS system. The typical sequence of events of the EMS system is reporting, dispatch, first response, EMS response, and hospital care.

- As a first responder, your primary goal is to provide immediate care for a sick or injured patient. As more highly trained personnel (EMTs or paramedics) arrive on the scene, you will assist them in treating and preparing the patient for transportation.

- Once your role in treating the patent is finished, it is important that you record your observations about the scene, the patient's condition, and the treatment you provided. Documentation should be clear, concise, accurate, and according to the accepted policies of your organization.

- Remember that medical information about a patient is confidential and should be shared only with other medical personnel who are involved in the care of that particular patient.

- The overall leader of the medical care team is the physician or medical director. To ensure that the patient receives appropriate medical treatment, it is important that first responders receive direction from a physician.

Vital Vocabulary

The Vital Vocabulary are the key terms for this chapter.

advanced life support (ALS) The use of specialized equipment such as cardiac monitors, defibrillators, intravenous fluids, drug infusion, and endotracheal intubation to stabilize the patient.

appropriate medical facility A hospital with adequate medical resources to provide continuing care to sick or injured patients who are transported after field treatment by first responders.

basic life support (BLS) Emergency lifesaving procedures performed without advanced emergency procedures to stabilize patients who have experienced sudden illness or injury.

defibrillation Delivery of an electric current through a person's chest wall and heart for the purpose of ending lethal heart rhythms such as ventricular fibrillation.

emergency medical technician-basic (EMT-B) A person who is trained and certified to provide basic life support and certain other noninvasive prehospital medical procedures.

emergency services dispatch center A fire, police, or emergency medical services (EMS) agency; a 9-1-1 center; or a seven-digit telephone number used by one or all of the emergency agencies to receive and dispatch requests for emergency care.

paramedics Emergency medical technicians who have completed an extensive course of 800 or more hours, successfully passed a national or state certification, and who can perform advanced life support skills.

Technology

- Interactivities
- Vocabulary Explorer
- Anatomy Review
- Web Links
- Online Review Manual

www.FirstResponder.EMSzone.com

Assessment in Action

Assessment in Action presents a fictitious scenario to help you review what you learned in this chapter.

As a first responder, you are often the first step in the process of a patient getting the necessary care needed in an emergency situation. You will work closely with a variety of other emergency and nonemergency personnel. Your role may vary greatly depending upon the scene and the additional resources available.

1. What are some of the responsibilities of a first responder?

2. What is your role in the initial treatment of a patient?

   A. Perform patient assessment.
   B. Administer emergency medical care and reassurance.
   C. Move patients only when necessary.
   D. All of the above.

3. In what way can you be of assistance to emergency medical providers of a higher level?

   A. Start an IV.
   B. Interpret cardiac rhythms.
   C. Help prepare the patient for transport.
   D. Give epinephrine.

4. What is your role in the continuing treatment and subsequent transportation of a patient?

5. What are some of the differences in the treatment that a first responder can provide versus that of an EMT-B or paramedic?

6. What are some of the standard components of an EMS system?

   A. Medical and support facilities
   B. Communications system
   C. Public information and education
   D. Medical direction
   E. All of the above

7. When documenting a scene, what information should you NOT include in your report?

   A. Condition of the patient when found
   B. The patient's description of the injury or illness
   C. The initial and later vital signs
   D. Patient's work history

The Well-Being of the First Responder

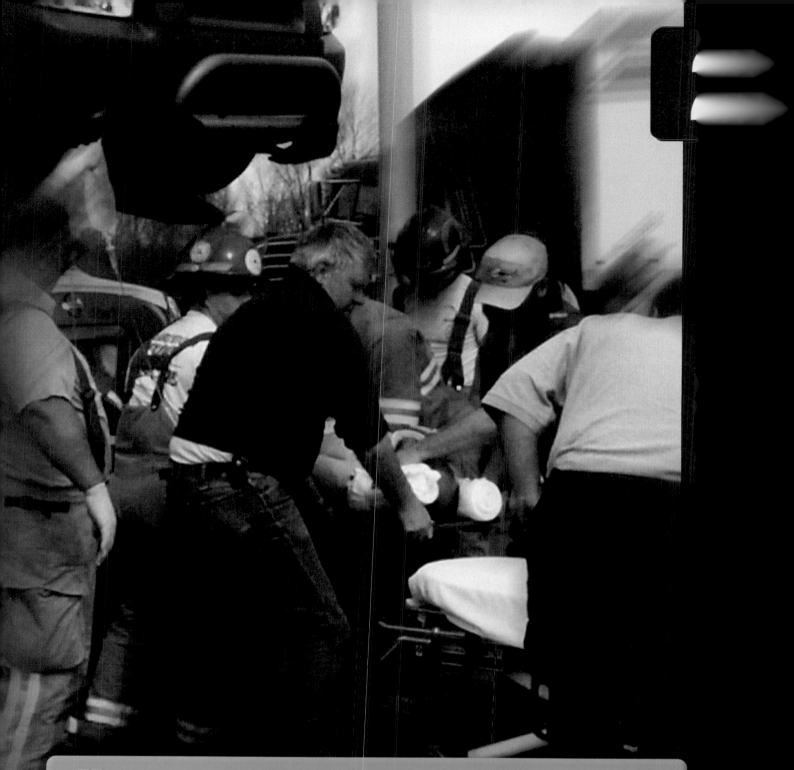

You are the Provider

As a new member of your public safety organization, you notice that some long-time veterans of your organization seem to be more relaxed and others seem to show more signs of stress during emergency responses.

1. What steps can you take to reduce stress during emergency responses?
2. How are your off-duty activities related to the level of stress you experience while on duty?
3. How can failing to follow universal precautions affect your health?

Introduction

This chapter is designed to help you understand the factors that may affect your physical or emotional well-being as a first responder. You, your patients, and their families will all experience stress, so this chapter addresses methods for preventing and reducing stress. It also discusses hazards you may encounter from infectious diseases and presents methods you must follow to reduce your risk of infection. Finally, this chapter covers scene safety and how to prevent injury to yourself and further injury to your patients.

Emotional Aspects of Emergency Medical Care

Providing emergency medical care as a first responder is a stress-producing experience. You will feel the stress, as will your patients, their families and friends, and bystanders. Because stress cannot be completely eliminated, you must learn how to avoid unnecessary stress and how to prevent your stress level from getting too high. Some of the same stress-reduction techniques that you will learn can also be used by your patients and their families and friends.

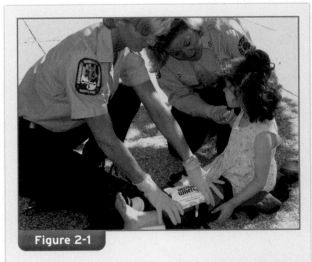

Figure 2-1

Certain kinds of patients may produce a high level of stress.

Although all emergency medical calls produce a certain level of stress, some types of calls are more stressful than others. Your past experiences may make it difficult for you to deal with certain types of calls. For example, if a patient with severe injuries reminds you of a close family member, you may have difficulty treating the patient without experiencing a high level of stress. This is especially true if an emergency call involves a very young or a very old patient Figure 2-1 ▲. Calls involving death, violence, or mass casualties are also likely to produce high levels of stress. Likewise, past experiences may also play a part in reducing stress during the care of a patient.

Because you work in a stressful environment, you must make a conscious effort to prevent and reduce unnecessary stress. You can do this in several different ways: learn to recognize the signs and symptoms of stress, adjust your lifestyle to

Technology

- Interactivities
- Vocabulary Explorer
- Anatomy Review
- Web Links
- Online Review Manual

Safety Tips

Do not underestimate the effect that stress can have on you. A fire fighter, EMS provider, or law enforcement official in a busy department can see more suffering in a year than many people will see in their entire lifetimes.

include stress-reducing activities, and learn what services and resources are available to help you.

Normal Reactions to Stress

You need to understand how stress can affect you and the people for whom you provide emergency medical services. Because dying is one of the most intense types of stress that people experience, the grief reaction to death and dying provides a basis for looking at stress. Everyone who is involved with a death or with a dying patient—the patient, the family, and the caregivers—goes through this grief process, even though each is involved with the patient in different ways.

One well-recognized model for people's reaction to death and dying defines five stages: denial, anger, bargaining, depression, and acceptance—but not all people move through the grief process in exactly the same way and at the same pace. When you first encounter someone, he or she may be experiencing any stage of grief.

1. **Denial** ("Not me!"). The first stage in the grief process is **denial**. A person experiencing denial cannot believe what is happening. This stage may serve as a protection for the person experiencing the situation, and it may also serve as a protection for you as the caregiver. Realize that this reaction is normal.

2. **Anger** ("Why me?"). The second stage of the grief process is **anger**. Understanding that anger is a normal reaction to stress can also help you deal with anger that is directed toward you by a patient or by a patient's family. Do not get defensive because this anger is a result of the situation and not a result of anything you do. This realization can enable you to tolerate the situation without letting the patient's anger distract you from performing your duties as an emergency medical provider.

3. **Bargaining** ("Okay, but . . ."). The third stage of the grief process is **bargaining**. Bargaining is the act of trying to make a deal to postpone death and dying. If you encounter a patient who is in this stage, try to respond with a truthful and helpful comment such as, "We are doing everything we can and the paramedics will be here in just a few minutes." Remember that bargaining is a normal part of the grief process.

4. **Depression.** The fourth stage of the grief process is **depression**. Depression is often characterized by sadness or despair. A person who is unusually silent or who seems to retreat into his or her own world may have reached this stage. This may also be the point at which a person begins to accept the situation. It is not surprising that patients and their families get depressed about a situation that involves death and dying—nor is it surprising that you as a rescuer also get depressed. American society tends to consider death a failure of medical care rather than a natural event that happens to everyone. A certain amount of depression is a natural reaction to a major threat or loss. The depression can be mild or severe; it can be of short duration or long lasting. If depression continues, it is important to contact qualified professionals who can help you.

5. **Acceptance.** The final stage of the grief process is **acceptance**. Acceptance does not mean that you are satisfied with the situation. It means that you understand that death and dying cannot be changed. It may require a lot of time to work through the grief process and arrive at this stage. As an emergency medical provider, you may see acceptance in family members who have had time to realize that

In the Field

As you go through the anger phase, you may direct your anger at the patient, the patient's family, your coworkers, or your own family. Anger is a normal reaction to unpleasant events. Sometimes it helps to talk out your anger with coworkers, family members, or a counselor. By talking through your anger, you avoid keeping it bottled up inside where it can cause unhealthy physical symptoms or emotional reactions. Directing the energy from your anger in positive ways to alleviate a bad situation may help you move forward. For example, at the scene of a motor vehicle crash, you may be angry that a child has been injured. Focusing your energy on providing the best medical care for the injured child may help you work through your feelings.

Signs and Symptoms

Stress

The following warning signs should help you recognize stress in coworkers or friends or in yourself:

- Irritability (often directed at coworkers, family, and friends)
- Inability to concentrate
- Change in normal disposition
- Difficulty in sleeping or nightmares (may be hard to recognize because many emergency care workers work a pattern of rotating hours that makes normal sleep patterns hard to maintain)
- Anxiety
- Indecisiveness
- Guilt
- Loss of appetite
- Loss of interest in sexual relations
- Loss of interest in work
- Isolation

Safety Tips

Because public safety services must be provided 24 hours a day, many law enforcement, fire, EMS, and security personnel work rotating shifts. Fire fighters may work 24-hour shifts with a variety of days off. Law enforcement personnel may be required to alternate between day and night shifts.

These work schedules disrupt normal sleep patterns. In addition, many people in public safety work overtime shifts or a second job. This combination of factors often means that many public safety providers do not get an adequate amount of sleep.

Scientific studies have documented that most people need about 8 hours of uninterrupted sleep per night. If you are not meeting this need, your mental and physical health may suffer and you will be less able to deal with stress. It is important to establish adequate sleep as a priority in your life.

their loved one's illness is a terminal event and that the patient is not going to recover. However, not all people who experience grief are able to work through it and accept the loss.

By understanding these five stages, you can better understand the grief reaction experienced by patients, their families, and their friends. You can also better understand your reaction to stressful situations. Some helpful techniques for dealing with patients in stressful situations are presented in Chapter 12. These techniques will help you to develop more comfort and skill when dealing with stressful situations.

Stress Management

Stress management has three components: recognizing stress, preventing stress, and reducing stress.

Recognizing Stress

An important step in managing stress in yourself and others is the ability to recognize its signs and symptoms. Then you can take steps to prevent or reduce stress.

Preventing Stress

Three simple-to-remember techniques that can prevent stress are: eat, drink, and be merry (in a healthy, stress-reducing manner).

1. **Eat.** A healthy, well-balanced diet helps prevent and reduce stress. A healthy daily diet should include 6 ounces of whole-grain cereal, breads, rice, or pasta; $2\frac{1}{2}$ cups of a variety of vegetables; 2 cups of fruit; 3 cups of low-fat or fat-free milk and yogurt; and $5\frac{1}{2}$ ounces of lean meats, poultry, fish, beans, and nuts. Limit your intake of fats, sugars, and salt. To illustrate this healthy variety of foods, the U.S. Department of Agriculture (USDA) created the MyPyramid food guidance system, which is shown in **Figure 2-2 ▶**.

   The amount of food you need is related to your size, your weight, and your level of physical activity. The steps you can take to plan a healthy diet are illustrated in **Figure 2-3 ▶**.

   Many people need to cut down on the amount of sweets in their diet. Eating large quantities of sweets puts your energy level on a roller coaster. Your blood sugar quickly rises, but in a couple of hours, the blood sugar drops and you crave more sweets. It is much better

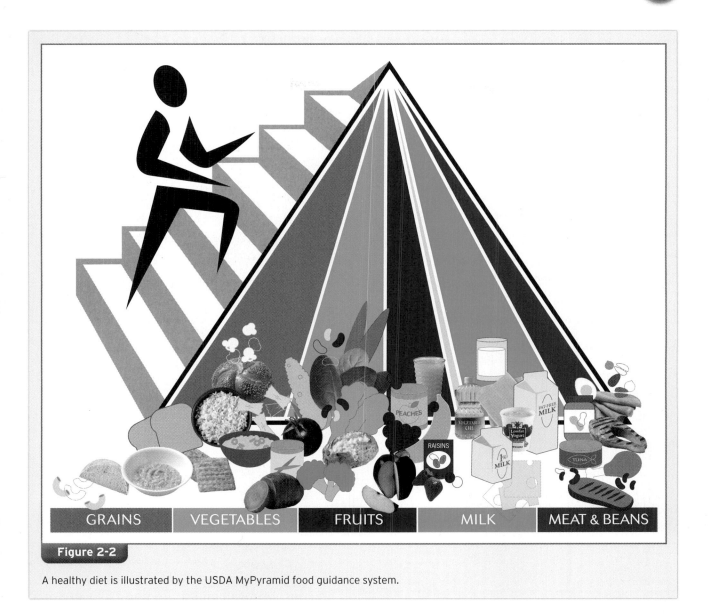

Figure 2-2

A healthy diet is illustrated by the USDA MyPyramid food guidance system.

| GRAINS | VEGETABLES | FRUITS | MILK | MEAT & BEANS |

to eat an adequate amount of breads, cereals, rice, and pasta. These provide energy over a longer period of time and help to reduce the highs and lows brought on by excess sugars.

EMS providers often find it hard to maintain regular meal schedules. By planning your food intake and having healthy foods available, you can improve your eating habits. Healthy eating not only helps to cut down on your stress level, it also helps reduce your risk of heart and blood vessel diseases, which are the most common causes of death in public safety workers. Keeping your weight at recommended levels helps your body deal better with stress.

2. **Drink.** Active EMS providers need to drink adequate amounts of fluids every day **Figure 2-4 ▶**. Dehydration is a special risk for law enforcement officers, fire fighters, and EMS providers who wear hot bunker gear or ballistic vests. The average adult loses about eight glasses of water a day through sweat, exhaling, and elimination. Water in adequate quantities is essential for maintaining proper body processes. Natural fruit juices are another good source of fluids. It is important to keep your body hydrated while you are on duty. When you are working in a hot environment or are involved in a strenuous incident, rehabilitate yourself by

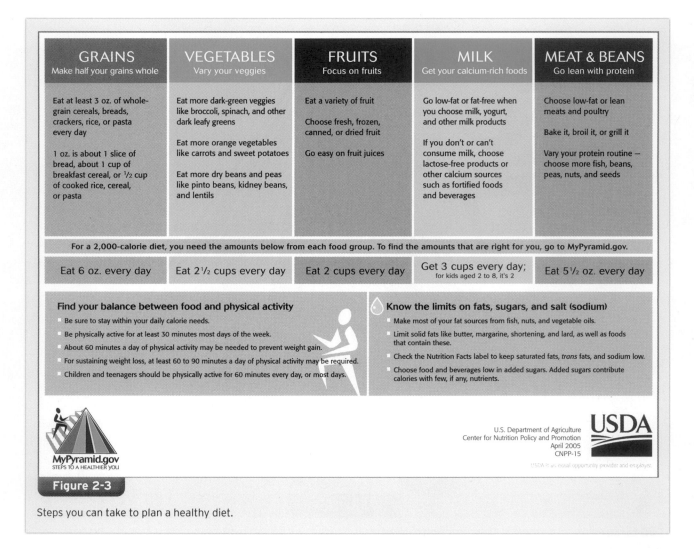

GRAINS Make half your grains whole	VEGETABLES Vary your veggies	FRUITS Focus on fruits	MILK Get your calcium-rich foods	MEAT & BEANS Go lean with protein
Eat at least 3 oz. of whole-grain cereals, breads, crackers, rice, or pasta every day 1 oz. is about 1 slice of bread, about 1 cup of breakfast cereal, or ½ cup of cooked rice, cereal, or pasta	Eat more dark-green veggies like broccoli, spinach, and other dark leafy greens Eat more orange vegetables like carrots and sweet potatoes Eat more dry beans and peas like pinto beans, kidney beans, and lentils	Eat a variety of fruit Choose fresh, frozen, canned, or dried fruit Go easy on fruit juices	Go low-fat or fat-free when you choose milk, yogurt, and other milk products If you don't or can't consume milk, choose lactose-free products or other calcium sources such as fortified foods and beverages	Choose low-fat or lean meats and poultry Bake it, broil it, or grill it Vary your protein routine — choose more fish, beans, peas, nuts, and seeds

For a 2,000-calorie diet, you need the amounts below from each food group. To find the amounts that are right for you, go to MyPyramid.gov.

| Eat 6 oz. every day | Eat 2½ cups every day | Eat 2 cups every day | Get 3 cups every day; for kids aged 2 to 8, it's 2 | Eat 5½ oz. every day |

Find your balance between food and physical activity
- Be sure to stay within your daily calorie needs.
- Be physically active for at least 30 minutes most days of the week.
- About 60 minutes a day of physical activity may be needed to prevent weight gain.
- For sustaining weight loss, at least 60 to 90 minutes a day of physical activity may be required.
- Children and teenagers should be physically active for 60 minutes every day, or most days.

Know the limits on fats, sugars, and salt (sodium)
- Make most of your fat sources from fish, nuts, and vegetable oils.
- Limit solid fats like butter, margarine, shortening, and lard, as well as foods that contain these.
- Check the Nutrition Facts label to keep saturated fats, *trans* fats, and sodium low.
- Choose food and beverages low in added sugars. Added sugars contribute calories with few, if any, nutrients.

MyPyramid.gov
STEPS TO A HEALTHIER YOU

U.S. Department of Agriculture
Center for Nutrition Policy and Promotion
April 2005
CNPP-15

USDA

USDA is an equal opportunity provider and employer.

Figure 2-3

Steps you can take to plan a healthy diet.

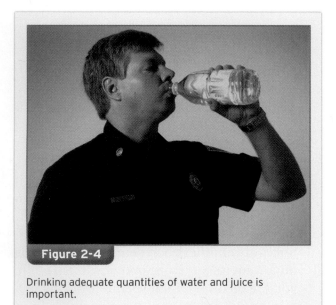

Figure 2-4

Drinking adequate quantities of water and juice is important.

consuming adequate amounts of water or a sports drink.

Avoid consuming excessive amounts of caffeine and alcohol. Caffeine is a drug that causes adrenaline to be released in your body; adrenaline raises your blood pressure and increases your stress level. By limiting your intake of caffeine-containing beverages such as coffee and cola drinks, you can reduce your tendency toward stress. Caffeine and alcohol also cause dehydration. Drinking alcoholic beverages is to be discouraged. Although alcoholic drinks seem to relax you, they cause depression and reduce your ability to deal with stress.

3. **Be cheerful.** A happy person is not suffering from elevated stress. It is important to bal-

ance your lifestyle. Assess both your work environment and your home environment. At work, address problems promptly before they produce major stress. Try to schedule your work to allow adequate off-duty time for sleep and personal activities. If you are working in a volunteer agency, avoid having everyone on call all the time.

Try to create a stress-reducing environment away from work. Spend time with your friends and family. In your recreational activities, include friends who are not coworkers. Develop hobbies or activities that are not related to your job. Exercise regularly. Exercise is a great stress reliever. Swimming, running, and bicycling are three types of excellent aerobic exercise. Avoid the use of tobacco products; they are stress producers, not stress relievers. Meditation or religious activities reduce stress for many people. People who can balance the pressures of work with relaxing activities at home usually enjoy life much more than people who can never leave the stories and stress of work behind. If you are feeling stress away from your job, consider seeking assistance from a mental health care professional.

Reducing Stress

If pressures at work or home cause continual stress, you may benefit from the help of a mental health professional. This person is trained to listen nonjudgmentally and to help you resolve the issues that are causing your stress. Mental health professionals include psychologists, psychiatrists, social workers, and specially trained clergy. A mental health professional may be connected with your department. Your medical insurance may cover this type of care.

Critical Incident Stress Management is a comprehensive program that is available through some public safety departments. It consists of preincident stress education, on-scene peer support, and critical incident stress debriefings (CISDs). You should contact CISD personnel whenever you are exhibiting signs or symptoms of stress.

1. **Preincident stress education** provides information about the stresses that you will encounter and the reactions you may experience.

It helps emergency responders understand the normal stress responses to the abnormal emergency situations they encounter.

2. **On-scene peer support** and disaster support services provide aid for you on the scene of especially stressful incidents such as major disasters or situations that involve the death of a coworker or a child.

3. A **critical incident stress debriefing (CISD)** is used to alleviate the stress reactions caused by high-stress emergency situations. Debriefings are meetings between emergency responders and specially trained leaders. The purpose of a debriefing is to allow an open discussion of feelings, fears, and reactions to the high-stress situation. A debriefing is not an investigation or an interrogation. Debriefings are usually held within 24 to 72 hours after a major incident. The CISD leaders offer suggestions and information on overcoming stress Figure 2-5 ▾ .

Find out if your department has a CISD program. Contact this team if you are involved in a high-stress incident such as a call that involves a very young or a very old patient, a mass-casualty incident, or a situation that involves unusual violence. If you think you might be experiencing signs or symptoms of stress from such an incident, contact your supervisor or a stress counselor. More information about critical incident stress debriefing is available in Chapter 12.

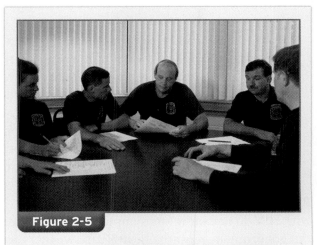

Figure 2-5

A critical incident stress debriefing (CISD) is a tool that may relieve stress.

Scene Safety

Infectious Diseases and Body Substance Isolation

In recent years, the acquired immunodeficiency syndrome (AIDS) epidemic and the growing concern about tuberculosis and hepatitis have increased awareness of infectious diseases. Some understanding of the most common infectious diseases is important so you can protect yourself from unnecessary exposure to these diseases and so you do not become unduly alarmed about them.

Federal regulations require all health care workers, including first responders, to assume that all patients in all settings are potentially infected with human immunodeficiency virus (HIV), the virus that can lead to AIDS; hepatitis B virus (HBV); or other bloodborne **pathogens**. These regulations require that all health care workers use protective equipment to prevent possible exposure to blood and certain bodily fluids of patients. This concept is known as **body substance isolation (BSI)**.

HIV is transmitted by direct contact with infected blood, semen, or vaginal secretions. There is no scientific documentation that the virus is transmitted by contact with sweat, saliva, tears, sputum, urine, feces, vomitus, or nasal secretions, unless these fluids contain visible signs of blood. Exposure can take place in the following ways:

- The patient's blood is splashed or sprayed into your eyes, nose, or mouth or into an open sore or cut.
- You have blood from the infected patient on your hands and then touch your own eyes, nose, mouth, or an open sore or cut.
- A needle that was used to inject the patient breaks your skin.
- Broken glass at a motor vehicle crash or other incident that is covered with blood from an infected patient penetrates your glove and skin.

Remember that many patients who are infected with HIV do not show any symptoms. This is why the government requires health care workers to wear certain types of gloves any time they are likely to come into contact with secretions or blood from any patient. You should also cover

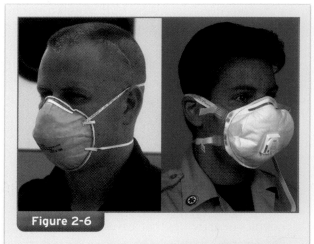

Figure 2-6

Two types of respirators that reduce the transmission of airborne diseases.

any open wounds that you have whenever you are on the job.

Hepatitis B is also spread by direct contact with infected blood, although it is far more contagious than HIV. First responders should follow the universal precautions described in the following section to reduce their chance of contracting hepatitis B. Check with your medical director about receiving injections of hepatitis vaccine to protect you against this infection. This vaccine should be made available to you.

Tuberculosis is also becoming a common problem, and the presence of drug-resistant strains makes this disease very dangerous to first responders. Tuberculosis is spread through the air whenever an infected person coughs or sneezes. Although tuberculosis is often hard to distinguish from other diseases, patients who pose the highest risk almost invariably have a cough. Wear a face mask or a high-efficiency particulate air (HEPA) respirator **Figure 2-6 ▲** and put an oxygen mask on the patient to minimize your exposure. If no oxygen mask is available, place a face mask on the patient. First responders should have a skin test for tuberculosis every year.

First responders may also encounter other diseases such as meningitis, syphilis, and whooping cough, as well as new diseases of concern such as West Nile Virus and SARS (severe acute respiratory syndrome). The best way to prevent exposure is to follow all BSI precautions with each patient.

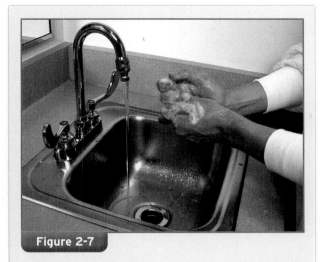

Figure 2-7

Wash your hands thoroughly if you are contaminated with blood or other bodily fluids.

Universal Precautions

You will not always be able to tell whether a patient's bodily fluids contain blood. Therefore, the Centers for Disease Control and Prevention (CDC) recommend that all health care workers use universal precautions, based on the assumption that all patients are potential carriers of bloodborne pathogens.

The CDC recommends that all health care workers use the following **universal precautions**:

1. Always wear gloves when handling patients and change gloves after contact with each patient (see Skill Drill 2-1). Wash your hands immediately after removing gloves. Note that leather gloves are not considered safe—leather is porous and traps fluids.
2. Always wear protective eyewear or a face shield when you anticipate that blood or other bodily fluids may splatter. Wear a gown or apron if you anticipate splashes of blood or other bodily fluids such as those that occur with childbirth and major trauma.
3. Wash your hands and other skin surfaces immediately and thoroughly if they become contaminated with blood and other bodily fluids Figure 2-7 ▲ . Change contaminated clothes and wash exposed skin thoroughly.
4. Do not recap, cut, or bend used needles. Place them directly in a puncture-resistant container designed for "sharps."

5. Even though saliva has not been proven to transmit HIV, you should use a face shield, pocket mask, or other airway adjunct if the patient needs resuscitation.

Proper removal of gloves is important to minimize the spread of pathogens Skill Drill 2-1 ▶ :

SKILL DRILL 2-1

1. Begin by partially removing one glove. With the other gloved hand, pinch the first glove at the wrist, being careful to touch only the outside of the glove, and start to roll it back off the hand, inside out Step 1 .
2. Remove the second glove by pinching the exterior with the partially gloved hand Step 2 .
3. Pull the second glove inside out toward the fingertips Step 3 .
4. Grasp both gloves with your free hand, touching only the clean interior surfaces Step 4 .

Federal agencies such as the Occupational Safety and Health Administration (OSHA) and state agencies such as state public health departments have regulations about BSI. Because these regulations are constantly changing, it is important for your department to keep up-to-date on

Safety Tips

Simple, portable safety equipment can help prevent injuries and illnesses.
- Medical gloves, masks, and eye protection prevent the spread of infectious diseases.
- Brightly colored clothing or vests make you more visible to traffic in the daytime; reflective striping or vests make you more visible in the dark.
- Heavy gloves can help prevent cuts at a motor vehicle accident scene.
- A hard hat or helmet is needed when you are at an industrial or motor vehicle collision scene.

Some situations require additional safety equipment. Do not hesitate to call for additional equipment as needed.

Skill DRILL 2-1

Proper Removal of Medical Gloves

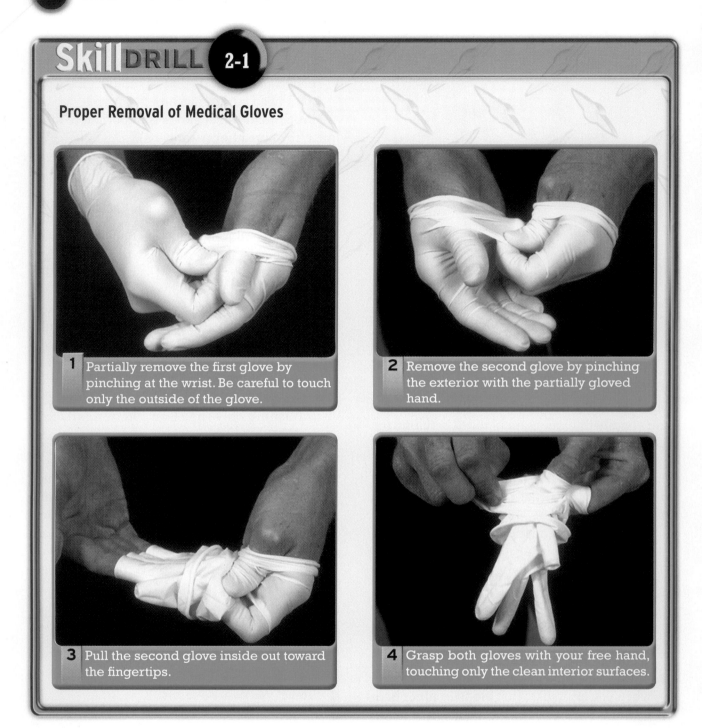

1 Partially remove the first glove by pinching at the wrist. Be careful to touch only the outside of the glove.

2 Remove the second glove by pinching the exterior with the partially gloved hand.

3 Pull the second glove inside out toward the fingertips.

4 Grasp both gloves with your free hand, touching only the clean interior surfaces.

these regulations and to provide continuing education to keep you current with the latest changes related to infectious disease precautions.

Immunizations

Certain immunizations are recommended for emergency medical care providers. These include tetanus prophylaxis and hepatitis B vaccine. Tuberculin testing is also recommended. Your medical director can determine what immunizations and tests are needed for members of your department.

Responding to the Scene

Scene safety is a most important consideration to you as a first responder. Safety considerations need to include your own safety and the safety of all the other people present at the scene of an emergency. An injured or killed first responder cannot help those in need, and becomes someone who needs help, increasing the difficulty of a rescue. Close attention to factors involving safety can prevent unnecessary illness, injuries, and death.

Dispatch

Safety begins when you are dispatched to an emergency. Use your dispatch information to anticipate what hazards may be present and to determine how to approach the scene of the emergency.

Response

Vehicle accidents are a major cause of death and disability of law enforcement officials, fire fighters, and EMS providers. As you respond to the scene of an emergency, remember the safety information that you have been taught in your driving courses. Fasten your safety belt, plan the best route, and drive quickly but safely to the scene.

Parking Your Vehicle

When you arrive at the emergency scene, park your vehicle so that it protects the area from traffic hazards. Check to be sure that the emergency warning lights are operating correctly. Be careful when getting out of your vehicle, especially if you must step into a traffic area. Brightly colored uniforms or vests enhance your visibility in the daytime; reflective material on your uniform or on a safety vest helps make you more visible in the dark **Figure 2-8 ▶** . If your vehicle is not needed to protect the incident scene, park it out of the way of traffic. Leave room for other arriving vehicles such as ambulances to be positioned near the patient. Above all else, make sure that you have protected the emergency scene from further accidents.

Assessing the Scene

As you approach the emergency scene, scan the entire area carefully to determine what hazards are present. Consider the following hazards based on the type of emergency; address them in what-

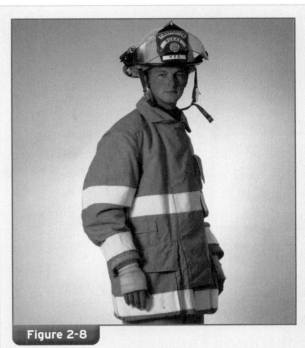

Figure 2-8

Reflective clothing helps to make you more visible.

ever order is most appropriate. For example, you should assess the scene of a motor vehicle accident for downed electrical wires before you check for broken glass.

Traffic

Is traffic a problem? Sometimes (for example, on a busy highway) your first action should be to control the flow of traffic so that additional accidents do not make the situation any worse. If you need more help to handle traffic, call for assistance before you get out of your vehicle.

Crime or Violence

If your dispatch information leads you to believe that the incident involves violence or a crime, approach carefully. If you are trained in law enforcement procedures, follow your local protocols. If you are not a law enforcement official, proceed very carefully. If you have any doubts about the safety of the scene, it is better to wait at a safe distance and request help from law enforcement officials. If the scene involves a crime, remember to take a mental picture of the scene and avoid disturbing anything at the scene unless it is absolutely necessary to move objects to provide patient care.

Voices of
Experience

Showing That You Care

"It will be some time before we can get any patients out." That is the transmission that we heard over the radio. It was a cold night, and two cars had been involved in a head-on collision on an icy road. There were five patients trapped in the cars.

> **We knew that we had to do our very best to keep them from going into shock as the fire department continued their attempt to free the patients from the vehicle.**

There was not much that we could do until the fire department gained access to the patients. Once access was gained, we were instructed to enter one vehicle and begin assessing the two patients trapped there.

My partner and I entered the vehicle and began to provide care. Much to our surprise, both of the occupants in this vehicle were members of our rescue squad. Once everyone on the scene figured out who the patients were, a sense of anxiety developed on the scene, and there was a rush to get them freed. Their level of consciousness was decreasing and they were beginning to be overcome by the cold. We knew that we had to do our very best to keep them from going into shock as the fire department continued their attempt to free the patients from the vehicle. I kept talking to them, explaining what was being done and how we would make sure that they would receive good care. I remembered from my EMS training that hearing is the last sense to be lost, so I knew that if I kept talking they might hear me.

Once the fire department was able to free the patients from the vehicle, we moved them quickly to the waiting ambulances. The paramedics took over, and they quickly began care and transport to the hospital.

We returned to the scene, where many members of our rescue squad had gathered. The mood was somber as we waited to hear from the hospital.

In a couple of hours we heard that both of our squad members were stable and improving. A few of us went to see them in the hospital the next day. Much to my surprise, they told me that what had kept them going was my constant talking and reassurance throughout the extrication, and that they had missed that during the ride to the hospital.

Later that day, I considered what my squad members had told me. I realized then that oftentimes the most important care you can give your patients is simply talking to them and showing that you care. Even after more than 20 years in EMS, it is a skill that I have never forgotten.

Jose V. Salazar, MPH, NREMT-P
Captain
Loudoun County Fire-Rescue
Leesburg, Virginia

Crowds

Crowds come in all sizes and have different personalities. Friendly neighborhood crowds may interfere very little with your duties. Unfriendly crowds may require a police presence before you are able to treat the patient. Assess the feeling of the crowd before you get in a position from which there is no exit. Request help from law enforcement officials before the crowd is out of control. Safety considerations may require you to wait for the arrival of police before you approach the patient.

Electrical Hazards

Electrical hazards can be present at many different types of emergency scenes. Patients located inside buildings may be in contact with a wide variety of electrical hazards, ranging from a faulty extension cord in a house to a high-voltage feeder line in an industrial setting. Patients located outside may be in contact with high-voltage electrical power lines that have fallen because of a motor vehicle accident or a storm. Assess the emergency scene for any indications of electrical problems. Inside a building, look for cords, electrical wires, or electrical appliances near or in contact with the patient; outside, look for damaged electrical poles and downed electrical wires. Do not approach an emergency scene if there are indications of electrical problems. Keep all other people away from the source of the hazard, too. Because electricity is invisible, make sure that the electrical current has been turned off by a qualified person before you get close to the source of the current. You should always wear a helmet with a chin strap and face shield in situations that may involve electrical hazards.

Fire

Fire is a hazard that can result in injury or death to you and to the patient. If there appears to be a fire, call at once for fire department assistance. If you are a trained fire fighter, follow rescue and firefighting procedures for your department. If you are not a trained fire fighter, do not exceed the limits of your training. Entering a burning building without proper turnout gear and self-contained breathing apparatus is an unwise course of action. Any attempt to rescue someone from a burning building is a high-risk undertaking. Vehicles that have been involved in accidents also may present a fire hazard from fuel or other spilled fluids. Keep all ignition sources such as cigarettes and road flares away. Carefully assess the fire hazard before you determine your course of action.

Hazardous Materials

Hazardous materials (sometimes referred to as HazMats) may be found almost anywhere. Some transportation accidents involve hazardous materials. They may also be found in homes, businesses, and industries. Federal regulations require vehicles that are transporting hazardous materials to be marked with specific placards **Figure 2-9 ▾**. If you believe that an accident may

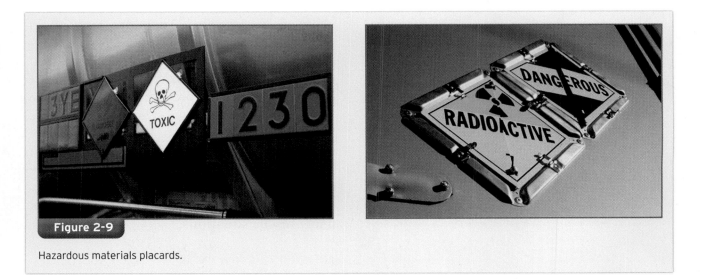

Figure 2-9

Hazardous materials placards.

involve hazardous materials, stop at some distance from the accident and determine if the vehicle is marked with a placard. A pair of binoculars in the life support kit is helpful for this. The placard indicates the class of material that is being carried. You should carry an emergency response guidebook to assist you in determining the hazard involved. The presence of odors or fumes may be the first indication of hazardous materials located in buildings. If you believe that a hazardous material is present, call for assistance from the agency that handles hazardous materials in your community. Remain far enough away from a suspected HazMat incident that you do not become an additional casualty. (See Chapter 18 for more information on handling HazMat incidents.)

Unstable Objects

Unstable objects may include vehicles, trees, poles, buildings, cliffs, and piles of materials. After an accident, a motor vehicle may be located in an unstable position. You may need to stabilize the vehicle before you can begin patient extrication. Do not attempt to enter or get under an unstable vehicle. Motor vehicle accidents may result in other unstable objects, including trees or poles that were hit in the accident. Fires and explosions can result in unstable buildings. Assess a building for stability before attempting to enter it. If you are in doubt about the safety of the building, call for trained personnel rather than attempt to enter an unsafe building alone.

Safety Tips

After working at a scene that involves potential infectious exposure, first responders should clean and disinfect their equipment. Cleaning refers to the removal of dirt, dust, blood, or other visible contaminants. Disinfection requires special chemicals that kill pathogenic agents when applied directly to a surface. It is also important to complete the appropriate documentation of the exposure.

Sharp Objects

Sharp objects are frequently present at an emergency scene. These range from broken glass at the scene of a motor vehicle crash to hypodermic needles in the pocket of a drug addict. Being aware of sharp objects can reduce the chance of injury to yourself and to your patients. Vinyl or latex medical gloves can help prevent the spread of disease from blood contamination, but they provide no protection against sharp objects. When glass or other sharp objects are present, you should wear heavy leather or firefighting gloves over your medical gloves to prevent injuries.

Animals

Animals, whether they are pets, farm stock, or wild, are present in a wide variety of indoor and outdoor settings. Pets can become very upset in the confusion of a medical emergency. If you need to enter a house to take care of a patient, be sure excited pets have been secured in a part of the house away from the patient. People often travel with their pets, so pets can be part of the scene of a motor vehicle crash. Service dogs may be possessive of their owners. Farm animals can be a safety hazard, too. Be careful when entering a field that may contain livestock. Animals may present hazards such as bites or stings. Careful assessment of the incident scene can prevent unnecessary injuries.

Environmental Conditions

Weather is one part of life that cannot be changed or controlled. Therefore, you should consider the effect it will have on rescue operations. Dress appropriately for the expected weather. Keep patients dry and at a comfortable temperature. Be prepared for temperature extremes. Avoid getting too hot or too cold. Be prepared for precipitation. Be alert to possible damage from high winds. Darkness makes it hard for you to see all the hazards that may be present. Use any emergency lighting that is present. A flashlight is a valuable tool to have in many rescue situations.

Special Rescue Situations

Special safety considerations are required in situations involving water rescue, ice rescue, confined space or below-grade rescue, terrorism, and mass-casualty incidents. These situations are covered in Chapters 18, 19, and 20. Do not enter an emergency situation that is unsafe unless you have the proper training and equipment.

Airborne and Bloodborne Pathogens

Because airborne and bloodborne pathogens cannot be seen directly, you should always remember the universal precautions described earlier and apply them as appropriate. It is important that you see your doctor immediately any time you are potentially exposed to an infectious disease.

You are the Provider   SUMMARY

Review the *You are the Provider* case study provided at the beginning of the chapter.

As a new member of your public safety organization, you notice that some long-time veterans of your organization seem to be more relaxed and others seem to show more signs of stress during emergency responses.

1. What steps can you take to reduce stress during emergency responses?

Carefully learning the material presented in this training course will help to reduce the level of stress you experience. Maintaining a good diet with adequate exercise and sleep will also serve to reduce the stress you feel in stressful situations.

2. How are your off-duty activities related to the level of stress you experience while on duty?

Your activities and lifestyle off duty have an impact on the way you are able to handle stress on duty. Maintaining healthy lifestyle choices off duty will help to reduce the stress you encounter on duty.

3. How can failing to follow universal precautions affect your health?

Failing to follow universal precautions increases your risk of contracting a contagious disease, which could result in a short-term or chronic illness.

Prep Kit

Ready for Review

The Ready for Review thoroughly summarizes the chapter.

- First responders should understand the role that stress plays in the lives of emergency care providers and patients who have suffered a sudden illness or accident. Stress is a normal part of a first responder's life.

- The five stages of the grief process are denial, anger, bargaining, depression, and acceptance. Patients and rescuers move through these stages at different rates.

- Stress management consists of recognizing, preventing, and reducing critical incident stress.

- Scene safety is an important part of your job. You should understand how airborne and bloodborne infectious diseases are spread and how body substance isolation prevents their spread.

- As you arrive on the scene of an accident or illness, you must assess the scene for a wide variety of hazards, including traffic, crime, crowds, unstable objects, sharp objects, electrical problems, fire, hazardous materials, animals, environmental conditions, special rescue situations, and infectious disease exposure. You should understand the safety equipment and precautions that are needed for first responder rescue situations.

Vital Vocabulary

The Vital Vocabulary are the key terms for this chapter.

acceptance The fifth stage of the grief process; when the person experiencing grief recognizes the finality of the grief-causing event.

anger The second stage of the grief reaction; when the person suffering grief becomes upset at the grief-causing event or other situation.

bargaining The third stage of the grief reaction; when the person experiencing grief barters to change the grief-causing event.

body substance isolation (BSI) An infection control concept that treats all bodily fluids as potentially infectious.

critical incident stress debriefing (CISD) A system of psychological support designed to reduce stress on emergency personnel after a major stress-producing incident.

denial The first stage of a grief reaction; when the person suffering grief rejects the grief-causing event.

depression The fourth stage of the grief reaction; when the person expresses despair—an absence of cheerfulness and hope—as a result of the grief-causing event.

on-scene peer support Stress counselors at the scene of stressful incidents to deal with stress reduction.

pathogens Microorganisms that are capable of causing disease.

preincident stress education Training about stress and stress reactions conducted for public safety providers before they are exposed to stressful situations.

universal precautions Procedures for infection control that treat blood and certain bodily fluids as capable of transmitting bloodborne diseases.

Technology

- Interactivities
- Vocabulary Explorer
- Anatomy Review
- Web Links
- Online Review Manual

Assessment in Action

Assessment in Action presents a fictitious scenario to help you review what you learned in this chapter.

As a new first responder, you and your partner are dispatched for a call at a residence. As you arrive, you determine that a 7-year-old girl has fallen from a tree and is unresponsive. Her right arm appears to be deformed.

1. Your partner seems to be disturbed as she starts to care for the patient. This call:
   - A. May be more stressful because a child is involved.
   - B. Should not be especially stressful for a first responder.

2. Other signs that might indicate that your partner is experiencing stress include:
   - A. Anger
   - B. Denial
   - C. Bargaining
   - D. All of the above

3. A stress-reducing diet includes all of the following EXCEPT:
   - A. Fruits
   - B. Vegetables
   - C. Milk, yogurt, and cheese
   - D. Caffeine

The following questions are not related to the scenario above.

4. Which of the following help prevent first responders from getting infectious diseases?
   - A. Practice good body substance isolation techniques.
   - B. Get recommended vaccinations.
   - C. Practice universal precautions.
   - D. All of the above.

5. The hazards at an emergency scene will vary from one scene to another.
   - A. True
   - B. False

6. One of the first hazards you need to handle at an emergency scene is:
   - A. Airborne pathogens
   - B. Environmental conditions
   - C. Sharp objects
   - D. Traffic

Medical, Legal, and Ethical Issues

National Standard Curriculum Objectives

Cognitive

1-3.1 Define the First Responder scope of care. (p 40)

1-3.2 Discuss the importance of Do Not Resuscitate [DNR] (advance directives) and local or state provisions regarding EMS application. (p 42)

1-3.3 Define consent and discuss the methods of obtaining consent. (p 41)

1-3.4 Differentiate between expressed and implied consent. (p 41)

1-3.5 Explain the role of consent of minors in providing care. (p 41)

1-3.6 Discuss the implications for the First Responder in patient refusal of transport. (p 42)

1-3.7 Discuss the issues of abandonment, negligence, and battery and their implications to the First Responder. (p 42)

1-3.8 State the conditions necessary for the First Responder to have a duty to act. (p 40)

1-3.9 Explain the importance, necessity, and legality of patient confidentiality. (p 45)

1-3.10 List the actions that a First Responder should take to assist in the preservation of a crime scene. (p 46)

1-3.11 State the conditions that require a First Responder to notify local law enforcement officials. (p 45)

1-3.12 Discuss issues concerning the fundamental components of documentation. (p 46)

Affective

1-3.13 Explain the rationale for the needs, benefits, and usage of advance directives. (p 42)

1-3.14 Explain the rationale for the concept of varying degrees of DNR. (p 42)

Psychomotor

None

Chapter Objectives*

Knowledge and Attitude Objectives

1. Define "duty to act" as it relates to a first responder. (p 40)
2. Describe the standard of care and the scope of care for a first responder. (p 40)
3. Describe and compare the following types of consent:
   - Expressed consent (p 41)
   - Implied consent (p 41)
   - Consent for minors (p 41)
   - Consent of mentally ill patients (p 42)
   - Refusal of care (p 42)
4. Explain the purpose of living wills and advance directives. (p 42)
5. Describe the importance of the following legal concepts:
   - Abandonment (p 42)
   - Death on the scene (p 43)
   - Negligence (p 43)
   - Confidentiality (p 45)
6. Explain the purpose of Good Samaritan laws. (p 45)
7. Describe the federal, state, and local regulations that apply to first responders. (p 45)
8. Describe reportable events in your local area. (p 45)
9. Describe the steps to be taken at a crime scene. (p 46)
10. Explain the reasons for documentation. (p 46)

*These are chapter learning objectives.

You are the Provider

As a first responder, you studied hard to gain the knowledge and master the skills needed to provide emergency medical care. You still have some concerns about the legal implications associated with providing emergency medical assistance.

1. What steps can you take to minimize these concerns?
2. How does the expression "treat every patient as if he or she were a family member" relate to your concerns?

Introduction

First responders need to know some basic legal principles that govern the way they provide care to patients. Knowing these principles can help you provide the best care for patients and prevent situations that could result in legal difficulties for you, your agency, or your department. Because some laws differ from one location to another, you will need to learn the specific laws of your state and your local jurisdiction.

Duty to Act

The first legal principle to consider is the duty to act. A citizen arriving on the scene of an automobile collision is not required by law to stop and give emergency care to victims. However, if you are employed by an agency that has designated you as a first responder and you are dispatched to the scene of an accident or illness, you do have a duty to act. You must proceed promptly to the scene and render emergency medical care within the limits of your training and available equipment ▶ Figure 3-1 ▶ . Any failure to respond or render necessary emergency medical care leaves both you and your agency vulnerable to legal action.

Technology

| Interactivities |
| Vocabulary Explorer |
| Anatomy Review |
| Web Links |
| Online Review Manual |

Standard of Care

What level of care are you expected to give to a patient? As a first responder, you obviously cannot provide the same level of care as a physician, but you are responsible for providing the level of care that a person with similar training would provide under similar circumstances. As a trained first responder, you are expected to use your knowledge and skills to the best of your ability under the circumstances. The circumstances under which you must provide care may affect the standard of care. The standard of care is the manner in which you must act or behave. To comply with the standard of care, you must meet two criteria: (1) You must treat the patient to the best of your ability and (2) you must provide care that a reasonable, prudent person with similar training would provide under similar circumstances. It is important to know exactly what the local standards of care are and what statutes pertain to your community.

Scope of Care

The scope of care you give as a first responder is defined on several levels. The National Curriculum for First Responders, developed by the U.S. Department of Transportation, specifies the skills taught in this course and the way those skills should be performed. States also have scope of care laws that may modify parts of the specifications in the national curriculum. The medical director for your department may use medical protocols or standing orders to specify your scope of care. In some cases, online medical direction is provided by two-way radio or wireless telephone.

Ethical Responsibilities and Competence

Your community and your department have entrusted you, as a first responder, with certain ethical responsibilities. You have a responsibility to conform to accepted professional standards of con-

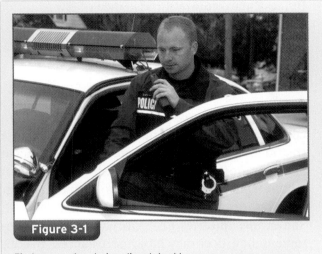
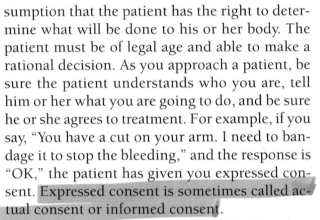

Figure 3-1

First responders being dispatched to an emergency scene.

duct. These include staying up-to-date on the first responder skills and knowledge needed to provide good patient care. You are also responsible for reviewing your performance and assessing the techniques you use. You should evaluate your response times and try to follow up patient care outcomes with your medical director or hospital personnel. Always look for ways to improve your performance. Continuing education classes and refresher courses are designed to keep you current; make the most of them. Participate in quality improvement activities within your department.

Ethical behavior requires honesty. Your reports should accurately reflect the conditions found. Give complete and correct reports to other EMS providers. If you make a mistake on the report or report information incorrectly, do not try to cover it up. Never change a report except to correct an error. Remember that the actions you take in the first few minutes of an emergency may make the difference between life and death for a patient. Your competence and your ethical behavior are valuable to you and to the patient.

Consent for Treatment

Consent simply means approval or permission. Legally, however, there are several types of consent. In expressed consent, the patient actually lets you know—verbally or nonverbally—that he or she is willing to accept the treatment you provide. Expressed consent is based on the as-

sumption that the patient has the right to determine what will be done to his or her body. The patient must be of legal age and able to make a rational decision. As you approach a patient, be sure the patient understands who you are, tell him or her what you are going to do, and be sure he or she agrees to treatment. For example, if you say, "You have a cut on your arm. I need to bandage it to stop the bleeding," and the response is "OK," the patient has given you expressed consent. Expressed consent is sometimes called actual consent or informed consent.

Any patient who does not specifically refuse emergency care can be treated under the principle of implied consent. The principle of implied consent is best understood in the situation of an unconscious patient. Because this patient is unable to communicate, the principles of law assume consent for treatment. Therefore, a first responder should never hesitate to treat an unconscious patient.

Consent for Minors

A minor is a person who has not yet reached the legal age designated by a particular state. Under the law, minors (who may be as old as 19) are not considered capable of speaking for themselves. In most cases, emergency treatment of a minor by a physician must wait until a parent or legal guardian consents to the treatment. If a minor requires emergency medical care in the field (out of the hospital) and the permission of a parent or legal guardian cannot be quickly obtained, do not

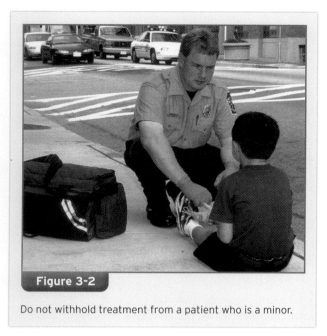

Figure 3-2

Do not withhold treatment from a patient who is a minor.

hesitate to give appropriate emergency medical care. Emergency medical treatment for a minor should never be delayed or withheld just to obtain permission from a parent or legal guardian **Figure 3-2 ▲**. Let hospital officials determine what treatment can be postponed until permission is obtained. Remember that good prehospital patient care is your first responsibility. By following the course of action that is best for the patient, you will stand on firm legal ground.

Consent of Mentally Ill

A rational adult may legally refuse to be treated. The legal issues are more complicated if the patient who refuses to be treated appears to be out of touch with reality and is a danger to self or others. The difficult part, even for highly trained medical personnel, is determining whether such a patient is rational. Generally, if the person appears to be a threat to self or others, arrangements need to be made to place this person under medical care. The legal means by which these arrangements are made vary from state to state. You and other members of the EMS system should know your state's legal mechanism for handling patients who refuse to be treated and who do not appear to be making rational and reasonable decisions. Do not hesitate to involve law enforcement agencies, because this

process may require the issuance of a warrant or an order of protective custody.

Patient Refusal of Care

Remember that any person who is mentally in control, or competent, has a legal right to refuse treatment from emergency medical personnel at any time. You can continue to talk with a person who refuses treatment and try to help him or her understand the consequences of this action. Sometimes another EMS provider or a law enforcement officer may have more success in convincing a patient that he or she needs to receive treatment.

Advance Directives

An advance directive, also commonly called a living will, is a written document drawn up by a patient, a physician, and a lawyer. Similar documents are also called advance directives to physicians, durable power of attorney for health care, or do not resuscitate (DNR) orders. Advance directives are often written when a patient has a terminal condition. For example, a terminally ill patient may request that no CPR be performed. If you are not able to determine if an advance directive is legally valid, you should begin appropriate medical care and leave the questions about advance directives to physicians. Some states have systems, such as bracelets, to identify patients with advance directives. You should know your local policies and protocols.

Legal Concepts

Abandonment

Abandonment occurs when a trained person begins emergency care and then leaves the patient before another trained person arrives to take over. Once you have started treatment, you must continue that treatment until a person who has the same or at least as much training arrives on the scene and takes over. Never leave a patient with-

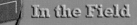

In the Field

Four Legal Concepts You Should Understand

1. Abandonment
2. Persons dead at the scene
3. Negligence
4. Confidentiality

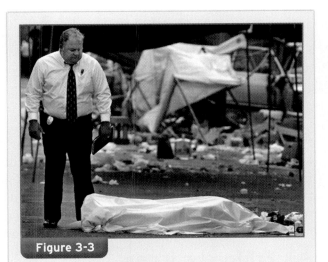

Figure 3-3

Learn the protocol for dealing with patients who are obviously dead at the scene.

out care after you begin treatment. The most common abandonment scenario occurs when an EMS provider responds to a call, examines the patient, assesses the patient's condition, fails to transport the patient to a hospital, and finds out later that the patient died. Treatment began, but the patient was abandoned.

Persons Dead at the Scene

If there is any indication that a person is alive when you arrive on the scene, you should begin providing necessary care. Persons who are obviously dead should be handled according to the laws of your state and the protocols of your service. Generally, you cannot assume a person is dead unless one or more of the following conditions exist:

1. **Decapitation.** Decapitation means that the head is separated from the body. When this occurs, there is obviously no chance of saving the patient.
2. **Rigor mortis.** Rigor mortis is the temporary stiffening of muscles that occurs several hours after death. The presence of this stiffening indicates that the patient is dead and cannot be resuscitated.
3. **Tissue decomposition.** Body tissue begins to decompose and flesh begins to decay only after a person has been dead for more than a day.
4. **Dependent lividity.** Dependent lividity is the red or purple color that occurs on the parts of the patient's body that are closest to the ground. It is caused by blood seeping into the tissues on the dependent, or lower, part of the person's body. Dependent lividity occurs after a person has been dead for several hours.

If any of these signs is present, you can usually consider the patient to be dead. It is important that you know the protocol your department uses in dealing with patients who are dead on the scene **Figure 3-3 ▲**. Chapter 9 covers these criteria as they relate to starting CPR.

Negligence

Negligence occurs when a patient suffers further injury or harm because the care that was administered did not meet the standards expected from a person with similar training in a similar situation. For negligence to occur, four conditions must be present:

1. Duty to act
2. Breach of duty
3. Resulting injuries
4. Proximate cause

As a first responder who has been called to a scene to provide patient care, you have a duty to help the patient. If you fail to provide care according to the level of your training, this could constitute a breach of duty. For negligence to be proved, the patient must sustain injuries as a result of your improper care. Injuries related to your negligent actions or failure to act properly constitute proximate cause. Examples of negligence include reckless or careless performance or care that does not meet the accepted standard for a first responder.

Voices of Experience

Do Their Parents Know Where They Are?

I was the attendant-in-charge dispatched to a rollover motor vehicle collision at about 2:30 AM one dreary, rainy night. Dispatch information told me that an SUV was involved and that our county sheriff's department was already at the scene. We were sent to direct aid with an adjoining fire department engine that arrived on scene first. We arrived at the scene a couple of minutes after the engine and discovered that there were multiple patients. I made contact with the engine company lieutenant and became the medical group supervisor.

> **Ethically, it can be a challenge to treat patients who act irresponsibly.**

The story was a sad one. The sheriff deputy already had taken the driver of the SUV into custody. He told me that there were four occupants in the SUV who were taking methamphetamines and drinking alcohol. They were not wearing any vehicle restraints. When the sheriff had tried to pull the vehicle over, the driver evaded the pursuit and in the ensuing chase, the SUV rolled over and ejected three of the four occupants.

I began triage and found one passenger on the roadside, screaming in pain from an open femur fracture. There were already EMTs preparing her for transport. I immediately called for a second EMS unit. The other two occupants had been thrown from the vehicle in opposite directions. They were approximately 25 feet from the vehicle, sustaining fatal injuries. These two patients were teenagers. To this day, I can recall thinking to myself that this was not what I had come into this profession to do. I didn't like the tremendous responsibility of declaring someone dead. I was there to save the lives of people. Look at this tragedy; these two young people had no futures ahead of them. Did their parents know where they were?

I persuaded the sheriff's department to release the driver into my care for evaluation at the emergency department. Due to the mechanism of injury and the deaths of the other occupants as risk factors, it was important to have the driver examined for any hidden injuries. As I transferred the patient to the bed in the emergency room, a vial of methamphetamines fell out of his pocket. He laid there laughing, displaying no remorse for the deaths of his "friends."

As an EMS provider, it is difficult to respond to situations like this one. Ethically, it can be a challenge to treat patients who act irresponsibly and put their own lives and the lives of others in unnecessary danger. However, we must put our own personal feelings aside and treat the patient regardless of our feelings. In situations like this one, it is helpful to have the assistance of a law enforcement official to ensure scene safety while the patients are triaged and treated. Police assistance is especially important in cases where drug and alcohol use may affect the behavior of the patients.

T.J. Bishop, NREMT-P
Clinical Officer
North Country EMS
Yacolt, Washington

Confidentiality

Most patient information is confidential. Confidential information includes patient circumstances, patient history, assessment findings, and patient care given. This information should be shared only with other medical personnel who are involved in the patient's care. Do not discuss this privileged information with your family or friends.

In certain circumstances, you may release confidential information to designated individuals. In most states, records may be released when a legal subpoena is presented or the patient signs a written release. The patient must be mentally competent and fully understand the nature of the release.

Some information about a patient's care may be classified as public information. You should learn what patient information is considered public information in your state. Public information can be released to the news media through your department's approved process.

HIPAA

HIPAA is the acronym for the Health Insurance Portability and Accountability Act of 1996. Although this act had many aims, including improving the portability and continuity of health insurance coverage and combating waste and fraud in health insurance and in the provision of health care, the section of the act that most affects EMS relates to patient privacy. The aim of this section was to strengthen laws for the protection of the privacy of health care information and to safeguard patient confidentiality. As such, it provides guidance on what type of information is protected, the responsibility of health care providers regarding that protection, and penalties for breaching that protection.

Most personal health information is protected and should not be released without the patient's permission. If you are not sure, do not give any information to anyone other than those directly involved in the care of the patient. For specific policies, each EMS service is required to have a manual and a privacy officer who can answer questions. You can expect to receive further training on how this act impacts your specific response agency and resource hospital.

Good Samaritan Laws

Most states have adopted Good Samaritan laws, which protect citizens from liability for errors or omissions in giving good faith emergency care. These laws vary considerably from state to state and they may or may not apply to first responders in your state. Recently, legal experts have noted that Good Samaritan laws may no longer be needed because they provide little or no legal protection for a rescuer or EMS provider.

Any properly trained first responder who practices the skills and procedures learned in a first responder course should not be overly concerned about lack of protection under Good Samaritan statutes.

Regulations

As a first responder, you are subject to a variety of federal, state, local, and agency regulations. You should become familiar with these regulations so you can follow them. The most important regulations govern your ability to work as a first responder. You may have to become registered or certified as a first responder through a state agency or you may have to register through the National Registry of Emergency Medical Technicians. It is your responsibility to keep any required certifications or registrations up-to-date.

Reportable Events

State and federal agencies have requirements for reporting certain events, including crimes and infectious diseases. Reportable crimes include knife wounds, gunshot wounds, motor vehicle accidents, suspected child abuse, domestic violence, elder abuse, dog bites, and rape. You must learn which crimes are reportable in your area. You also need to know your agency's procedures on reporting these crimes. Certain infectious diseases are also reportable. It is important that you learn how this process is handled in your agency and what you are required to do.

Crime Scene Operations

Many emergency medical situations are also crime scenes. As a first responder, you should keep the following considerations in mind:

1. Protect yourself. Be sure the scene is safe before you try to enter.
2. If you determine that a crime scene is unsafe, wait until law enforcement personnel signal that the scene is safe for entry.
3. Your first priority is patient care. Nothing except your personal safety should interfere with that effort.
4. Move the patient only if necessary, such as for rapid transport to the hospital, for administration of CPR, or for treatment of severe shock. If you must move the patient, take a mental "snapshot" of the scene.
5. Touch only what you need to touch to gain access to the patient.
6. Preserve the crime scene for further investigation **Figure 3-4** ▸. Do not move furniture unless it interferes with your ability to provide care. If you must move anything out of the way, move it no further than necessary to provide care.
7. Be careful where you put your equipment. You could alter or destroy evidence if you put your equipment on top of it.
8. Keep nonessential personnel such as curious neighbors away from the scene.
9. After you have attended to a patient at a crime scene, write a short report about the incident and make a sketch of the scene that shows how and where you found the patient. This may be useful if you are required to recall the incident 2 or 3 years later.

Documentation

After you have finished treating the patient, record your observations about the scene, the patient's condition, and the treatment you pro-

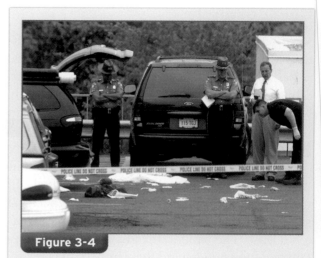

Figure 3-4

Crime scene operations require you to change the scene as little as possible.

vided. Documentation should be done according to the policies of your organization. These policies should follow appropriate local and state laws. Your documentation is important because it is the initial account describing the patient's condition and the care administered. You will not be able to remember the treatment you provide to each patient without documentation. It also serves as a legal record of your treatment and will be required in the event of a lawsuit. Documentation also provides a basis for evaluating the quality of care provided. Documentation should be clear, concise, accurate, and readable. More information on documentation is presented in Chapter 8.

Documentation should include the following information:

1. The condition of the patient when found
2. The patient's description of the injury or illness
3. The patient's initial and repeat vital signs
4. The treatment you gave the patient
5. The agency and personnel who took over treatment of the patient
6. Any reportable conditions present
7. Any infectious disease exposure
8. Anything unusual regarding the case

You are the Provider   SUMMARY

Review the *You are the Provider* case study provided at the beginning of the chapter.

As a first responder, you studied hard to gain the knowledge and master the skills needed to provide emergency medical care. You still have some concerns about the legal implications associated with providing emergency medical assistance.

1. What steps can you take to minimize these concerns?

You can minimize your concerns about the legal liability of providing emergency medical care by understanding the concepts of standard of care, scope of care, and consent for treatment. Following these concepts while rendering emergency medical care provides significant protection from legal problems.

2. How does the expression "treat every patient as if he or she were a family member" relate to your concerns?

The expression "treat every patient as if he or she were a family member" serves to remind you that the best protection from legal problems is to render the best care you can while treating each patient with the respect you would give to a family member.

Prep Kit

Ready for Review

The Ready for Review thoroughly summarizes the chapter.

- This chapter introduces the legal principles you need to know as a first responder.

- As a first responder, you have a duty to act when you are dispatched on a medical call as a part of your official duties.

- You are held to a certain standard of care, which is related to your level of training, and you are expected to perform to the level a similarly trained person would perform under similar circumstances.

- You should understand the differences between expressed consent, implied consent, consent for minors, consent of mentally ill persons, and the right to refuse care.

- Advance directives give a patient the right to have care withheld. Because first responders cannot determine the validity of these documents, it is best to begin treatment for these patients.

- This chapter also covers the concepts of abandonment, negligence, and confidentiality, as well as the purpose of Good Samaritan laws, even though they are not needed for first responders.

- You must understand the importance of federal and state regulations that govern your performance as a first responder. You must also understand your department's operational regulations. Certain events that deal with contagious diseases or with illegal acts must be reported to the proper authorities. You should know how to deal with these reportable events.

- Crime scene operations are a complex environment. Following proper procedures assures that the patient receives good medical care and that the crime scene is not compromised for the law enforcement investigation.

- Your job is not complete until the paperwork is done. It is important that first responders document their findings and treatment. This provides good patient care and adequate legal documentation.

- By understanding and following these legal concepts, you will build the foundation for the skills you need to be a good first responder.

Vital Vocabulary

The Vital Vocabulary are the key terms for this chapter.

abandonment Failure of the first responder to continue emergency medical treatment until relieved by someone with the same or higher level of training.

advance directive A legal document with specific instructions that the patient does not want to be resuscitated or kept alive by mechanical support systems. Also called a living will.

competent Able to make rational decisions about personal well-being.

duty to act A first responder's legal responsibility to respond promptly to an emergency scene and provide medical care (within the limits of training and available equipment).

expressed consent Consent actually given by a person authorizing the first responder to provide care or transportation.

Good Samaritan laws Laws that encourage individuals to voluntarily help an injured or suddenly ill person by minimizing the liability for any errors or omissions in rendering good faith emergency care.

implied consent Consent to receive emergency care that is assumed because the individual is unconscious, underage, or so badly injured or ill that he or she cannot respond.

negligence Deviation from the accepted standard of care resulting in further injury to the patient.

standard of care The manner in which an individual must act or behave when giving care.

Technology

- Interactivities
- Vocabulary Explorer
- Anatomy Review
- Web Links
- Online Review Manual

Assessment in Action

Assessment in Action presents a fictitious scenario to help you review what you learned in this chapter.

You and your partner are dispatched to the local supermarket. When you arrive on scene, you find a 2-year-old boy lying on the floor next to an overturned grocery cart. The boy is bleeding profusely from his head but appears to be conscious, alert, and oriented. You inquire about the boy's parents only to find that the boy is at the store with his 16-year-old sister.

1. What type of consent—if any—do you have to treat this patient?

   A. Expressed
   B. Implied
   C. Informed
   D. None

2. To what level must you provide care to this patient?

   A. You cannot treat this patient because there is not a parent on scene to give you the needed permission.
   B. You must treat the patient to the best of your ability and you must provide care that a reasonable, prudent person with similar training would provide under similar circumstances.

3. If you were to refuse to treat this patient and left the scene, you would be guilty of:

   A. HIPAA
   B. Abandonment
   C. Scope of care
   D. Duty to act

4. For negligence to occur, what four conditions must be present?

   A. Duty to act, breach of duty, resulting injuries, proximate cause
   B. Duty to act, breach of duty, abandonment, resulting injuries

5. If this child had been bitten by a dog, this would be considered a reportable event.

   A. True
   B. False

The Human Body

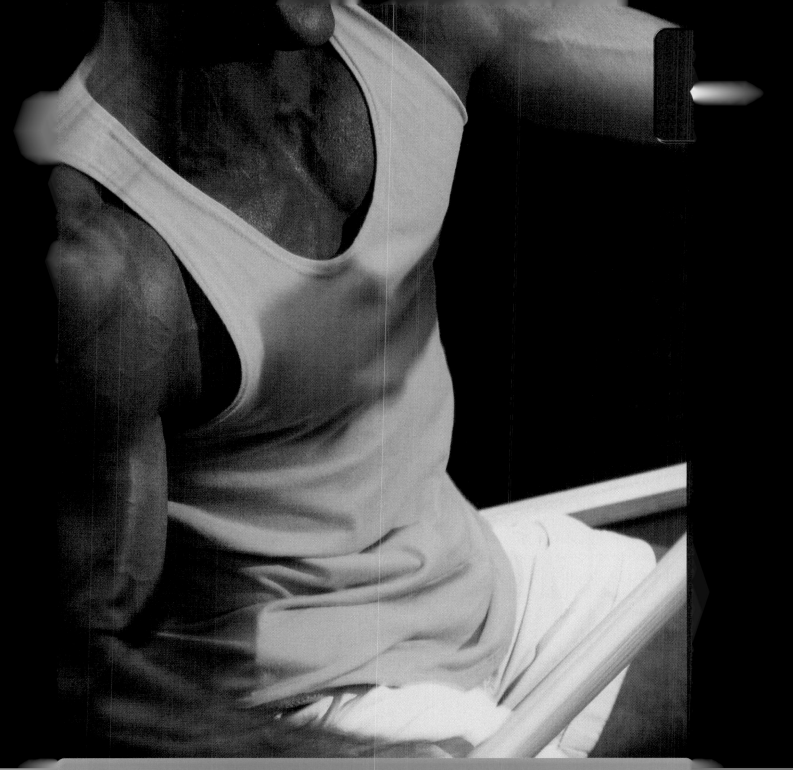

You are the Provider

You are dispatched to 114 Foster Center Road for a 47-year-old man who is complaining of back pain. When you arrive, you find an alert and oriented middle-aged man lying on the floor of his bedroom. He states that when he bent down to pick up his belt, his back tightened up. Now the pain is so bad that he cannot move. When you ask him where the pain is, he points to his lower back.

1. Why is some knowledge of anatomy and some understanding of the function of body systems so important in cases like this?

Introduction

To be an effective first responder, you must understand the basic structure and functions of the human body. This knowledge will help you understand the problem the patient is experiencing, perform an adequate patient examination, communicate your findings to the other members of the emergency medical team, and provide appropriate emergency treatment for the patient's condition. This chapter describes human anatomy and the relationships among eight body systems.

Topographic Anatomy

The anatomic terms in this section are used to describe the location of injury or pain. Knowing the basic anatomic terms for human body parts is important because all members of the emergency medical team must be able to speak the same language when treating a patient. However, if you cannot remember the proper anatomic term for a certain body location, you can use lay terms.

Visualize a person standing and facing you, with arms at the sides and thumbs pointing outward (palms toward you). This is the standard anatomic position; you should keep it in

mind when describing a location on the body. **Figure 4-1 ▾** identifies <u>topographic anatomy</u>.

The first terms that should be clarified are left and right. These terms always refer to the patient's left and right. **Anterior** and **posterior** simply mean front and back, respectively. The **midline** refers to an imaginary vertical line drawn from head to toe that separates the body into a left half and a right half.

Two other useful terms are medial and lateral. **Medial** means closer to the midline of the body; **lateral** means away from the midline. In this context, the eyes are lateral to the nose.

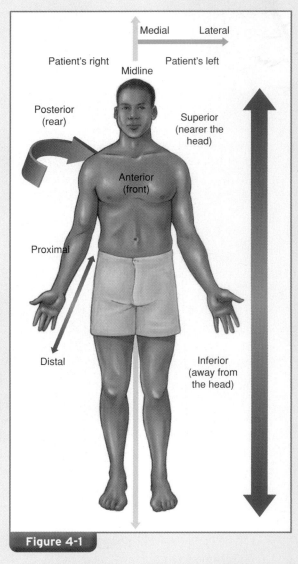

Figure 4-1

Topographic anatomy terms for describing a location on the body.

The term **proximal** means close and **distal** means distant. On the body, proximal means close to the point where an arm or leg is attached. Distal means distant from the point of attachment. For example, if the thigh bone (femur) is broken, the break can be either proximal (the end closer to the hip) or distal (the end farther away from the hip).

The term **superior** means closer to the head and **inferior** means closer to the feet. For example, the hips are inferior to the chest and the chest is superior to the hip.

Body Systems

Body systems work together to perform common functions. By studying these body systems, you will have a better background for understanding illnesses and injuries.

The Respiratory System

Because airway maintenance is one of the most important skills you will learn as a first responder, the **respiratory system** is the first of the body systems reviewed.

The respiratory system consists of all the structures of the body that contribute to normal breathing Figure 4-2 ▶ . The respiratory system brings oxygen into the body and removes the waste gas, carbon dioxide.

The airway consists of the nose (nasopharynx), mouth (oropharynx), throat, **larynx** (voicebox), trachea (windpipe), and the passages within the lungs Figure 4-3 ▶ .

At the upper end of the larynx is a tiny flapper valve called the **epiglottis**. The epiglottis keeps food from entering the larynx. The airway within the lungs branches into narrower and narrower passages that end in tiny air sacs called alveoli. These air sacs are surrounded by tiny blood vessels.

Oxygen (O_2) in inhaled air passes through the thin walls that separate the air sacs from the blood vessels and is absorbed by the blood. **Carbon dioxide (CO_2)** passes from the blood across the same thin walls into the air sacs and is exhaled. This exchange of carbon dioxide for oxygen occurs 12 to 16 times per minute,

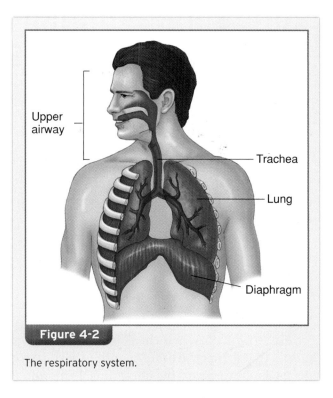

Figure 4-2

The respiratory system.

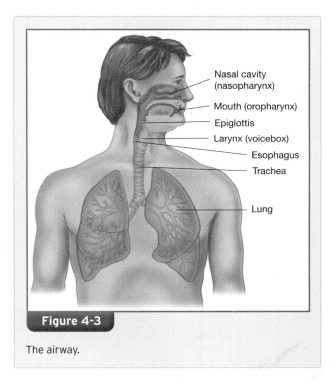

Figure 4-3

The airway.

24 hours a day, without any conscious effort on your part Figure 4-4 ▶ . The rate of breathing increases when the body needs more oxygen or when it generates additional carbon dioxide. Blood transports the inhaled oxygen to all parts of the body through the circulatory system.

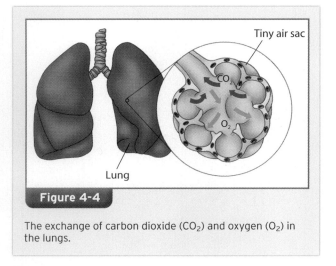

Figure 4-4

The exchange of carbon dioxide (CO_2) and oxygen (O_2) in the lungs.

Infants and children have somewhat different respiratory systems than adults:

- A child's airway is smaller and more flexible. When you perform rescue breathing on a child, do not apply as much force as for an adult.
- Because of its smaller size, a child's airway is more easily blocked by a foreign object.

Very young infants can breathe only through their noses. Therefore, if an infant's nose becomes blocked, the infant will show signs of respiratory distress.

Air is inhaled when the **diaphragm**, a large muscle that forms the bottom of the chest cavity, moves downward and the chest muscles contract to expand the size of the chest. Air is exhaled when these muscles relax, thus decreasing the size of the chest **Figure 4-5 ▼**.

The Circulatory System

The **circulatory system** is responsible for pumping blood through the body. The circulatory system consists of the heart, which pumps blood through a network of blood vessels to all parts of the body.

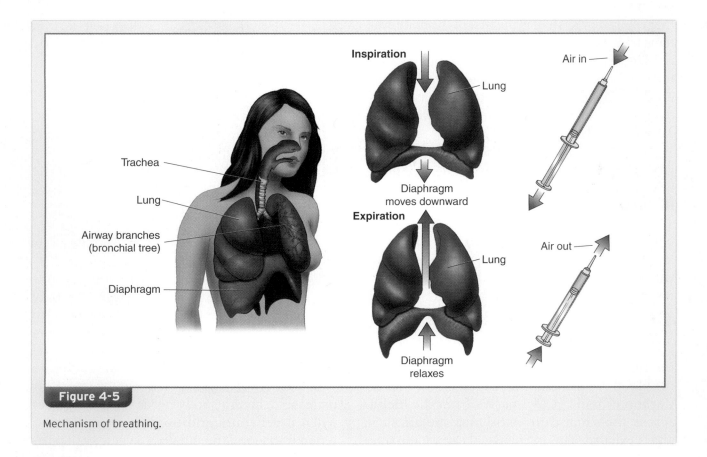

Inspiration

Lung

Air in

Diaphragm moves downward

Expiration

Lung

Air out

Diaphragm relaxes

Trachea

Lung

Airway branches (bronchial tree)

Diaphragm

Figure 4-5

Mechanism of breathing.

After blood picks up oxygen in the lungs, it goes to the heart, which pumps it to the rest of the body. The cells of the body absorb oxygen and nutrients from the blood and release waste products (including carbon dioxide), which the blood carries back to the lungs and kidneys. In the lungs, the blood exchanges the carbon dioxide for more oxygen and the cycle begins again **Figure 4-6 ▾**.

The human heart consists of four chambers, two on the right side and two on the left side. Each upper chamber is called an **atrium**. The right atrium receives blood from the veins of the body; the left atrium receives blood from the lungs. The bottom chambers are the right and left ventricles. The right ventricle pumps blood to the lungs; the left ventricle pumps blood throughout the body and is the most muscular chamber of the heart. The four chambers of the heart work together in a well-ordered sequence to pump blood to the lungs and to the rest of the body **Figure 4-7 ▸**.

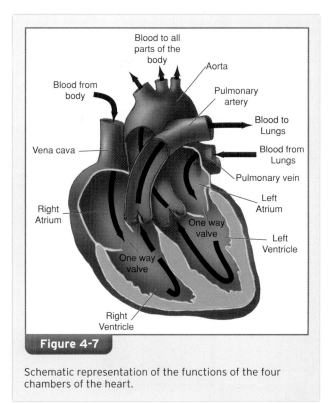

Figure 4-7

Schematic representation of the functions of the four chambers of the heart.

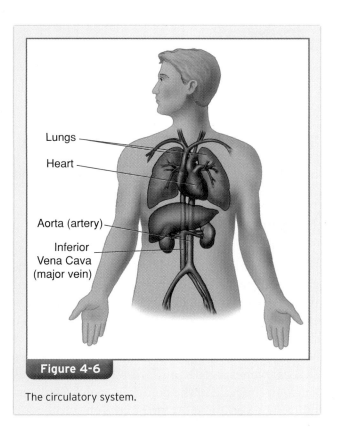

Figure 4-6

The circulatory system.

One-way check valves in the heart and the veins allow the blood to flow in only one direction through the circulatory system. The arteries carry blood away from the heart at high pressure and therefore have thick walls. The arteries closest to the heart are quite large (about 1 inch in diameter) but become smaller farther away from the heart.

Three major arteries are the neck (or carotid) artery, the groin (or femoral) artery, and the wrist (or radial) artery. The locations of these arteries are shown in **Figure 4-8 ▸**. Because these arteries lie between a bony structure and the skin, they are used as locations to measure the patient's **pulse**, or the wave of pressure that is created by the heart as it forces blood into the arteries.

The capillaries are the smallest vessels in the system. Some capillaries are so small that only one blood cell at a time can go through them. At the capillary level, oxygen and nutrients pass from the blood cells into the cells of body tissues, and carbon dioxide and other waste products pass from the tissue cells to the blood cells, which then return to the lungs.

Veins are the thin-walled vessels of the circulatory system that carry blood back to the heart.

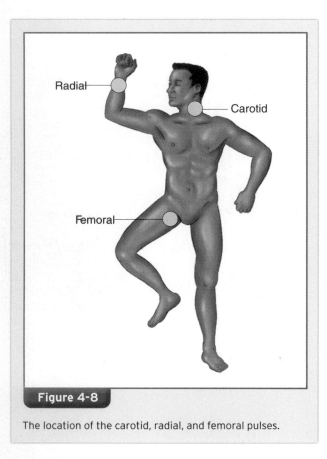

Figure 4-8

The location of the carotid, radial, and femoral pulses.

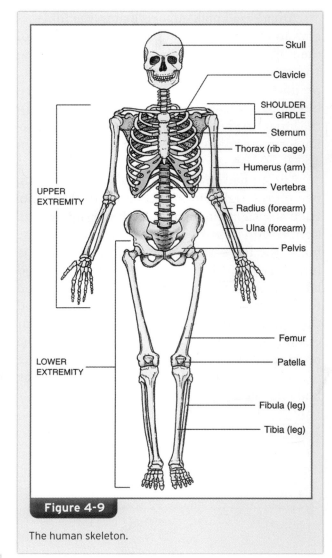

Figure 4-9

The human skeleton.

Blood has several components: <u>plasma</u> (a clear, straw-colored fluid), red blood cells, white blood cells, and <u>platelets</u>. Blood gets its red color from the red blood cells, which carry oxygen from the lungs to the body and bring carbon dioxide back to the lungs. The white blood cells are called infection fighters because they devour bacteria and other disease-causing organisms. Platelets start the blood-clotting process.

The Skeletal System

The skeletal system consists of bones and is the supporting framework for the body. The three functions of the skeletal system are to:

1. Support the body
2. Protect vital structures
3. Manufacture red blood cells

The skeletal system is divided into seven areas beginning with the head **Figure 4-9** ▶.

The Skull

The bones of the head include the <u>skull</u> and the lower jawbone. The skull consists of many bones fused together to form a hollow sphere that contains and protects the brain. The jawbone is a movable bone that is attached to the skull and completes the structure of the head.

The Spine

The spine is the second area of the skeletal system and consists of a series of 33 separate bones called <u>vertebrae</u>. The spinal vertebrae are stacked on top of each other and are held together by muscles, <u>tendons</u> (cords that attach muscles to bones), disks, and <u>ligaments</u> (fibrous bands that connect bone to bone). The spinal cord, a group of nerves that carry messages to and from the brain, passes through the hole in the center of each spinal vertebra. The vertebrae provide excellent protection for the spinal cord. In addition to protecting the spinal cord, the spine is the primary support structure for the entire body. The spine has five sections Figure 4-10 ▾ :

1. **Cervical spine** (neck)
2. **Thoracic spine** (upper back)
3. **Lumbar spine** (lower back)
4. **Sacrum** (base of spine)
5. **Coccyx** (tailbone)

The Shoulder Girdles

The **shoulder girdles** form the third area of the skeletal system. Each shoulder girdle supports an arm and consists of the collarbone (clavicle), the shoulder blade (scapula), and the upper arm bone (humerus).

The Upper Extremity

The fourth major area of the skeletal system is the upper extremity, which consists of three major bones. The arm has one bone (the **humerus**) and the forearm has two bones (the **ulna** and the **radius**). The radius is located on the thumb or lateral side of the arm and the ulna is located on the little-finger or medial side. The wrist and hand are considered part of the upper extremity and consist of several bones, whose names you do not need to learn. You can consider these bones as one unit for the purposes of emergency treatment.

The Rib Cage

The fifth area of the skeletal system is the rib cage (chest). The twelve sets of **ribs** protect the heart, lungs, liver, and spleen. All of the ribs attach to the spine Figure 4-11 ▾ . The upper five sets of ribs connect directly to the **sternum** (breastbone). The ends of the sixth through tenth rib sets are connected to each other and to the sternum by a bridge of **cartilage**. The eleventh and twelfth rib sets are attached to the spine but not attached to the sternum in any way and are called **floating ribs**.

The sternum is located in the front of the chest. The pointed structure at the bottom of the sternum is called the **xiphoid process**.

The Pelvis

The sixth area of the skeletal system is the **pelvis**. The pelvis serves as the link between the body and the lower extremities. In addition, the pelvis protects the reproductive organs and the other organs located in the lower abdominal cavity.

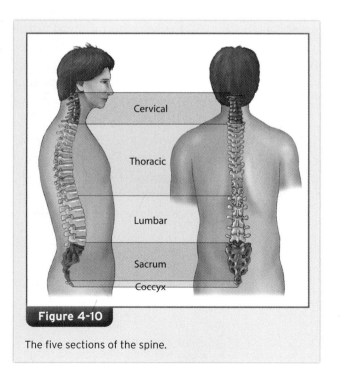

Figure 4-10

The five sections of the spine.

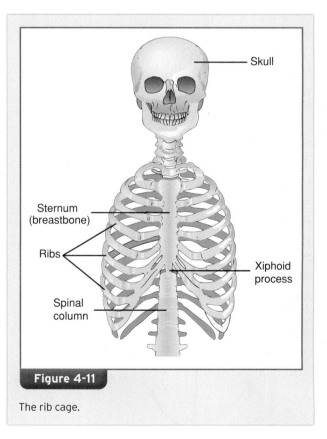

Figure 4-11

The rib cage.

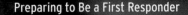

Voices of Experience

Taking the Time

It was around 3:00 AM when my partner and I responded to a call from a 75-year-old woman who had visited her physician the previous day. Upon arrival at the residence, the patient greeted us and led us to the kitchen table where she had several new prescriptions. The patient was very frightened and stated, "The doctor just said take these pills, and I feel shaky now." Unfortunately, the doctor hadn't explained what all these medications were for.

> **Sometimes, it is not the high-stress trauma cases that teach you the most, but rather the calls where you can help patients by explaining the situation in a way that eases their fear.**

After taking a look at the prescriptions and obtaining the patient's medical history, my partner and I developed a plan to help the patient understand how the medications worked and why her doctor had prescribed them to assist with her hypertension and non–insulin-dependent diabetes. After 20 minutes of sitting with the patient and illustrating on a piece of paper how the body systems work, the patient had a better understanding of why the new medications were prescribed and how they would improve her health.

One of the most important aspects of patient care is having a basic understanding of the human body and its functions. In order to properly care for any patient, the provider must know how body systems work and be able to convey that knowledge to the most important person in the EMS process—the patient.

When I entered the field of EMS, I had the goal of making a difference in the life of at least one person; this experience allowed me to achieve my goal. Sometimes, it is not the high-stress trauma cases that teach you the most, but rather the calls where you can help patients by explaining the situation in a way that eases their fear. Approximately one week after this call, the patient's daughter arrived at the EMS substation and delivered a plate of homemade chocolate chip cookies. She explained that her mother had lived alone for several years and was very frightened of any and all medical treatment prior to that evening. According to the patient's daughter, after discussing her medications with us, her mother was much more comfortable with medical appointments and procedures, which led to a more positive relationship with professional health care providers.

As a first responder, you will be faced with a wide variety of cases that all involve a basic understanding of the human body. Some of them will require you to show that understanding through lifesaving actions, while others will require you to take the time to discuss with your patients how they might take a more active role in their own medical treatment. No matter what kind of call you get, a basic understanding of the human body is key to determining what the problem is and how best to handle it.

Michael Hay, MHA, LP, NREMT-P
Texas Department of State Health Services
EMS Compliance
San Antonio, Texas

You can see that a protective bony structure encases each of the essential organs of the body:

- The skull protects the brain.
- The vertebrae protect the spinal cord.
- The ribs protect the heart and lungs.
- The pelvic bones protect the lower abdominal and reproductive organs.

The Lower Extremities

The lower extremities form the seventh area of the skeletal system. Each lower extremity consists of the thigh and the leg. The thighbone (femur) is the longest and strongest bone in the entire body. The leg has two bones, the tibia and fibula. The kneecap (patella) is a small, relatively flat bone that protects the front of the knee joint. Like the wrist and hand, the ankle and foot contain a large number of smaller bones that you can consider as one unit.

Joints

Where two bones come in contact with each other, a <u>joint</u> is formed. Supporting tissues called tendons and ligaments help to hold the joint together. Joints are lubricated by a thin fluid that is contained in a sac surrounding the joint.

There are three types of joints. Fused joints do not permit any movement between the bone ends. The skull is an example of a fused joint. Hinge joints allow movement in one plane. The knee, elbow, and fingers are examples of hinge joints. Ball-and-socket joints allow movement in more than one plane. The shoulder and the hip are examples of ball-and-socket joints. **Figure 4-12 ▼** shows different types of joints.

Moveable joints are designed to permit a certain amount of movement. If movement occurs beyond these limits, injury and damage to the joint will occur.

The Muscular System

Your body contains three different types of muscles: skeletal, smooth, and cardiac. Skeletal muscles provide both support and movement. They are attached to bones by tendons. These muscles cause movement by alternately contracting (shortening) and relaxing (lengthening). To move bones, skeletal muscles are usually paired in opposition: as one member of the pair contracts, the other relaxes. This mechanical opposition enables you to open and close your hand, turn your head, and bend and straighten your elbow. For example, when the biceps relaxes, an opposing muscle on the back of the arm contracts, straightening the elbow. Because skeletal muscles can be contracted or relaxed whenever you want, they are also called voluntary muscles.

Smooth muscles carry out many of the automatic functions of the body, such as propelling food through the digestive system. You have no control over smooth muscles, so they are also called involuntary muscles.

Cardiac muscle is found only in the heart. Cardiac muscle is adapted to its special function of working all the time. It has a rich blood supply and can live only a few minutes without an adequate supply of oxygen.

Sometimes the skeletal and muscular systems are considered together. In this case, the

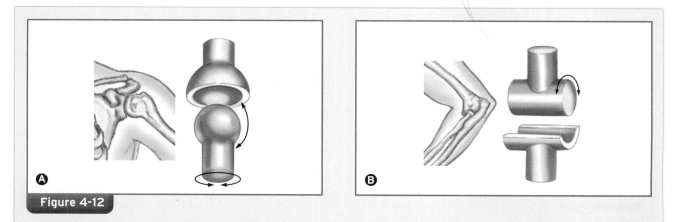

Figure 4-12

Different types of joints. **A.** The shoulder is a ball-and-socket joint. **B.** The elbow joints are hinge joints, which allow motion only in one plane.

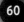

two systems are referred to as the muscu-loskeletal system.

The Nervous System

The **nervous system** governs the body's functioning. The nervous system consists of the brain, the spinal cord, and the individual **nerves** that extend throughout the body   Figure 4-13 ▾ . The brain and spinal cord are called the central nervous system. The cables of nerve fibers outside the central nervous system are called the peripheral nervous system.

The brain is the body's "central computer" and controls the functions of thinking, voluntary actions (things you do consciously), and involuntary (automatic) functions such as breathing, heartbeat, and digestion.

The spinal cord is a long, tube-like structure that extends from the base of the brain. It con-

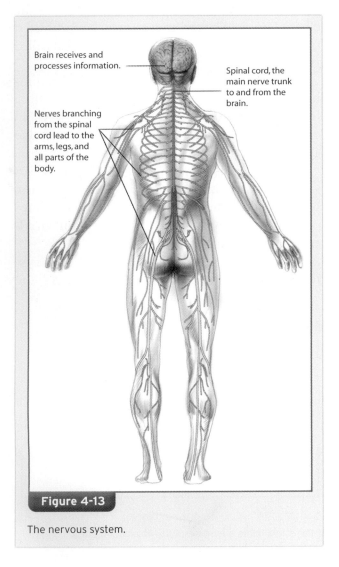

Brain receives and processes information.

Spinal cord, the main nerve trunk to and from the brain.

Nerves branching from the spinal cord lead to the arms, legs, and all parts of the body.

Figure 4-13

The nervous system.

sists of a complex network of nerves that make up a two-way communication system between the brain and the rest of the body. Nerves branch out from the spinal cord to every part of the body (like telephone lines, Internet connections, and television cables going into houses and individual rooms). Some nerves send signals to the brain about what is happening to the body; for example, whether it is feeling heat, cold, pain, or pleasure. Other nerves carry signals to muscles that cause the body to move in response to the sensory signals it has received. Without the nervous system, you would not have such sensations nor would you be able to control the movement of your muscles.

The Digestive System

The **digestive system** breaks down food into a form that can be carried by the circulatory system to the cells of the body. Food that is not used is eliminated as solid waste from the body.

The major organs of the digestive system are located in the abdomen. The digestive tract is about 35 feet long. It begins at the mouth and continues through the throat, esophagus (tube through which food passes), stomach, small intestine, large intestine, rectum, and anus. Besides the digestive tract, the digestive system also includes the liver, gallbladder, and pancreas   Figure 4-14 ▸ .

The liver performs several digestive functions, including the production of bile. Bile is stored in the gallbladder and released into the small intestine to help digest fats.

The pancreas also has several digestive functions. Probably its best-known function is the production of **insulin**. Insulin is released directly into the bloodstream and aids in the body's use of sugar. Disruption of insulin production causes diabetes.

The Genitourinary System

The **genitourinary system** is responsible for the body's reproductive functions and for the removal of waste products from the bloodstream.

The major organs of male reproduction are the testes, which produce sperm, and the penis, which delivers sperm to fertilize the female egg. The major female reproductive organs are the

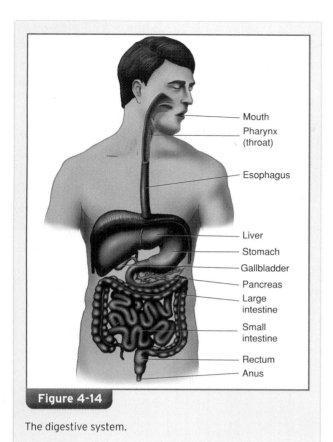

Figure 4-14

Mouth
Pharynx (throat)
Esophagus
Liver
Stomach
Gallbladder
Pancreas
Large intestine
Small intestine
Rectum
Anus

The digestive system.

ovaries, which produce eggs, and the uterus, which holds the fertilized egg as it develops during pregnancy. The egg released by the ovaries travels to the uterus through the fallopian tubes. The external opening of the female reproductive system is called the birth canal (vagina).

The removal of waste products by the genitourinary system begins in the kidneys, which filter the blood to form urine. The urine flows down from the kidneys through tubes (ureters) into the bladder. The bladder collects and stores the urine before it passes out of the body through the urethra.

Skin

Skin covers all parts of the body and has three major functions:

1. Protecting against harmful substances
2. Regulating temperature
3. Receiving information from the outside environment.

Figure 4-15 ▾ identifies the layers of the skin. The dermis is the deeper or inner layer of the

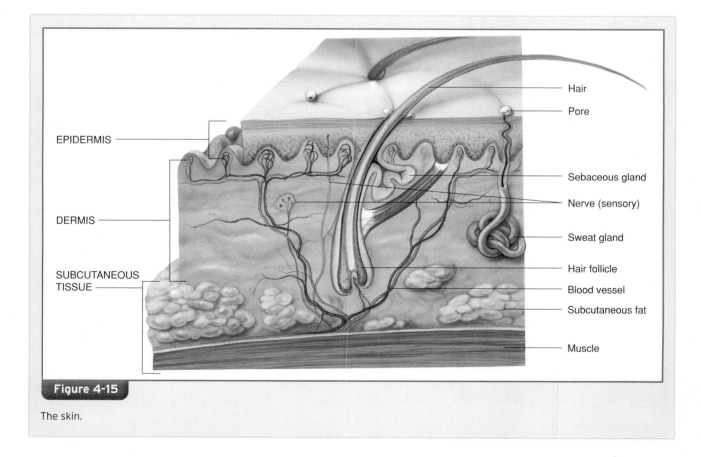

Figure 4-15

EPIDERMIS
DERMIS
SUBCUTANEOUS TISSUE

Hair
Pore
Sebaceous gland
Nerve (sensory)
Sweat gland
Hair follicle
Blood vessel
Subcutaneous fat
Muscle

The skin.

skin. The prefix *epi-* means upon. Therefore the epidermis is the outer layer of skin that is located upon the dermis.

Skin protects the body from the environment. Because skin provides an intact layer of cells that serves as a barrier to most foreign substances, it prevents harmful materials from getting into the body. The skin is an effective barrier to bacteria and viruses as long as it is not damaged.

Skin regulates the internal temperature of the body. If the body gets too hot, the small blood vessels close to the skin open up (dilate) and bring more body heat to the surface of the skin, where the heat can be transferred to the air. Another source of cooling occurs as the sweat released by the skin evaporates. If the body becomes cold, the blood vessels near the skin surface constrict, transferring more body heat to the inside or core part of the body.

Skin receives information from the environment. The skin can perceive touch, pressure, and pain; it can sense degrees of heat or cold. These perceptions are picked up by special sensors in the skin and transmitted through the nerves and the spinal cord to the brain. The brain serves as the computer to interpret these sensations.

You are the Provider   SUMMARY

Review the *You are the Provider* case study provided at the beginning of the chapter.

You are dispatched to 114 Foster Center Road for a 47-year-old man who is complaining of back pain. When you arrive, you find an alert and oriented middle-aged man lying on the floor of his bedroom. He states that when he bent down to pick up his belt, his back tightened up. Now the pain is so bad that he cannot move. When you ask him where the pain is, he points to his lower back.

1. **Why is some knowledge of anatomy and some understanding of the function of body systems so important in cases like this?**

   Having some knowledge of anatomy and the function of body systems can help you understand the source of an injury or illness and can improve patient care. Understanding terminology helps you to communicate with other members of the medical care team. Using proper terminology also helps to avoid misunderstandings.

Prep Kit

Ready for Review

The Ready for Review thoroughly summarizes the chapter.

- This chapter covers human anatomy and the function of body systems. To understand the location of specific signs or symptoms, it is necessary to examine topographic anatomy.

- The chapter presents a brief explanation of body systems. The respiratory system consists of the lungs and the airway. This system functions to take in air through the airway and transport it to the lungs. In the lungs, red blood cells absorb the oxygen and release carbon dioxide so it can be expelled from the body.

- The circulatory system consists of the heart (the pump), the blood vessels (the pipes), and blood (the fluid). Its role is to transport oxygenated blood to all parts of the body and to remove waste products, including carbon dioxide.

- The skeletal system consists of the bones of your body. These bones function to provide support, to protect vital structures, and to manufacture red blood cells. The muscular system consists of three kinds of muscles: voluntary (skeletal) muscles, smooth (involuntary) muscles, and cardiac (heart) muscles. Muscles provide both support and movement. The skeletal system works with the muscular system to provide motion. Sometimes these two systems together are called the musculoskeletal system.

- The nervous system consists of the brain, the spinal cord, and individual nerves. The brain serves as the central computer and the nerves transmit messages between the brain and the body.

- The digestive system consists of the mouth, esophagus, stomach, intestines, liver, gallbladder, and pancreas. It breaks down usable food and eliminates solid waste.

- The genitourinary system consists of the organs of reproduction together with the organs involved in the production and excretion of urine.

- The skin covers all parts of the body. It protects the body from the environment, regulates the internal temperature of the body, and transmits sensations from the skin to the nervous system.

- A basic understanding of the body systems provides you with the background you need to treat the illnesses and injuries you will encounter as a first responder.

Vital Vocabulary

The Vital Vocabulary are the key terms for this chapter.

anterior The front surface of the body.

carbon dioxide (CO_2) The gas formed in respiration and exhaled in breathing.

cartilage A tough, elastic form of connective tissue that covers the ends of most bones to form joints; also found in some specific areas such as the nose and the ears.

cervical spine That portion of the spinal column consisting of the seven vertebrae located in the neck.

circulatory system The heart and blood vessels, which together are responsible for the continuous flow of blood throughout the body.

coccyx The tailbone; the small bone below the sacrum formed by the final four vertebrae.

diaphragm A muscular dome that separates the chest from the abdominal cavity. Contraction of the diaphragm and the chest wall muscles brings air into the lungs; relaxation expels air from the lungs.

digestive system The gastrointestinal tract (stomach and intestines), mouth, salivary glands, pharynx, esophagus, liver, gallbladder, pancreas, rectum, and anus, which together are responsible for the absorption of food and the elimination of solid waste from the body.

Technology

- Interactivities
- Vocabulary Explorer
- Anatomy Review
- Web Links
- Online Review Manual

www.FirstResponder.EMSzone.com

distal Describing structures that are nearer to the free end of an extremity; any location that is farther from the midline than the point of reference named.

epiglottis The valve located at the upper end of the voicebox that prevents food from entering the larynx.

floating ribs The eleventh and twelfth ribs, which do not connect to the sternum.

genitourinary system The organs of reproduction, together with the organs involved in the production and excretion of urine.

humerus The upper arm bone.

inferior That portion of the body or body part that lies nearer the feet than the head.

insulin A hormone produced by the pancreas that enables sugar in the blood to be used by the cells of the body; supplementary insulin is used in the treatment and control of diabetes mellitus.

joint A place where two bones come into contact.

larynx A structure composed of cartilage in the neck that guards the entrance to the windpipe and functions as the organ of voice; also called the voicebox.

lateral Away from the midline of the body.

ligaments Fibrous bands that connect bones to bones and support and strengthen joints.

lumbar spine The lower part of the back formed by the lowest five nonfused vertebrae.

medial Toward the midline of the body.

midline An imaginary vertical line drawn from the mid-forehead through the nose and the navel to the floor.

nerves Fiber tracts or pathways that carry messages from the spinal cord and brain to all body parts and back; sensory, motor, or a combination of both.

nervous system The brain, spinal cord, and nerves.

pelvis The closed bony ring, consisting of the sacrum and the pelvic bones, that connects the trunk to the lower extremities.

plasma The fluid part of the blood that carries blood cells, transports nutrients, and removes cellular waste materials.

platelets Microscopic disk-shaped elements in the blood that are essential to the process of blood clot formation; the mechanism that stops bleeding.

posterior The back surface of the body.

proximal Describing structures that are closer to the trunk.

pulse The wave of pressure that is created by the heart as it contracts and forces blood out of the heart and into the major arteries.

radius The bone on the thumb side of the forearm.

respiratory system All body structures that contribute to normal breathing.

ribs The paired arches of bone, 12 on either side, that extend from the thoracic vertebrae toward the anterior midline of the trunk.

sacrum One of three bones (sacrum and two pelvic bones) that make up the pelvic ring; forms the base of the spine.

shoulder girdles The proximal portions of the upper extremity; each is made up of the clavicle, the scapula, and the humerus.

skull The bones of the head, collectively; serves as the protective structure for the brain.

sternum The breastbone.

superior Toward the head; lying higher in the body.

tendons Tough, rope-like cords of fibrous tissue that attach muscles to bones.

thoracic spine The 12 vertebrae that attach to the 12 ribs; the upper part of the back.

topographic anatomy The superficial landmarks on the body that serve as location guides to the structures that lie beneath them.

ulna The bone on the little-finger side of the forearm.

vertebrae The 33 bones of the spinal column: 7 cervical, 12 thoracic, 5 lumbar, 5 sacral, and 4 coccygeal vertebrae.

xiphoid process The flexible cartilage at the lower tip of the sternum.

Assessment in Action

Assessment in Action presents a fictitious scenario to help you review what you learned in this chapter.

You and your partner are dispatched to the scene of a pedestrian struck. As you arrive on scene, you find a 32-year-old man who was struck by a car. As you examine your patient, you find bruising on his chest, swelling in his abdomen, and note difficulty breathing. You also find a small cut on his forearm that is bleeding slightly.

1. What body systems may be affected from this injury?

   A. Respiratory system
   B. Circulatory system
   C. Digestive system
   D. All of the above

2. Of what significance is your patient's difficulty breathing?

3. What structures of the respiratory system might be damaged?

4. What are the components that make up the blood?

5. The bleeding in this scenario is most likely coming from:

   A. arteries.
   B. veins.
   C. capillaries.

Lifting and Moving Patients

Skill Objectives

1. Place a patient in the recovery position. (p 71)
2. Lift and move patients using good body mechanics. (p 71)
3. Perform the following emergency patient drags:
   - Clothes drag (p 71)
   - Blanket drag (p 72-73)
   - Arm-to-arm drag (p 73)
   - Fire fighter drag (p 73)
   - Cardiac arrest patient drag (p 72)
   - Emergency drag from a vehicle (p 74)
4. Perform the following patient carries:
   - Two-person extremity carry (p 74-75)
   - Two-person seat carry (p 75)
   - Cradle-in-arms carry (p 76)
   - Two-person chair carry (p 76)
   - Pack-strap carry (p 77)
   - Direct ground lift (p 77-78)
   - Transfer from a bed to a stretcher (p 78-79)
5. Perform the following walking assists for ambulatory patients:
   - One-person assist (p 77)
   - Two-person assist (p 77)

6. Assist other EMS providers with the following devices:
   - Wheeled ambulance stretcher (p 78)
   - Portable stretcher (p 79)
   - Stair chair (p 79)
   - Long backboard (p 79)
   - Short backboard (p 80)
   - Scoop stretcher (p 80)
7. Assist other EMS providers with the following procedures for patients with suspected spinal injuries:
   - Applying a cervical collar (p 84, 85)
   - Moving a patient using a backboard (p 84)
   - Applying short backboard devices (p 84)
   - Log rolling a patient onto a long backboard (p 85, 87)
   - Straddle lift (p 88)
   - Straddle slide (p 88-89)
   - Strapping techniques (p 89)
   - Head immobilization (p 90)

*These are chapter learning objectives.

AUTHOR'S NOTE: Some instructors may prefer to cover the material in this chapter after presenting the skills in Section 5.

Lifting and Moving Patients

You and your partner are dispatched to the Fair Oaks Mall. The dispatcher informs you that a patron has fallen near the east escalator. Dispatch has no further information on the condition of the patient. They notify you that the nearest EMS transport unit is about 8 minutes away.

1. Under what circumstances would it be necessary to move the patient before the EMS transport unit arrives?
2. Why is it often better for first responders to delay moving a patient until the arrival of an EMS transport unit?

Introduction

As a first responder, you must analyze a situation, quickly evaluate a patient's condition (under stressful circumstances and often by yourself), and carry out effective, lifesaving emergency medical procedures. These procedures sometimes include lifting, moving, or positioning patients as well as assisting other EMS providers in moving patients and preparing them for transport.

Usually you will not have to move patients. In most situations, you can treat the patient in the position found and later assist other EMS personnel in moving the patient. In some cases, however, the patient's survival may depend on your knowledge of emergency movement techniques. You may have to move patients for their own protection (for example, to remove a patient from a burning building), or you may have to move patients before you can provide needed emergency care (for example, to administer CPR to a cardiac arrest patient found in a bathroom).

General Principles

Every time you move a patient, keep the following general guidelines in mind:

1. Do no further harm to the patient.
2. Move the patient only when necessary.
3. Move the patient as little as possible.
4. Move the patient's body as a unit.
5. Use proper lifting and moving techniques to ensure your own safety.
6. Have one rescuer give commands when moving a patient (usually the rescuer at the patient's head).

You should also consider the following recommendations:

- Delay moving the patient, if possible, until additional EMS personnel arrive.
- Treat the patient before moving him or her unless the patient is in an unsafe environment.
- Try not to step over the patient (your shoes may drop sand, dirt, or mud onto the patient).
- Explain to the patient what you are going to do and how. If the patient's condition permits, he or she may be able to assist you.
- Move the patient as few times as possible.

Unless you must move patients for treatment or protection, leave them in the position you found them. There is usually no reason to hurry the moving process. If you suspect the patient has suffered trauma to the head or spine, keep the patient's head and spine immobilized so he or she does not move.

Technology

- Interactivities
- Vocabulary Explorer
- Anatomy Review
- Web Links
- Online Review Manual

Safety Tips

Whatever technique you use for moving patients, keep these rules of good body mechanics in mind:

1. Know your own physical limitations and capabilities. Do not try to lift too heavy a load.
2. Keep yourself balanced when lifting or moving a patient.
3. Maintain a firm footing.
4. Lift and lower the patient by bending your legs, not your back. Keep your back as straight as possible at all times and use your large leg muscles to do the work.
5. Try to keep your arms close to your body for strength and balance.
6. Move the patient as little as possible.

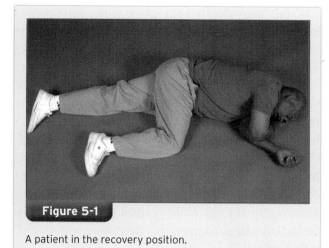

Figure 5-1

A patient in the recovery position.

Recovery Position

Unconscious patients who have not suffered trauma should be placed in a sidelying or <u>recovery position</u> to help keep the airway open Figure 5-1 ▲.

Body Mechanics

Your top priority as a first responder is to ensure your own safety. Improperly lifting or moving a patient can result in injury to you or to the patient. By exercising good body mechanics, you reduce the possibility of injuring yourself Figure 5-2 ▶. Good body mechanics means using the strength in the large muscles in your legs to lift patients instead of your back muscles. This prevents strains and injuries to weaker muscles, especially in your back. Get as close to the patient as possible so that your back is in a straight and upright position, and keep your back straight as you lift. Do not lift when your back is bent over a patient. Lift without twisting your body. Keep your feet in a secure position and be sure you have a firm footing before you start to lift or move a patient.

To lift safely, you must keep certain guidelines in mind. Before attempting to move a patient, assess the weight of the patient. Know your physical limitations and do not attempt to lift or move a patient who is too heavy for you to handle safely. Call for additional personnel if needed for your

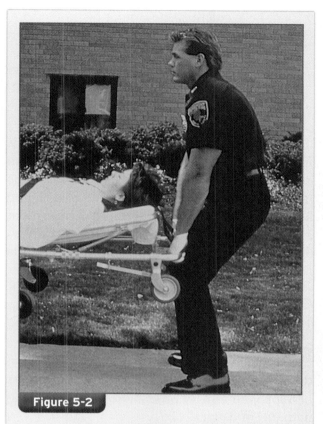

Figure 5-2

A first responder demonstrates good body mechanics while lifting a patient. His back is straight and he is lifting using his leg muscles.

safety and the safety of the patient. Because you will sometimes need to assist other EMS providers, you should practice with them so that lifts are handled in a coordinated and helpful manner.

As you are lifting, make sure you communicate with the other members of the lifting team. Failure to give clear commands or failure to lift at the same time can result in serious injuries to rescuers and patients. Practice makes perfect! Practice lifts and moves until they become smooth for you and your partner and for the patient.

Emergency Movement of Patients

When is emergency movement of a patient necessary? Move a patient immediately in the following situations:

- Danger of fire, explosion, or structural collapse exists.
- Hazardous materials are present.

- The accident scene cannot be protected.
- It is otherwise impossible to gain access to other patients who need lifesaving care.
- The patient has suffered cardiac arrest and must be moved so that you can begin CPR.

Emergency Drags

If the patient is on the floor or ground during an emergency situation, you may have to drag the person away from the scene instead of trying to lift and carry. Make every effort to pull the patient in the direction of the long axis of the body in order to provide as much spinal protection for the patient as possible.

Clothes Drag

The <u>clothes drag</u> is the simplest way to move the patient in an emergency Figure 5-3 ▾ . If the patient is too heavy for you to lift and carry, grasp the clothes just behind the collar, rest the patient's head on your arm for protection, and drag the patient out of danger.

FYI

Cardiac Patients and the Clothes Drag   In most situations, you can easily determine whether emergency movement is necessary. Cases of cardiac arrest are the exception. Cardiac arrest patients are often found in a bathroom or small bedroom. You will have to judge whether basic life support (BLS) or advanced life support (ALS) can be ad-

FYI. cont.

equately provided in that space. If the room is not large enough, you should move the patient as soon as you have determined that he or she has suffered cardiac arrest.

Drag the cardiac arrest patient from the tight space to a larger room (such as a living or dining room) that has space for two people to perform CPR and ALS procedures Figure 5-4 ▾ . Quickly move furniture out of the way so you have room to work. You will be able to deliver BLS and ALS with increased efficiency, more than making up for the time it took to move the patient. Take time to provide adequate room before you begin CPR!

Blanket Drag

If the patient is not dressed or is dressed in clothing that could tear easily during the clothes drag (for example, a nightgown), move the patient by using a large sheet, blanket, or rug. Place the blanket, rug, sheet, or similar item on the floor and roll the patient onto it. Pull the patient to safety by dragging the sheet or blanket. The <u>blanket drag</u> can also be used to move a patient who weighs more than you do Figure 5-5 ▸ .

Arm-to-Arm Drag

If the patient is on the floor, you can place your hands under the patient's armpits from the back of the patient and grasp the patient's forearms. The <u>arm-to-arm drag</u> allows you to move the pa-

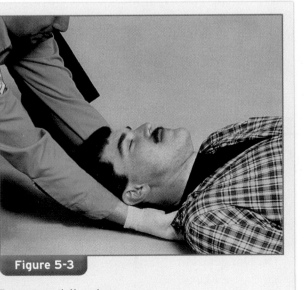

Figure 5-3

Emergency clothes drag.

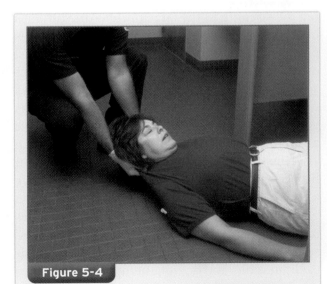

Figure 5-4

Remove the patient from a tight space to administer CPR.

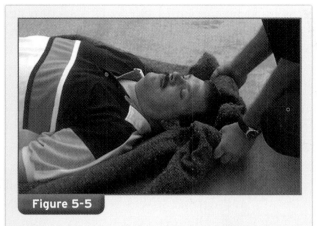

Figure 5-5

Blanket drag.

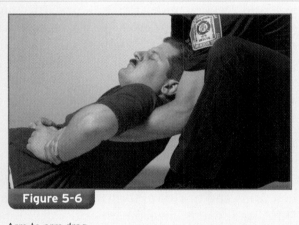

Figure 5-6

Arm-to-arm drag.

tient by carrying the weight of the upper part of the patient's body as the lower trunk and legs drag on the floor Figure 5-6 ◀ . This drag can be used to move a heavy patient with some protection for the patient's head and neck.

Fire Fighter Drag

The fire fighter drag enables you to move a patient who is heavier than you are because you do not have to lift or carry the patient. Tie the patient's wrists together with anything that is handy: a cravat (a folded triangular bandage), gauze, belt, or necktie, being careful not to impair circulation. Then get down on your hands and knees and straddle the patient. Pass the patient's tied hands around your neck, straighten your arms, and drag the patient across the floor by crawling on your hands and knees Figure 5-7 ▼ .

Emergency Drag From a Vehicle

One Rescuer   Sometimes you have to use emergency movement techniques to remove a patient from a wrecked vehicle (for example, when the vehicle is on fire or the patient needs CPR). All the basic movement principles apply, but the techniques need to be slightly modified because the patient is not lying down.

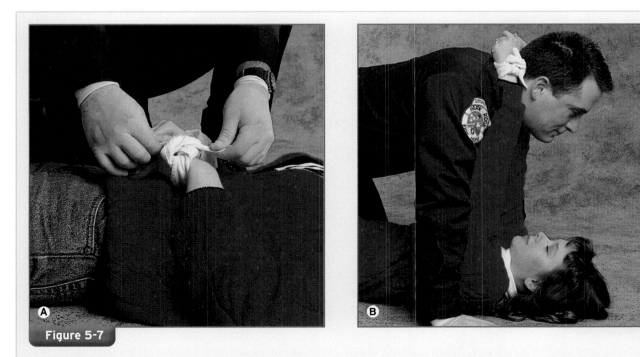

Ⓐ Ⓑ

Figure 5-7

Fire fighter drag. **A.** Tie the patient's wrists together. **B.** Drag the patient across the floor by crawling on your hands and knees with the patient's arms around your neck.

Grasp the patient under the arms and cradle the patient's head between your arms ▐ Figure 5-8 ▾ ▌. Pull the patient down into a horizontal position as you ease him or her from the vehicle. Although there is no effective way to remove a patient from a vehicle by yourself without causing some movement, it is important to prevent excess movement of the patient's neck.

Two or More Rescuers   If you must immediately remove a patient from a vehicle and two or more rescuers are present, have one rescuer support the patient's head and neck, while the second rescuer moves the patient by lifting under the arms. The patient can then be removed in line with the long axis of the body, with the head and neck stabilized in a neutral position. If time permits and if you have one available, use a long backboard for patient removal. Procedures for using a long backboard are covered later in this chapter.

Carries for Nonambulatory Patients

Many patients are not able or should not be allowed to move without your assistance. Patients who are unable to move because of injury or ill-ness must be carried to safety. This section describes several useful carrying techniques for non-ambulatory patients. Whatever technique you use, remember to follow the rules of good body mechanics.

Two-Person Extremity Carry

The <u>two-person extremity carry</u> can be done by two rescuers with no equipment in tight or narrow spaces, such as mobile home corridors, small hallways, and narrow spaces between buildings ▐ Figure 5-9 ▸ ▌. The focus of this carry is on the patient's <u>extremities</u>. The rescuers help the patient sit up. Rescuer One kneels behind the patient and reaches under the patient's arms and grasps the patient's wrists. Rescuer Two then backs in between the patient's legs, reaches around, and grasps the patient behind the knees. At a command from Rescuer One, the two rescuers stand up and carry the patient away, walking straight ahead.

▐ FYI ▌
Two-Person Seat Carry

With the <u>two-person seat carry</u>, two rescuers use their arms and bodies to form a seat for the patient. The rescuers kneel on opposite sides of the

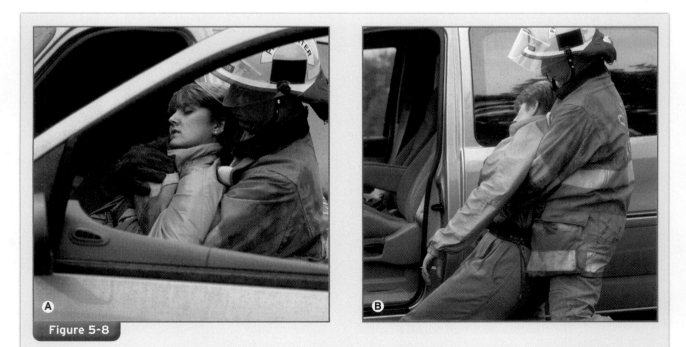

Figure 5-8

Emergency removal from a vehicle. **A.** Grasp the patient under the arms. **B.** Pull the patient down into a horizontal position.

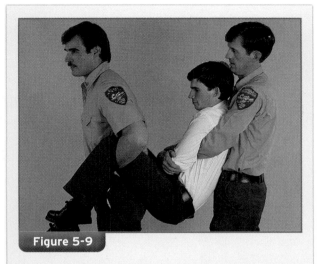

Figure 5-9

Two-person extremity carry.

FYI cont.

Cradle-in-Arms Carry

The **cradle-in-arms carry** can be used by one rescuer to carry a child. Kneel beside the patient and place one arm around the child's back and the other arm under the thighs. Lift slightly and roll the child into the hollow formed by your arms and chest. Be sure to use your leg muscles to stand **Figure 5-11 ▶**.

Two-Person Chair Carry

In the **two-person chair carry**, two rescuers use a chair to support the weight of the patient. A folding chair cannot be used. The chair carry is especially useful for taking patients up or down stairways or through a narrow hallway. An additional benefit is that because the patient is able to hold on to the chair (and should be encour-

FYI cont.

patient near the patient's hips. The rescuers then raise the patient to a sitting position and link arms behind the patient's back. The rescuers then place the other arm under the patient's knees and link with each other. If possible, the patient puts his or her arms around the necks of the rescuers for additional support. Although the two-person seat carry needs two rescuers, it does not require any equipment **Figure 5-10 ▼**.

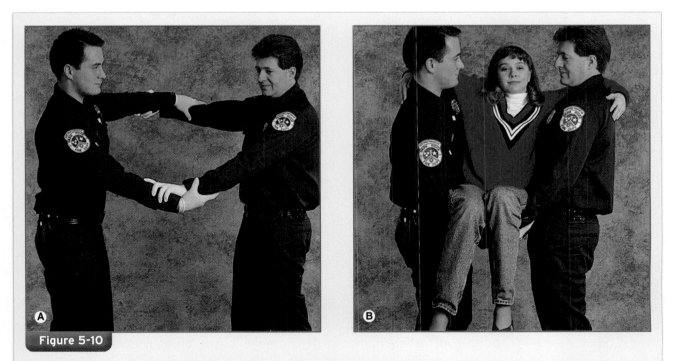

Figure 5-10

Two-person seat carry. **A.** Link arms. **B.** Raise the patient to a sitting position.

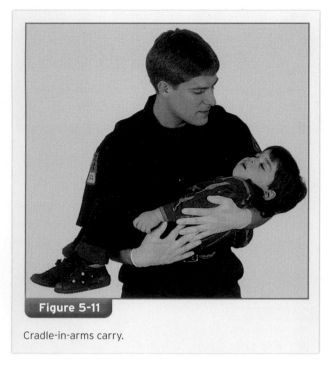

Figure 5-11

Cradle-in-arms carry.

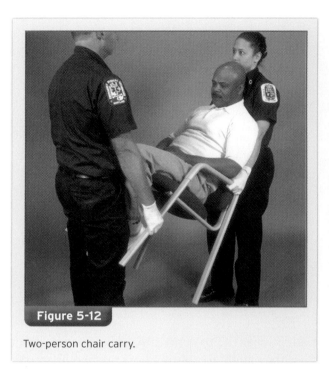

Figure 5-12

Two-person chair carry.

FYI cont.

aged to do so), he or she feels much more secure than with the two-person seat carry.

Rescuer One stands behind the seated patient, reaches down, and grasps the back of the chair close to the seat, as shown in Figure 5-12 ▶. Rescuer One then tilts the chair slightly backward on its rear legs so that Rescuer Two can step back in between the legs of the chair and grasp the chair's front legs. The patient's legs should be between the legs of the chair. When both rescuers are correctly positioned, Rescuer One gives the command to lift and walk away.

Pack-Strap Carry

The **pack-strap carry** is a one-person carry that allows you to carry a patient while keeping one hand free. Have the patient stand (or have other rescue personnel support the patient) and back into the patient so your shoulders fit into the patient's armpits. Grasp the patient's wrists and cross the arms over your chest Figure 5-13 ▶. Now you can hold both wrists in one hand and your other hand remains free.

Optimal weight distribution occurs when the patient's armpits are over your shoulders. Squat deeply to avoid potential injury to your back and

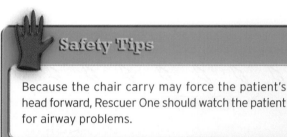

Safety Tips

Because the chair carry may force the patient's head forward, Rescuer One should watch the patient for airway problems.

FYI cont.

pull the patient onto your back. Once the patient is positioned correctly, bend forward to lift the patient off the ground, stand up, and walk away.

Direct Ground Lift

The direct ground lift is used to move a patient who is on the ground or the floor to an ambulance cot. It should be used only for those patients who have not suffered a traumatic injury. The direct ground lift requires you to bend over the patient and lift with your back in a bent position. Because the use of the direct ground lift results in poor body mechanics, its use is to be discouraged. Using a long backboard or portable cot is much better for your back and may be more comfortable for the patient. The steps for per-

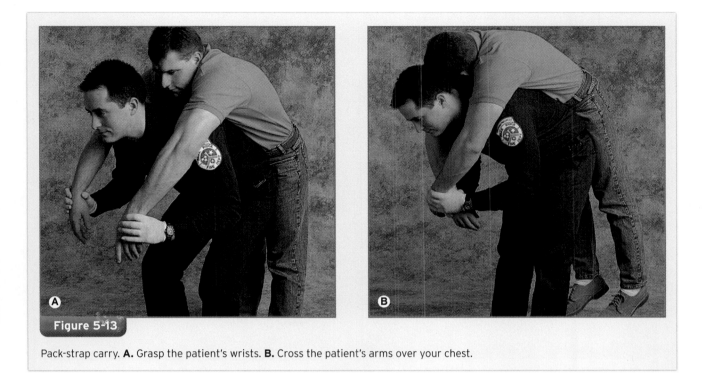

Figure 5-13

Pack-strap carry. **A.** Grasp the patient's wrists. **B.** Cross the patient's arms over your chest.

forming the direct ground lift are as follows
Skill Drill 5-1 ▸ :

SKILL DRILL 5-1

1. Assess the patient. Do not use this lift if there is any chance of head, spine, or leg injuries.
2. Rescuer One kneels at the patient's chest on the right or left side. Rescuer Two kneels at the patient's hips on the same side as Rescuer One **Step 1**.
3. Place the patient's arms on the chest.
4. Rescuer One places one arm under the patient's neck and shoulder to cradle the patient's head and then places the other arm under the patient's lower back. Rescuer Two places one arm under the patient's knees and the other arm above the buttocks **Step 2**.
5. Rescuer One gives the command: "Ready? Roll!" and both rescuers roll their forearms up so that the patient is as close to them as possible.
6. Rescuer One gives the command: "Ready? Lift!" and both rescuers lift the patient to their knees and roll the patient as close to their bodies as possible.

7. Rescuer One gives the command: "Ready? Stand!" and both rescuers stand and move the patient to the ambulance cot or bed **Step 3**.
8. To lower the patient to the cot or bed, the rescuers reverse the steps just listed **Step 4**.

Transferring a Patient from Bed to Stretcher

Many times patients who are ill will be found in their beds. If the EMS personnel need to transport these patients to the hospital, they may request your assistance with a patient transfer from the bed to the ambulance cot using the draw-sheet method **Figure 5-14 ▸**.

Place the cot next to the bed, making sure it is at the same height as the bed and that the

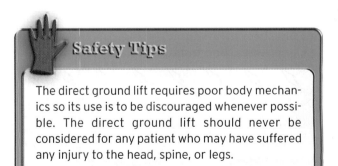

Safety Tips

The direct ground lift requires poor body mechanics so its use is to be discouraged whenever possible. The direct ground lift should never be considered for any patient who may have suffered any injury to the head, spine, or legs.

Skill DRILL 5-1

Direct Ground Lift

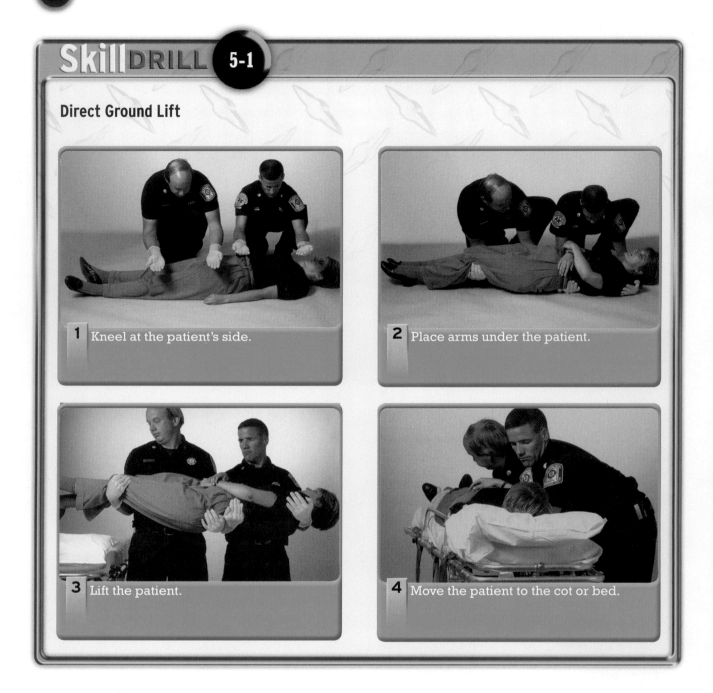

1 Kneel at the patient's side.

2 Place arms under the patient.

3 Lift the patient.

4 Move the patient to the cot or bed.

rails are lowered and straps unbuckled. Be sure to hold the cot to keep it from moving. Loosen the bottom sheet underneath the patient or log roll the patient onto a blanket. Reach across the cot and grasp the sheet and blanket firmly at the patient's head, chest, hips, and knees. Gently slide the patient onto the cot.

An alternate method for moving a patient is to loosen the bottom sheet of the patient's bed, place the ambulance cot parallel to the bed, and reach across the cot to pull the sheet and the pa-

tient onto the cot. This method must be used with caution because it requires the rescuers to reach across the cot to get to the patient. This results in poor body mechanics and therefore is to be discouraged.

Walking Assists for Ambulatory Patients

Frequently, many patients simply need assistance to walk to safety. Either one or two rescuers can

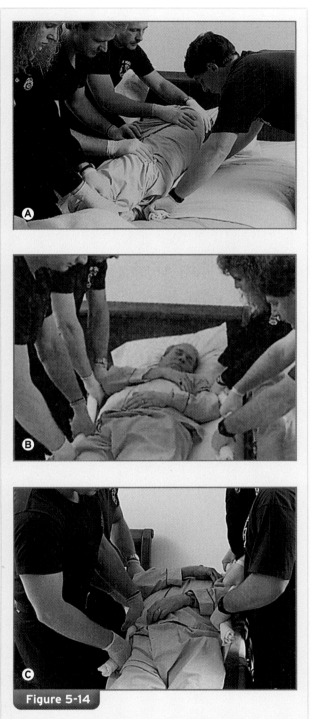

Figure 5-14

The draw-sheet method. **A.** Log roll the patient onto a sheet or blanket. **B.** Bring the cot in parallel to the bed. Gently pull the patient to the edge of the bed. **C.** Transfer the patient to the cot.

One-Person Walking Assist

The <u>one-person walking assist</u> can be used if the patient is able to bear his or her own weight. Help the patient stand. Have the patient place one arm around your neck and hold the patient's wrist (which should be draped over your shoulder). Put your free arm around the patient's waist and help the patient to walk **Figure 5-15 ▶**.

Two-Person Walking Assist

The <u>two-person walking assist</u> is the same as the one-person walking assist, except that two rescuers are needed. This technique is useful if the patient cannot bear weight. The two rescuers completely support the patient **Figure 5-16 ▶**.

Equipment

Most of the lifts and moves described in the previous section are done without any specialized equipment. However, EMS services commonly use various types of patient-moving equipment. To be able to assist other EMS providers, you should be familiar with this equipment.

Wheeled Ambulance Stretchers

Wheeled ambulance stretchers are carried by ambulances and are one of the most commonly used EMS devices **Figure 5-17 ▶**. These stretchers are also called cots. Most of them can be raised or lowered to several different heights. The head end of the cot can be raised to elevate the patient's head. These stretchers have belts to secure the patient. Each type of stretcher has its own set of levers and controls for raising and lowering. If

do this. Choose a technique after you have assessed the patient's condition and the incident scene. The technique you might use to help a patient to a chair is probably not appropriate to help a patient up a highway embankment.

Safety Tips

Do not use any of the lifts or carries explained in this chapter if you suspect that the patient has a spinal injury—unless, of course, it is necessary to remove the patient from a life-threatening situation.

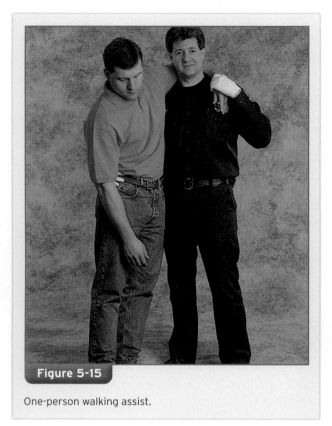

Figure 5-15

One-person walking assist.

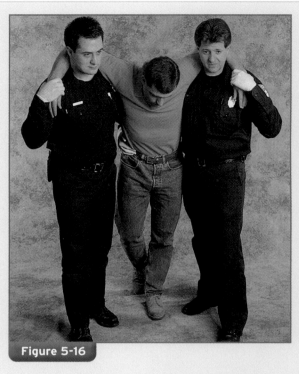

Figure 5-16

Two-person walking assist.

you regularly work with the same EMS unit, it will be helpful to learn how their particular type of stretcher operates.

Stretchers can be rolled or they can be carried by two or four people. If the surface is smooth, a wheeled stretcher can be rolled with one person guiding the head end and one person pulling the foot end. If the loaded stretcher must be carried, it is best to use four people, one person at each corner. This gives stability and requires less strength

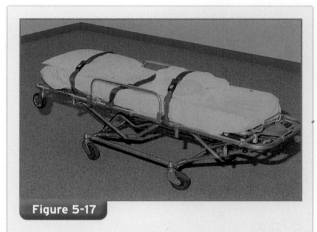

Figure 5-17

A wheeled ambulance stretcher.

than carrying with fewer people. If the stretcher must be carried through a narrow area, only two people will be able to carry it. The two rescuers should face each other from opposite ends of the stretcher. Carrying with two people requires that each be stronger and it is harder to balance the stretcher than when carrying with four people. As

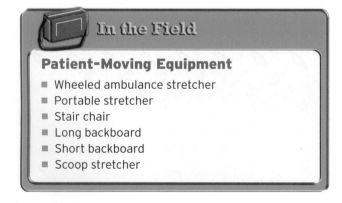

In the Field

Patient-Moving Equipment

- Wheeled ambulance stretcher
- Portable stretcher
- Stair chair
- Long backboard
- Short backboard
- Scoop stretcher

a first responder, you may also be asked to assist with loading a patient into the ambulance. You need to learn the method of loading ambulance stretchers that your EMS provider uses and practice this procedure with the EMS provider unit. It is important to lift as a team in a uniform way or else you can injure yourself or the other rescuers.

Portable Stretchers

A **portable stretcher** is used when the wheeled cot cannot be moved into a small space. They are smaller and lighter to carry than wheeled stretchers. Portable cots can be carried in the same ways that a wheeled cot is carried. An example of one type of portable stretcher is shown in Figure 5-18 ▸.

Stair Chair

A **stair chair** is a portable moving device used to carry a patient in a sitting position. They are good for patients who are short of breath or who are more comfortable in a sitting position. They are small, light, and easy to carry in narrow spaces. The stair chair is not intended for use with patients who have suffered any type of trauma. When carrying a stair chair, the rescuers must face each other and lift on a set command. If you are going to be assisting your local EMS provider with this device, you should learn how to unfold it and how to assist with carrying it. One type of stair chair is shown in Figure 5-19 ▸.

Backboards

Long Backboards

Long backboards are used for moving patients who have suffered trauma, especially if they may have suffered neck or back injuries. They are also useful for lifting and moving patients who are in small places or who need to be moved off the ground or floor. Long backboards are often used because they make lifting a patient much easier for the rescuers. Long backboards are made of varnished plywood or various types of plastic. Patients placed on long backboards must be secured with straps; if the patient has suffered back or neck injuries, the head should be im-

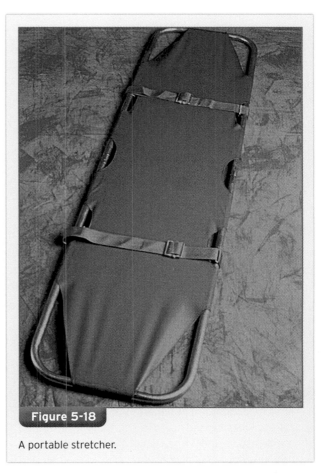

Figure 5-18

A portable stretcher.

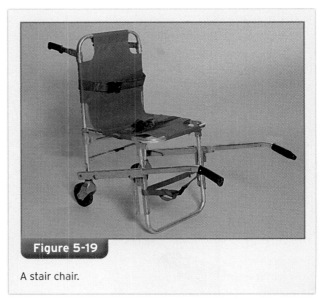

Figure 5-19

A stair chair.

mobilized. Procedures for assisting EMS providers with these devices are covered later in this chapter. One type of long backboard is pictured in Figure 5-20 ▸.

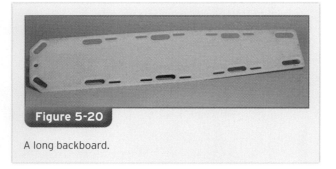

Figure 5-20

A long backboard.

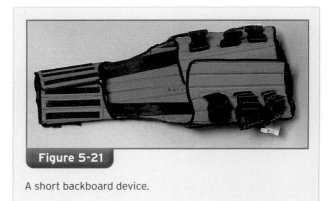

Figure 5-21

A short backboard device.

Short Backboard Devices

Short backboard devices are used to immobilize the head and spine of patients found in a sitting position who may have suffered possible head or spine injuries. Short backboard devices are made of wood or plastic. Some of these devices are in the form of a vest-like garment that wraps around the patient. Procedures to help you assist other EMS providers in applying these devices are covered later in this chapter. A short backboard device is pictured in **Figure 5-21 ▲**.

Scoop Stretchers

A **scoop stretcher** or orthopedic stretcher is a rigid device that separates into a right half and a left half. These devices are applied by placing one half on each side of the patient and then attaching the two halves together. These devices are helpful in moving patients out of small spaces. They should not be used if the patient has suffered head or spine injuries. You should practice using these devices if you will be assisting your local EMS provider with them. One type of scoop stretcher is shown in **Figure 5-22 ▼**.

In the Field

Moving Deceased Persons

First responders may be asked to assist with the removal of deceased persons, especially in cases of mass-casualty incidents. Usually deceased persons are placed in specially designed body bags before removal. Body bags are flexible and difficult to carry. Removal of deceased persons is much easier for rescuers if the body is placed on a backboard or portable stretcher after being placed in a body bag. This process makes patient movement much easier for the rescuer and greatly reduces the chance of injury to rescuers. It also creates a more respectful image of the deceased person for family members, bystanders, and members of the media.

In the Field

Improvise

Some devices that you can use as backboards include:

- Wide, sturdy planks
- Doors
- Ironing boards
- Sturdy folding tables
- Full-length lawn chair recliners
- Surfboards
- Snowboards

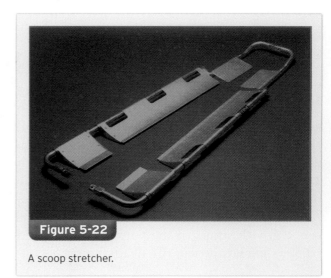

Figure 5-22

A scoop stretcher.

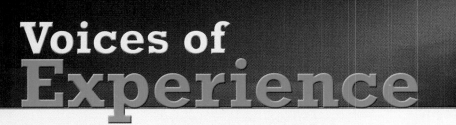

Voices of Experience

Do No Harm

My partner and I responded to a call for a patient in respiratory distress. When we entered the room, we found the patient in the tripod position—leaning forward on outstretched arms with the head and chin thrust slightly forward—the most common position for patients experiencing severe respiratory distress. He was very short of breath, using his accessory muscles to breathe. He looked tired and his color was dusky. He was able to respond to questions with only one- or two-word answers.

> **" One of the important decisions you will have to make as an emergency responder is whether or not to move the patient. "**

We decided that the patient needed to be transported to the hospital. Because even the smallest exertions can cause a patient who is experiencing respiratory distress to go into cardiac or respiratory arrest, we decided to move him on a stretcher. The patient was adamant he was going to move to the stretcher without our help. My partner and I explained the risks to the patient, but he would not be convinced. We finally decided it would be best to allow him to move himself, instead of arguing, which was not getting us anywhere. The patient moved himself and went into respiratory arrest. Despite our efforts to resuscitate him, the patient expired.

After the call, my partner and I felt terrible because we felt that we had not delivered the best care to this patient. We discussed the incident with the emergency physician at the hospital. The physician explained that, due to his low oxygen level, the patient may have been so short of breath that he was not thinking clearly. This was the last time I would allow a patient to move himself when the complaint was respiratory distress.

One of the important decisions you will have to make as an emergency responder is whether or not to move the patient. If you are going to move the patient, you have to consider the best way to move the patient without causing additional injury or aggravating the illness. Always keep in mind the first rule of medicine: Do no harm.

Terry Pool, EMT-P
EMS System Coordinator
Galesburg Area EMS System
Galesburg, Illinois

Treatment of Patients With Suspected Head or Spine Injury

Any time a patient has suffered a traumatic injury, you should suspect injury to the head, neck, or spine. Improper treatment can lead to permanent damage or paralysis. The patient's head should be kept in a neutral position and immobilized. It is also important that you be able to assist other EMS personnel in caring for patients who may have suffered head or spine injuries. The following sections show you how to immobilize a patient's head and neck and how to assist other EMS providers in placing a patient on a backboard. More information on spinal cord injuries is presented in Chapter 14.

Applying a Cervical Collar

A **cervical collar** is used to prevent excess movement of the head and neck Figure 5-23 ▼. These collars do not prevent head and neck movement; rather, they minimize the movement. When cervical collars are used, it is still necessary to immobilize the head and neck with your hands, a blanket roll, or foam blocks.

Soft cervical collars do not provide sufficient support for trauma patients. Many different types of rigid cervical collars for trauma patients are available. Figure 5-24 ▶ shows how one common style of rigid cervical collar is applied. A cer-

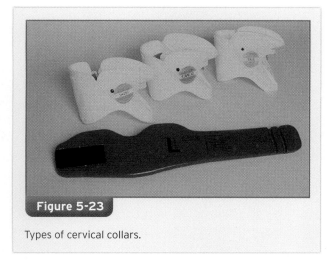

Figure 5-23

Types of cervical collars.

vical collar should be applied before the patient is placed on a backboard.

Movement of Patients Using Backboards

Placing a patient on a backboard is not your primary responsibility, but you may be required to assist other EMS personnel. Therefore, you must be familiar with the proper handling of patients who must be moved on backboards. Any patient who has suffered spinal trauma in a motor vehicle accident or fall and any victim of gunshot wounds to the trunk should be transported on a backboard. Although the specific technique used depends on the circumstances, the general principles described in the remainder of this chapter are relevant in nearly all cases.

The following principles of patient movement are especially important if you suspect spinal injury:

1. Move the patient as a unit.
2. Transport the patient face up (supine), the only position that gives adequate spinal stabilization. However, because patients secured to backboards often vomit, be prepared to turn the patient and backboard quickly as a unit to permit the vomitus to drain from the patient's mouth.
3. Keep the patient's head and neck in the neutral position.
4. Be sure that all rescuers understand what is to be done before attempting any movement.
5. Be sure that one rescuer is responsible for giving commands.

Assisting With Short Backboard Devices

Short backboard devices are used to immobilize patients found in a sitting position who have suffered trauma to the head, neck, or spine. Short backboard devices allow rescuers to immobilize the patient before moving. After the short backboard device is applied, the patient is carefully placed on a long backboard. As a first responder, you will not be applying a short backboard device by yourself. However, you may need to assist with the application of this device. Figure 5-25 ▶ illustrates how one common short backboard device is applied.

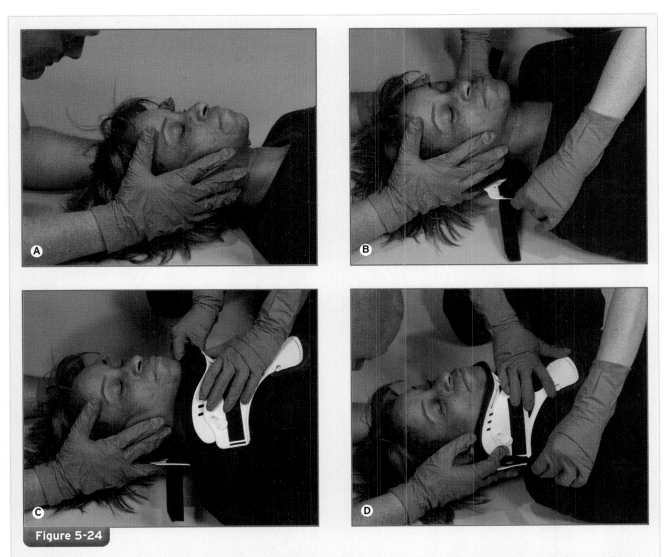

Figure 5-24

Applying a cervical collar. **A.** Stabilize head and neck. **B.** Insert back part of collar. **C.** Apply front part of collar. **D.** Secure collar together.

Log Rolling

Log rolling is the primary technique used to move a patient onto a long backboard. It is usually easy to accomplish, but it usually requires a team of four rescuers for safety and effectiveness—three to move the patient and one to maneuver the backboard. Log rolling is the movement technique of choice in all cases of suspected spinal injury. Because the log-rolling maneuver requires sufficient space for four rescuers, it is not always possible to perform it correctly. That is why the principles of movement rather than specific rules are stressed here. The procedure for the four-person log roll is shown in **Skill Drill 5-2** :

SKILL DRILL 5-2

1. All rescuers get into position to roll the patient Step 1 .
2. Once Rescuer One gives the command, rescuers roll the patient onto his or her side Step 2 .
3. The fourth person slides the backboard toward the patient Step 3 .
4. Once Rescuer One gives the command, rescuers roll the patient onto the backboard Step 4 .
5. Center the patient on the backboard. Secure the patient before moving Step 5 .

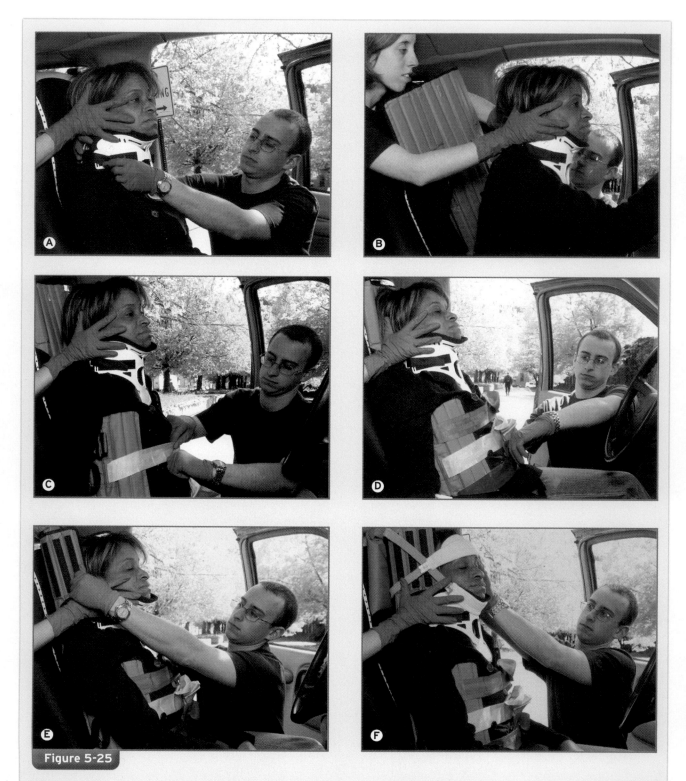

Figure 5-25

Applying a short backboard device. **A.** Stabilize the head and apply a cervical collar. **B.** Insert the device head first. **C.** Apply the middle strap. **D.** Apply the other straps. **E.** Place wings around head. **F.** Secure the head strap.

Skill DRILL 5-2

Four-Person Log Roll

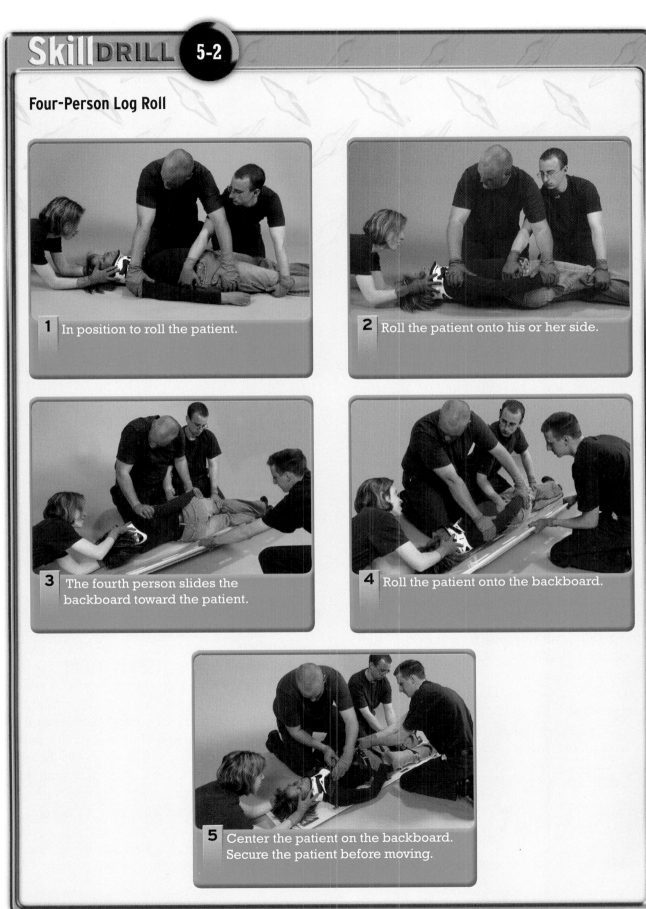

1 In position to roll the patient.

2 Roll the patient onto his or her side.

3 The fourth person slides the backboard toward the patient.

4 Roll the patient onto the backboard.

5 Center the patient on the backboard. Secure the patient before moving.

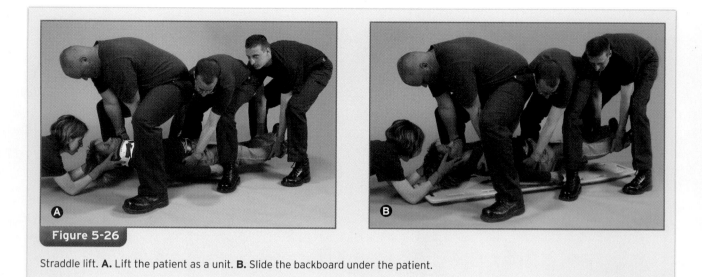

Figure 5-26

Straddle lift. **A.** Lift the patient as a unit. **B.** Slide the backboard under the patient.

In any patient-movement technique, and especially if spinal injury is suspected, everyone must understand who is directing the maneuver. The rescuer holding the patient's head (Rescuer One) should always give the commands so that all rescuers can better coordinate their actions. The specific wording of the command is not important, as long as every team member understands what the command is. Each member of the team must understand his or her specific position and function.

All patient-movement commands have two parts: a question and the order for movement. Rescuer One says, "The command will be 'Ready? Roll!'" When everyone is ready to roll the patient, Rescuer One says, "Ready? (followed by a short pause to allow for response from the team) Roll!"

In any log-rolling technique, you must move the patient as a unit. Keep the patient's head in a neutral position at all times. Do not allow the head to rotate, move backward (extend), or move forward (flex). Sometimes this is simply stated as, "Keep the nose in line with the belly button at all times."

Straddle Lift

The **straddle lift** can be used to place a patient on a backboard if you do not have enough space to perform a log roll. Modified versions of the straddle lift are commonly used to remove pa-

tients from automobiles. The straddle lift requires five rescuers: one at the head and neck, one to straddle the shoulders and chest, one to straddle the hips and thighs, one to straddle the legs, and one to insert the backboard under the patient after the other four have lifted the patient $1/2$ inch to 1 inch off the ground **Figure 5-26 ▲**.

The hardest part of the straddle-lift technique is coordinating the lifting so that the patient is raised just enough to slide the backboard under the patient. Because such team coordination can be difficult, it is important to practice this lift frequently.

Straddle Slide

In the **straddle slide**, a modification of the straddle-lift technique, the patient, rather than the backboard, is moved **Figure 5-27 ▶**. The rescuers' positions are the same as for the straddle lift. Each rescuer should have a firm grip on the patient (or the patient's clothing). Lift the patient as a unit just enough to be able to slide (break the resistance with the ground) him or her forward onto the waiting backboard. Slide the patient forward about 10 inches each time. Distances greater than 10 to 12 inches cause team coordination problems.

Do not lift the patient off the ground. Instead, slide the patient along the ground and onto the

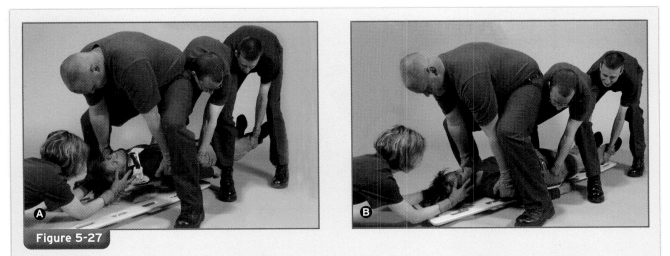

Figure 5-27

Straddle slide. **A.** Slide the patient about 10 inches at a time onto the backboard. **B.** Center the patient on the backboard.

Safety Tips

Make the up-and-forward movement in a single, smooth action. Lifting the patient up and then forward can strain your muscles.

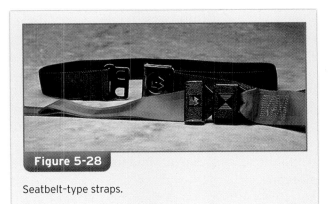

Figure 5-28

Seatbelt-type straps.

backboard. Lift the patient just enough to slide the patient onto the backboard.

Each rescuer should lean forward slightly and use a swinging motion to bring the patient onto the board. Rescuer One (who is at the patient's head) faces the other rescuers and moves backward during each movement. Rescuer One must not allow the patient's head to be driven into his or her knees!

Straps and Strapping Techniques

Every patient who is on a backboard should be strapped down to avoid sliding or slipping off the backboard. There are many ways to strap a patient to a backboard. The straps should be long enough to go around the board and a large patient. Straps 6 feet to 9 feet long with seatbelt-type buckles work well Figure 5-28 ▸ .

Once the patient is centered on the board, secure the upper torso with straps. Consider padding voids between the patient and the backboard. Next, secure the pelvis and upper legs, using padding as needed. Securing the straps around the wrist and hip area and the knees before securing the head to the backboard reduces the chance of head movement. Strap placement is shown in Figure 5-29 ▸ . Because there are many different types of straps and strapping techniques, learn the method used by your EMS system.

Head Immobilization

Once a patient has been secured to the backboard, the head and neck must be immobilized using commercially prepared devices (such as

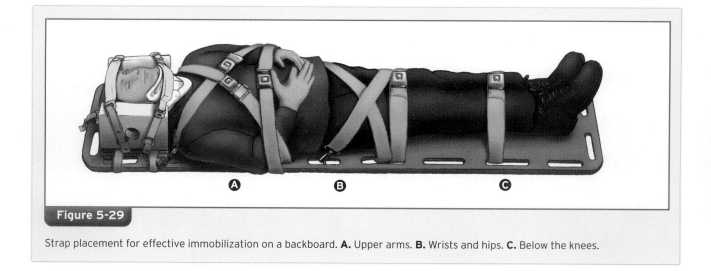

Figure 5-29

Strap placement for effective immobilization on a backboard. **A.** Upper arms. **B.** Wrists and hips. **C.** Below the knees.

foam blocks) or improvised devices (such as a blanket roll). The use of a blanket roll is explained here because it works well and because a blanket is almost always available. The blanket roll should be assembled ahead of time. Fold and roll the blanket (with towels as bulk filler) as shown in **Skill Drill 5-3 ▸**. Because there are many different types of straps and strapping techniques, learn the method used by your EMS system.

SKILL DRILL 5-3

1. Fold the blanket into a long rectangular shape Step 1 .
2. Insert a rolled towel and roll the blanket from each end Step 2 .
3. Roll the ends together Step 3 .
4. Place extra cravats in between the two rolled ends Step 4 .
5. Tie the rolled ends together with two cravats Step 5 and Step 6 .

To place the blanket roll under a patient's head, one rescuer should unroll it enough to fit around the head as another rescuer maintains head stabilization. The rescuer holding the patient's head (Rescuer One) carefully slides his or her hands out from between the blanket and stabilization is maintained by the blanket roll **Skill Drill 5-4 ▸** :

SKILL DRILL 5-4

1. Rescuer One stabilizes the patient's head Step 1 .
2. Both rescuers apply a cervical collar Step 2 .
3. Place straps around the backboard and the patient Step 3 .
4. Insert the blanket roll under the patient's head Step 4 .
5. Roll the blanket snugly against the patient's neck and shoulders Step 5 .
6. Tie two cravats around the blanket roll and around the backboard Step 6 .
7. Continue to stabilize the patient's head.
8. Tie two cravats around the backboard.
9. Assess sensory and motor function after immobilization.

Head stabilization must be maintained throughout the entire procedure (first by manually stabilizing the patient's head, then by using the blanket roll). The blanket roll must be fitted securely against the patient's shoulders in order to widen the base of support for the patient's head. Secure the blanket roll to the head with two cravats tied around the blanket roll; one over the patient's forehead and the other under the chin. Use two more cravats in the same positions to bind the head and the blanket roll to the backboard. The patient's head and neck are now adequately

Skill DRILL 5-3

Preparing a Blanket Roll

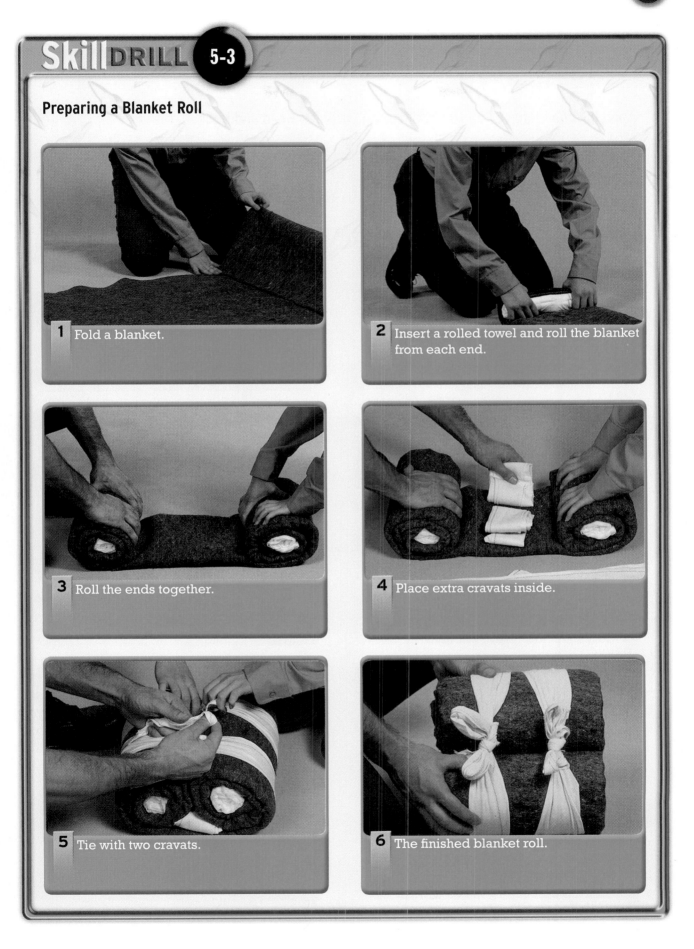

1 Fold a blanket.

2 Insert a rolled towel and roll the blanket from each end.

3 Roll the ends together.

4 Place extra cravats inside.

5 Tie with two cravats.

6 The finished blanket roll.

Skill DRILL 5-4

Applying the Blanket Roll to Stabilize the Patient's Head and Neck

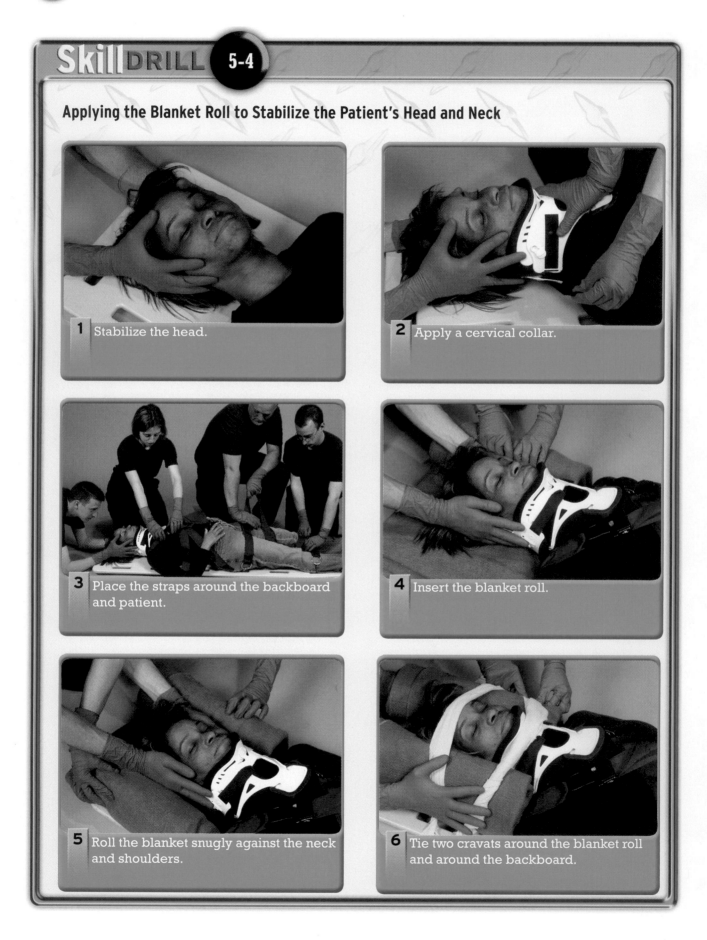

1 Stabilize the head.

2 Apply a cervical collar.

3 Place the straps around the backboard and patient.

4 Insert the blanket roll.

5 Roll the blanket snugly against the neck and shoulders.

6 Tie two cravats around the blanket roll and around the backboard.

stabilized against the backboard. This head-immobilization technique, coupled with proper placement of straps around the backboard, adequately immobilizes the spine of an injured patient and packages the patient for movement as a unit. Foam blocks are quick to apply and provide good stabilization of the patient's head and neck. The use of one type of foam blocks is shown in **Figure 5-30 ▼** .

In an extreme emergency where a patient must be moved from a dangerous environment and a commercially prepared backboard is not available, you should improvise. Make sure that the improvised backboard is strong enough to carry the pa-tient without breaking. Improvised devices should be used only when a patient must be moved to prevent further injury or death and when a commercially prepared backboard is not available.

Treatment Tips

Carefully monitor all immobilized patients for airway problems.

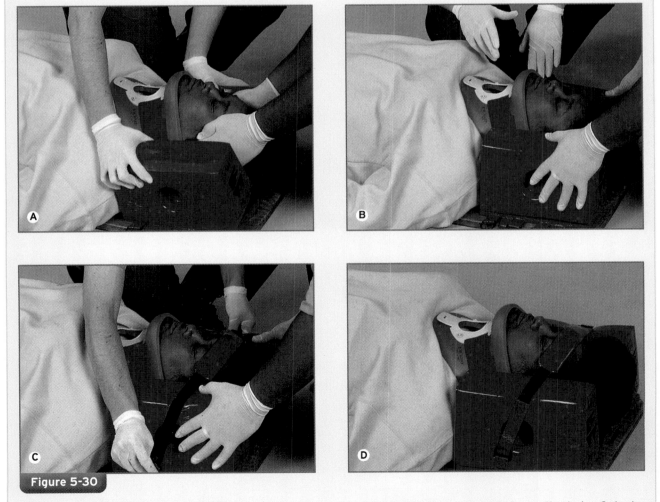

Figure 5-30

Application of a commercial device to stabilize a patient's head and neck. **A.** Apply the head blocks. **B.** Secure the device. **C.** Apply the immobilization straps. **D.** The head is immobilized.

You are the Provider

SUMMARY

Review the *You are the Provider* case study provided at the beginning of the chapter.

You and your partner are dispatched to the Fair Oaks Mall. The dispatcher informs you that a patron has fallen near the east escalator. Dispatch has no further information on the condition of the patient. They notify you that the nearest EMS transport unit is about 8 minutes away.

1. Under what circumstances would it be necessary to move the patient before the EMS transport unit arrives?

One of the most important decisions facing you as a first responder is whether to move a patient. Generally you should not move a patient unless there is a compelling reason to do so. However, patients do require moving in certain emergency situations. These include fires, explosions, structural collapse, the presence of hazardous materials, unsafe vehicle collision scenes, and cases where you need to move a patient to perform CPR. In general, when an imminent threat to the patient's safety exists that can be eliminated by moving the patient, it is better to do so. However, unless one of these conditions exists, it is usually better to wait for additional personnel before moving a patient.

2. Why is it often better for first responders to delay moving a patient until the arrival of an EMS transport unit?

There are several reasons why it is usually better to wait for additional EMS providers before moving a patient. EMTs and paramedics have more training in lifting and moving patients. EMS transport units carry a variety of equipment for lifting and moving patients. The expression "Many hands make light work" is certainly true here. Injuries to rescuers are less likely when there are adequate people to move a patient. Patient safety is enhanced when an adequate number of people are available. Because first responders usually do not transport patients, there is no hurry to move patients before the arrival of an EMS transport unit.

Prep Kit

Ready for Review

The Ready for Review thoroughly summarizes the chapter.

- In most situations, you can treat the patient in the position found and later assist other EMS personnel in moving the patient. In some cases, however, the patient's survival may depend on your knowledge of emergency movement techniques.

- Every time you move a patient, keep the following general guidelines in mind:
  - Do no further harm to the patient.
  - Move the patient only when necessary.
  - Move the patient as little as possible.
  - Move the patient's body as a unit.
  - Use proper lifting and moving techniques to ensure your own safety.
  - Have one rescuer give commands when moving a patient.

- Always use good body mechanics when you move patients, including:
  - Know your own physical limitations and capabilities.
  - Keep yourself balanced when lifting or moving a patient.
  - Maintain a firm footing.
  - Lift and lower the patient by bending your legs, not your back. Keep your back as straight as possible at all times and use your leg muscles to do the work.
  - Try to keep your arms close to your body for strength and balance.
  - Move the patient as little as possible.

Technology

- Interactivities
- Vocabulary Explorer
- Anatomy Review
- Web Links
- Online Review Manual

- Unconscious patients who have not suffered trauma should be placed in the recovery position.

- If a patient is on the floor or ground during an emergency situation, you may have to drag the person away from the scene instead of trying to lift and carry. Make every effort to pull the patient in the direction of the long axis of the body in order to provide spinal protection.

- Do not lift or move a patient if you suspect a spinal injury, unless it is necessary to remove the patient from a life-threatening situation.

- EMS services typically use wheeled ambulance stretchers, portable stretchers, stair chairs, long backboards, short backboards, or scoop stretchers to move patients.

- Any time a patient has suffered a traumatic injury, you should suspect injury to the head, neck, or spine. The patient's head should be kept in a neutral position and immobilized. A cervical collar is used to prevent excess movement of the head and neck.

- Log rolling is the primary technique used to move a patient onto a backboard. Every patient who is on a backboard should be strapped down to avoid sliding or slipping off the backboard.

- Once a patient has been secured to the backboard, the head and neck must be immobilized using commercially prepared devices or improvised devices.

Vital Vocabulary

The Vital Vocabulary are the key terms for this chapter.

arm-to-arm drag An emergency-patient move that consists of the rescuer grasping the patient's arms from behind; used to remove a patient from a hazardous place.

blanket drag An emergency-patient move in which a rescuer encloses a patient in a blanket and drags the patient to safety.

cervical collar A neck brace that partially stabilizes the neck following injury.

clothes drag An emergency-patient move used to remove a patient from a hazardous environment; performed by grasping the patient's clothes and moving the patient head first from the unsafe area.

cradle-in-arms carry A one-rescuer patient movement technique used primarily for children; the patient is cradled in the hollow formed by the rescuer's arms and chest.

extremities The arms and legs.

fire fighter drag A method of moving a patient without lifting or carrying him or her; used when the patient is heavier than the rescuer.

log rolling A technique used to move a patient onto a long backboard.

one-person walking assist A method used if the patient is able to bear his or her own weight.

pack-strap carry A one-person carry that allows the rescuer to carry a patient while keeping one hand free.

portable stretcher A lightweight nonwheeled device for transporting a patient; used in small spaces where the wheeled ambulance stretcher cannot be used.

recovery position A sidelying position that helps an unconscious patient maintain an open airway.

scoop stretcher A firm patient-carrying device that can be split into halves and applied to the patient from both sides.

stair chair A small portable device used for transporting patients in a sitting position.

straddle lift A method used to place a patient on a backboard if there is not enough space to perform a log roll.

straddle slide A method of placing a patient on a long backboard by straddling both the board and patient and sliding the patient onto the board.

two-person chair carry Two rescuers use a chair to support the weight of the patient.

two-person extremity carry A method of carrying a patient out of tight quarters using two rescuers and no equipment.

two-person seat carry A method of carrying a patient in which two rescuers link arms behind the patient's back and under the patient's knees; requires no equipment.

two-person walking assist Used when a patient cannot bear his or her own weight; two rescuers completely support the patient.

Assessment in Action

Assessment in Action presents a fictitious scenario to help you review what you learned in this chapter.

You and your partner have been called to an assisted-living facility to help evacuate patients because floodwaters caused by a hurricane are threatening to cut off the access road to the facility. The officer in charge assigns you and your partner to one wing that has four patients. He asks that you bring the patients to the front lobby where they will be assigned to vehicles for evacuation.

1. The first gentleman tells you he can walk slowly, but he is weak. What technique could you use to help this man?

   A. Straddle slide
   B. One-person walking assist
   C. Two-person extremity carry
   D. Pack-strap carry

2. The second room is occupied by a woman who has a brace on her ankle. She is not supposed to put weight on her sprained ankle. Which of the following carries would you consider using for this patient?

   A. Two-person extremity carry
   B. Pack-strap carry
   C. Two-person seat carry
   D. Direct ground lift

3. In the third room is an 82-year-old woman who says she has a heart condition and gets short of breath if she walks very far. How would you move this person?

   A. One-person walking assist
   B. Two-person extremity carry
   C. Pack-strap carry
   D. Two-person chair carry

4. The fourth person is confined to bed because she suffered a stroke 2 years ago. A nurse asks you to transfer this woman to a stretcher she furnishes for you. How would you move this woman to the stretcher?

   A. Direct ground lift
   B. Log roll
   C. Clothes drag
   D. Patient transfer technique

The following questions do not relate to the above scenario but test general knowledge.

5. The most commonly used technique for placing a patient on a backboard is:

   A. Straddle slide
   B. Log roll
   C. Straddle lift
   D. Direct ground lift

6. If you need to move a heavy unconscious person from a life-threatening emergency, which of the following would you use?

   A. Straddle slide
   B. Straddle lift
   C. Fire fighter drag
   D. Clothes drag

7. Which is the correct order of steps to secure a patient with a possible head and neck injury to a backboard?

   1. Immobilize the head to the backboard
   2. Manually stabilize the head
   3. Immobilize the torso and legs
   4. Apply a cervical collar

      A. 4,2,1,3
      B. 2,4,3,1
      C. 3,2,4,1
      D. 2,4,1,3

Airway

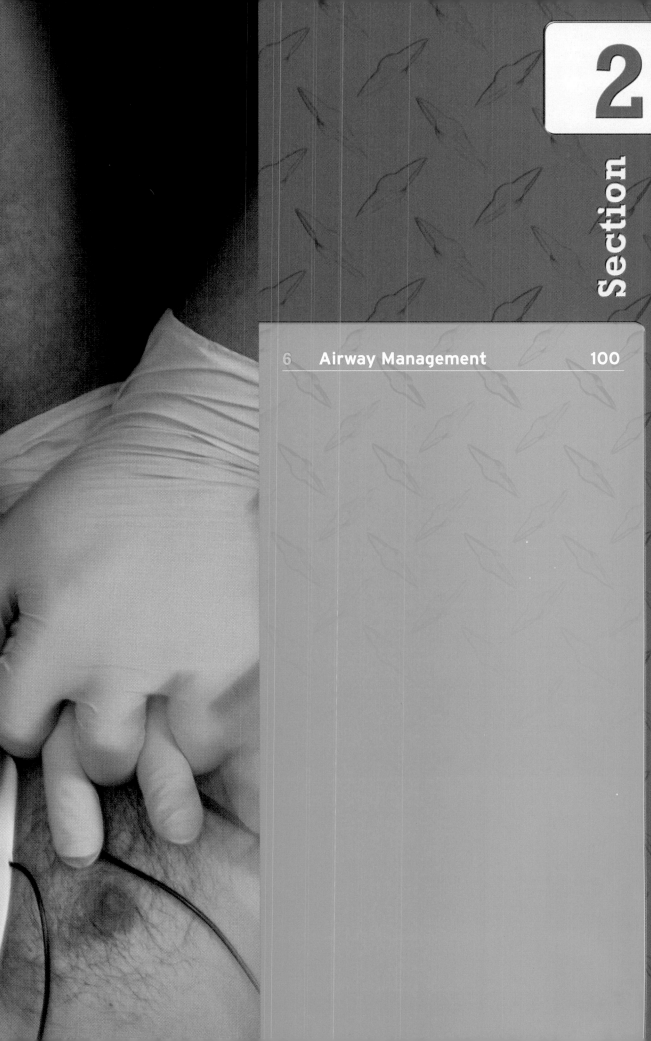

Airway Management

National Standard Curriculum Objectives

Cognitive

2-1.1   Name and label the major structures of the respiratory system on a diagram. (p 105-106)

2-1.2   List the signs of inadequate breathing. (p 116)

2-1.3   Describe the steps in the head-tilt chin-lift. (p 108)

2-1.4   Relate mechanism of injury to opening the airway. (p 108)

2-1.5   Describe the steps in the jaw thrust. (p 108-109)

2-1.6   State the importance of having a suction unit ready for immediate use when providing emergency medical care. (p 109)

2-1.7   Describe the techniques of suctioning. (p 110-111)

2-1.8   Describe how to ventilate a patient with a resuscitation mask or barrier device. (p 119-121)

2-1.9   Describe how ventilating an infant or child is different from an adult. (p 113)

2-1.10 List the steps in providing mouth-to-mouth and mouth-to-stoma ventilation. (p 121, 131-132)

2-1.11 Describe how to measure and insert an oropharyngeal (oral) airway. (p 113)

2-1.12 Describe how to measure and insert a nasopharyngeal (nasal) airway. (p 115)

2-1.13 Describe how to clear a foreign body airway obstruction in a responsive adult. (p 129)

2-1.14 Describe how to clear a foreign body airway obstruction in a responsive child with complete obstruction or partial airway obstruction and poor air exchange. (p 126-127)

2-1.15 Describe how to clear a foreign body airway obstruction in a responsive infant with complete obstruction or partial airway obstruction and poor air exchange. (p 129-130)

2-1.16 Describe how to clear a foreign body airway obstruction in an unresponsive adult. (p 129)

2-1.17 Describe how to clear a foreign body airway obstruction in an unresponsive child. (p 129)

2-1.18 Describe how to clear a foreign body airway obstruction in an unresponsive infant. (p 130)

Affective

2-1.19 Explain why basic life support ventilation and airway protective skills take priority over most other basic life support skills. (p 105)

2-1.20 Demonstrate a caring attitude toward patients with airway problems who request emergency medical services. (p 104)

2-1.21 Place the interests of the patient with airway problems as the foremost consideration when making any and all patient care decisions. (p 104)

2-1.22 Communicate with empathy to patients with airway problems, as well as with family members and friends of the patient. (p 104)

Psychomotor

2-1.23 Demonstrate the steps in the head-tilt chin-lift. (p 108)

2-1.24 Demonstrate the steps in the jaw thrust. (p 108)

2-1.25 Demonstrate the techniques of suctioning. (p 110)

2-1.26 Demonstrate the steps in mouth-to-mouth ventilation with body substance isolation (barrier shields). (p 119-121)

2-1.27 Demonstrate how to use a resuscitation mask to ventilate a patient. (p 120)

2-1.28 Demonstrate how to ventilate a patient with a stoma. (p 131-132)

2-1.29 Demonstrate how to measure and insert an oropharyngeal (oral) airway. (p 114)

2-1.30 Demonstrate how to measure and insert a nasopharyngeal (nasal) airway. (p 115)

2-1.31 Demonstrate how to ventilate infant and child patients. (p 122-125)

2-1.32 Demonstrate how to clear a foreign body airway obstruction in a responsive adult. (p 128)

2-1.33 Demonstrate how to clear a foreign body airway obstruction in a responsive child. (p 129)

2-1.34 Demonstrate how to clear a foreign body airway obstruction in a responsive infant. (p 130)

2-1.35 Demonstrate how to clear a foreign body airway obstruction in an unresponsive adult. (p 129)

2-1.36 Demonstrate how to clear a foreign body airway obstruction in an unresponsive child. (p 129)

2-1.37 Demonstrate how to clear a foreign body airway obstruction in an unresponsive infant. (p 130)

Chapter Objectives*

Knowledge and Attitude Objectives

1. Identify the anatomic structures of the respiratory system and state the function of each structure. (p 105-106)
2. State the differences in the respiratory systems of infants, children, and adults. (p 106)
3. Describe the process used to check a patient's responsiveness. (p 107)
4. Describe the steps in the head tilt-chin lift technique. (p 108)
5. Describe the steps in the jaw-thrust technique. (p 108-109)
6. Describe how to check for fluids, solids, and dentures in a patient's mouth. (p 109)
7. State the steps needed to clear a patient's airway using finger sweeps and suction. (p 109)
8. Describe the steps required to maintain a patient's airway using the recovery position, oral airways, and nasal airways. (p 112-113)
9. Describe the signs of adequate breathing, the signs of inadequate breathing, the causes of respiratory arrest, and the major signs of respiratory arrest. (p 116)
10. Describe how to check a patient for the presence of breathing. (p 118)
11. Describe how to perform rescue breathing using a mouth-to-mask device, a mouth-to-barrier device, and mouth-to-mouth techniques. (p 119-121)
12. Describe, in order, the steps for recognizing respiratory arrest and performing rescue breathing in infants, children, and adults. (p 122)
13. Describe the differences between the signs and symptoms of a mild airway obstruction and those of a severe or complete airway obstruction. (p 126-127)
14. List the steps in managing a foreign-body airway obstruction in infants, children, and adults. (p 127-131)
15. List the special considerations needed to perform rescue breathing in patients with stomas. (p 131-132)
16. Describe the special considerations of airway care and rescue breathing in children and infants. (p 123)
17. Describe the hazards that dental appliances present during the performance of airway skills. (p 133)
18. Describe the steps in providing airway care to a patient in a vehicle. (p 133-134)

Skill Objectives

1. Demonstrate the head tilt-chin lift and jaw-thrust techniques for opening blocked airways. (p 108-109)
2. Check for fluids, solids, and dentures in a patient's airway. (p 109)
3. Correct a blocked airway using finger sweeps and suction. (p 109)
4. Place a patient in the recovery position. (p 112)
5. Insert oral and nasal airways. (p 114-115)
6. Check for the presence of breathing. (p 118)
7. Perform rescue breathing using a mouth-to-mask device, a mouth-to-barrier device, and mouth-to-mouth techniques. (p 119-121)
8. Demonstrate the steps in recognizing respiratory arrest and performing rescue breathing on an adult patient, a child, and an infant. (p 122)
9. Perform the steps needed to remove a foreign-body airway obstruction in an infant, a child, and an adult. (p 128-131)
10. Demonstrate rescue breathing on a patient with a stoma. (p 131-132)
11. Perform airway management on a patient in a vehicle. (p 133-134)

*These are chapter learning objectives.

rway Management

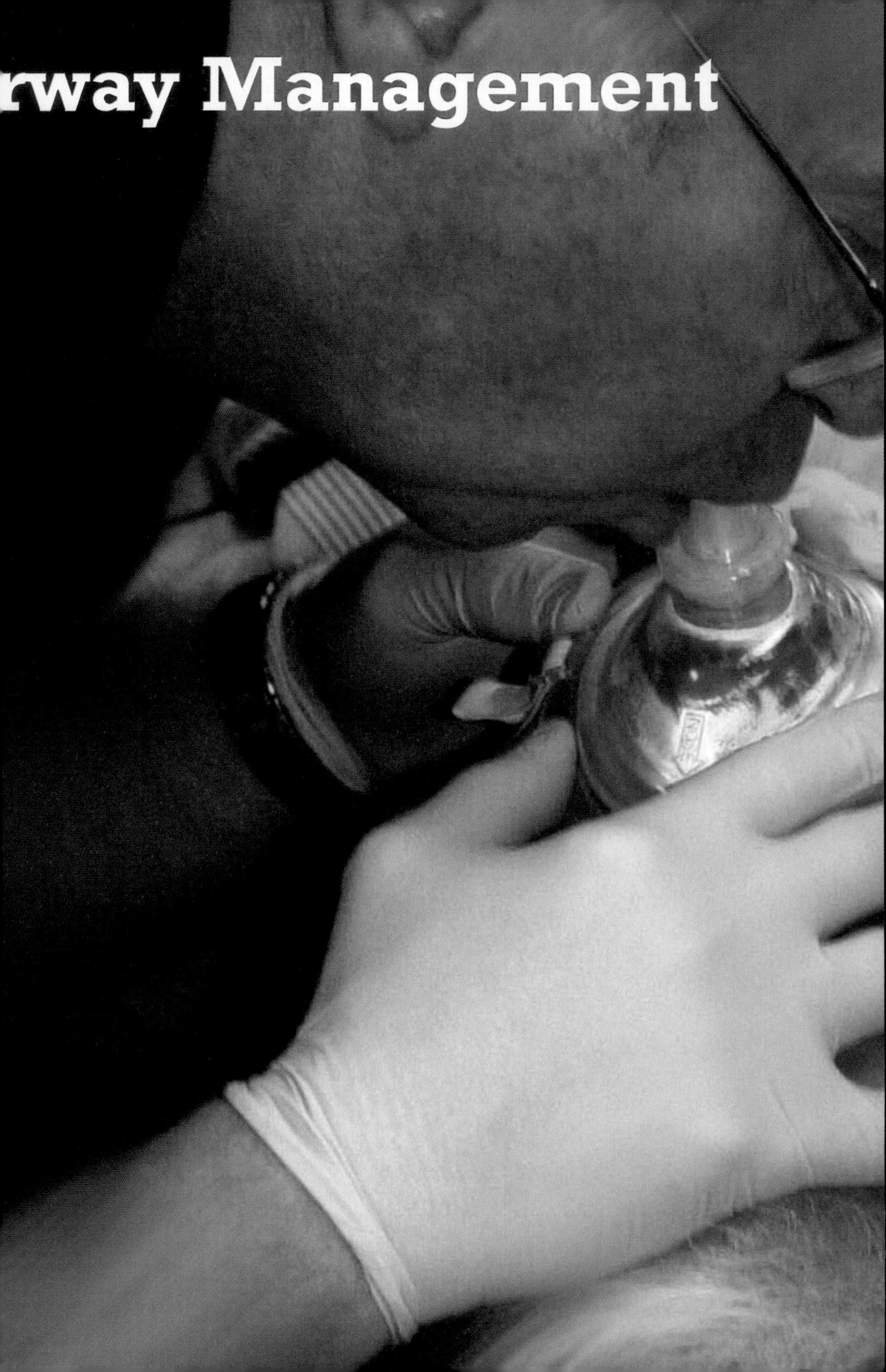

You are the Provider

At 4:35 PM, your dispatcher alerts you and requests that you respond to Pleasant High School to assist a teacher. A 63-year-old female is reportedly having difficulty breathing. Two minutes into your 4-mile response, your dispatcher reports that the teacher is in respiratory arrest.

1. How would your method of opening the patient's airway change depending on whether the patient had fallen or blacked out?
2. What equipment do you need to open a patient's airway?
3. How can you determine if a patient has a foreign body occluding the airway?

Introduction

This chapter introduces the two most important lifesaving skills: airway care and rescue breathing. Patients must have an open airway passage and must maintain adequate breathing to survive. By learning and practicing the simple skills in this chapter, you can often make the difference between life and death for a patient.

A review of the major structures of the respiratory system is needed before you practice airway and rescue breathing skills. Once you learn the functions of these structures, you will be a long way down the road to becoming proficient in performing these skills.

The skills of airway care and rescue breathing are as easy as A and B—the "A" stands for airway, and the "B" stands for breathing. Because you must assess and correct the airway before you turn your attention to the patient's breathing status, it is helpful to remember the AB sequence. In Chapter 9, "C" will be added for the assessment and correction of the patient's circulation. As you learn the skills presented in this chapter and in Chapter 9, remember the ABC sequence. A second mnemonic that will be used throughout both this chapter and Chapter 9 is "check and correct." By using this two-step sequence for each of the ABCs, you will be able to remember the steps needed to check and correct problems involving the patient's airway, breathing, and circulation.

The "A" or airway section presents airway skills, including how to check the level of consciousness (responsiveness) and manually correct a blocked airway by using the head tilt–chin lift and jaw-thrust techniques. You must check the patient's airway for foreign objects. If you find foreign objects, you must correct the problem and remove the objects by using either a manual technique or a suction device. You will learn when and how to use oral and nasal airways to keep the patient's airway open.

The "B" or breathing section describes how to check patients to determine whether they are breathing adequately. You will learn how to correct breathing problems by using three rescue breathing techniques: mouth-to-mask, mouth-to-barrier device, and mouth-to-mouth.

You will learn how to check patients to determine if they have an airway obstruction that can cause death in only a few minutes. You will learn how to correct this condition using manual techniques that require no special equipment.

Remember that patients with airway problems will likely be extremely anxious during the episode. It is your responsibility as a first responder to treat these patients and their families with compassion while you provide care.

As you study this chapter, remember the check-and-correct process for both airway and breathing skills. Do not forget that the A and B skills presented in this chapter will be followed by C (for circulation) skills in Chapter 9. After you have learned the airway, breathing, and circulation skills (the ABCs), you will be able to perform **cardiopulmonary resuscitation (CPR)**. CPR is used to save the lives of people suffering from cardiac arrest.

Anatomy and Function of the Respiratory System

To maintain life, all organisms must receive a constant supply of certain substances. In human beings, these basic life-sustaining substances are food, water, and **oxygen (O$_2$)**. A person can live several weeks without food because the body can

Technology

- Interactivities
- Vocabulary Explorer
- Anatomy Review
- Web Links
- Online Review Manual

use nutrients it has stored. Although the body does not store as much water, it is possible to live several days without fluid intake. However, lack of oxygen, even for a few minutes, can result in irreversible damage and death.

The most sensitive cells in the human body are in the brain. If brain cells are deprived of oxy-gen and nutrients for 4 to 6 minutes, they begin to die. Brain death is followed by the death of the entire body. Once brain cells have been destroyed, they cannot be replaced. This is why it is impor-tant to understand the anatomy and function of the respiratory system.

The main purpose of the respiratory system is to provide oxygen and to remove carbon diox-ide from the red blood cells as they pass through the lungs. This action forms the basis for your study of the lifesaving skill of CPR.

The parts of the body used in breathing are shown in   Figure 6-1 ◄   and include the mouth (**oropharynx**), the nose (**nasopharynx**), the throat, the **trachea** (windpipe), the lungs, the diaphragm (the dome-shaped muscle between the chest and the abdomen), and numerous chest muscles. Air enters the body through the nose and mouth. In an unconscious patient lying on his or her back, the passage of air through both nose and mouth may be blocked by the tongue   Figure 6-2 ▼ .

The tongue is attached to the lower jaw (**mandible**). When a person loses consciousness, the jaw relaxes and the tongue falls backward into the rear of the mouth, effectively blocking the pas-sage of air from both nose and mouth to the lungs. A partially blocked airway often produces a snor-ing sound. At the bottom of the throat are two pas-sages: the **esophagus** (the tube through which food passes) and the trachea. The epiglottis is a thin

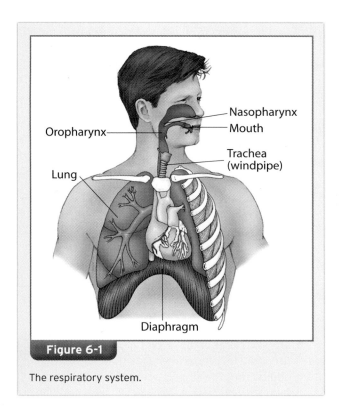

Figure 6-1

The respiratory system.

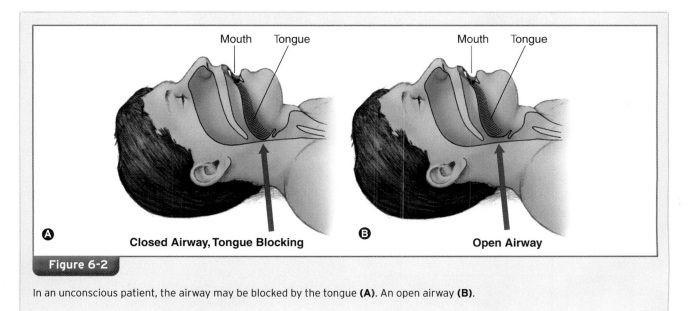

Figure 6-2

In an unconscious patient, the airway may be blocked by the tongue **(A)**. An open airway **(B)**.

flapper valve that allows air to enter the trachea but helps prevent food or water from doing so. Air passes from the throat to the larynx (voicebox), which can be seen externally as the Adam's apple in the neck. Below the trachea, the **airway** divides into the **bronchi** (two large tubes). The bronchi branch into smaller and smaller airways in the **lungs**. The lungs are located on either side of the heart and are protected by the sternum at the front and by the rib cage at the sides and back ` Figure 6-3 ▾ `.

The airways branch into smaller and smaller passages, which end as tiny air sacs called **alveoli**. The alveoli are surrounded by very small blood vessels, the **capillaries**. The actual exchange of gases takes place across a thin membrane that separates the capillaries of the circulatory system from the alveoli of the lungs ` Figure 6-4 ▸ `. The incoming oxygen passes from the alveoli into the blood, and the outgoing carbon dioxide passes from the blood into the alveoli.

The lungs consist of soft, spongy tissue with no muscles. Therefore, movement of air into the lungs depends on movement of the rib cage and the diaphragm. As the rib cage expands, air is drawn into the lungs through the trachea. The diaphragm, a muscle that separates the abdominal cavity from the chest, is dome shaped when it is relaxed. When the diaphragm contracts, it flattens and moves downward. This action increases the size of the chest cavity and draws air into the lungs through the trachea. In normal breathing, the combined actions of the diaphragm and the rib cage automatically produce adequate inhalation and exhalation ` Figure 6-5 ▸ `.

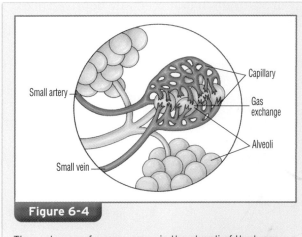

Figure 6-4

The exchange of gases occurs in the alveoli of the lungs.

Special Populations

- The structures of the respiratory systems in children and infants are smaller than they are in adults. Thus the air passages of children and infants may be more easily blocked by secretions or by foreign objects.
- In children and infants, the tongue is proportionally larger than it is in adults. Thus, the tongue of these smaller patients is more likely to block their airway than it would in an adult patient.
- Because the trachea of an infant or child is more flexible than that of an adult, it is more likely to become narrowed or blocked than that of an adult.
- The head of a child or an infant is proportionally larger than the head of an adult. You will have to learn slightly different techniques for opening the airways of children.
- Children and infants have smaller lungs than adults. You need to give them smaller breaths when you perform rescue breathing.
- Most children and infants have healthy hearts. When a child or infant suffers cardiac arrest (stoppage of the heart), it is usually because the patient has a blocked airway or has stopped breathing, not because there is a problem with the heart.

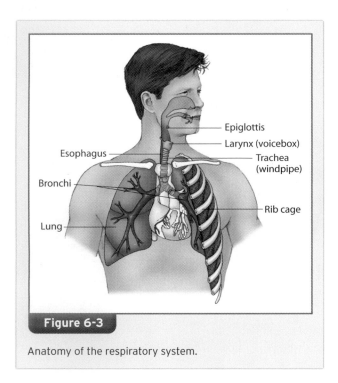

Figure 6-3

Anatomy of the respiratory system.

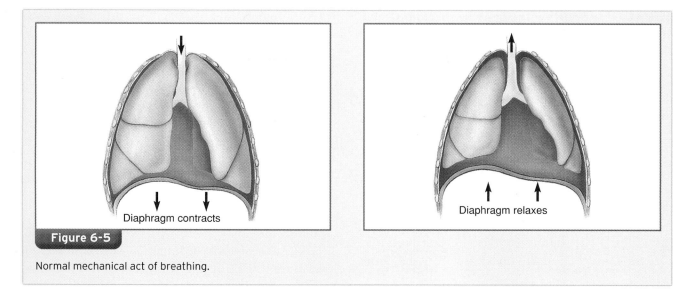

Diaphragm contracts

Diaphragm relaxes

Figure 6-5

Normal mechanical act of breathing.

"A" Is for Airway

The patient's airway is the pipeline that transports life-giving oxygen from the air to the lungs and transports the waste product, carbon dioxide, from the lungs to the air. In healthy individuals, the airway automatically stays open. An injured or seriously ill person, however, may not be able to protect the airway and it may become blocked.

If a patient cannot protect his or her airway, you, as a first responder, must take certain steps to check the condition of the patient's airway and correct the problem to keep the patient alive.

Check for Responsiveness

The first step in assessing a patient's airway is to check the patient's level of responsiveness. When you first approach a patient, you immediately can determine whether the patient is responsive (conscious) or unconscious (unresponsive) by asking, "Are you okay? Can you hear me?" **Figure 6-6 ▶** . If you get a response, you can assume that the patient is conscious and has an open airway.

If there is no response, grasp the patient's shoulder and gently shake the patient. Then repeat your question. If the patient still does not respond, you can assume the patient is unconscious and that you will need more help. Before doing anything for the patient, call 9-1-1 ("phone first") if the EMS system has not already been activated, especially if you are the only rescuer. Position the

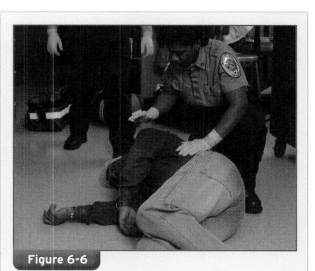

Figure 6-6

Establish the level of consciousness.

Treatment Tips

Airway Assessment
- Check for responsiveness.
- Correct the blocked airway using the head tilt-chin lift or jaw-thrust technique.
- Check the airway for fluids, foreign bodies, or dentures.
- Correct the airway using finger sweeps or suction.
- Maintain the airway manually, with an oral or nasal airway, or with the recovery position.

patient by supporting the patient's head and neck and placing the patient on his or her back.

Correct the Blocked Airway

An unconscious patient's airway is often blocked (occluded) because the tongue has dropped back and is obstructing it. In this case, simply opening the airway may enable the patient to breathe spontaneously.

Head Tilt–Chin Lift Technique

To open the airway, place one hand on the forehead and place the fingers of the other hand under the bony part of the lower jaw near the chin.

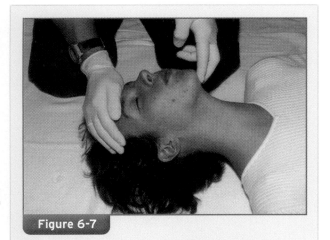

Figure 6-7

Open the patient's airway using the head tilt-chin lift technique.

Push down on the forehead and lift up and forward on the chin. Be certain you are not merely pushing the mouth closed when you use this technique. This method of opening the airway is called the **head tilt–chin lift technique** (or maneuver) **Figure 6-7 ◀**.

Follow these steps to perform the head tilt–chin lift technique:

1. Place the patient on his or her back and kneel beside the patient.
2. Place one hand on the patient's forehead and apply firm pressure backward with your palm. Move the patient's head back as far as possible.
3. Place the tips of the fingers of your other hand under the bony part of the lower jaw near the chin.
4. Lift the chin forward to help tilt the head back.

Jaw-Thrust Technique

The **jaw-thrust technique** (or maneuver) is another way to open a patient's airway. If a patient was injured in a fall, diving mishap, or automobile collision and has a neck injury, tilting the head may cause permanent paralysis. If you suspect a neck injury, first try to open the airway using the jaw-thrust technique. Open the airway by placing your fingers under the angles of the jaw and pushing upward. At the same time, use your thumbs to open the mouth slightly. The jaw-thrust technique should open the airway without extending the neck **Figure 6-8 ▾**.

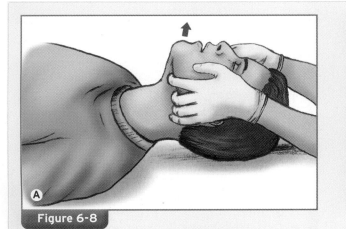
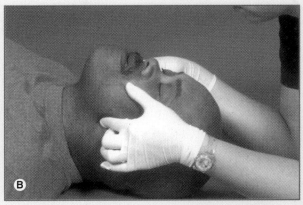

Figure 6-8

The jaw-thrust technique should open the patient's airway without extending the neck. **A.** Kneeling above the patient's head, place your fingers behind the angles of the lower jaw and move the jaw upward. Use your thumbs to help position the lower jaw. **B.** The completed maneuver should look like this.

Follow these steps to perform the jaw-thrust technique:

1. Place the patient on his or her back and kneel at the top of the patient's head. Place your fingers behind the angles of the patient's lower jaw and move the jaw forward with firm pressure.
2. Tilt the head backward to a neutral or slight sniffing position. Do not extend the cervical spine in a patient who has suffered an injury to the head or neck.
3. Use your thumbs to pull the patient's lower jaw down, opening the mouth enough to allow breathing through the mouth and nose.

If you are not able to open the patient's airway using the jaw-thrust technique, try the head tilt–chin lift technique as a secondary attempt to open the patient's airway.

Check for Fluids, Foreign Bodies, or Dentures

After you have opened the patient's airway by using either the head tilt–chin lift or the jaw-thrust techniques, look in the patient's mouth to see if anything is blocking the patient's airway. Potential blocks include secretions, such as vomitus, mucus, or blood; foreign objects, such as candy, food, or dirt; and dentures or false teeth that may have become dislodged and are blocking the patient's airway. If you find anything in the patient's mouth, remove it by using one of the techniques noted in the following sections. If the patient's mouth is clear, consider using one of the devices described in the section on airway devices.

Correct the Airway Using Finger Sweeps or Suction

Vomitus, mucus, blood, and foreign objects must be cleared from the patient's airway. This can be done by using finger sweeps, suctioning, or by placing the patient in the recovery position.

Finger Sweeps

Finger sweeps can be done quickly and require no special equipment except a set of medical gloves. To perform a finger sweep, follow the steps in **Skill Drill 6-1 ▶**:

SKILL DRILL 6-1

1. Turn the patient onto his or her side Step 1.
2. Insert your gloved fingers into the patient's mouth Step 2.
3. Curve your fingers into a C-shape and sweep it from one side of the back of the mouth to the other Step 3. Scoop out as much of the material as possible. A gauze pad wrapped around your gloved fingers may help remove the obstructing materials. Repeat the finger sweeps until you have removed all the foreign material in the patient's mouth. Finger sweeps should be your first attempt at clearing the airway even if suction equipment is available.

Suctioning

Sometimes just sweeping out the mouth is not enough to clear the materials completely from the mouth and upper airway. Suction machines can be helpful in removing secretions such as vomitus, blood, and mucus from the patient's mouth. Two types of suction devices are available: manual and mechanical. Suctioning the airway (either manually or mechanically) is a lifesaving technique. Although a gauze pad and your gloved fingers can do most of the work, the use of supplementary suction devices enables you to remove a greater amount of obstructing material from the patient's airway.

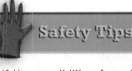

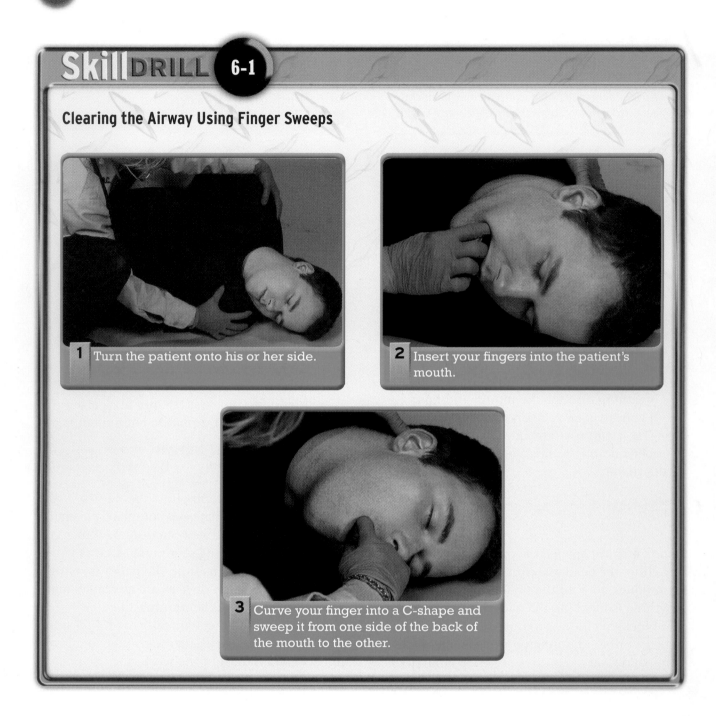

SkillDRILL 6-1

Clearing the Airway Using Finger Sweeps

1 Turn the patient onto his or her side.

2 Insert your fingers into the patient's mouth.

3 Curve your finger into a C-shape and sweep it from one side of the back of the mouth to the other.

Manual Suction Devices Several **manual suction devices** are available to first responders **Figure 6-9 ▶** . These devices are relatively inexpensive and are compact enough to fit into first responder life support kits. With most manual suction devices, you insert the end of the suction tip into the patient's mouth and squeeze or pump the hand-powered pump. Be sure that you do not insert the tip of the suction device farther than you can see. Manual suction devices are used in the same way as the mechanical suction devices described in the

following section. The only difference is the power source. Be sure to follow local medical protocols on first responders' authorization to use suction devices in the field.

Mechanical Suction Devices A **mechanical suction device** uses either a battery-powered pump or an oxygen-powered **aspirator** to create a vacuum that will draw the obstructing materials from the patient's airway **Figure 6-10 ▶** . Usually, both a rigid suction tip and a flexible whistle-tip catheter can be used with mechani-

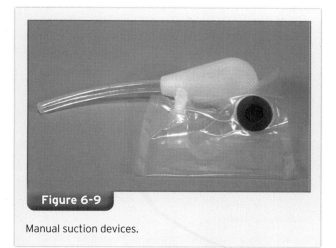

Figure 6-9

Manual suction devices.

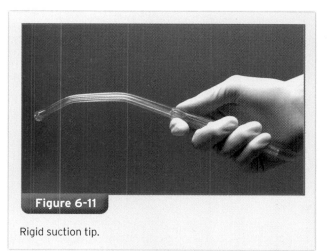

Figure 6-11

Rigid suction tip.

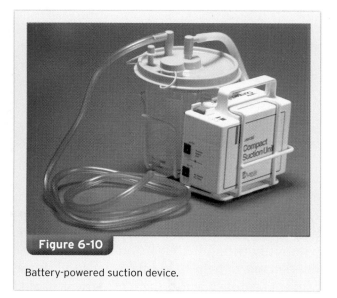

Figure 6-10

Battery-powered suction device.

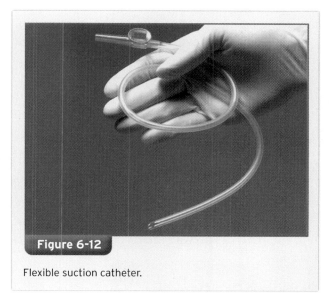

Figure 6-12

Flexible suction catheter.

cal suction devices. To use this type of suction machine, you must first learn how to operate the device and control the force of the suction. When using mechanical suction, first clear the mouth of large pieces of material with your gloved fingers. After the mouth is clear, turn the suction device on and use the rigid tip to remove most of the remaining material   **Figure 6-11 ▶** . Do not suction for more than 15 seconds at a time because the suction draws air out of the patient's airway, as well as any obstructing material. If the rigid tip has a suction control port (a small hole located close to the tip's handle), place a finger over the hole to create the suction. Do not keep your finger over this control port for longer than 15 seconds at a time because you may rob the patient of oxygen.

After you have cleared most of the obstructing material out of the patient's mouth and upper airway with the rigid tip, change to the flexible tip and clear out material from the deeper parts of the patient's throat   **Figure 6-12 ▲** . Flexible whistle-tip catheters also have suction control ports, which are located close to the end of the catheter that attaches to the suction machine. Again, place a finger over the control port to achieve suction.

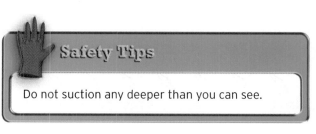

Safety Tips

Do not suction any deeper than you can see.

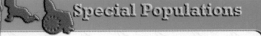
Maintain the Airway

If a patient is unable to keep the airway open, you must open the airway manually. You have learned how to do this by using the head tilt–chin lift or jaw-thrust maneuvers to open the airway. Unconscious patients will not be able to keep their airway open. You can continue to keep the airway open by using the head tilt–chin lift or jaw-thrust maneuvers. To do this, you must continue holding the patient's head to maintain the head tilt or the jaw-thrust positions.

If the patient is breathing adequately, you can keep the airway open by placing the patient in the recovery position. You can also insert an oral or nasal airway to keep the patient's airway open. These two mechanical airway devices will maintain the patient's airway after you have opened it manually.

Recovery Position

If an unconscious patient is breathing and the patient has not suffered trauma, one way to keep the airway open is to place the patient in the recovery position **Figure 6-13 ▶**. The recovery position helps keep the patient's airway open by allowing secretions to drain out of the mouth instead of draining into the trachea. It also uses gravity to help keep the patient's tongue and lower jaw from blocking the airway.

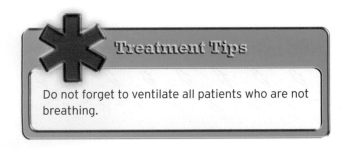

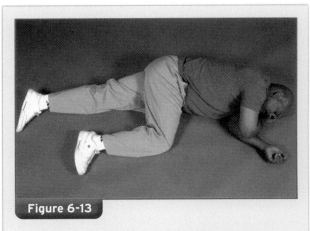

Figure 6-13

Recovery position for an unconscious patient.

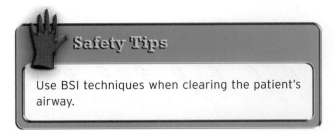
To place a patient in the recovery position, carefully roll the patient onto one side as you support the patient's head. Roll the patient as a unit without twisting the body. You can use the patient's hand to help hold his or her head in the proper position. Place the patient's face on its side so any secretions drain out of the mouth. The head should be in a position similar to the tilted back position of the head tilt–chin lift technique.

Oral Airway

An **oral airway** has two primary purposes: It is used to maintain the patient's airway after you have manually opened the airway, and it functions as a pathway through which you can suction the patient **Figure 6-14 ▶**. Oral airways can be used for unconscious patients who are breathing or who are in **respiratory arrest** (sudden stoppage of breathing). An oral airway can be used in any unconscious patient who does not have a **gag reflex**. Oral airways cannot be used in conscious patients because they have a gag reflex. These airways can be used with mechanical breathing devices such as the **pocket mask**.

Respiratory Arrest
- No chest movement
- No breath sounds
- No air movement
- Blue skin (cyanosis), especially around the lips

The roof of a child's mouth is more fragile than that of an adult. This means you must be especially careful to avoid injuring it as you insert the oral airway. The technique for inserting an oral airway in a child is almost the same as for an adult patient. However, to make it easier to insert the airway, use two or three stacked tongue blades and depress the tongue. This will press the tongue forward and away from the roof of the mouth so you can insert the airway.

There are two styles of oral airways: One has an opening down the center and the other has a slot along each side. The opening or slot permits the free flow of air and allows you to suction through the airway. Before you insert the oral airway, you need to select the proper size. Choose the proper size by measuring from the earlobe to the corner of the patient's mouth. When properly inserted, the airway will rest inside the mouth. The curve of the airway should follow the contour of the tongue. The flange should rest against the lips. The other end should be resting in the back of the throat.

Follow these steps to insert an oral airway **Skill Drill 6-2 ▶** :

SKILL DRILL 6-2

1. Select the proper size airway by measuring from the patient's earlobe to the corner of the mouth **Step 1** .
2. Open the patient's mouth with one hand after manually opening the patient's airway with a head tilt–chin lift or jaw-thrust maneuver.
3. Hold the airway upside down with your other hand. Insert the airway into the patient's mouth and guide the tip of the airway along the roof of the patient's mouth, advancing it until you feel resistance **Step 2** .
4. Rotate the airway 180° until the flange comes to rest on the patient's teeth or lips **Step 3** .

Be especially careful when you insert the airway. You could injure the roof of the patient's mouth by the rough insertion of an oral airway. Remember that an oral airway does not open the patient's airway. It will maintain the open airway after you have opened it with a manual technique.

Nasal Airway

A second type of device you can use to keep the patient's airway open is a **nasal airway** **Figure 6-15 ▶** . This device is inserted into the patient's nose. Nasal airways can be used in both unconscious and conscious patients who are not able to maintain an open airway. Usually a patient will tolerate a nasal airway better than an oral airway. It is not as likely to cause vomiting. One disadvantage of a nasal airway is that you cannot suction through it because the inside diameter of the airway is too small for the standard whistle-tip catheter suction tip.

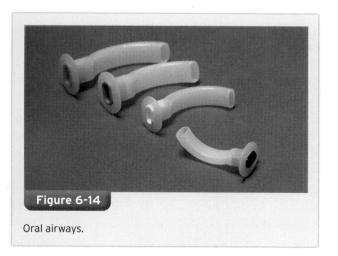

Figure 6-14

Oral airways.

Skill DRILL 6-2

Inserting an Oral Airway

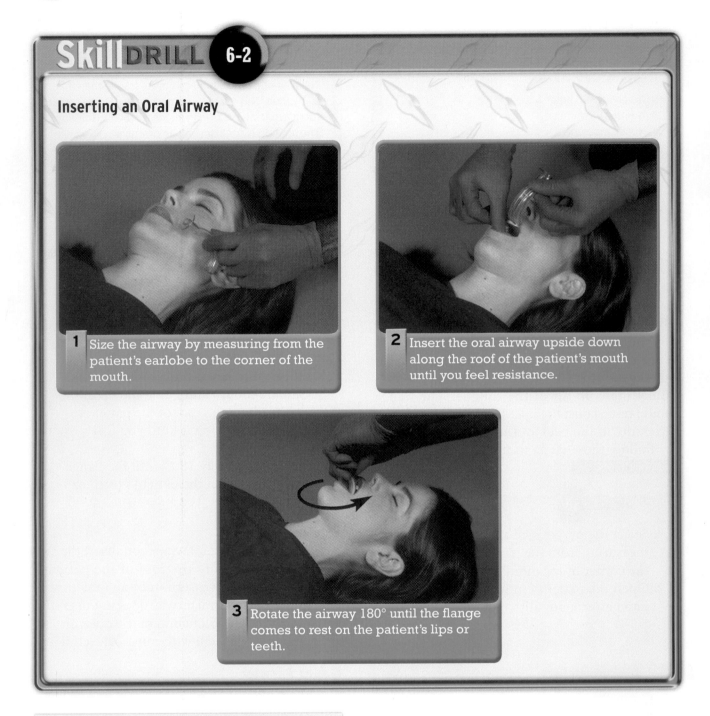

1 Size the airway by measuring from the patient's earlobe to the corner of the mouth.

2 Insert the oral airway upside down along the roof of the patient's mouth until you feel resistance.

3 Rotate the airway 180° until the flange comes to rest on the patient's lips or teeth.

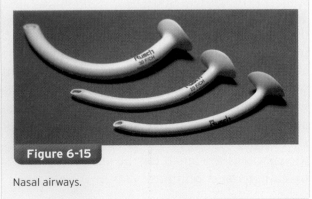

Figure 6-15

Nasal airways.

You will have to select the proper size nasal airway for the patient. Measure from the tip of the patient's nose to the earlobe. Coat the airway with a water-soluble lubricant before inserting it. This makes it easier for you to insert the airway and reduces the chance of trauma to the patient's airway. Insert the airway in the larger nostril. As you insert the airway, follow the curvature of the floor of the nose. The airway is fully inserted when the flange or trumpet rests against the patient's nostril. At this point, the other end

Skill DRILL 6-3

Inserting a Nasal Airway

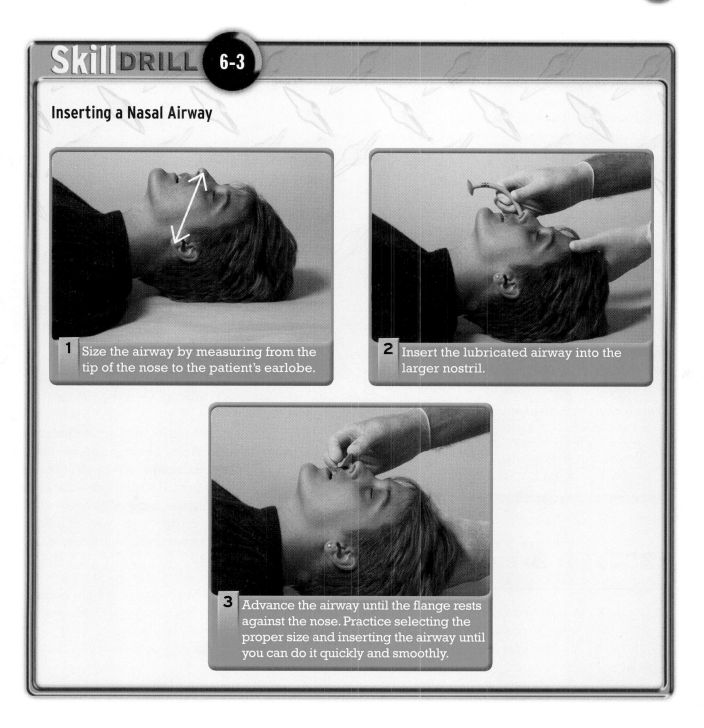

1 Size the airway by measuring from the tip of the nose to the patient's earlobe.

2 Insert the lubricated airway into the larger nostril.

3 Advance the airway until the flange rests against the nose. Practice selecting the proper size and inserting the airway until you can do it quickly and smoothly.

of the airway will reach the back of the patient's throat and an open airway for the patient can be maintained.

Follow these steps to insert a nasal airway **Skill Drill 6-3** :

Skill DRILL 6-3

1. Select the proper size airway by measuring from the tip of the patient's nose to the earlobe **Step 1** .

2. Coat the airway with a water-soluble lubricant.
3. Select the larger nostril.
4. Gently stretch the nostril open by using your thumb.
5. Gently insert the airway until the flange rests against the nose **Step 2** and **Step 3** . Do not force the airway. If you feel any resistance, remove the airway and try to insert it in the other nostril.

In the Field

To open the patient's airway:
1. Perform the head tilt-chin lift maneuver, or
2. Perform the jaw-thrust maneuver.

To maintain the patient's airway:
1. Continue to apply the head tilt-chin lift or jaw-thrust maneuver, and
   A. Insert an oral airway, or
   B. Insert a nasal airway, or
2. Place the patient in the recovery position.

After you open and maintain the patient's airway, you need to continue to monitor the status of the patient's breathing.

Treatment Tips

If a patient has suffered severe head trauma, there is some chance that a nasal airway may further damage the brain. You should check with your local medical control to determine the protocol for using a nasal airway in these patients.

"B" Is for Breathing

After you have checked and corrected the patient's airway, check and correct the patient's breathing. To do this, you must understand the signs of adequate breathing, the signs of inadequate breathing, and the signs and causes of respiratory arrest.

Signs of Adequate Breathing

To check for adequate breathing, look, listen, and feel at the same time. If a patient is breathing adequately, look for the rise and fall of the patient's chest, listen for the sounds of air passing into or out of the patient's nose and mouth, and feel the air moving on the side of your face. Place the side of your face close to the patient's nose and mouth and watch the patient's chest. In this way, you can look for chest movements, listen for the sounds of air moving, and feel the air as it moves in and out of the patient's nose and mouth.

A normal adult has a resting breathing rate of approximately 12 to 20 breaths per minute. Remember that one breath includes both an inhalation and an exhalation.

Signs of Inadequate Breathing

If a patient is breathing inadequately, you will detect signs of abnormal respirations. Noisy respirations, wheezing, or gurgling indicate partial blockage or constriction somewhere along the respiratory tract. Rapid or gasping respirations may indicate that the patient is not receiving an adequate amount of oxygen due to illness or injury. The patient's skin may be pale or even blue, especially around the lips or fingernail beds.

The most critical sign of inadequate breathing is respiratory arrest (total lack of respirations). This critical state is characterized by lack of chest movements, lack of breath sounds, and lack of air against the side of your face. In patients with severe hypothermia, respirations can be slowed (and/or shallow) to the point that the patient does not appear to be breathing.

There are many causes of respiratory arrest. A common cause is heart attack, which claims more than 500,000 lives each year. Other major causes of respiratory arrest include:

- Mechanical blockage or obstruction caused by the tongue
- Vomitus, particularly in a patient weakened by an illness such as a stroke
- Foreign objects such as broken teeth, dentures, balloons, marbles, pieces of food, or pieces of hard candy (especially in small children)
- Illness or disease such as severe stroke
- Drug overdose
- Poisoning
- Severe loss of blood
- Electrocution by electrical current or lightning

Voices of Experience

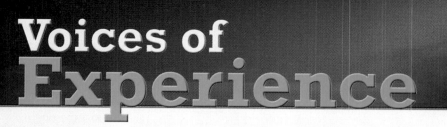

Making a Difference

It was a dark and stormy night—really, it was! My family and I were traveling on Interstate 5 to my parent's house to spend Christmas. It was cold and getting icy on some of the overpasses. As my car crested the top of one of the overpasses, I saw six headlights in my lane pointing in various directions. I may not know much about cars, but I did know that this wasn't right.

I walked up to the three cars that had obviously slid on the ice coming over the overpass. They had struck each other and spun around so that all three were facing the wrong way on the freeway. Two people were getting out of one of the cars; this car looked the worst. The second car looked a little better, but the driver was still inside. I walked up to the door, thinking that if the people in the more damaged car were all right, this driver would be all right also.

> **The patient was breathing, and all I could think was: "Did I do that?"**

Well, math doesn't always work like it should and patients *never* read the textbook. I remember asking if he was OK as I looked up and saw the lights of a fire engine approaching. I thought it was strange that the man didn't answer me, so I looked down and froze; the man didn't talk, he didn't move—he wasn't breathing. The next thing I knew I was yelling for help, but the fire fighters didn't come. They couldn't hear me over the traffic.

Even while I was panicking, I saw my hand reach in and lift the patient's head. Just that fast, he changed from a man to a patient. Without even realizing what I was doing, my hand reached in and lifted his head; my other hand also entered the car and I was doing a jaw thrust on the patient. While I was wondering if I had actually done the airway maneuver or just imagined it, I heard something. It sounded like thunder bursting out of the patient's chest and mouth. It was a breath! The patient was breathing, and all I could think was: "Did I do that?" I must have, although I didn't remember doing anything. Then I looked down at my hands and the patient (my instructors would be proud); I was doing a perfect jaw-thrust maneuver.

I felt a hand on my back. I looked and it was a paramedic telling me he would take over the airway. I let go and watched as the paramedics packaged "my" patient and put him in the ambulance. Later, I was told that I had done a good job and that I had probably saved the patient's life. I think I told that story to everyone I knew—and a few people I didn't know—that Christmas.

The night of that accident, I wasn't a paramedic; I wasn't even an EMT. I was a first responder. I was debating whether I wanted to go on to EMT training or do other things. I hadn't even used my skills on a real person, except for my "victim" during my practical exam. That night the training took over; it worked as if it was the most natural thing in the world. I was a first responder and I had helped someone and saved his life. Anyone who tells you that you are "just" a first responder is wrong! If a first responder hadn't been there on that dark and stormy night, that man would have died. As a first responder, you can and will make a difference.

Fifteen years later, I look back and smile. I made a difference that night.

David K. Anderson, BS, EMT-P
Director of Paramedic Education
Northwest Regional Training Center
Vancouver, Washington

Check for the Presence of Breathing

After establishing the loss of consciousness and opening the airway of the unconscious patient, check for breathing by looking, listening, and feeling (Figure 6-16 ▾):

- Look for the rising and falling of the patient's chest.
- Listen for the sound of air moving in and out of the patient's nose and mouth.
- Feel for the movement of air on the side of your face and ear. Continue to look, listen, and feel for at least 5 seconds; if you do not scrutinize the patient for a period of time, you risk checking between breaths and missing any signs of breathing that are present. Your breathing check should take no more than 10 seconds. If there are no signs of breathing, proceed to the next step and correct the lack of breathing by beginning rescue breathing. If the patient is breathing adequately (about 12 to 20 times a minute with adequate depth), you can continue to maintain the airway and monitor the rate and depth of respirations to ensure adequate breathing continues.

Correct the Breathing

You must breathe for any patient who is not breathing. As you perform **rescue breathing**, keep the patient's airway open by using the head tilt–chin lift maneuver (or the jaw-thrust maneuver for patients with head or neck injuries). To perform rescue breathing, blow your air into the patient's mouth. Pinch the patient's nose with your thumb and forefinger, take a deep breath, and blow slowly for 1 second (Figure 6-17 ▾). Use slow, gentle, sustained breathing and just enough breath to make the patient's chest rise. This minimizes the amount of air blown into the stomach. Remove your mouth and allow the lungs to deflate. Breathe for the patient a second time. After these first two breaths, breathe once into the patient's mouth every 5 to 6 seconds. The rate of breaths should be 10 to 12 per minute for an adult.

Rescue breathing can be done by using a mouth-to-mask device, a barrier device, or just your mouth. The mouth-to-mask and barrier devices prevent you from putting your mouth directly on the patient's mouth. These devices should be available to you as a first responder. If a rescue breathing device is not available, you must weigh the potential good to the patient against the limited chance that you will contract an infectious disease if you perform mouth-to-mouth rescue breathing.

Mouth-to-Mask Rescue Breathing

Your first responder life support kit should contain an artificial ventilation device that enables you to perform rescue breathing without mouth-

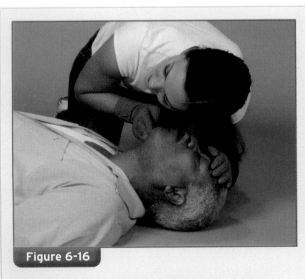

Figure 6-16

Check for breathing by looking, listening, and feeling.

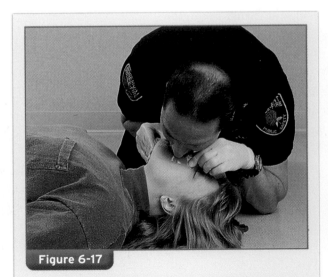

Figure 6-17

To perform rescue breathing, pinch the patient's nose with your thumb and forefinger.

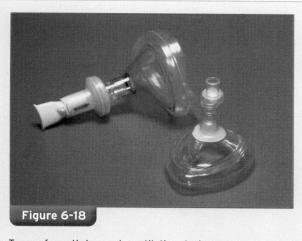

Figure 6-18

Types of mouth-to-mask ventilation devices.

to-mouth contact with the patient. This simple piece of equipment is called a mouth-to-mask ventilation device. A **mouth-to-mask ventilation device** consists of a mask that fits over the patient's face, a one-way valve, and a mouthpiece through which the rescuer breathes **Figure 6-18 ▲**. It may also have an inlet port for supplemental oxygen and a tube between the mouthpiece and the mask. Because mouth-to-mask devices prevent direct contact between you and the patient, they reduce the risk of transmitting infectious diseases.

To use a mouth-to-mask ventilation device for rescue breathing, follow the steps in **Skill Drill 6-4 ▶** :

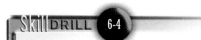

SKILL DRILL 6-4

1. Position yourself at the patient's head.
2. Use the head tilt–chin lift or jaw-thrust technique to open the patient's airway **Step 1** and **Step 2** .
3. Place the mask over the patient's mouth and nose. Make sure that the mask's nose notch is on the nose and not the chin.
4. Grasp the mask and the patient's jaw, using both hands. Use the thumb and forefinger of each hand to hold the mask tightly against the face. Hook the other three fingers of each hand under the patient's jaw and lift up to seal the mask tightly against the patient's face **Step 3** .

5. Maintain an airtight seal as you pull up on the jaw to maintain the proper head position.
6. Take a deep breath and then seal your mouth over the mouthpiece.
7. Breathe slowly into the mouthpiece for 1 second **Step 4** . Breathe until the patient's chest rises.
8. Monitor the patient for proper head position, air exchange, and vomiting.

Practice this technique frequently on a manikin until you can do it well.

Mouth-to-Barrier Rescue Breathing

Mouth-to-barrier devices also provide a barrier between the rescuer and the patient **Figure 6-19 ▼**. Some of these devices are small enough to carry in your pocket. Although a wide variety of devices is available, most of them consist of a port or hole that you breathe into and a mask or plastic film that covers the patient's face. Some also have a one-way valve that prevents backflow of secretions and gases. These devices provide variable degrees of infection control.

To perform mouth-to-mouth rescue breathing with a barrier device, follow the steps in **Skill Drill 6-5 ▶** :

SKILL DRILL 6-5

1. Open the airway with the head tilt–chin lift technique. Press on the

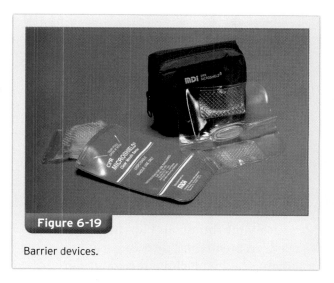

Figure 6-19

Barrier devices.

Skill DRILL 6-4

Performing Mouth-to-Mask Rescue Breathing

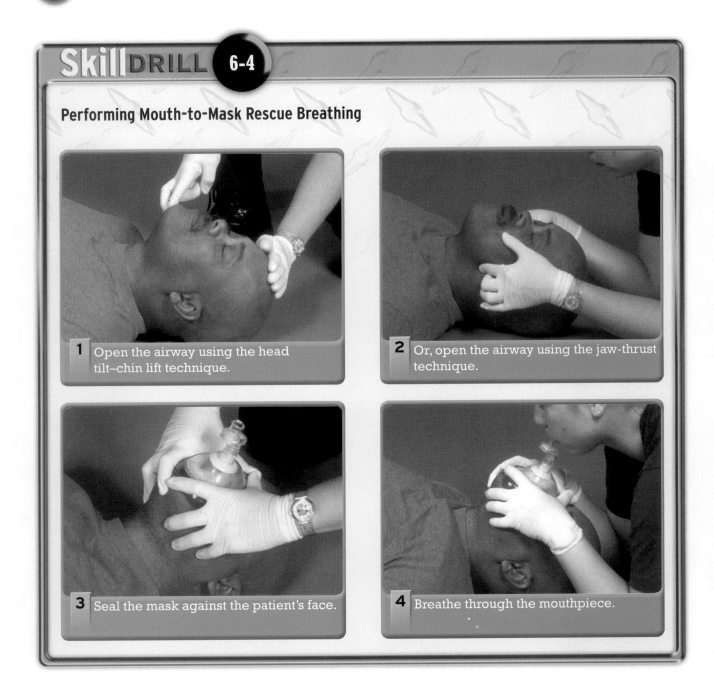

1 Open the airway using the head tilt–chin lift technique.

2 Or, open the airway using the jaw-thrust technique.

3 Seal the mask against the patient's face.

4 Breathe through the mouthpiece.

forehead to maintain the backward tilt of the head Step 1 .

2. Keep the patient's mouth open with the thumb of whichever hand you are using to lift the patient's chin.

3. Place the barrier device over the patient's mouth Step 2 .

4. Pinch the patient's nostrils together with your thumb and forefinger. Take a deep breath and then make a tight seal by placing your mouth on the

barrier device around the patient's mouth.

5. Breathe slowly into the patient's mouth for 1 second. Breathe until the patient's chest rises Step 3 .

6. Remove your mouth and allow the patient to exhale passively. Check to see that the patient's chest falls after each exhalation.

7. Repeat this rescue breathing sequence 10 to 12 times per minute (one breath every 5 to 6 seconds) for an adult.

Skill DRILL 6-5

Performing Mouth-to-Barrier Rescue Breathing

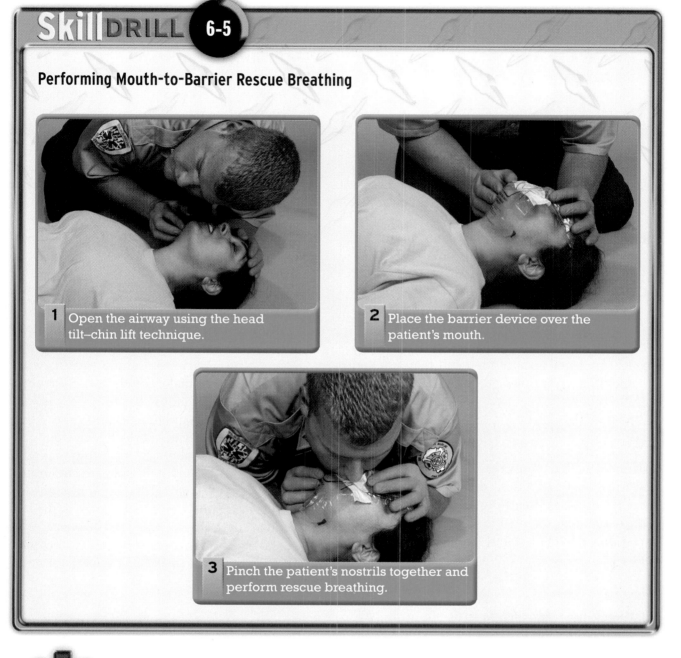

1 Open the airway using the head tilt–chin lift technique.

2 Place the barrier device over the patient's mouth.

3 Pinch the patient's nostrils together and perform rescue breathing.

Treatment Tips

The three methods for performing rescue breathing are all potentially lifesaving. You should use a mouth-to-mask or mouth-to-barrier breathing device whenever possible. If a rescue breathing device is not available, you must weigh the potential good to the patient against the limited chance that you will contract an infectious disease from mouth-to-mouth breathing.

Mouth-to-Mouth Rescue Breathing

Mouth-to-mouth rescue breathing is an effective way of providing artificial ventilation for non-breathing patients. It requires no equipment except you. However, because there is a somewhat higher risk of contracting a disease when using this method, you should use a mask or barrier breathing device if available. If a rescue breathing device is not available, you must weigh the potential good to the patient against the limited chance that you will contract an infectious disease from mouth-to-mouth breathing.

To perform mouth-to-mouth rescue breathing, follow these steps:

1. Open the airway with the head tilt–chin lift maneuver. Press on the forehead to maintain the backward tilt of the head.

2. Pinch the patient's nostrils together with your thumb and forefinger.

3. Keep the patient's mouth open with the thumb of whichever hand you are using to lift the patient's chin.

4. Take a deep breath and then make a tight seal by placing your mouth over the patient's mouth.

5. Breathe slowly into the patient's mouth for 1 second. Breathe until the patient's chest rises.

6. Remove your mouth and allow the patient to exhale passively. Check to see that the patient's chest falls after each exhalation.

7. Repeat this rescue breathing sequence 10 to 12 times per minute for adult patients and about 12 to 20 times per minute for children and infants.

Airway and Breathing Review

Assume that all patients may be in respiratory arrest until you can assess them and determine whether they are breathing adequately. A summary of the steps required to recognize respiratory arrest and perform rescue breathing in adults follows.

Airway

1. Check for responsiveness by shouting "Are you okay?" and gently shaking the patient's shoulder. If the patient is unresponsive and the EMS system has not been notified, activate the EMS system. Place the patient on his or her back.

2. Correct a closed airway by using the head tilt–chin lift maneuver or, if the patient has suffered any injury to the head or neck, the jaw-thrust maneuver.

3. Check the mouth for secretions, vomitus, or solid objects.

4. Correct a blocked airway, if needed, by using finger sweeps or suction to remove foreign substances.

5. Maintain the airway by manually holding it open or by using an oral or nasal airway.

Breathing

1. Check for the presence of breathing:
   - Look for the rising and falling of the patient's chest.
   - Listen for the sound of air moving in and out of the patient's nose and mouth.
   - Feel for air moving on the side of your face and ear. Continue to look, listen, and feel for at least 5 seconds but no more than 10 seconds. If the patient is breathing adequately, place him or her in the recovery position. If the patient is not breathing, go to the next step.

2. Correct the lack of breathing by performing rescue breathing using a mouth-to-mask or mouth-to-barrier device, if available. Blow slowly into the patient's mouth for 1 second, using slow, gentle, sustained breaths with enough force to make the chest rise. Remove your mouth and allow the lungs to deflate. Breathe for the patient a second time. After these first two breaths, breathe once into the patient's mouth about every 5 to 6 seconds.

Generally, when mouth-to-mouth rescue breathing is necessary, **external cardiac compressions** are also required. External cardiac compressions, the "C" part of the ABCs, are explained in Chapter 9.

A skill performance sheet titled One-Rescuer Adult CPR is shown in **Figure 6-20 ▶** for your review and practice.

Performing Rescue Breathing on Children and Infants

The "A" steps required to check and correct the patient's airway and the "B" steps needed to check and correct the patient's breathing are similar for adults, children, and infants. However, there are some differences. You must learn and practice the different airway and breathing sequences for children and infants.

Rescue Breathing for Children

For purposes of performing rescue breathing, a child is a person between 1 year of age and the beginning of puberty (12–14 years of age). The steps

One-Rescuer Adult CPR

Steps	Adequately Performed
1. Establish unresponsiveness. Activate the EMS system.	
2. Open airway using head tilt–chin lift maneuver. (If trauma is present, use jaw-thrust maneuver.) Check breathing (look, listen, and feel).*	
3. Give two slow breaths at 1 second per breath. If chest does not rise, reposition head and try to ventilate again. Watch for chest rise; allow for exhalation between breaths.	
4. Check for signs of circulation. Check carotid pulse and look for signs of coughing and movement. If breathing is absent but pulse is present, provide rescue breathing (one breath every 5 to 6 seconds [10 to 12 breaths per minute]).	
5. If no pulse, give cycles of 30 chest compressions (rate, 100 compressions per minute) followed by two slow breaths.	
6. After five cycles of 30 to 2 (about 2 minutes), check pulse.* If no pulse, continue CPR and recheck patient in 2 minutes.	

*If victim is unresponsive but breathing, place in the recovery position.
Source: Based on the 2005 CPR and ECC guidelines.

Figure 6-20

Skill performance sheet.

for determining responsiveness, checking and correcting airways, and checking and correcting a child's breathing are essentially the same as for an adult patient, but you should keep the following differences in mind:

1. Children are smaller and you will not have to use as much force to open their airways and tilt their heads.
2. The rate of rescue breathing is slightly faster for children. Give 1 rescue breath every 3 to 5 seconds (about 12 to 20 rescue breaths per minute) instead of the adult rate of 1 rescue breath every 5 to 6 seconds (10 to 12 rescue breaths per minute).

A skill performance sheet titled One-Rescuer Child CPR is shown in **Figure 6-21 ▶** for your review and practice.

Rescue Breathing for Infants

If the patient is an infant (under 1 year of age), you must vary rescue breathing techniques slightly. Keep in mind that an infant is tiny and must be treated extremely gently. The steps in rescue breathing for an infant are shown in **Skill Drill 6-6 ▶**:

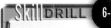 **SKILL DRILL 6-6**

Airway

1. Check for responsiveness by gently shaking the infant's shoulder or tapping the bottom of the foot **Step 1**. If the infant is unresponsive, place the infant on his or her back and proceed to the next step.
2. Open the airway, if it is closed, by using the head tilt–chin lift maneuver. Do not

One-Rescuer Child CPR

Steps	Adequately Performed
1. Establish unresponsiveness. If a second rescuer is available, have him or her activate the EMS system.	
2. Open airway using head tilt-chin lift maneuver. (If trauma is present, use jaw-thrust maneuver.) Check breathing (look, listen, and feel).*	
3. Give two effective breaths (1 second per breath); if airway is obstructed, reposition head and try to ventilate again. Watch for chest rise; allow for exhalation between breaths.	
4. Check for signs of circulation. Check carotid pulse and look for signs of coughing or movement. If breathing is absent but pulse is present, provide rescue breathing (one breath every 3 to 5 seconds [12 to 20 breaths per minute]).	
5. If no pulse, give 30 chest compressions (rate 100 compressions per minute), followed by two slow breaths.	
6. After five cycles of CPR (about 2 minutes), check pulse.* If rescuer is alone, activate the EMS system and return to the patient. If no pulse, continue CPR.	

*If victim is unresponsive but breathing, place in the recovery position.
Source: Based on the 2005 CPR and ECC guidelines.

Figure 6-21

Skill performance sheet.

tip the infant's head back too far because this may block the infant's airway. Tilt it only enough to open the airway Step 2 .

3. The rate of rescue breathing for infants is the same as for children. Give one rescue breath every 3 to 5 seconds (about 12 to 20 rescue breaths per minute).

4. Do not overinflate an infant's lungs. Use small puffs of air.

Breathing

1. Check for the presence of breathing:
   - Look for the rising and falling of the infant's chest.
   - Listen for the sound of air moving in and out of the infant's mouth and nose.

- Feel for the movement of air on the side of your face and ear Step 3 . Continue to look, listen, and feel for at least 5 seconds but no more than 10 seconds. If there is adequate breathing, place the patient in the recovery position. If there is no breathing, go to the next step.

2. Correct the lack of breathing by performing rescue breathing Step 4 . Cover the infant's mouth and nose with your mouth. Blow gently into the infant's mouth and nose for 1 second. Watch the chest rise with each breath. Remove your mouth and allow the lungs to deflate. Breathe for the infant a second time. After these first two breaths, breathe into the infant's mouth

Skill DRILL 6-6

Performing Infant Rescue Breathing

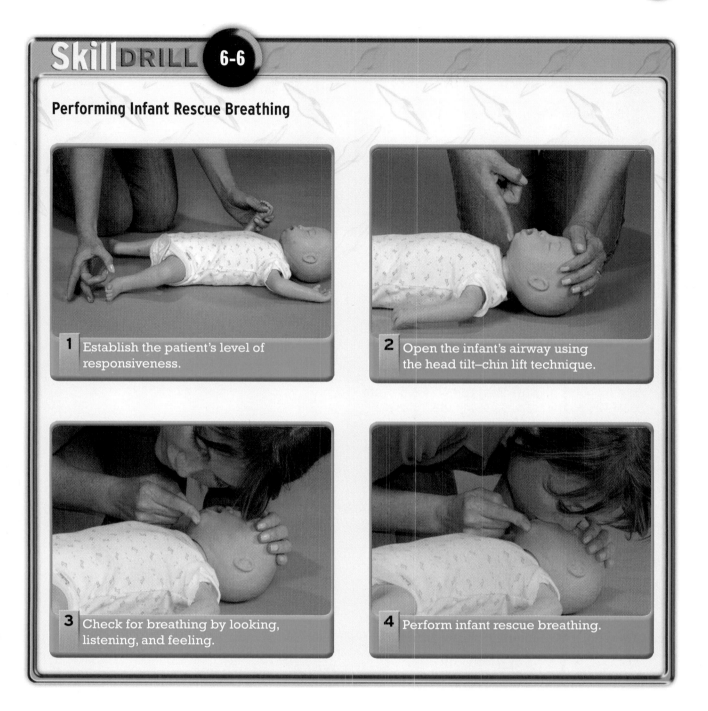

1 Establish the patient's level of responsiveness.

2 Open the infant's airway using the head tilt–chin lift technique.

3 Check for breathing by looking, listening, and feeling.

4 Perform infant rescue breathing.

and nose every 3 to 5 seconds (12 to 20 rescue breaths per minute).

Often when mouth-to-mouth rescue breathing is necessary, external cardiac compressions are also required. External cardiac compressions, the "C" part of the ABCs, are explained in Chapter 9. A skill performance sheet titled One-Rescuer Infant CPR is shown in **Figure 6-22** ▶ for your review and practice.

Foreign Body Airway Obstruction

Causes of Airway Obstruction

Your attempt to perform rescue breathing may not be effective because of an **airway obstruction**. The most common airway obstruction is the tongue. If the tongue is blocking the airway, the

One-Rescuer Infant CPR

Steps	Adequately Performed
1. Establish unresponsiveness. If a second rescuer is available, have him or her activate the EMS system.	
2. Open airway using the head tilt–chin lift maneuver. (If trauma is present, use jaw-thrust maneuver.) Check breathing (look, listen, and feel).*	
3. Give two effective breaths (1 second per breath); if chest does not rise, reposition head and try to ventilate again. Watch for chest rise; allow for exhalation between breaths.	
4. Check for signs of circulation. Check brachial pulse and look for signs of coughing or movement. If breathing is absent but pulse is present, provide rescue breathing (one breath every 3 to 5 seconds [12 to 20 breaths per minute]).	
5. If no pulse, give 30 chest compressions (rate of 100 compressions per minute) followed by two slow breaths.	
6. After five cycles of CPR (about 2 minutes), check pulse and return to the patient.* If rescuer is alone, activate the EMS system. If no pulse, continue CPR.	

*If victim is unresponsive but breathing, place in the recovery position.
Source: Based on the 2005 CPR and ECC guidelines.

Figure 6-22

Skill performance sheet.

head tilt–chin lift maneuver or jaw-thrust maneuver should open the airway. However, if a foreign body is lodged in the air passage, you must use other techniques.

Food is the most common foreign object that causes an airway obstruction. An adult may choke on a large piece of meat; a child may inhale candy, a peanut, or a piece of a hot dog. Children may put small objects in their mouths and inhale such things as tiny toys or balloons. Vomitus may obstruct the airway of a child or an adult **Figure 6-23 ▶**.

Types of Airway Obstruction

Airway obstruction may be partial (a mild obstruction) or complete (a severe obstruction). The first step in caring for a conscious person who may have an obstructed airway is to ask, "Are you choking?" If the patient can reply to your question, the airway is not completely blocked. If the patient is unable to speak or cough, the airway is completely blocked.

Mild Airway Obstruction

In partial or mild airway obstruction, the patient coughs and gags. This indicates that some air is passing around the obstruction. The patient may even be able to speak, although with difficulty.

To treat a mildly obstructed airway, encourage the patient to cough. Coughing is the most effective way of expelling a foreign object. If the patient is unable to expel the object by coughing (if, for example, a bone is stuck in the throat),

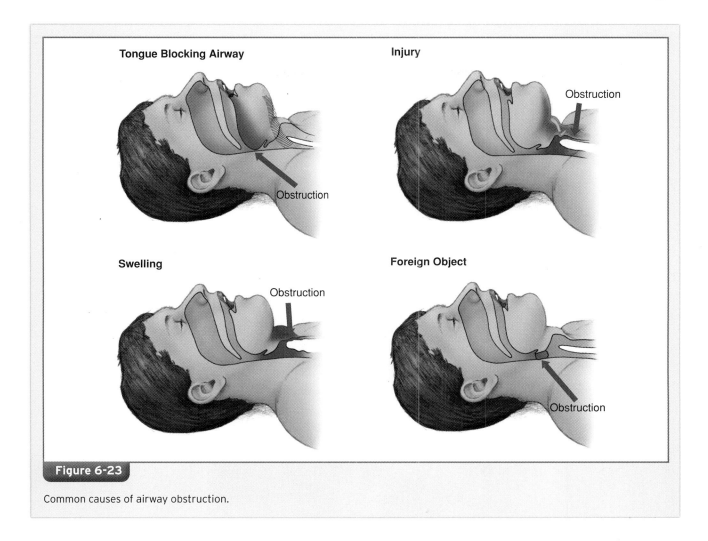

Figure 6-23

Common causes of airway obstruction.

you should arrange for the patient's **prompt transport** to an appropriate medical facility. Such a patient must be monitored carefully while awaiting transport and during transport because a mild obstruction can become a severe (complete) obstruction at any moment.

Severe Airway Obstruction

A patient with a severe (complete) airway obstruction will have different signs and symptoms. The body quickly uses all the oxygen breathed in with the last breath. The patient is unable to breathe in or out and, because he or she cannot exhale air, speech is impossible. Other symptoms of a severe airway obstruction may include poor air exchange, increased breathing difficulty, and a silent cough. If the airway is completely obstructed, the patient will lose consciousness in 3 to 4 minutes.

The currently accepted treatment for a completely obstructed airway in an adult or child involves abdominal thrusts. This technique is also called the <u>Heimlich maneuver</u>. Abdominal thrusts compress the air that remains in the lungs, pushing it upward through the airway so that it exerts pressure against the foreign object. The pressure pops the object out, in much the same way that a cork pops out of a bottle after the bottle has been shaken to increase the pressure. Many rescuers report that abdominal thrusts can cause an obstructing piece of food to fly across the room. A person who has had an obstruction removed from their airway by the Heimlich maneuver should be transported to a hospital for examination by a physician.

Management of Foreign Body Airway Obstructions

Airway Obstruction in an Adult

The steps to treat severe airway obstruction vary, depending on whether the patient is conscious or unconscious. If the patient is conscious, stand

Skill DRILL 6-7

Managing Airway Obstruction in a Conscious Patient

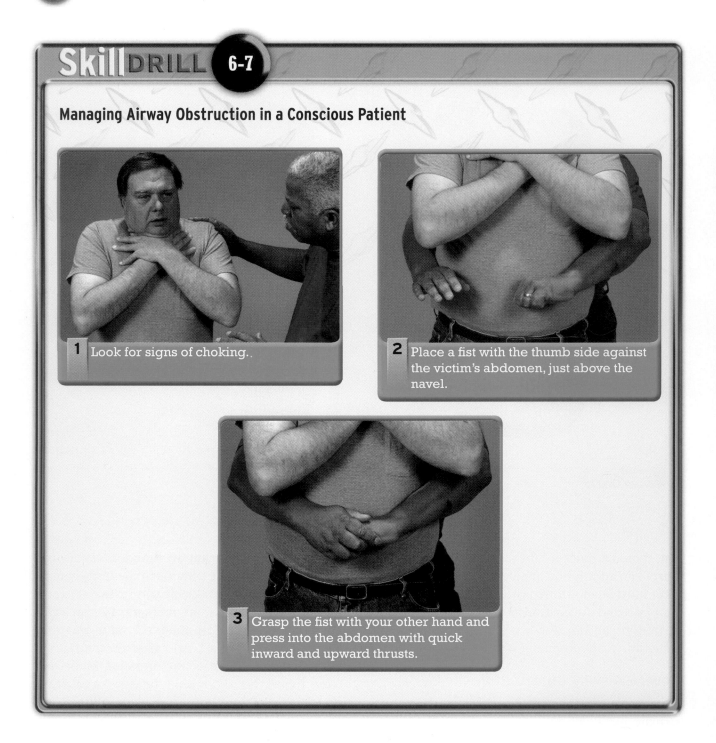

1 Look for signs of choking..

2 Place a fist with the thumb side against the victim's abdomen, just above the navel.

3 Grasp the fist with your other hand and press into the abdomen with quick inward and upward thrusts.

behind the patient and perform the abdominal thrusts while the patient is standing or seated in a chair.

Locate the xiphoid process (the bottom of the sternum) and the navel. Place one fist above the navel and well below the xiphoid process, thumb side against the patient's abdomen. Grasp your fist with your other hand. Then apply abdominal thrusts sharply and firmly, bringing your fist in and slightly upward. Do not give the patient a bear hug; rather, apply pressure at the point where your fist contacts the patient's abdomen. Each thrust should be distinct and forceful. Repeat these abdominal thrusts until the foreign object is expelled or until the patient becomes unresponsive. Review the steps in **Skill Drill 6-7 ▲** until you can carry them out automatically. To assist a conscious patient with a complete airway obstruction, you must:

SKILL DRILL 6-7

1. Ask, "Are you choking? Can you speak?" If there is no response, assume that the airway obstruction is complete **Step 1**.
2. Stand behind the patient and position the thumb side of your fist just above the patient's navel **Step 2**.
3. Press into the patient's abdomen with a quick upward thrust **Step 3**. Repeat the abdominal thrusts until either the foreign body is expelled or the patient becomes unresponsive.
4. If the patient is obese or in the late stages of pregnancy, use chest thrusts instead of abdominal thrusts. Chest thrusts are done by standing behind the patient and placing your arms under the patient's armpits to encircle the patient's chest. Press with quick backward thrusts.

If the patient becomes unresponsive, continue with the following steps.

5. Ensure that the EMS system has been activated.
6. Begin CPR:
   - Open the airway by using the head tilt–chin lift maneuver.
   - Look into the mouth for any foreign object. Use finger sweeps only if you can see a foreign object.
   - Give two rescue breaths.
   - Begin chest compressions. (This part of the CPR sequence is covered in Chapter 9.)
7. Continue these steps of CPR until more advanced EMS personnel arrive.

Recent studies have shown that performing chest compressions on an unresponsive patient increases the pressure in the chest similar to performing abdominal thrusts and may relieve an airway obstruction. Therefore performing CPR on a patient who has become unresponsive has the same effect as performing the Heimlich maneuver on a conscious patient.

A skill performance sheet titled Adult: Foreign Body Airway Obstruction is shown in **Figure 6-24 ▶** for your review and practice.

Airway Obstruction in a Child

The steps for relieving an airway obstruction in a conscious child (1 year of age to the onset of puberty) are the same as for an adult patient. The anatomic differences between adults and children/infants require that you make some adjustments in your technique. When opening the airway of a child or infant, tilt the head back just past the neutral position. Tilting the head too far back (hyperextending the neck) can actually obstruct the airway of a child or infant. If you are by yourself and a child with an airway obstruction becomes unresponsive, perform CPR for five cycles (about 2 minutes) before activating the EMS system.

A skill performance sheet titled Child: Foreign Body Airway Obstruction is shown in **Figure 6-25 ▶** for your review and practice.

Airway Obstruction in an Infant

The process for relieving an airway obstruction in an infant (less than 1 year of age) must take into consideration that an infant is extremely fragile. An infant's airway structures are very small, and they are more easily injured than those of an adult. If you suspect an airway obstruction, assess the infant to determine if there is any air exchange. If the infant has an audible cry, the airway is not completely obstructed. Ask the person who was with the infant what was happening when the episode began. This person may have seen the infant put a foreign body into his or her mouth.

If there is no movement of air from the infant's mouth and nose, a sudden onset of severe breathing difficulty, a silent cough, or a silent cry, suspect a severe airway obstruction. To relieve an airway obstruction in an infant, use a combination of back slaps and chest thrusts. You must have a good grasp of the infant in order to alternate the back slaps and the chest thrusts. Review the following sequence until you can carry it out

Adult: Foreign Body Airway Obstruction

Steps	Adequately Performed
1. Ask "Are you choking?"	
2. Give abdominal thrusts (chest thrusts for pregnant or obese victim).	
3. Repeat thrusts until foreign body is dislodged or until patient becomes unresponsive.	
If the patient becomes unresponsive:	
4. Ensure that the EMS system has been activated.	
5. Begin CPR: ■ Open the airway by using the head tilt-chin lift maneuver. ■ Look into the mouth for any foreign object. Use finger sweeps only if you can see a foreign object. ■ Give two rescue breaths. ■ Begin chest compressions. (This part of the CPR sequence is covered in Chapter 9.)	
6. Continue these CPR steps until more advanced EMS personnel arrive.	

Source: Based on the 2005 CPR and ECC guidelines.

Figure 6-24

Skill performance sheet.

automatically. To assist a conscious infant with a severe airway obstruction, you must:

1. Assess the infant's airway and breathing status. Determine that there is no air exchange.
2. Place the infant in a face-down position over one arm so that you can deliver five back slaps. Support the infant's head and neck with one hand and place the infant face down with the head lower than the trunk. Rest the infant on your forearm and support your forearm on your thigh. Use the heel of your hand and deliver up to five back slaps forcefully between the infant's shoulder blades.
3. Support the head and turn the infant face up by sandwiching the infant between your hands and arms. Rest the infant on his or her back with the head lower than the trunk.
4. Deliver five chest thrusts in the middle of the sternum. Use two fingers to deliver the chest thrusts in a firm manner.
5. Repeat the series of back slaps and chest thrusts until the foreign object is expelled or until the infant becomes unresponsive.

If the infant becomes unresponsive, continue with the following steps:

6. Ensure that the EMS system has been activated.
7. Begin CPR:
   ■ Open the airway by using the head tilt–chin lift maneuver.
   ■ Look into the mouth for any foreign object. Use finger sweeps only if you can see a foreign object.
   ■ Give two rescue breaths.
   ■ Begin chest compressions. (This part of the CPR sequence is covered in Chapter 9.)

Child: Foreign Body Airway Obstruction

Steps	Adequately Performed
1. Ask "Are you choking?"	
2. Give abdominal thrusts.	
3. Repeat thrusts until foreign body is dislodged or until patient becomes unresponsive.	
If the patient becomes unresponsive:	
4. If a second rescuer is available, have him or her activate the EMS system.	
5. Begin CPR: ■ Open the airway by using the head tilt-chin lift maneuver. ■ Look into the mouth for any foreign object. Use finger sweeps only if you can see a foreign object. ■ Give two rescue breaths. ■ Begin chest compressions. (This part of the CPR sequence is covered in Chapter 9.)	
6. Continue CPR for five cycles (about 2 minutes) and then activate the EMS system if you are by yourself.	
7. Continue CPR until more advanced EMS personnel arrive.	

Source: Based on the 2005 CPR and ECC guidelines.

Figure 6-25

Skill performance sheet.

8. Continue these CPR steps until more advanced EMS personnel arrive.

NOTE: If you are by yourself, perform CPR for five cycles (about 2 minutes) and then activate the EMS system.

Recent studies have shown that performing chest compressions on an unresponsive patient increases the pressure in the chest similar to performing chest thrusts and may relieve an airway obstruction. Therefore performing CPR on an infant who has become unresponsive has the same effect as performing the chest thrusts on a conscious patient.

A skill performance sheet titled Infant: Foreign Body Airway Obstruction is shown in **Figure 6-26** ▶ for your review and practice.

Special Considerations

Rescue Breathing for Patients With Stomas

Some individuals have had surgery that removed part or all of the larynx. In these patients, the upper airway has been rerouted to open through a **stoma** (hole) in the neck. These patients are called neck breathers. Rescue breathing must therefore be given through the stoma in the patient's neck. The technique is called **mouth-to-stoma breathing**.

The steps in performing mouth-to-stoma breathing are:

1. Check every patient for the presence of a stoma.

Infant: Foreign Body Airway Obstruction

Steps	Adequately Performed
1. Confirm severe airway obstruction. Check for sudden onset of serious breathing difficulty, ineffective cough, silent cough or cry.	
2. Give up to five back slaps and up to five chest thrusts.	
3. Repeat Step 2 until foreign body is dislodged or until infant becomes unresponsive.	
If the infant becomes unresponsive:	
4. If a second rescuer is available, have him or her activate the EMS system.	
5. Begin CPR: ▪ Open the airway by using the head tilt-chin lift maneuver. ▪ Look into the mouth for any foreign object. Use finger sweeps only if you can see a foreign object. ▪ Give two rescue breaths. ▪ Begin chest compressions. (This part of the CPR sequence is covered in Chapter 9.)	
6. Continue CPR for five cycles (about 2 minutes) and then activate the EMS system if you are by yourself.	
7. Continue CPR until more advanced EMS personnel arrive.	

Source: Based on the 2005 CPR and ECC guidelines.

Figure 6-26

Skill performance sheet.

2. If you locate a stoma, keep the patient's neck straight; do not hyperextend the patient's head and neck.

3. Examine the stoma and clean away any mucus in it.

4. To determine if a stoma tube is clear, you must asssess the patient's breathing status. If the patient is breathing adequately, the tube is clear and does not need to be touched. If the patient is in distress, suction the tube to clear any secretions.

5. Place your mouth directly over the stoma and use the same procedures as in mouth-to-mouth breathing. It is not necessary to seal the mouth and nose of most people who have a stoma.

6. If the patient's chest does not rise, he or she may be a partial neck breather. In these patients, you must seal the mouth and nose with one hand and then breathe through the stoma. A bag-mask or pocket-mask device can also be used to ventilate a patient with a stoma **Figure 6-27 ▸**.

Gastric Distention

Gastric distention occurs when air is forced into the stomach instead of the lungs. This makes it harder to get an adequate amount of air into the patient's lungs, and it increases the chance that

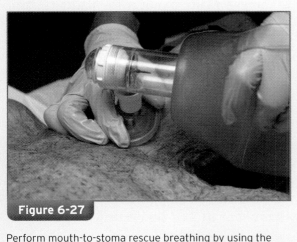

Figure 6-27

Perform mouth-to-stoma rescue breathing by using the same procedure as in mouth-to-mouth breathing, by breathing through the stoma.

the patient will vomit. Breathe slowly into the patient's mouth just enough to make the chest rise. Remember that the lungs of children and infants are smaller and require smaller breaths during rescue breathing. The excess air may enter the stomach and cause gastric distention. Preventing gastric distention is much better than trying to cure the results of it.

Dental Appliances

Do not remove dental appliances that are firmly attached. They may help keep the mouth fuller so you can make a better seal between the patient's

mouth and your mouth or a breathing device. Loose dental appliances, however, may cause problems. Partial dentures may become dislodged during trauma or while you are performing airway care and rescue breathing. If you discover loose dental appliances during your examination of the patient's airway, remove the dentures to prevent them from occluding the airway. Try to put them in a safe place so they will not get damaged or lost.

Airway Management in a Vehicle

If you arrive on the scene of an automobile accident and find that the patient has airway problems, how can you best assist the patient and maintain an open airway? If the patient is lying on the seat or floor of the car, you can apply the standard jaw-thrust maneuver. Use the jaw-thrust maneuver if there is any possibility that the accident could have caused a head or spinal injury.

When the patient is in a sitting or semi-reclining position, approach him or her from the side by leaning in through the window or across the front seat. Grasp the patient's head with both hands. Put one hand under the patient's chin and the other hand on the back of the patient's head just above the neck, as shown in **Figure 6-28 ▼**. Maintain a slight upward pressure to support the head and cervical spine and to ensure that the

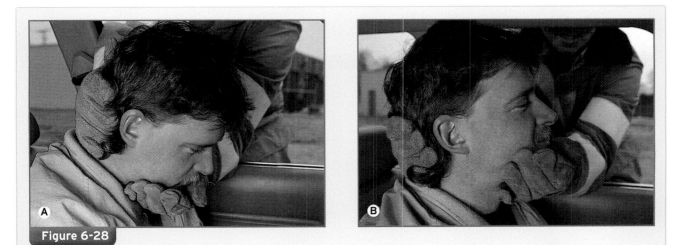

A **B**

Figure 6-28

Airway management in a vehicle. **A.** To open the airway, place one hand under the chin and the other hand on the back of the patient's head. **B.** Raise the head to neutral position to open the airway.

airway remains open. This technique will often enable you to maintain an open airway without moving the patient. This technique has several advantages:

1. You do not have to enter the automobile.

2. You can easily monitor the patient's carotid pulse and breathing patterns by using your fingers.

3. It stabilizes the patient's cervical spine.

4. It opens the patient's airway.

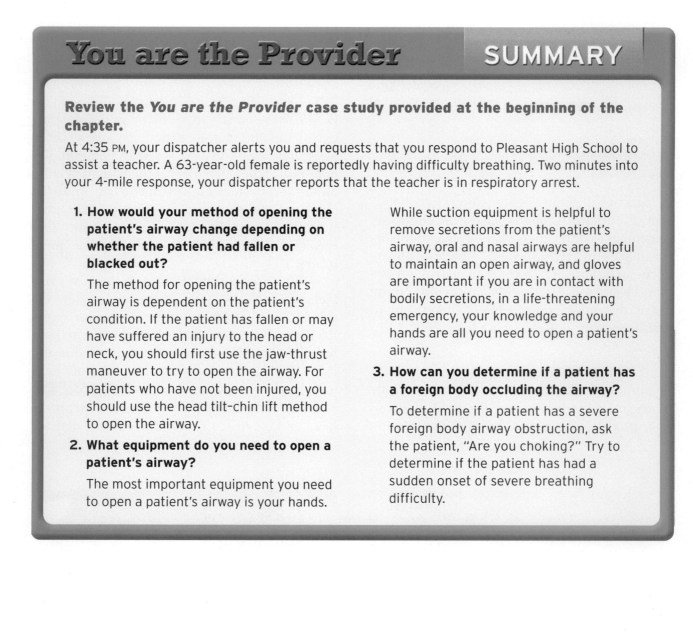

You are the Provider   SUMMARY

Review the *You are the Provider* case study provided at the beginning of the chapter.

At 4:35 PM, your dispatcher alerts you and requests that you respond to Pleasant High School to assist a teacher. A 63-year-old female is reportedly having difficulty breathing. Two minutes into your 4-mile response, your dispatcher reports that the teacher is in respiratory arrest.

1. How would your method of opening the patient's airway change depending on whether the patient had fallen or blacked out?

The method for opening the patient's airway is dependent on the patient's condition. If the patient has fallen or may have suffered an injury to the head or neck, you should first use the jaw-thrust maneuver to try to open the airway. For patients who have not been injured, you should use the head tilt–chin lift method to open the airway.

2. What equipment do you need to open a patient's airway?

The most important equipment you need to open a patient's airway is your hands.

While suction equipment is helpful to remove secretions from the patient's airway, oral and nasal airways are helpful to maintain an open airway, and gloves are important if you are in contact with bodily secretions, in a life-threatening emergency, your knowledge and your hands are all you need to open a patient's airway.

3. How can you determine if a patient has a foreign body occluding the airway?

To determine if a patient has a severe foreign body airway obstruction, ask the patient, "Are you choking?" Try to determine if the patient has had a sudden onset of severe breathing difficulty.

Prep Kit

Ready for Review

The Ready for Review thoroughly summarizes the chapter.

■ The main purpose of the respiratory system is to provide oxygen and to remove carbon dioxide from the red blood cells as they pass through the lungs. The structures of the respiratory systems in children and infants are smaller than they are in adults. Thus the air passages of children and infants may be more easily blocked by secretions or by foreign objects.

■ When a patient experiences possible respiratory arrest, check for responsiveness; open the blocked airway using the head tilt-chin lift or jaw-thrust maneuver; check for fluids, solids, or dentures in the mouth; and correct the airway, if needed, using finger sweeps or suction.

■ Maintain the airway by continuing to manually hold the airway open, or by placing the patient in the recovery position, or by inserting an oral or a nasal airway. Check for breathing by looking, listening, and feeling for air movement, and correct any problems by using mouth-to-mask or mouth-to-barrier device or by performing mouth-to-mouth rescue breathing. It is important to use the correct sequence for adults, children, and infants.

■ If the airway is obstructed in a conscious adult or child, kneel or stand behind the patient and perform the Heimlich maneuver. Give abdominal thrusts until the obstruction is relieved or the patient becomes unconscious. For an unconscious adult or child with an airway obstruction, perform chest compressions. Move to the head, open the airway, and look in the patient's mouth. Do not perform a finger sweep—regardless of the patient's age—unless you can see the object. Attempt rescue breathing again. If the airway is still obstructed, repeat chest compressions, visualization of the mouth, and ventilation attempts until the obstruction is relieved.

Technology

Interactivities

Vocabulary Explorer

Anatomy Review

Web Links

Online Review Manual

Vital Vocabulary

The Vital Vocabulary are the key terms for this chapter.

airway The passages from the openings of the mouth and nose to the air sacs in the lungs through which air enters and leaves the lungs.

airway obstruction Partial (mild) or complete (severe) obstruction of the respiratory passages resulting from blockage by food, small objects, or vomitus.

alveoli The air sacs of the lungs where the exchange of oxygen and carbon dioxide takes place.

aspirator A suction device.

bronchi The two main branches of the windpipe that lead into the right and left lungs. Within the lungs, they branch into smaller airways.

capillaries The smallest blood vessels that connect small arteries and small veins. Capillary walls serve as the membrane to exchange oxygen and carbon dioxide.

cardiopulmonary resuscitation (CPR) The artificial circulation of the blood and movement of air into and out of the lungs in a pulseless, nonbreathing patient.

esophagus The tube through which food passes. It starts at the throat and ends at the stomach.

external cardiac compressions A means of applying artificial circulation by applying rhythmic pressure and relaxation on the lower half of the sternum.

gag reflex A strong involuntary effort to vomit caused by something being placed or caught in the throat.

head tilt–chin lift technique Opening the airway by tilting the patient's head backward and lifting the chin forward, bringing the entire lower jaw with it.

Heimlich maneuver A series of manual thrusts to the abdomen to relieve an upper airway obstruction.

jaw-thrust technique Opening the airway by bringing the patient's jaw forward without extending the neck.

lungs The organs that supply the body with oxygen and eliminate carbon dioxide from the blood.

mandible The lower jaw.

manual suction devices Hand-powered devices used for clearing the upper airway of mucus, blood, or vomitus.

mechanical suction device An electrically or battery-powered device used for clearing the upper airway of mucus, blood, or vomitus.

mouth-to-mask ventilation device A piece of equipment that consists of a mask, a one-way valve, and a mouthpiece. Rescue breathing is performed by breathing into the mouthpiece after placing the mask over the patient's mouth and nose.

mouth-to-stoma breathing Rescue breathing for patients who, because of surgical removal of the larynx, have a stoma.

nasal airway An airway adjunct that is inserted into the nostril of a patient who is not able to maintain a natural airway. It is also called a nasopharyngeal airway.

nasopharynx The posterior part of the nose.

oral airway An airway adjunct that is inserted into the mouth to keep the tongue from blocking the upper airway. It is also called an oropharyngeal or nasopharyngeal airway.

oropharynx The posterior part of the mouth.

oxygen (O$_2$) A colorless, odorless gas that is essential for life.

pocket mask A mechanical breathing device used to administer mouth-to-mask rescue breathing.

rescue breathing Artificial means of breathing for a patient.

respiratory arrest Sudden stoppage of breathing.

stoma An opening in the neck that connects the windpipe (trachea) to the skin.

trachea The windpipe.

Assessment in Action

Assessment in Action presents a fictitious scenario to help you review what you learned in this chapter.

You are called to a day care center for the report of a child choking. As you arrive you find a four-year-old child lying on the floor. The day care worker tells you that the child may have put something in his mouth. The child does not respond to your verbal stimuli or your touch on the shoulder. (Questions 1–5 are based on this scenario.)

1. Your next step should be:

    A. Perform rescue breathing.
    B. Open the airway.
    C. Check for foreign bodies.
    D. Place the child in the recovery position.

2. When you need to open the airway you should use the:

    A. Jaw-thrust technique
    B. Cross finger technique
    C. Head tilt–chin lift technique
    D. Mouth-to-nose technique

3. How would you recognize an airway obstruction in this patient?

    A. By looking, listening, and feeling for breathing
    B. By not being able to ventilate when attempting to give the initial two breaths
    C. By checking the pulse
    D. By looking for signs of respirations and circulations

4. You should perform a finger sweep:

    A. After giving chest thrusts
    B. In all patients
    C. Only when you can see the obstruction
    D. Only when the abdominal thrusts do not work

5. If you are not able to ventilate this patient, you should:

    A. Use the jaw-thrust technique and ventilate.
    B. Reposition the head and try to ventilate again.
    C. Give a bigger rescue breath.
    D. Give abdominal thrusts.

Questions 6–9 are based on the following scenario. You are called to a city park for a reported accident. You find a 25-year-old woman who has hit a tree while in-line skating.

6. Your first step in assessing this patient should be:

    A. Shake her shoulder.
    B. Check her pulse.
    C. Check for breathing.
    D. Establish her level of responsiveness.

7. To open the airway, you should use:

    A. Head tilt–chin lift technique
    B. Tongue-jaw lift technique
    C. Jaw-thrust technique
    D. An oral airway

8. As you open this patient's airway, you should also:

    A. Check the carotid pulse.
    B. Stabilize the patient's neck.
    C. Check the patient's level of responsiveness.
    D. Perform rescue breathing.

9. After determining the patient is not breathing you should begin rescue breathing by giving ___ slow breath(s) at ___ second(s) per breath.

    A. 1, 2
    B. 2, 1
    C. 1, 3
    D. 2, 2

Patient Assessment

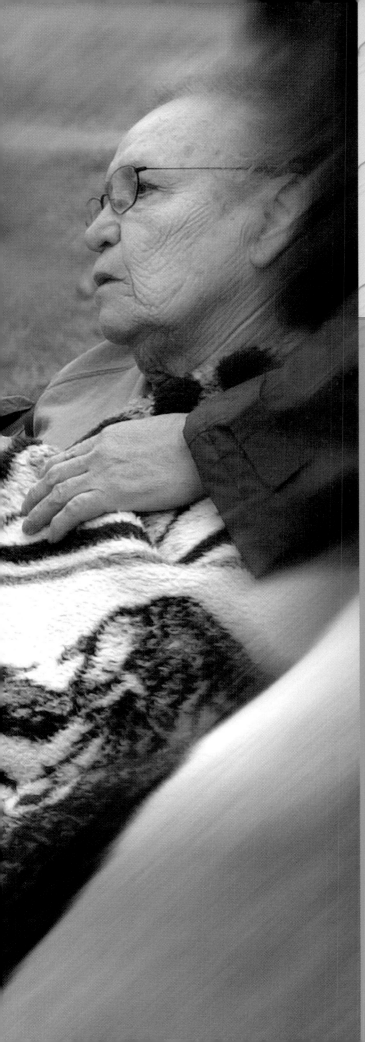

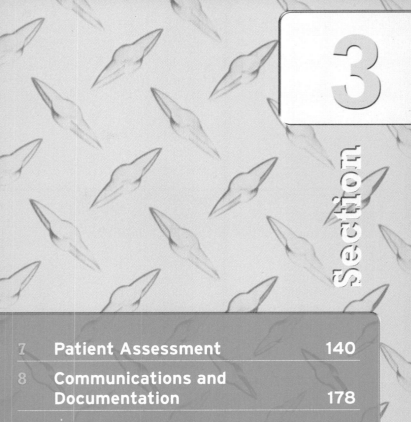

Patient Assessment

National Standard Curriculum Objectives

Cognitive

3-1.1 Discuss the components of scene size-up. (p 147-149)

3-1.2 Describe common hazards found at the scene of a trauma and a medical patient. (p 147-148)

3-1.3 Determine if the scene is safe to enter. (p 148)

3-1.4 Discuss common mechanisms of injury/nature of illness. (p 148)

3-1.5 Discuss the reason for identifying the total number of patients at the scene. (p 149)

3-1.6 Explain the reason for identifying the need for additional help or assistance. (p 149)

3-1.7 Summarize the reasons for forming a general impression of the patient. (p. 151)

3-1.8 Discuss methods of assessing mental status. (p 152)

3-1.9 Differentiate between assessing mental status in the adult, child, and infant patient. (p 152)

3-1.10 Describe methods used for assessing if a patient is breathing. (p 152)

3-1.11 Differentiate between a patient with adequate and inadequate breathing. (p 152)

3-1.12 Describe the methods used to assess circulation. (p 153)

3-1.13 Differentiate between obtaining a pulse in an adult, child, and infant patient. (p 153)

3-1.14 Discuss the need for assessing the patient for external bleeding. (p 153)

3-1.15 Explain the reason for prioritizing a patient for care and transport. (p 149)

3-1.16 Discuss the components of the physical exam. (p 157)

3-1.17 State the areas of the body that are evaluated during the physical exam. (p 160-165)

3-1.18 Explain what additional questioning may be asked during the physical exam. (p 160)

3-1.19 Explain the components of the SAMPLE history. (p 167-168)

3-1.20 Discuss the components of the ongoing assessment. (p 171)

3-1.21 Describe the information included in the First Responder "hand-off" report. (p 171)

Affective

3-1.22 Explain the rationale for crew members to evaluate scene safety prior to entering. (p. 147)

3-1.23 Serve as a model for others by explaining how patient situations affect your evaluation of the mechanism of injury or illness. (p 151)

3-1.24 Explain the importance of forming a general impression of the patient. (p 151)

3-1.25 Explain the value of an initial assessment. (p 151)

3-1.26 Explain the value of questioning the patient and family. (p 154)

3-1.27 Explain the value of the physical exam. (p 157)

3-1.28 Explain the value of an ongoing assessment. (p 171)

3-1.29 Explain the rationale for the feelings that these patients might be experiencing. (p 154)

3-1.30 Demonstrate a caring attitude when performing patient assessments. (p 151)

3-1.31 Place the interests of the patient as the foremost consideration when making any and all patient care decisions during patient assessment. (p 154)

3-1.32 Communicate with empathy during patient assessment to patients as well as with family members and friends of the patient. (p 151)

Psychomotor

3-1.33 Demonstrate the ability to differentiate various scenarios and identify potential hazards. (p 147)

3-1.34 Demonstrate the techniques for assessing mental status. (p 152)

3-1.35 Demonstrate the techniques for assessing the airway. (p 152)

3-1.36 Demonstrate the techniques for assessing if the patient is breathing. (p 152, 157)

3-1.37 Demonstrate the techniques for assessing if the patient has a pulse. (p 153, 157)

3-1.38 Demonstrate the techniques for assessing the patient for external bleeding. (p 153)

3-1.39 Demonstrate the techniques for assessing the patient's skin color, temperature, condition, and capillary refill (infants and children only). (p 158-159)

3-1.40 Demonstrate questioning a patient to obtain a SAMPLE history. (p 167)

3-1.41 Demonstrate the skills involved in performing the physical exam. (p 157-165)

3-1.42 Demonstrate the ongoing assessment. (p 171)

Chapter Objectives*

Knowledge and Attitude Objectives

1. Discuss the importance of each of the following steps in the patient assessment sequence:
   - Scene size-up (p 147)
   - Initial patient assessment (p 151)
   - Examining the patient from head to toe (p 157)
   - Obtaining the patient's medical history (p 167)
   - Performing an ongoing assessment (p 171)
2. Discuss the components of a scene size-up. (p 147-149)
3. Describe why it is important to get an idea of the number of patients at an emergency scene as soon as possible. (p 149)
4. List and describe the importance of the following steps of the initial patient assessment:
   - Forming a general impression of the patient (p 151)
   - Assessing the patient's responsiveness and stabilizing the spine if necessary (p 151)
   - Assessing the patient's airway (p 152)
   - Assessing the patient's breathing (p 152)
   - Assessing the patient's circulation (p 153)
   - Updating responding EMS units (p 154)
5. Describe the differences in checking airway, breathing, and circulation when the patient is an adult, a child, or an infant. (p 152-153)
6. Explain the significance of the following signs: respiration, circulation, skin condition, pupil size and reactivity, level of consciousness. (p 157-159)
7. Describe the sequence used to perform a head-to-toe physical examination. (p 160-165)
8. State the areas of the body that you should examine during a physical examination. (p 160-165)
9. Describe the importance of obtaining the patient's medical history. (p 167)
10. State the information that you should obtain when taking a patient's medical history. (p 167-168)
11. List the information that should be addressed in your hand-off report about the patient's condition. (p 171)
12. List the differences between performing a patient assessment on a trauma patient and performing one on a medical patient. (p 172)
13. Describe the components of the ongoing assessment. (p 171-172)

Skill Objectives

1. Perform the following five steps of the patient assessment sequence given a real or simulated incident:
   - Scene size-up (p 147)
   - Initial patient assessment, including:
     - Forming a general impression of the patient (p 151)
     - Assessing the patient's responsiveness and stabilizing the patient's spine if necessary (p 151)
     - Assessing the patient's airway (p 152)
     - Assessing the patient's breathing (p 152)
     - Assessing the patient's circulation (including severe bleeding) and stabilizing those functions if necessary (p 153)
     - Updating responding EMS units (p 154)
   - Examination of the patient from head to toe (p 160-165)
   - Obtaining the patient's medical history using the SAMPLE format (p 167-168)
   - Performing an ongoing assessment (p 171)
2. Identify and measure the following signs on adult, child, and infant patients: respiration, pulse, capillary refill, skin color, skin temperature, skin moisture, pupil size and reactivity, level of consciousness. (p 157-159)

*These are chapter learning objectives.

Patient Assessment

You are the Provider

It is one of those rare days when spring has sprung and everyone wants to enjoy the great outdoors. As you are returning to your station after completing a call, your dispatcher announces that there is a report of a person who is short of breath at a local park. Your unit is the closest to the scene. As you begin to respond, the dispatcher informs you that the information is from a third-party call and there is no further information about the patient.

1. As you arrive at the location of your patient, you find a 14-year-old male who has been hit in the chest with a baseball and is experiencing shortness of breath and pain when breathing. What are the steps of the patient assessment you should use in examining this patient?
2. If instead you arrive on the scene and find a 76-year-old female sitting on a park bench experiencing shortness of breath, how would you change the steps of the patient assessment from the steps used in Question 1?

Patient Assessment

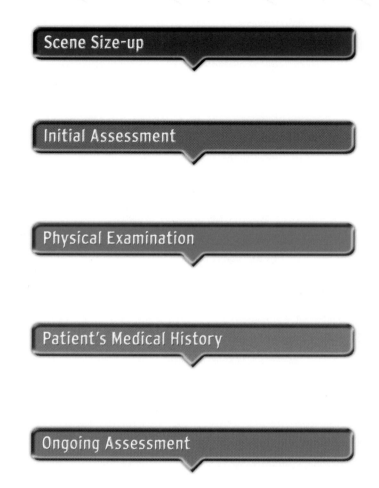

Scene Size-up

Initial Assessment

Physical Examination

Patient's Medical History

Ongoing Assessment

Introduction

As a first responder, you will be the first trained EMS person on many emergency scenes. Your initial actions will affect not only you, but also the patient and other responders. Your assessment of the scene and the patient will affect the level of care requested for the patient.

It is important that you are able to perform a systematic patient assessment to determine what injuries or illness the patient has suffered. The patient assessment sequence consists of the following steps:

1. Perform a scene size-up.
2. Perform an initial patient assessment to identify immediate threats to life.
3. Examine the patient from head to toe.
4. Obtain the patient's medical history.
5. Perform an ongoing assessment.

By performing these five steps, you can systematically gather the information you need. After you have learned these steps, you will discover that you can modify them to gather needed information about a patient who is suffering from a medical problem as opposed to a patient who is suffering from trauma (a wound or injury).

FYI

The skills and knowledge presented in this chapter follow an **assessment-based care** model. With assessment-based care, the treatment rendered is based on the patient's symptoms. Assessment-based care requires a careful and thorough evaluation of the patient to provide appropriate care. If a given condition has already been diagnosed by a physician and is known to the patient, you will sometimes know the patient's diagnosis. Other times, you will have to respond to the signs and symptoms you find during the assessment process. Throughout this text, you will find signs and symptoms of certain medical conditions. Careful and thorough study of the skills and knowledge related to patient assessment will go a long way in helping you perform as a valuable member of the EMS team in your community.

Patient Assessment

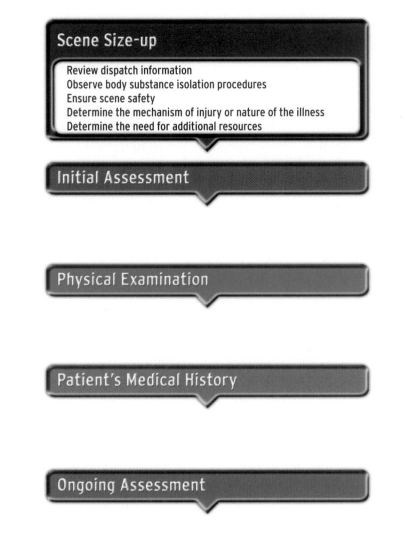

Scene Size-up

Review dispatch information
Observe body substance isolation procedures
Ensure scene safety
Determine the mechanism of injury or nature of the illness
Determine the need for additional resources

Initial Assessment

Physical Examination

Patient's Medical History

Ongoing Assessment

Patient Assessment Sequence

The patient assessment sequence is designed to give a framework so you can safely approach an emergency scene, determine the need for additional help, examine the patient to determine if injuries or illnesses are present, obtain the patient's medical history, and report the results of your assessment to other EMS personnel. A complete patient assessment consists of five steps.

Perform a Scene Size-Up

The scene size-up is a general overview of the incident and its surroundings. Based on this information, you can make decisions about the safety of the scene, what type of incident is present, any mechanism of injury, and the need for additional resources.

FYI

Review Dispatch Information

Your scene size-up begins before you arrive at the actual scene of the emergency. You can anticipate possible conditions by reviewing and understanding dispatch information. Your dispatcher should have obtained the following information: the location of the incident, the main problem or type of incident, the number of people involved, and the safety level of the scene. As you receive the dispatcher's information, you should begin to assess it **Figure 7-1 ▶**.

In addition to the information obtained from the dispatcher, other factors could affect your actions. Consider, for example, the time of day, the day of the week, and weather conditions. A call from a school during school hours may require a different response than a call during the weekend. Finally, think about the resources that may be needed and mentally prepare for other situations you may find when you arrive on the scene.

If you happen on a medical emergency, notify the emergency medical dispatch center by using your two-way radio. If you do not have a two-way radio, send someone to call for help. Re-

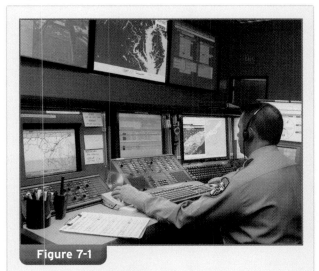

Figure 7-1

Review dispatch information.

FYI cont.

lay the following information: the location of the incident, the main problem or type of incident, the number of people involved, and the safety of the scene.

Observe Body Substance Isolation

Before arriving at the scene, prepare yourself by anticipating the types of body substance isolation (BSI) that may be required. You should always have gloves readily available. Consider whether the use of additional protection, such as eye protection, gowns, or masks, may be necessary. In other words, try to anticipate your needs for equipment to ensure good BSI.

Ensure Scene Safety

When you arrive at the scene, remember to park your vehicle so that it helps secure the scene and minimizes traffic blockage.

As you approach the scene, scan the area to determine the extent of the incident, the possible number of people injured, and the presence of possible hazards **Figure 7-2 ▶**. It is important to scan the scene to ensure that you are not putting yourself in danger.

Hazards can be visible or invisible. Visible hazards include such things as the scene of a crash, fallen electrical wires, traffic, spilled gasoline, unstable buildings, a crime scene, and crowds.

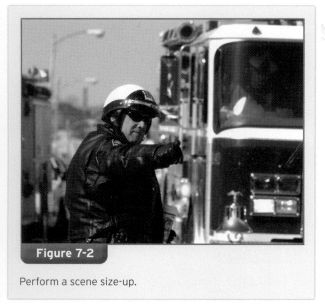

Figure 7-2

Perform a scene size-up.

Unstable surfaces such as slopes, ice, and water pose potential hazards. Invisible hazards include electricity, hazardous materials, and poisonous fumes. Downed electrical wires or broken poles may indicate an electrical hazard. Never assume a downed electrical wire is safe. Confined spaces such as farm silos, industrial tanks, and below-ground pits often contain poisonous gases or lack enough oxygen to support life. Hazardous materials placards may indicate the presence of a chemical hazard.

Note the hazards, consider your ability to manage them, and decide whether to call for assistance. This assistance may include the fire department, additional EMS units, law enforcement officers, heavy-rescue equipment, hazardous materials teams, electric or gas company personnel, or other special resources. If a hazardous condition exists, make every effort to ensure that bystanders, rescuers, and patients are not exposed to it unnecessarily. If possible, see to it that any hazardous conditions are corrected or minimized as soon as possible. Noting such conditions early keeps them from becoming part of the problem later.

Some emergency scenes will not be safe for you to enter. These scenes will require personnel with special training and equipment. If a scene is unsafe, keep people away until specially trained teams arrive. It is also important to identify potential exit routes from the scene in case a hazard becomes life threatening to you or your patients.

Mechanism of Injury or Nature of Illness

As you approach the scene, look for clues that may indicate how the accident happened **Figure 7-3 ▶**. This is called the mechanism of injury. If you can determine the mechanism of injury or the nature of the illness, you can sometimes predict the patient's injuries. For example, a ladder lying on the ground next to a spilled paint bucket probably indicates that the patient fell from the ladder and may have broken bones. If the incident is an automobile accident, knowing what type of accident occurred makes it possible to anticipate the types of injuries that may be present. For example, a rollover accident results in different injuries than a car-tree collision. It is also possible to anticipate injuries by examining the extent of damage to an automobile. If the windshield is broken, look for head and spine injuries; if the steering wheel is bent, check for a chest injury. (See Chapter 14 for more information on mechanisms of injury that result in musculoskeletal injuries.) Ask the patient (if conscious) or family members or bystanders for additional information about the mechanism of injury. The same type of overview that gives you information at the scene of an accident can also help provide information about a patient's condition. Again, ask the patient, family, or bystanders why you were called.

Do not, however, rule out any injury without conducting a head-to-toe physical exami-

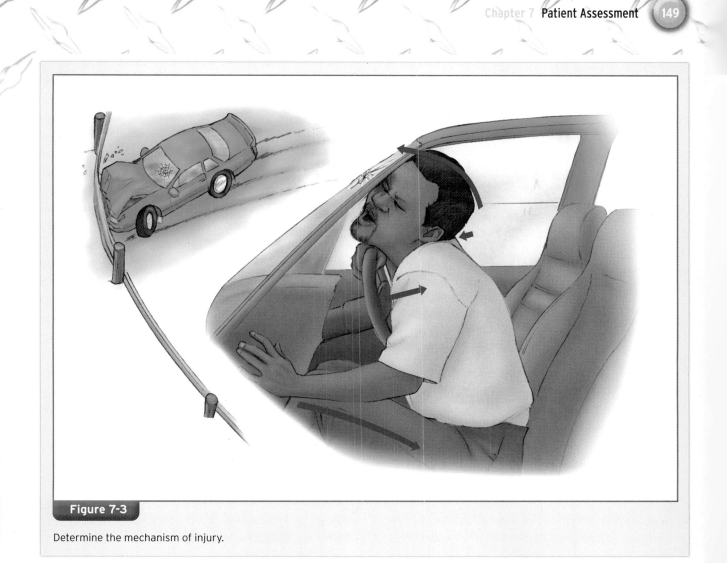

Figure 7-3

Determine the mechanism of injury.

nation of the patient. The mechanism of the accident may provide clues, but it cannot be used to determine what injuries are present in a particular patient. In the previous example, the painter may have had a heart attack while climbing the ladder.

Determine the Need for Additional Resources

If there is more than one patient, count the total number of patients. Call for additional assistance if you think you will need help. It may be necessary to sort patients into groups according to the severity of their injuries to determine which pa-

In the Field

Call for additional assistance before beginning to treat the patient(s). It will take time for more help to arrive, so the sooner you request aid, the better. In addition, you are less likely to call for help if you first become involved in patient care, and this can be detrimental to the patient's chance for recovery.

tients should be treated and transported first. The topic of triage, or patient sorting, is covered more thoroughly in Chapter 18.

Patient Assessment

Scene Size-up

Initial Assessment

Form a general impression of the patient
Assess responsiveness (AVPU)
Check the patient's airway
Check the patient's breathing
Check the patient's circulation (including severe bleeding)
Acknowledge the patient's primary complaint
Update responding EMS units

Physical Examination

Patient's Medical History

Ongoing Assessment

Perform an Initial Patient Assessment

The second step in the patient assessment sequence is the <u>initial patient assessment</u>. During the initial patient assessment, determine and correct any life-threatening conditions. Do all steps in the initial patient assessment quickly as you make contact with the patient.

Form a General Impression of the Patient

As you approach the patient, form a general impression. Note the sex and the approximate age of the patient. Your scene survey and general impressions may help determine whether the patient has experienced trauma or illness. (If you cannot determine whether the patient is suffering from an illness or an injury, treat the patient as a trauma patient.) The patient's position or the sounds he or she is making may also be indicators of the problem. You may get some impression of the patient's level of consciousness. Although your first impression is valuable, do not let it block out later information that may lead you in another direction.

Assess Responsiveness

The first part of determining the patient's responsiveness is to introduce yourself. Many patients will be conscious and able to interact with you. As you approach the patient, tell the patient your name and function Figure 7-4 ▾ . For example, "I'm Chris Smith from the sheriff's department, and I'm here to help you." This simple introduction helps establish:

- Your reason for being at the accident
- The fact that you will be helping the patient
- The level of consciousness of the patient

The introduction is your first contact with the patient. It should put the patient at ease by conveying that you are a trained person ready to help. Next, ask the patient's name, and then use it when talking with the patient, family, or friends. The patient's response helps you determine the patient's level of consciousness. Avoid telling the patient that everything will be all right.

Even if the patient appears to be unconscious, introduce yourself and talk with the patient as you conduct the rest of the patient assessment. Many patients who appear to be unconscious can hear your voice and need the reassurance it carries. Do not say anything you do not want the patient to hear!

If a patient appears to be unconscious, call to the patient in a tone of voice that is loud enough for the patient to hear. If the patient does not respond to the sound of your voice, gently touch the patient or shake the patient's shoulder.

The patient's level of consciousness can range from fully conscious to unconscious.

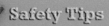

Safety Tips

Remember that performing a patient assessment may bring you in contact with the patient's blood, body fluids, waste products, and mucous membranes. You need to wear approved gloves and take other precautions to ensure that you maintain BSI to prevent any exposure to infected body fluids. Follow the latest standards from the Centers for Disease Control and Prevention and Occupational Safety and Health Administration.

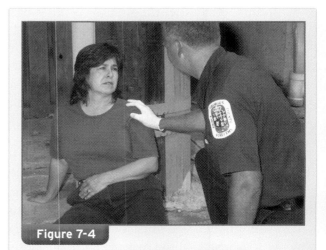

Figure 7-4

As you approach the patient, introduce yourself. If a patient appears unconscious, gently touch or shake the patient's shoulder to get a response.

Initial Assessment

Initial Assessment

Infants and children may not have the verbal skills to answer the questions used to assess responsiveness in adults. Therefore, you should assess the interaction of children and infants with their environment and with their parents.

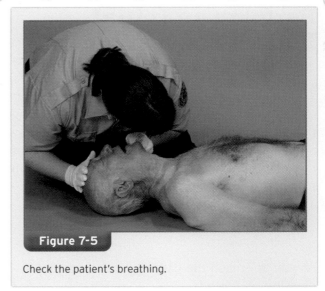

Figure 7-5

Check the patient's breathing.

Describe the patient's level of consciousness using the four-level **AVPU scale**:

A **Alert**. An alert patient is able to answer the following questions accurately and appropriately: What is your name? Where are you? What is today's date? A patient who can answer these questions is said to be "alert and oriented."

V **Verbal**. A patient is said to be "responsive to verbal stimulus" even if the patient only reacts to loud sounds.

P **Pain**. A patient who is responsive to pain will not respond to a verbal stimulus but will move or cry out in response to pain. Response to pain is tested by pinching the patient's earlobe or pinching the patient's skin over the collarbone. If the patient withdraws from the painful stimulus, he or she is said to be "responsive to painful stimuli."

U **Unresponsive**. An unresponsive patient will not respond to either a verbal or a painful stimulus. This patient's condition is described as "unresponsive."

If the patient has suffered any type of major trauma, provide manual stabilization of the patient's neck as soon as possible. This will prevent any further injury to the neck and spinal column.

Check the Patient's Airway

The third part of the initial assessment is to check the patient's airway. If the patient is alert and able to answer questions without difficulty, then the airway is open. If the patient is not responsive to verbal stimuli, then you must assume that the airway may be closed. In the case of an unconscious patient, open the airway by using the head tilt–chin lift technique for patients with medical problems and the jaw-thrust technique (without tilting the

patient's head) for patients who have suffered trauma. After the airway is open, inspect it for foreign bodies or secretions. Clear the airway as needed. You may need to insert an airway adjunct to keep the airway open. (See Chapter 6 for information about airway adjuncts.)

Check the Patient's Breathing

If the patient is conscious, assess the rate and quality of the patient's breathing. Does the chest rise and fall with each breath or does the patient appear to be short of breath? If the patient is unconscious, check for breathing by placing the side of your face next to the patient's nose and mouth. You should be able to hear the sounds of breathing, see the chest rise and fall, and even feel the movement of air on your cheek Figure 7-5 ▲ . If breathing is difficult or if you hear unusual sounds, you may have to remove an object from the patient's mouth, such as food, vomitus, dentures, gum, chewing tobacco, or broken teeth.

If you cannot detect any movement of the chest and no sounds of air are coming from the nose and mouth, breathing is absent. Take immediate steps to open the patient's airway and perform rescue breathing. If trauma is suspected, protect the cervical spine by keeping the patient's head in a neutral position and using the jaw-thrust maneuver to open the airway. Maintain cervical stabilization until the head and neck are immobilized (these procedures are covered in Chapter 5).

Check the Patient's Circulation

Next, check the patient's circulation (heartbeat). If the patient is unconscious, take the carotid pulse **Figure 7-6 ▾**. Place your index and middle fingers together and touch the larynx (Adam's apple) in the patient's neck. Then slide your two fingers off the larynx toward the patient's ear until you feel a slight notch. Practice this maneuver until you are able to find a carotid pulse within 5 seconds of touching the patient's larynx. If you cannot feel a pulse with your fingers in 5 to 10 seconds, begin cardiopulmonary resuscitation (CPR), which is covered in Chapter 9.

If the patient is conscious, assess the radial pulse rather than the carotid pulse **Figure 7-7 ▸**. Place your index and middle fingers on the patient's wrist at the thumb side. You should practice taking the radial pulse often to develop this skill.

Next, quickly check the patient for severe external bleeding. If you discover severe bleeding, you must take immediate action to control it by applying direct pressure over the wound. These procedures are covered in Chapter 13.

Quickly assess the patient's skin color and temperature. This assessment will give an idea of whether the patient is suffering from internal bleeding and shock. It is important to check the color of the patient's skin when you

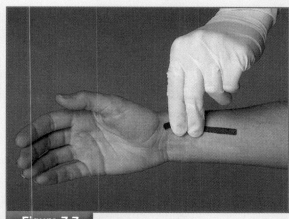

Figure 7-7

Take the radial pulse if the patient is conscious.

arrive on the scene so that you can tell if the color changes as time goes on.

Skin color is described as:
- **Pale** (whitish, indicating decreased circulation to that part of the body or to all of the body)
- **Flushed** (reddish, indicating excess circulation to that part of the body)

Special Populations

To assess circulation in an infant, check the brachial pulse, located on the inside of the upper arm. You can feel the brachial pulse by placing your index and middle fingers on the inside of the infant's arm halfway between the shoulder and the elbow **Figure 7-8 ▾**. Check for 5 to 10 seconds.

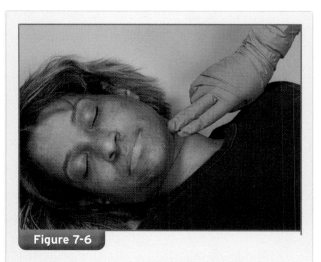

Figure 7-6

Check an unconscious patient's circulation by taking the carotid pulse.

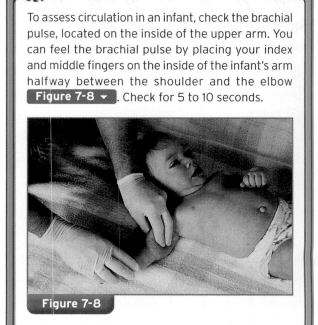

Figure 7-8

Take the brachial pulse if the patient is an infant.

Initial Assessment

- **Blue** (also called <u>cyanosis</u>, indicating lack of oxygen and possible airway problems)
- **Yellow** (indicating liver problems)
- **Normal**

Patients with deeply pigmented skin may show color changes in the fingernail beds, in the whites of the eyes, or inside the mouth.

Acknowledge the Patient's Chief Complaint

As you perform the initial patient assessment, you will often form an impression of the patient's <u>chief complaint</u>. It is important to acknowledge the patient's primary or chief complaint and provide reassurance **Figure 7-9 ▸**. A conscious patient will often complain of an injury that causes great pain or results in obvious bleeding. However, the injury that the patient complains of may not be the most serious injury. Do not allow a conscious patient's comments to distract you from completing the patient assessment sequence. Acknowledge the patient's chief complaint by saying something like, "Yes, I can see that your

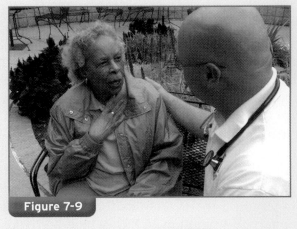

Figure 7-9

Acknowledge the patient's chief complaint.

arm appears to be broken, but let me finish checking you completely in case there are any other injuries. I will then treat your injured arm." In an unconscious patient, the primary "complaint" is unconsciousness.

Update Responding EMS Units

In some EMS systems, you will be expected to update responding EMS units about the condition of your patient. This report should include age and sex of the patient, the chief complaint, level of responsiveness, and status of airway, breathing, and circulation. This update helps them know what to expect when they arrive on the scene.

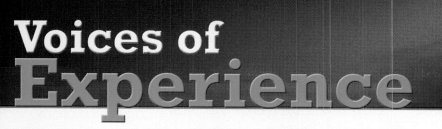

Voices of Experience

First Responders Are Vital to Positive Outcomes

"There's another one down!" someone yelled from outside.

I was in the back of the parked ambulance tending to a man who had been injured at the dirt-bike race-track where my volunteer ambulance company was on standby. As the ranking officer, it was my job to coordinate all EMS operations at the track. As the only EMT on the scene, it was also my job to provide hands-on care as needed. When I heard that there was another patient, I looked down at the patient on the cot in front of me and my heart dropped to my feet.

The man I was treating had suffered a dramatic crash. I could feel a deformity in his right ribs and he was having difficulty breathing. He was also beginning to exhibit signs of shock. I radioed for another ambulance to transport him, but they had not arrived yet. I couldn't leave this patient.

> " The ability of the first responders to perform a quick and accurate patient assessment is what allowed us to have such a positive outcome. "

The first responders immobilized the second patient, an 8-year-old boy, on a backboard and they were bringing him toward the ambulance. He was complaining of severe pain in his right lower leg. I instructed one of the first responders to radio for a second transporting unit, and then I looked around, frantically searching my mind for a way to care for both patients until more help arrived.

I may have been the only EMT on the scene, but I was lucky enough to have two trained and capable first responders available to assist me. They carried the boy in and placed him on a picnic table behind the ambulance. They performed a head-to-toe assessment of the boy and obtained his vital signs and SAMPLE history. They quickly and correctly determined that his only injury was an open fracture to his right lower leg.

By the time the transporting units arrived, both patients had been stabilized. The first responders had controlled the boy's bleeding and applied a dressing over his wound. They had determined that his vital signs were stable, made sure that he was securely immobilized on the backboard, and reported their assessment findings and interventions to the transporting crew. Both patients were transported and treated without incident and both recovered quickly.

The ability of the first responders to perform a quick and accurate patient assessment is what allowed us to have such a positive outcome—rather than the nightmare it could have been. Looking back on this particular call, I am proud that even with a limited number of personnel, we were able to treat both patients effectively. First responders play a vital role on the emergency scene, and on this particular scene, the training and skills of the first responders were truly indispensable.

Sheri Polley, NREMT-B
Linesville Volunteer Fire Department Ambulance
Linesville, Pennsylvania

Patient Assessment

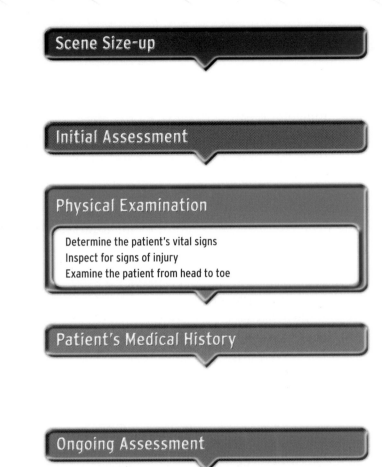

Scene Size-up

Initial Assessment

Physical Examination

Determine the patient's vital signs
Inspect for signs of injury
Examine the patient from head to toe

Patient's Medical History

Ongoing Assessment

Perform a Physical Examination

The **physical examination** of the patient from head to toe is done to assess non–life-threatening conditions after you have completed the initial assessment and stabilized life-threatening conditions. This exam helps you locate and begin initial management of the signs and symptoms of illness or injury. After you complete the physical examination, review any positive signs and symptoms of injury or illness. This review will help you to get a better picture of the patient's overall condition.

Signs and Symptoms

In a careful and systematic patient assessment, you need to understand the difference between a **sign** and a **symptom**. You need to be able to assess selected signs and report them systematically. You also need to be able to understand and report the symptoms that the patient reports. Simply put, a sign is something about the patient you can see or feel for yourself. A symptom is something the patient tells you about his or her condition, such as "My back hurts" or "I think I am going to vomit."

The first step of the physical examination is to determine the patient's **vital signs**. These consist of respiration, pulse, and temperature. (Blood pressure, a fourth vital sign, is not routinely taken by first responders; however, your EMS service may include it as an optional skill. It is covered in Chapter 21.)

Respiration

The **respiratory rate** is a vital sign that indicates how fast the patient is breathing. It is measured as breaths per minute. In a normal adult, the resting respiratory rate is between 12 and 20 breaths per minute. One cycle of inhaling (breathing in) and exhaling (breathing out) is counted as one breath (respiration). Count the patient's breaths for 1 minute to determine the respiratory rate.

Respirations may be rapid and shallow (characteristic of shock) or slow (characteristic of a stroke or drug overdose). Respirations may also be described as deep, wheezing, gasping, panting, snoring, noisy, or labored. If the patient is not breathing, respiration is described as "absent," a condition that would have been addressed during the initial assessment.

When you are checking the rate or noting the quality of respirations, make sure that your face or hand is close enough to the patient's face to feel the exhaled air on your skin. Also watch for the rise and fall of the chest. When counting respirations in a conscious patient, try not to let the patient know that you are counting. If the patient knows you are counting respirations, you may not get an accurate count.

Pulse

The second vital sign is the **pulse**, which indicates the speed and force of the heartbeat. A pulse can be felt anywhere on the body where an artery passes over a hard structure such as a bone. Although there are many such places on the body, the four most common pulse points are the radial (wrist), the carotid (neck), the brachial (arm), and the posterior tibial (ankle).

The most commonly taken pulse is the **radial pulse**, located at the wrist where the radial artery passes over one of the forearm bones, the radius (see Figure 7-7). The **carotid pulse** is taken over a **carotid artery**, located on either side of the patient's neck just under the jawbone (see Figure 7-6). The **brachial pulse** is taken on the inside of the arm, halfway between the shoulder and the elbow (see Figure 7-8). The **posterior tibial pulse** is located on the inner aspect of the ankle just behind the ankle bone Figure 7-10 ▸.

In general, take the radial pulse of a conscious patient and the carotid pulse of an unconscious patient. When examining an infant, use the brachial pulse. The posterior tibial pulse is used to assess the circulatory status of a leg. To check a patient's pulse, determine three things: rate, rhythm, and quality. To determine the pulse rate (heartbeats per minute), find the patient's pulse with your fingers, count the beats for 30 seconds, and multiply by two. In a normal adult, the resting pulse rate is about 60 to 100 beats per minute, although in a physically fit person (such as a

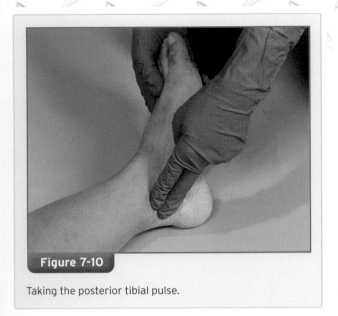

Figure 7-10

Taking the posterior tibial pulse.

jogger) the resting rate may be lower (about 40 to 60 beats per minute). In children, the pulse rate is normally faster (about 70 to 150 beats per minute; see Chapter 16). A very slow pulse (fewer than 40 beats per minute) can be the result of a serious illness, whereas a very fast pulse (more than 120 beats per minute) can indicate that the patient is in shock. Remember, however, that a person who is in excellent physical condition may have a pulse rate of less than 50 beats per minute, and a person who is simply anxious or worried could have a fast pulse rate (more than 110 beats per minute).

You should also be able to determine the rhythm and describe the quality of the pulse. Note whether the pulse is regular or irregular. A strong pulse is often referred to as a **bounding pulse**. This is similar to the heart rate that follows physical exertion such as running or lifting heavy objects. The beats are very strong and well defined. A weak pulse is often called a **thready pulse**. The pulse is present, but the beats are not easily detected. A thready pulse is a more dangerous sign than a bounding pulse. A bounding pulse can be dangerous if the patient has high blood pressure and is at risk for a stroke.

Capillary Refill

Capillary refill is the ability of the circulatory system to return blood to the capillary vessels after the blood has been squeezed out. The capillary refill test is done on the patient's fingernails or toenails. To perform this test, squeeze the patient's nail bed firmly between your thumb and forefinger Figure 7-11 ▾ . The patient's nail bed will look pale. Release the pressure. Count 2 seconds by saying "capillary refill." The patient's nail bed should become pink. This indicates a normal capillary refill time.

If the patient has lost a lot of blood and is in shock or if the blood vessels supplying that limb have been damaged, the capillary refill will be delayed or entirely absent. Capillary refill will be delayed in a cold environment and should not be used as the sole means for assessing the circulatory status of an extremity. Check with your medical director to determine if you should use the capillary refill test.

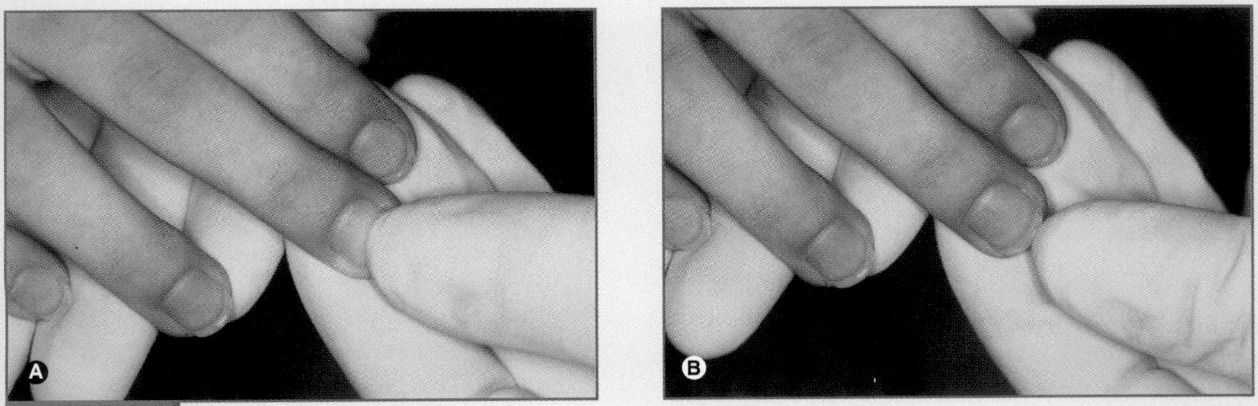

Figure 7-11

Checking capillary refill time. **A.** Squeeze the nail bed between your thumb and forefinger. **B.** Release the pressure.

Skin Condition

The patient's skin should be checked for color and moisture. Normal body temperature is about 98.6°F (37°C). Precise body temperature is taken with a thermometer, but you can estimate a patient's body temperature by placing the back of your hand on the patient's forehead. The patient's skin temperature is judged, in relation to your skin temperature, as hot or cold.

Some illnesses can cause the skin to become excessively moist or excessively dry. Therefore, together with its relative temperature, the patient's skin might be described as hot and dry, hot and moist, cold and dry, or cold and moist.

After determining the patient's vital signs, you should also be able to identify and measure these other important signs: pupil size and reactivity and level of consciousness.

FYI

Pupil Size and Reactivity

It is important to examine each eye to detect signs of head injury, stroke, or drug overdose. Look to see whether the **pupils** (the circular openings in the middle of the eyes) are of equal size and whether they both react (contract) when light is shone into them Figure 7-12 ▾ . The following findings are abnormal:

■ **Pupils of unequal size.** Unequal pupils can indicate a stroke or injury to the brain

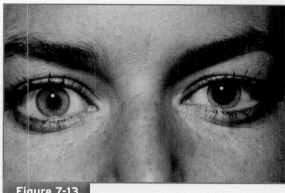

Figure 7-13

Unequal pupils may indicate a stroke or injury to the brain.

FYI cont.

 Figure 7-13 ▲ . A small percentage of people normally have unequal pupils, but in an unconscious patient, unequal pupils are often a sign of serious illness or injury.

■ **Pupils that remain constricted.** Constricted pupils are often present in a person who is taking narcotics. They are also a sign of certain central nervous system diseases.

■ **Pupils that remain dilated (enlarged).** Dilated pupils indicate a relaxed or unconscious state. Pupils will dilate within 30 to 60 seconds of cardiac arrest. Head injuries and the use of certain drugs such as barbiturates can also cause dilated pupils.

Level of Consciousness

You will usually assess the patient's level of consciousness as part of your initial assessment. However, it is important to observe and note any changes that occur between the time of your arrival and the time you turn over the patient's care to personnel at the next level of the EMS system. Report any changes from one level of consciousness to another, using the AVPU scale (see page 152).

Signs Review

Signs are indicators of illness or injury that a first responder can observe in a patient. They help to determine what is wrong with the patient and the

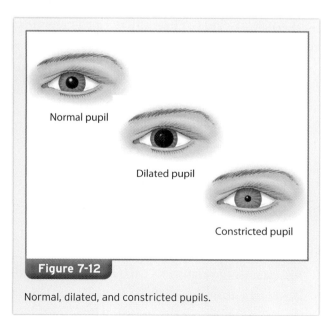

Normal pupil

Dilated pupil

Constricted pupil

Figure 7-12

Normal, dilated, and constricted pupils.

severity of the patient's condition. Vital signs include the patient's respirations (respiratory status), pulse (circulatory status), skin condition, and temperature. Other signs include pupil size and reaction and level of consciousness.

To assess a patient's respiratory status, determine the patient's breathing rate and whether breaths are rapid or slow, shallow or deep, noisy or quiet. In assessing a patient's circulatory status, determine the rate, rhythm, and quality of the victim's pulse. You can also determine if the patient's capillary refill is normal, slow, or absent. Although you may not be able to determine the patient's exact temperature, you will be able to state whether the patient is hot or cold. Skin condition is measured by color and moisture and can be described as pale, flushed, blue, yellow, normal, dry, or moist. To assess the patient's pupils, check to see whether the pupils are equal or unequal in size and whether they remain constricted or dilated. Use the AVPU scale to assess the patient's level of consciousness: alert, responsive to verbal stimuli, responsive to pain, or unresponsive.

Inspect for Signs of Injury

As you perform the patient examination, look and feel for the following signs of injury: deformities, open injuries, tenderness, and swelling. Use the acronym DOTS to remember these signs Table 7-1 ▾ .

Examine the Patient From Head to Toe

Conduct a thorough, hands-on, head-to-toe examination in a logical, systematic manner. It is important to conduct the examination the same way each time to be sure you search all areas of the body for injuries. Use a clear, concise format to communicate your findings to other medical personnel.

The head-to-toe examination can be done whether the patient is conscious or unconscious. Watch the reactions of a conscious patient to your examination. You may want to ask what the patient is feeling as you proceed with your examination. Remember that your examination is the main focus of this part of the assessment. Do not ask the patient so many questions that you are not doing a thorough physical examination.

If the patient is unconscious, it is vitally important that you assess the airway, breathing, and circulation during the initial assessment. After you have established breathing and pulse, begin a head-to-toe examination of the unconscious patient. Examining an unconscious patient is difficult because the patient cannot cooperate or tell you where something hurts—although your examination often will elicit grimaces or moans from an unconscious patient.

Assume that all unconscious, injured patients have spinal injuries. Stabilize the head and spine to minimize movement during the patient examination. It is essential to fully immobilize all injured, unconscious patients on a **backboard** before transporting them (see Chapter 5). You should also be cautious when treating a patient who is unconscious because of illness.

Examine the Head

Use both hands to examine thoroughly all areas of the scalp Figure 7-14 ▾ . Do not move the patient's head! This is especially important if the patient is unconscious or has suffered a spinal injury.

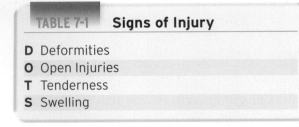

TABLE 7-1	Signs of Injury
D	Deformities
O	Open Injuries
T	Tenderness
S	Swelling

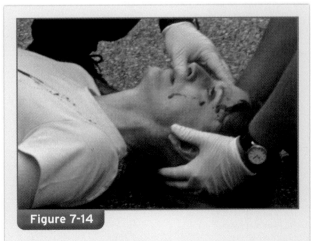

Figure 7-14

Examine the patient's head.

Injuries to the head bleed a lot. Be sure to find the actual wound; do not be fooled by globs of matted, bloody hair.

If necessary, remove the patient's eyeglasses and put them in a safe place. Many patients who need glasses become upset if their glasses are taken away. Use your judgment in each case. Be considerate of the patient. If the patient is wearing a wig, it may be necessary to remove the hairpiece to complete the head examination. Be sure to check the entire head for bumps, areas of tenderness, and bleeding.

Examine the Eyes

Cover one of the patient's eyes for 5 seconds. Then quickly open the eyelid and watch the pupil, the dark part at the center of the eye. The normal reaction of the pupil is to contract (get smaller). This should happen in about 1 second. If you are examining a patient's eyes at night or in the dark, use a flashlight and aim the light at the closed eye **Figure 7-15 ▾**.

A pupil that fails to react to light or pupils that are unequal in size may be important diagnostic signs and should be reported to personnel at the next level of medical care.

Examine the Nose

Examine the nose for tenderness or deformity, which may indicate a broken nose. Check to see if there is any blood or fluid coming from the nose.

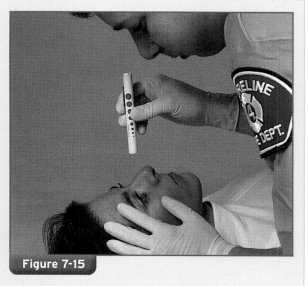

Figure 7-15

Examine the patient's eyes.

Examine the Mouth

Your first examination of the mouth should have taken place when you checked to see whether the patient was breathing. Now recheck the mouth for foreign objects such as food, vomitus, dentures, gum, chewing tobacco, and loose teeth. Be sure to carefully clear away any material that obstructs the patient's breathing. In addition, you should be ready to deal with vomiting. It is important to prevent **aspiration** (inhalation) of vomitus into the lungs.

Use your sense of smell to determine whether any unusual odors are present. A patient who is sick with diabetes may have a fruity breath odor. Do not allow the presence of alcohol on the patient's breath to change the way you treat the patient. In fact, if you detect alcohol, you should conduct an especially careful physical examination, particularly if the patient appears to be severely injured. Remember to place any unconscious patient who has not suffered trauma in the recovery position. This helps keep the patient's airway open and prevents aspiration of vomitus into the airway or lungs.

Examine the Neck

Examine the neck carefully using both hands, one on each side of the patient's neck **Figure 7-16 ▾**. Be sure to touch the vertebrae (the bony part of the back of the neck) to see whether gentle pressure produces pain. Check the neck veins. Swollen (distended) neck veins may indicate heart problems or major trauma to the chest.

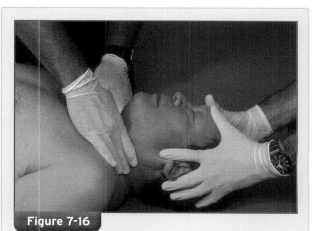

Figure 7-16

Use both hands to examine the patient's neck.

Physical Examination

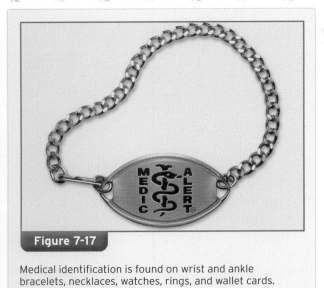

Figure 7-17

Medical identification is found on wrist and ankle bracelets, necklaces, watches, rings, and wallet cards.

TABLE 7-2		Skin Color
Color	**Term**	**Sign of:**
Red	Flushed	Fever or sunburn
White	Pale	Shock
Blue	Cyanotic	Airway obstruction
Yellow	Jaundiced	Liver disease

Examine the neck for a stoma (opening), which indicates that the patient is a "neck breather." A neck breather is a person who has undergone major surgery in which the airway above the stoma has been removed. The stoma may be the patient's only means of breathing, and the patient may not be able to speak normally. The stoma is usually concealed behind an article of clothing or a bib.

As your hands move down the patient's scalp and onto the neck, check for the presence of an emergency medical identification neck chain. You should look for MedicAlert® emblems as an indication of the patient's past medical history. The internationally recognized symbol shown in Figure 7-17 ▲ is found on necklaces, arm bracelets, ankle bracelets, watches, rings, and wallet cards and is carried by people who have a medical condition that warrants special attention if they become ill or injured. This is a patient directive that allows EMS personnel to access the patient's stored medical information by calling the MedicAlert Foundation. Each MedicAlert member has a unique, secure patient identifier engraved at

the bottom of his or her emblem. By wearing this emblem, the patient has consented to the release of information to attending medical personnel. The stored patient history can include conditions, allergies, medications and dosages, and implanted devices. If you find such a warning on a patient, it is your responsibility to give this information to the next person in the EMS system.

Examine the Face

While you are performing the hands-on examination of the head and neck, be sure to note the color of the facial skin, its temperature, and whether it is moist or dry Table 7-2 ▲ . After you have completed the head examination, be sure to note any bumps, bruises, cuts, or other abnormalities.

Examine the Chest

If the patient is conscious, ask him or her to take a deep breath and tell you whether there is any pain on **inhalation** or **exhalation**. Note whether the patient breathes with difficulty. Look and listen for signs of difficult breathing such as coughing, wheezing, or foaming at the mouth. It is important to look at both sides of the chest completely, noting any injuries, bleeding, or sections of the chest that move abnormally, unequally, or painfully. Unequal motion of one side or section may be a sign of a serious condition, called a **flail chest**, that can result from multiple rib **fractures** (breaks). Be sure to run your hands over all parts of the chest Figure 7-18 ▶ . Like the head and neck examinations, this must be accomplished with minimal patient movement.

Apply firm but gentle pressure to the collarbone (**clavicle**) to check for fractures. Check the chest for fractured ribs by placing your hands on the chest and pushing down gently but firmly. Then put your hands on each side of the chest and push inward, squeezing the chest.

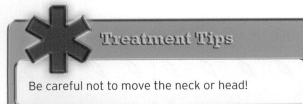

Treatment Tips

Be careful not to move the neck or head!

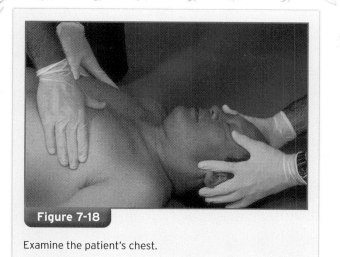

Figure 7-18

Examine the patient's chest.

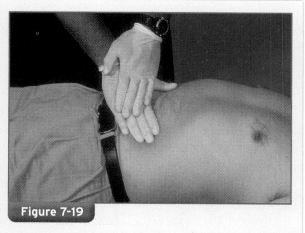

Figure 7-19

Examine the patient's abdomen.

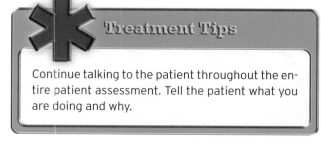

Figure 7-20

Examine the patient's pelvis by gently pressing on the pelvic bones. Place your hands on both sides of the pelvis and push downward and inward.

Treatment Tips

Continue talking to the patient throughout the entire patient assessment. Tell the patient what you are doing and why.

Examine the Abdomen

Continue your examination downward to the **abdomen** (stomach and groin). Look for any signs of external bleeding, penetrating injuries, or protruding parts, such as intestines Figure 7-19 ▲.

Ask the patient to relax the stomach muscles and observe whether the stomach remains rigid. Rigidity is often a sign of abdominal injury. Swelling is also a sign of abdominal injury.

Note whether the clothing has been soiled with urine or feces. This may be an important diagnostic sign for certain illnesses or injuries, such as stroke. Make sure you check the genital area for external injuries. Although both the patient and you may be socially uncomfortable during this examination, it must be done if there is any suspicion of injury.

Examine the Pelvis

Next check for fractures of the pelvis. First check for signs of obvious bruising, bleeding, or swelling. If no pain is reported by the patient, then gently press on the pelvic bones. If the patient reports pain or tenderness or if you note any movement, a severe injury may be present in this region Figure 7-20 ▲.

Examine the Back

The patient's back should be checked one side of the back at a time, using one hand to gently lift the patient's shoulder and the other to slide downward in the examination Figure 7-21 ▶. In cases where a patient has been injured, stabilize the head and neck to prevent movement while you examine the patient.

As you check each side of the back, be sure that your hands go all the way to the midline of the patient's body so you can feel the spinal column. Check half the back from one side; then switch and check the other side in the same

Physical Examination

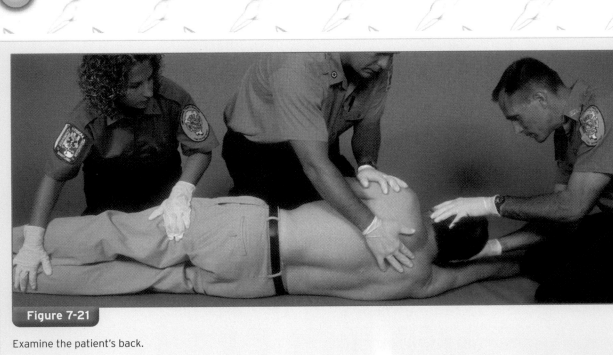

Figure 7-21

Examine the patient's back.

manner. This ensures that no part of the back is missed during the examination. If the patient is lying on his or her side or stomach, it will be much easier to examine the patient's back. If the patient must be rolled onto a backboard, you can examine the patient's back while the patient is on his or her side. Do not wait for a backboard if this will delay your examination of the patient.

Examine the Extremities

Do a systematic examination of each extremity to determine if there are any injuries. This examination consists of the following five steps:

1. Observe the extremity to determine if there is any visible injury. Look for bleeding and deformity.
2. Examine for tenderness in each extremity by encircling it with both hands and gently, but firmly, squeezing each part of the limb. Watch the patient's face and listen to see if the patient shows any signs of pain.
3. Ask the patient to move the extremity. Check for normal movement. Determine if there is any pain when the patient moves the extremity.
4. Check for sensation by touching the bare skin of each extremity. See if the patient can feel your touch.
5. Assess the circulatory status of each extremity by checking for the presence of a pulse in

that extremity and by checking for capillary refill.

Each upper extremity consists of the **arm**, the forearm, the wrist, and the hand. The arm extends from the shoulder to the elbow; the forearm extends from the elbow to the wrist.

Examine one upper extremity at a time **Figure 7-22 ▾**.

1. **Observe the extremity**. Start by looking at its position. Is it in a normal or an abnormal position? Does it look broken (deformed) to you?

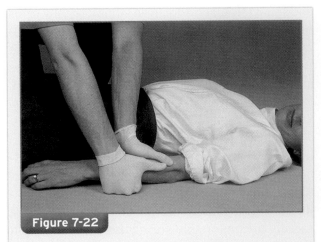

Figure 7-22

Examine the upper extremities one at a time.

Physical Examination

2. **Examine for tenderness.** Encircle the upper extremity with your hands. Work from the shoulder downward to the hand. Firmly squeeze the limb to locate any possible fractures.

3. **Check for movement.** Take the patient's hand in yours and ask the patient to squeeze your hand. Squeezing is usually painful for the patient if there is a fracture or other injury. If a conscious patient cannot squeeze your hand, you should assume that the extremity is seriously injured or paralyzed.

4. **Check for sensation.** Ask the patient if he or she feels any tingling or numbness in the extremity. Such tingling or numbness may be a sign of a spine injury. Check for sensation by touching the palm of the patient's hand. See if the patient can feel your touch.

5. **Assess the circulatory status.** Check the patient's radial pulse. Absence of a radial pulse indicates blood vessel damage. Check the fingers for capillary refill. Check the color, temperature, and moisture of the hand.

Repeat this examination for the other upper extremity.

Each lower extremity consists of the thigh, the **leg**, the ankle, and the foot. The thigh extends from the hip to the knee. The leg extends from the knee to the ankle. Examine one lower extremity at a time **Figure 7-23 ▶**:

1. **Observe the extremity.** Look at the position and shape of the lower extremity. Is it deformed? Is the foot rotated inward or outward?

2. **Examine for tenderness.** Encircle the lower extremity with your hands, as you did with the

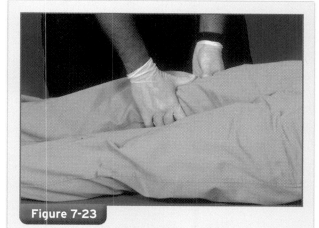

Figure 7-23

Examine the lower extremities one at a time.

upper extremities. Move from the groin to the foot. Be sure to make contact with all surfaces of the limb. Use firm but gentle pressure to identify tender (injured) areas. You are not handling eggs but are attempting to locate injuries.

3. **Check for movement.** Ask the patient to move the limb only if you have found no signs of injury in the first two steps. If there is a significant injury, movement will probably be painful. If a conscious patient cannot move the foot or toes, the limb is seriously injured or paralyzed.

4. **Check for sensation.** Ask the patient whether he or she can feel your touch as you examine the extremity. Tingling or numbness in a limb is a sign of spinal injury.

5. **Assess circulatory status.** Check the posterior tibial pulse, located just behind the ankle bone on the medial (inner) side of the ankle. Absence of this pulse indicates blood vessel damage, which is sometimes caused by fractures. Check the toes for capillary refill. Check the skin color, temperature, and moisture of the extremity. Repeat this examination for the other lower extremity.

Patient Assessment

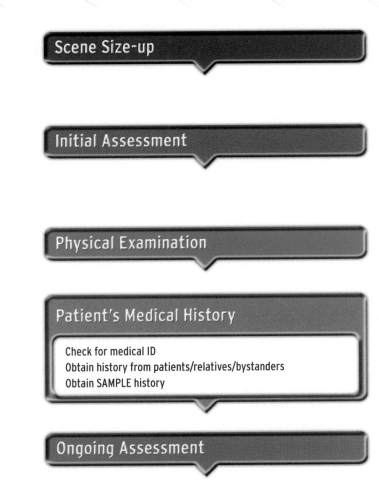

Scene Size-up

Initial Assessment

Physical Examination

Patient's Medical History

Check for medical ID
Obtain history from patients/relatives/bystanders
Obtain SAMPLE history

Ongoing Assessment

Obtain the Patient's Medical History

The purpose of obtaining a medical history is to gather a systematic account of the patient's past medical conditions, illnesses, and injuries, to determine the events leading up to the present medical situation and to determine the signs and symptoms of the current condition Figure 7-24 ▾ . It is important to question the patient in a clear and systematic manner in order to gain as much information as possible. Do not underestimate the importance of a good medical history. Physicians are taught that they can diagnose a patient's problem about 80% of the time after completing a thorough medical history. You are not expected to have the knowledge and training of a physician, but you should be able to gain a thorough medical history from a patient. Performing a medical history is an important part of the patient assessment sequence for injured patients and for ill patients.

Learn the relevant facts about the patient's past medical history. Ask the patient about any serious injuries, illnesses, or surgeries. Ask the patient what prescription medicines they are currently taking. Ask them what over-the-counter medicines and herbal medicines they are taking. Find out if the patient is allergic to any medicines, foods, or seasonal allergens such as ragweed.

Ask the patient about the medical situation that caused him or her to call EMS. Ask the patient to describe the events that led up to the current medical situation. Listen to how the patient describes these events. Ask the patient to describe the symptoms that he or she is currently experiencing. Ask the patient about the symptoms when the illness or injury began as well the symptoms the patient is experiencing now. A patient may have noticed certain signs you can observe. For instance, the patient may have noticed that his or her ankles are swollen. Ask when the patient last ate and what the patient has had to drink recently.

In order to perform a patient medical history in a consistent and thorough manner, remember the acronym SAMPLE. By using this easy-to-remember acronym, you can gain the information you need about past medical history as well as the events leading to the current episode of illness or injury.

It is important to use a systematic approach when obtaining a patient's medical history. The **SAMPLE history** provides a framework to ask needed questions of the patient. Remember to ask the patient one question at a time. Give the patient time to answer before you ask the next question. Listen carefully and use good eye contact to let the patient know that you are listening to the response. Designate one caregiver to ask questions to avoid confusing the patient.

S   **Signs and symptoms**. Ask the patient what signs and symptoms occurred at the beginning of the episode. Ask the patient what signs and symptoms he or she is experiencing now. Ask the patient if he or she is feeling any pain. If the patient is experiencing pain, ask him or her to describe the pain.

A   **Allergies**. Ask if the patient is allergic to any medications, any foods, or has seasonal allergies. Ask the patient to describe his or her reactions to any allergies. If the patient states that he or she has no allergies, communicate this to other EMS personnel.

M   **Medications**. Ask the patient if he or she is taking any medications prescribed by a physician. If the patient is taking prescription medications, ask the patient the purpose of these medicines. Ask the patient if he or she is taking over-the-counter medications or herbal remedies.

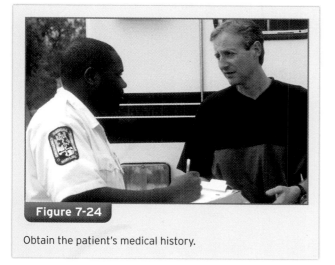

Figure 7-24

Obtain the patient's medical history.

Patient's Medical History

P   **Pertinent past medical history.** Ask if the patient is currently under the care of a physician. Ask the patient if he or she has any existing medical conditions such as diabetes or a heart condition. Ask the patient if he or she has had a serious illness or a serious injury. Ask the patient if he or she has been hospitalized recently. Try to keep this part of the history relevant to the current condition. A cardiac bypass operation is probably very relevant to a patient experiencing chest pains because it indicates cardiovascular disease. An operation to remove an inflamed appendix 10 years ago is probably not relevant to an illness today.

L   **Last oral intake.** Ask when the patient last had something to eat; ask the patient when he or she last had something to drink. If the patient is experiencing abdominal pain, ask the patient what he or she had to eat and drink in the last few hours.

E   **Events leading up to this illness or injury.** Ask the patient to describe what he or she was doing when the symptoms of this event started. Ask the patient if they noticed anything unusual in the hours before this episode started or if the patient was doing anything unusual just before he or she got sick.

See **Table 7-3 ▸** for an illustration of the SAMPLE acronym.

If the patient is unconscious or senile, a family member, friend, or coworker may be able to answer your questions. Important information can often be found on a medical identification necklace, bracelet, or card. The information you gain will help to determine what steps you need to take to treat the patient. This information needs to be communicated to other EMS personnel to help them in their assessment and treatment of the patient.

TABLE 7-3   **SAMPLE Medical History**

S Signs and symptoms of the injury or illness. These should be the reasons that caused the patient to call for emergency medical services. Patients should describe signs and symptoms in their own words.

A Allergies. Patients may be allergic to medications, food, or airborne particles.

M Medications. What medications is the patient taking? Ask about medications prescribed by the patient's physician, over-the-counter (nonprescription) medications, and herbal remedies.

P Pertinent past medical history. What events or symptoms might be related to the patient's current illness? For example, it would be important to know whether a patient experiencing severe chest pain had a previous heart attack.

L Last oral intake. When was the last time the patient had anything to eat or drink? Find out what the patient last ate or drank and how much he or she consumed.

E Events associated with or leading to this injury or illness. Knowing these events will help you put together the pieces of the medical history puzzle. Let patients describe these events in their own words.

Patient's Medical History

Patient Assessment

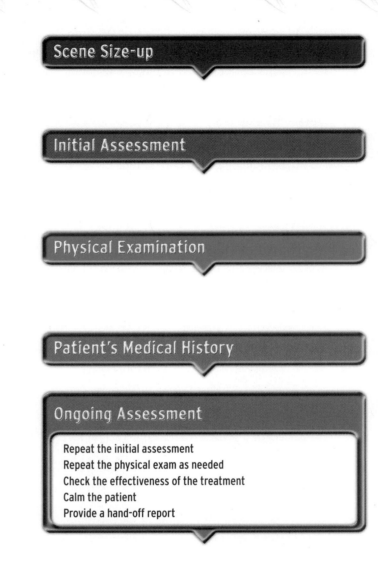

Scene Size-up

Initial Assessment

Physical Examination

Patient's Medical History

Ongoing Assessment

Repeat the initial assessment
Repeat the physical exam as needed
Check the effectiveness of the treatment
Calm the patient
Provide a hand-off report

Provide Ongoing Assessment

The patient assessment sequence helps determine each patient's initial condition. Patients who appear stable can become unstable quickly. Therefore, it is essential that you watch all patients carefully for changes in status. As a general rule, monitor the patient's vital signs every 10 minutes. Continue to maintain an open airway, monitor breathing and pulse for rate and quality, and observe the patient's skin color and temperature. If the patient is unstable, take the patient's vital signs every 5 minutes. If the patient's condition changes, repeat the physical examination. Check to see if the interventions you took were effective. Continue to talk with the patient. Tell the patient what you are doing and give reassurance.

Providing a Hand-Off Report

It is important that you describe your findings concisely and accurately to the emergency medical personnel who take over the care of your patients in a hand-off report **Figure 7-25 ▾**.

The easiest way to report your patient assessment results is to use the same systematic approach you followed during the patient assessment:

1. Provide the age and sex of the patient.
2. Describe the history of the incident.

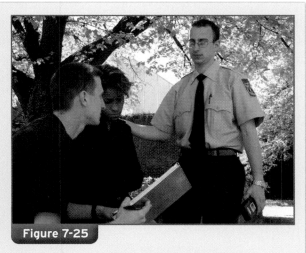

Figure 7-25

Report your findings in a hand-off report.

Treatment Tips

Serious changes can occur rapidly!

---

3. Describe the patient's primary or chief complaint.
4. Describe the patient's level of responsiveness.
5. Report the status of the vital signs: airway, breathing, and circulation (including severe bleeding).
6. Describe the results of the physical examination.
7. Report any pertinent medical conditions using the SAMPLE format.
8. Report the interventions provided.

Working in a systematic manner will help ensure that you do not overlook any significant symptoms, signs, or injuries and will help to make the hand-off report complete and accurate. For example, a hand-off report on a 23-year-old man injured in an automobile accident might include the following information:

1. The patient is a 23-year-old man.
2. He was involved in a two-car, head-on collision.
3. He is complaining of stomach pain and has a 2-inch cut on his forehead.
4. He is conscious and alert.
5. His pulse is 78 beats per minute and strong. His respirations are 16 breaths per minute and are regular and deep.
6. Examination revealed a 2-inch cut on his forehead, marks on his stomach, and moderate pain midway between his right knee and ankle.
7. He has no known medical conditions.
8. The patient is on his back, covered with a blanket to preserve his body heat. We have bandaged his laceration and immobilized his leg with an inflatable splint.

More information on the hand-off report is included in Chapter 8.

Remember that the purpose of the patient assessment sequence is to:

- Assist in finding the patient's injuries so you can treat them.

- Obtain information about the patient's condition, which you provide to the EMS personnel at the next level of medical care.

With practice, you can complete the entire patient assessment sequence in about 2 minutes. This is not a complete medical examination but, as the name implies, is a patient assessment by first responders.

Examine every patient involved in an incident before you begin major treatment of any single patient. The exceptions to this rule are airway, breathing, and circulatory problems (severe bleeding or shock), which you must treat as you encounter them during patient assessment. Except for these life-threatening conditions, begin no treatment until you have examined all patients to determine the extent and severity of injuries and to make sure that you treat injuries in their order of severity.

A Word About Trauma and Medical Patients

Patients can generally be divided into two main categories: those who suffer from trauma and those who have a sudden illness. Trauma is the term used for an injury to a patient. The injury may be major or minor. Some incidents that cause trauma include falls, motor-vehicle crashes, and sports-related injuries. Examples of sudden illnesses include heart attacks, strokes, asthma, and gallbladder problems. The patient assessment sequence you have learned can be used to examine patients who have suffered from trauma, illnesses, or both.

When examining trauma patients, follow the sequence as you learned it:

1. Size up the scene.
2. Perform an initial patient assessment:
   A. Form a general impression of the patient.
   B. Assess the patient's responsiveness and stabilize the patient's spine if necessary.
   C. Assess the patient's airway.
   D. Assess the patient's breathing.
   E. Assess the patient's circulation (including severe bleeding) and stabilize if necessary.
   F. Update the responding EMS units.
3. Examine the patient from head to toe.
4. Obtain the patient's medical history using the SAMPLE format.
5. Provide ongoing assessment.

This sequence gives the information about the trauma patient in a logical order. It allows you to assess the most critical factors first. Although you may have to vary the order of the steps somewhat for certain patients, you should try to generally follow this order. When dealing with a patient with a sudden illness, modify the preceding sequence slightly. The first two steps of the patient assessment sequence are the same for both illness and injury. However, when dealing with an illness, change the sequence to obtain the patient's medical history before you perform the head-to-toe examination. In a conscious patient, the most important thing is to make sure you gather all the information needed to perform a complete patient assessment.

Although it is often helpful to consider whether the patient's problem is caused by trauma or sudden illness, avoid jumping to conclusions. Some patients need to be treated for both trauma and sudden illness. (For example, a person who has a heart attack while driving a car needs to be treated for the heart attack and for any trauma suffered in the motor-vehicle crash.) The most important factor to remember is to follow a system of patient assessment that will gather all the information needed.

Ongoing Assessment

You are the Provider

SUMMARY

Review the *You are the Provider* case study provided at the beginning of this chapter.

It is one of those rare days when spring has sprung and everyone wants to enjoy the great outdoors. As you are returning to your station after completing a call, your dispatcher announces that there is a report of a person who is short of breath at a local park. Your unit is the closest to the scene. As you begin to respond, the dispatcher informs you that the information is from a third-party call and there is no further information about the patient.

1. As you arrive at the location of your patient, you find a 14-year-old male who has been hit in the chest with a baseball and is experiencing shortness of breath and pain when breathing. What are the steps of the patient assessment you should use in examining this patient?

Calls where you have a limited amount of dispatch information are challenging for EMS personnel. In a case like this, you have to keep an open mind until you are with the patient and can begin your patient assessment sequence. In this situation, your patient is a 14-year-male who has been hit in the chest and is experiencing shortness of breath and pain when breathing. For this patient who has suffered trauma, the five-step patient assessment should be:

1. Scene size-up
2. Initial patient assessment
3. Physical examination
4. Patient's medical history
5. Ongoing assessment

2. If instead you arrive on the scene and find a 76-year-old female sitting on a park bench experiencing shortness of breath, how would you change the steps of the patient assessment from the steps used in Question 1?

In this situation, you find a 76-year-old female who is sitting on a park bench and is experiencing shortness of breath. In assessing this patient with a medical complaint and no trauma, you should follow the five-step patient assessment as in Question 1, except you should complete the patient's medical history before you conduct the physical examination. The five-step patient assessment sequence for this patient with a medical condition should be:

1. Scene size-up
2. Initial patient assessment
3. Patient's medical history
4. Physical examination
5. Ongoing assessment

Remember that patients who have suffered trauma can have medical conditions, too!

Prep Kit

Ready for Review

The Ready for Review thoroughly summarizes the chapter.

- A complete patient assessment consists of five steps: perform a scene size-up, perform an initial patient assessment, perform a physical examination, obtain a patient's medical history, and provide an ongoing assessment.

- The scene size-up is a general overview of the incident and its surroundings. Based on this information, you can make decisions about the safety of the scene, what type of incident is present, any mechanism of injury, and the need for additional resources.

- During the initial patient assessment, determine and correct any life-threatening conditions. The steps of initial patient assessment are: form a general impression of the patient, assess responsiveness, check the patient's airway, check the patient's breathing, check the patient's circulation, acknowledge the patient's chief complaint, and update responding EMS units.

- The physical examination of the patient from head to toe is done to assess non-life-threatening conditions after completing the initial assessment and after stabilizing any life-threatening conditions. This exam helps you locate and begin initial management of the signs and symptoms of illness or injury. After completing the physical examination, review any positive signs and symptoms of illness or injury.

- The purpose of obtaining a medical history is to gather a systematic account of the patient's past medical conditions, illnesses, and injuries to determine the signs and symptoms of the current condition. The SAMPLE history provides a framework to ask needed questions of the patient.

- It is essential that you watch all patients carefully for changes in status. If the patient is stable, monitor vital signs every 10 minutes. If the patient is unstable, monitor vital signs every 5 minutes. If the patient's condition changes, repeat the physical examination.

- Provide a concise and accurate hand-off report to emergency medical personnel.

- Patients can generally be divided into two main categories: medical and trauma. When examining trauma patients, follow the patient assessment sequence:

1. Size up the scene.
2. Perform an initial patient assessment:
   - Form a general impression of the patient.
   - Assess the patient's responsiveness and stabilize the spine if necessary.
   - Assess the airway.
   - Assess breathing.
   - Assess circulation and stabilize if necessary.
   - Update responding EMS units.
3. Examine the patient from head to toe.
4. Obtain the patient's medical history using the SAMPLE format.
5. Provide ongoing assessment.

Technology

- Interactivities
- Vocabulary Explorer
- Anatomy Review
- Web Links
- Online Review Manual

Vital Vocabulary

The Vital Vocabulary are the key terms for this chapter.

abdomen The body cavity between the thorax and the pelvis that contains the major organs of digestion and excretion.

arm Part of the upper extremity that extends from the shoulder to the elbow.

aspiration Breathing in foreign matter such as food, drink, or vomitus into the airway or lungs.

assessment-based care A system of patient evaluation in which the chief complaint of the patient and other signs and symptoms are gathered. The care given is based on this information rather than on a formal diagnosis.

AVPU scale A scale to measure a patient's level of consciousness. The letters stand for Alert, Verbal, Pain, and Unresponsive.

backboard A straight board used for splinting, extricating, and transporting patients with suspected spinal injuries.

bounding pulse A strong pulse (similar to the pulse that follows physical exertion like running or lifting heavy objects).

brachial pulse Pulse located in the arm between the elbow and shoulder; used for checking pulse in infants.

capillary refill The ability of the circulatory system to restore blood to the capillary blood vessels after it has been squeezed out by the examiner.

carotid artery The principal arteries of the neck. They supply blood to the face, head, and brain.

carotid pulse A pulse that can be felt on each side of the neck where the carotid artery is close to the skin.

chief complaint The patient's response to questions such as "What happened?" or "What's wrong?".

clavicle The collarbone.

cyanosis Bluish coloration of the skin resulting from poor oxygenation of the circulating blood.

exhalation Breathing out.

flail chest A condition that occurs when three or more ribs are each broken in two places, and the chest wall lying between the fractures becomes a free-floating segment.

fractures Breaks in a bone.

inhalation Breathing in.

initial patient assessment The first actions taken to form an impression of the patient's condition; to determine the patient's responsiveness and introduce yourself to the patient; to check the patient's airway, breathing, and circulation; and to acknowledge the patient's chief complaint.

leg The lower extremity; specifically, the lower portion, from the knee to the ankle.

physical examination The step in the patient assessment sequence in which the first responder carefully examines the patient from head to toe, looking for additional injuries and other problems.

posterior tibial pulse Ankle pulse.

pulse The wave of pressure that is created by the heart as it contracts and forces blood out of the heart and into the major arteries.

pupils The circular openings in the middle of the eye.

radial pulse Wrist pulse.

respiratory rate The speed at which a person is breathing (measured in breaths per minute).

sign A condition that you observe in a patient, such as bleeding or the temperature of a patient's skin.

SAMPLE history A patient's medical history. The letters stand for Signs/symptoms, Allergies, Medications, Pertinent past history, Last oral intake, Events associated with the illness or injury.

symptom A condition the patient tells you, such as "I feel dizzy."

thready pulse A weak pulse.

trauma A wound or injury.

vital signs Signs of life, specifically pulse, respiration, blood pressure, and temperature.

Assessment in Action

Assessment in Action presents a fictitious scenario to help you review what you learned in this chapter.

You are dispatched to the local grocery store for a fall injury. Upon arrival, you find a 63-year-old male lying on the ground complaining of hip pain.

1. There are five steps of a patient assessment. Place the following in the correct order.
   1. Physical examination
   2. Initial patient assessment
   3. Patient's medical history
   4. Scene size-up
   5. Ongoing assessment

   A. 4, 2, 3, 1, 5,
   B. 3, 1, 4, 2, 5
   C. 4, 2, 1, 3, 5
   D. 1, 3, 2, 5, 4

2. Of the following, what is your first step of the scene size-up?

   A. Body substance isolation
   B. Scene safety
   C. Determine the need for additional assistance
   D. Determine the mechanism of injury

3. Place the following parts of the second step of the patient assessment sequence in the order that you should perform them.
   1. Check the patient's airway.
   2. Assess responsiveness.
   3. Check the patient's circulation.
   4. Update the responding EMS units.
   5. Form a general impression of the patient.
   6. Check the patient's breathing.

   A. 5, 2, 1, 6, 3, 4
   B. 6, 5, 3, 4, 1, 2
   C. 3, 2, 1, 5, 6, 4
   D. 2, 6, 3, 4, 5, 1

4. There are six steps of the initial assessment. Place them in the correct order.
   A. Assess the patient's breathing and correct any life-threatening conditions.
   B. Assess the patient's airway and correct any life-threatening conditions.
   C. Update the responding EMS units.
   D. Form a general impression of the patient.
   E. Assess the patient's circulation, including severe bleeding.
   F. Assess the patient's responsiveness and stabilize the spine if necessary.

   1. _____
   2. _____
   3. _____
   4. _____
   5. _____
   6. _____

5. How often do you need to repeat the initial assessment of a stable patient?

   A. Every 3 to 5 minutes
   B. Every 5 to 10 minutes
   C. Every 10 to 15 minutes
   D. Only when you see a change in the patient's condition

Communications and Documentation

National Standard Curriculum Objectives

Cognitive

1-3.12 Discuss issues concerning the fundamental components of documentation. (p 190-191)

3-1.21 Describe the information included in the First Responder "hand-off" report. (p 191)

Affective

3-1.30 Demonstrate a caring attitude when performing patient assessments. (p 184, 185)

3-1.31 Place the interests of the patient as the foremost consideration when making any and all patient care decisions during patient assessment. (p 184, 185)

3-1.32 Communicate with empathy during patient assessment to patients as well as with family members and friends of the patient. (p 184, 185)

Psychomotor

None

Chapter Objectives*

Knowledge and Attitude Objectives

1. Describe the importance of communications and documentation for first responders. (p 180)
2. Describe the different types of equipment used by first responders in voice radio and data systems. (p 180-181)
3. Describe the importance of data systems for first responders. (p 181)
4. Explain the functions of radio communications during the following phases of a response:
   - Dispatch (p 182)
   - Response to the scene (p 182)
   - Arrival at the scene (p 182)
   - Update of responding EMS units (p 183)
   - Transfer of patient care to other EMS personnel (p 183)
   - Postrun activities (p 183)
5. Describe guidelines for effective communication with patients. (p 185)
6. Explain the skills that will help you communicate with:
   - Hearing-impaired patients (p 188)
   - Visually impaired patients (p 189)
   - Geriatric patients (p 189)
   - Pediatric patients (p 189-190)
7. Describe the legal significance of documentation. (p 191)
8. List the areas (topics) that should be included in a run report to ensure proper documentation. (p 191)

There are no skill objectives for this chapter.

*These are chapter learning objectives.

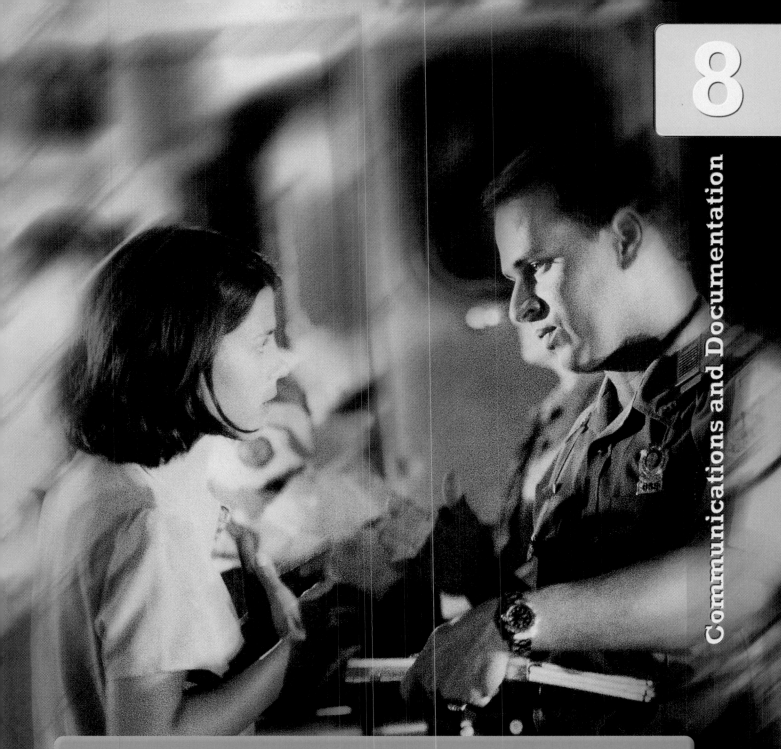

You are the Provider

Just as you are finishing your lunch, you hear the alert tones on your mobile radio. Your dispatcher announces, "Unit 403, respond to a vehicle collision with injuries at the corner of Main Street and University Drive. Your time out is thirteen forty-seven. Your run number is three-two-six-five."

1. How do the functions of the radio communications system change during different phases of an emergency medical call?
2. Why is it important to have protocols for the use of a radio communications system?
3. Why is it important to document your observations, assessments, and treatments for each call?

Introduction

A vital part of your role as a medical first responder involves communications and documentation. Communications are important during every phase of a call. The dispatcher must communicate the location and type of call to designated responders. First responders need to communicate with patients, bystanders, family members, dispatchers, and other members of the public safety community. Once you have completed a call, it is important to document the condition of the patient and the treatment given to the patient.

Communications Systems and Equipment

The purpose of a communications system is to relay information from one location to another when it is impossible to communicate face to face. The results of using a communications system will only be as accurate as the information that is put into the system. It is important for you as a first responder to have a basic idea of how your department's communications system works. Communications systems can be divided into two categories: those that transmit voice communications and those that transmit data.

Technology

- Interactivities
- Vocabulary Explorer
- Anatomy Review
- Web Links
- Online Review Manual

In the Field

Interoperability

It is important for different agencies that are working together to have the ability to communicate with one another. This concept is called interoperability.

Voice Systems

Voice communication systems transmit the spoken word from one location to another. The two types of voice systems most commonly used in public safety agencies are radio systems and phone systems.

Radio Systems

Most first responders use some type of radio communication system. It is important that you understand the basics of a radio communication system and that you understand how to properly operate the radio system used by your department. Radio communications are regulated by the Federal Communications Commission (FCC). Frequencies are assigned according to the function of your organization. First responders who are part of a law enforcement agency are usually assigned different frequencies than first responders who are part of a fire department.

Several different types of radios exist. A **base station** is a powerful stationary two-way radio that is attached to one or more fixed antennas. A base station is used by dispatchers to send and receive messages to and from all parts of the service area. A base station may be attached to several different antennas in order to reach all parts of a geographic service area. They may be designed to transmit and receive on multiple frequencies. Some systems are designed so that different frequencies are used for different functions of communications.

A **mobile radio** is mounted in a vehicle and draws electricity from the electrical system of the vehicle. It has an external antenna, which is usually mounted on the roof or cab of the vehicle. The operating console is mounted so the driver or passenger of the vehicle can conveniently operate the radio. Mobile radios are used primarily to send and receive voice messages.

A **portable radio** is designed to be carried by rescuers 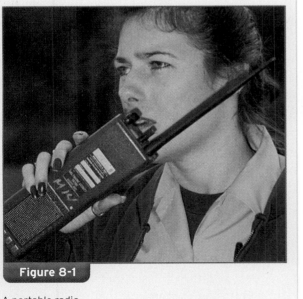. These self-contained units incorporate a two-way radio with a self-contained battery, a built-in microphone, and a built-in antenna. Most portable radios are capable of operating on multiple channels. One drawback of many portable radios is that the controls are small and hard to see in darkness; therefore, rescuers who use these radios must become extremely familiar with the controls and operation. Portable radios are low-powered devices and are often used with a repeater system. A **repeater** is a device that receives a weak radio signal, amplifies that signal, and then rebroadcasts it. Repeaters are used to cover geographic areas where radio signals are weak. These geographic areas are called dead spots.

Telephone Systems

Telephone systems primarily convey voice communications. Public safety agencies may use phone systems to relay dispatch information or to handle routine administrative communications. Landline phone systems are tied together through an above-ground or below-ground hardwired system. Cellular phones rely on radio waves between a cellular phone and a cellular tower to propagate and receive phone messages. The advantage of cell phones is that they can be taken with you wherever you go. Many cellular systems make equipment and air time available to EMS services at little or no cost as a public service.

Data Systems

Communication systems are also used to send and receive data. Data can be transmitted through radio systems or through phone systems. Many different types of data can be sent between emergency responders and communication centers. Computer-generated routing information is an example of data that are useful for emergency responders. A wide variety of devices exists for transmitting data, including portable computers and personal digital assistants (PDAs).

Paging systems can transmit text messages or voice communications. Pagers are radio receivers that are silent unless activated by a dispatcher. Many departments use paging systems to alert members to emergency incidents.

A **mobile data terminal (MDT)** transmits data messages through a radio system **Figure 8-2** and is frequently incorporated into a mobile radio system. MDTs reduce the amount of time the radio frequency is tied up to send or receive a message.

A **fax machine** uses a phone line or radio system to send written data. Some public safety providers use fax machines to transmit dispatch information.

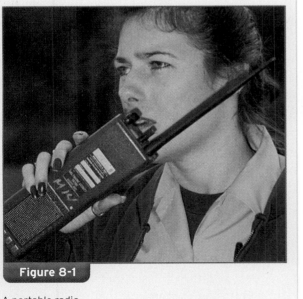

Figure 8-1

A portable radio.

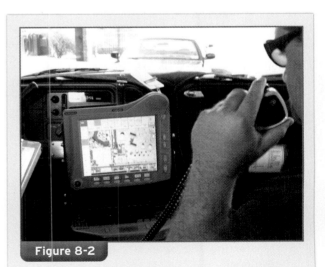

Figure 8-2

A mobile data terminal (MDT) can be used to display routing information transmitted from the dispatch center.

Telemetry is used by advanced life support providers to transmit electrocardiograms (EKGs) and other patient data to online medical control. Telemetry can operate through a phone system or through a radio system.

E-mail is used to transmit a wide variety of messages. It can be transmitted over wires or through a wireless system.

As a first responder, you will not be involved in using all these types of communications, but you should have some understanding of how these various communication devices operate. It is more important for you to understand how to send and receive data in your department than it is to understand how the system is constructed.

The Functions of Radio Communications

Throughout the different phases of an EMS call, communication systems are used for different functions. Calls for medical assistance can be divided into different phases, including dispatch, response to the scene, arrival at the scene, transferring the care of the patient to other EMS personnel, and postrun activities. During these phases, it is important to communicate certain findings to other members of the EMS or public safety team.

Dispatch

The function of dispatch can be accomplished using a phone system, a paging system, a fax, or a radio system. Dispatch may use voice, text messaging, or an MDT to alert responders to an emergency. It is your duty to keep your equipment

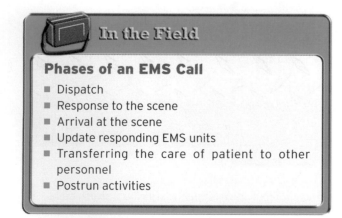

In the Field

Phases of an EMS Call

- Dispatch
- Response to the scene
- Arrival at the scene
- Update responding EMS units
- Transferring the care of patient to other personnel
- Postrun activities

In the Field

Do not start responding to a call until you are sure where you are going because you may be going out of your way.

ready to receive a call whenever you are on duty. Listen carefully to voice messages to ensure that you are receiving the information correctly. If you are not sure that you have received all the dispatch information correctly, ask the dispatcher to repeat it. If you receive dispatch information via an MDT, text messaging, or a fax, you can refer to the message to verify the location and type of call.

Response to the Scene

While responding to the scene of an emergency, your dispatcher may give you further information about the location of the call or the condition of the patient. Be alert for any additional information that the dispatcher gives you. In the event that you are delayed in responding because your vehicle would not start or you encounter unexpected traffic, a blocked railroad crossing, or other unexpected traffic delays, notify your dispatch of the situation. Your message will enable the dispatch to start another unit to the same call if necessary **Figure 8-3 ▶** .

Arrival at the Scene

As you arrive at the scene, perform a visual survey—an overview of the scene. Your visual survey of the entire scene gives you an impression of the overall situation, including the number of patients involved and the severity of their injuries. Once you have performed an initial visual survey, try to give the communications center a concise verbal picture of the scene. For a simple call with one patient, this report will be more concise than the report for a more complex call. Your report should verify the location of the incident, the type of incident, any hazards present, the number of victims, and any additional assistance required. It is better to request additional assistance and find you do not need it than to wait and then call for help after the need is more acute **Figure 8-4 ▶** .

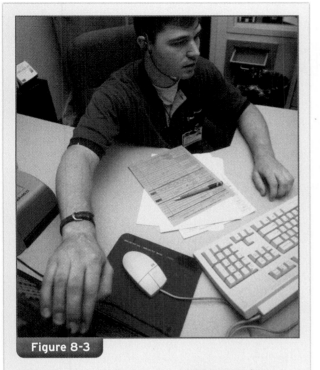

Figure 8-3

Notify your dispatch if you encounter any problems while en route to the scene.

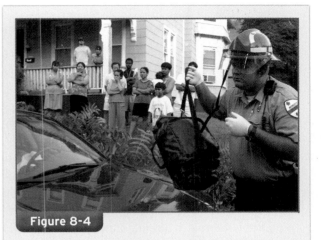

Figure 8-4

Arrival of a first responder at an emergency scene.

Update Responding EMS Units

In some EMS systems, you will be expected to update responding EMS units about the condition of your patient. This report should include the age and sex of the patient, the chief complaint, level of responsiveness, and the status of airway, breathing, and circulation. This update helps them know what to expect when they arrive on the scene.

Transferring the Care of the Patient to Other EMS Personnel

With many EMS incidents, you will be the first trained person to arrive on the scene. You will have performed a patient assessment and some treatment before EMTs or paramedics arrive. When EMTs or paramedics arrive, it is important to provide them with a "hand-off" report. Describe your findings concisely and accurately.

The easiest way to report your patient assessment results is to use the same systematic approach you follow during patient assessment:

1. Provide the age and sex of the patient.
2. Describe the history of the incident.
3. Describe the patient's chief complaint.
4. Describe the patient's level of responsiveness.
5. Report the status of the vital signs, airway, breathing, and circulation (including severe bleeding).
6. Describe the results of the physical examination.
7. Report any pertinent medical conditions using the SAMPLE format.
8. Report the interventions provided.

Working in a systematic manner will help ensure that you do not overlook any significant symptoms, signs, or injuries and will help to make the hand-off report complete and accurate.

EMTs and paramedics contact online medical control to secure permission to perform certain skills, to get direction regarding patient care, and to give the hospital patient-care reports. As a first responder, you may be present when these EMS providers contact medical control through their radio or cellular phone system. In most EMS systems, first responders are not required to contact medical control for the basic skills they are permitted to perform. If your EMS system utilizes online medical control for first responders, you will need to learn when to contact medical control and how to contact them.

Postrun Activities

After you have turned over the care of the patient to other EMS providers, you need to report this status to your communications center. It is important that the communications center knows how long it will take you to get your unit ready

TABLE 8-1	Guidelines for Effective Radio Communication

- **Monitor the channel before transmitting** to avoid interfering with other radio traffic.
- **Plan your message before pushing the transmit switch.** This will keep your transmissions brief and precise. You should use a standard format for your transmissions.
- **Press the push-to-talk (PTT) button** on the radio, then wait for 1 second before starting your message. Otherwise, you might cut off the first part of your message before the transmitter is working at full power.
- **Hold the microphone 2″ to 3″ from your mouth.** Speak clearly, but never shout into the microphone. Speak at a moderate, understandable rate, preferably in a clear, even voice.
- **Identify the person or unit you are calling first**, then identify your unit as the sender. You will rarely work alone, so say "we" instead of "I" when describing yourself.
- **Acknowledge a transmission** as soon as you can by saying "Go ahead" or whatever is commonly used in your area. You should say, "Over and out," or whatever is commonly used in your area when you are finished. If you cannot take a long message, simply say "Stand by" until you are ready.
- **Use plain English.** Avoid meaningless phrases ("Be advised"), slang, or complex codes. Avoid words that are difficult to hear, such as "yes" and "no." Use "affirmative" and "negative."
- **Keep your message brief.** If your message takes more than 30 seconds to send, pause after 30 seconds and say, "Do you copy?" The other party can then ask for clarification if needed. Also, someone else with emergency traffic can break through if necessary.
- **Avoid voicing negative emotions**, such as anger or irritation, when transmitting. Courtesy is assumed, making it unnecessary to say "please" and "thank you," which wastes air time. Listen to other communications in your system to get a good idea of the common phrases and their uses.
- **When transmitting a number with two or more digits**, say the entire number first and then each digit separately. For example, say "sixty-seven," followed by "six-seven."
- **Do not use profanity on the radio.** It is a violation of FCC rules and can result in substantial fines and even loss of your organization's radio license.
- **Use EMS frequencies for EMS communications.** Do not use these frequencies for any other type of communications.
- **Reduce background noise as much as possible.** Move away from wind, noisy motors, or tools. Close the window if you are in a moving ambulance. When possible, shut off the siren during radio transmissions.

for service and when you are available for another call. Providing a written report of a call is covered under the section on documentation.

The protocols for communicating with others during each phase of an EMS call may vary from one system to another. It is important that you learn and follow the standard procedures and protocols of your department Table 8-1 ▲.

Verbal Communications

As an EMS provider, you need to be proficient in effective verbal communications. Most verbal communications occur through face-to-face conversations. Good communication means that the

person receiving the message will understand exactly what the person who sent the message meant. Effective communication requires feedback; the receiver needs to communicate to the sender that the message has been received and understood.

Both external and internal distractions can hinder effective communication. Noise and other people talking constitute external distractions. Internal distractions such as letting yourself think about a personal matter while on scene can also negatively affect your ability to communicate. A first responder who lacks empathy for a patient may have a harder time communicating than a first responder who cares. Prejudice against a certain type or group of people can also hinder effective communication. Good communication requires careful thinking and patience.

As a first responder, you should master a number of communication skills that will enable you to effectively communicate with EMS personnel and other public safety providers. Verbal communications with the patient, the family, and the rest of the health care team are an essential part of high-quality patient care. First responders must be able to determine what the patient needs and then relay this information to others. The following section includes guidelines for effective communication with patients. Most of these guidelines will also foster effective communication with other public safety personnel.

Guidelines for Effective Communication With Patients

Your communication skills will be put to the test when you communicate with patients and/or family members in emergency situations. Remember that someone who is sick or injured is scared and might not understand what you are doing and saying. Therefore, your gestures, body movements, and attitude toward the patient are critically important in gaining the trust of both the patient and family. The following guidelines for communication will help you calm and reassure your patients.

Introduce Yourself

Introduce yourself by name and by title. This gives the patient, family members, and bystanders an idea of who you are and lets them know your qualifications. Many citizens in your community may not understand that trained first responders arrive in variety of vehicles: fire trucks, police cars, and private vehicles. Introducing yourself helps to put the patient at ease and makes your job of assessing and treating the patient easier **Figure 8-5 ▶** .

Ask the Patient's Name and Use It

Ask the patient what he or she wishes to be called. Knowing the patient's name helps you to establish contact with him or her. Use the patient's first name only if the patient is a child or the patient asks you to use his or her first name. For example, if a young man says his name is "Ron," he probably wants to be called "Ron." Otherwise, it is preferable to use

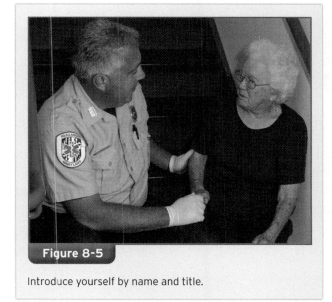
Figure 8-5
Introduce yourself by name and title.

a courtesy title such as "Mrs. Smith" or "Mr. Jones." Avoid using terms such as "Pops" or "Dear"; these are demeaning and irritating to many patients.

Make and Keep Eye Contact

Look into the patient's eyes as you talk. Doing so indicates to the patient that you are focused on his or her needs and that you are speaking to the patient. You should also maintain eye contact as you listen to the patient. Emergency scenes can be very noisy and confusing. By maintaining good eye contact, you help the patient focus on communicating with you.

Use Language the Patient Can Understand

Use language that is clear and that accurately conveys your questions and information. Avoid using technical medical terms that may frighten or confuse the patient. It is disrespectful to talk down to a patient. Use feedback to determine if the level of your language is appropriate for the patient.

Speak Slowly, Clearly, and Distinctly

In the middle of an emergency call, it is easy for both EMS providers and patients to get rushed. It is important to slow down and speak in a clear, distinct voice. By slowing down and speaking distinctly, you can avoid having to repeat questions and explanations. This will save you time in the long run and reduce errors in communications.

Voices of Experience

Take Credit for the Care You Provide

The voice transmission on the radio was filled with anxiety. "Oh, please send me some help, and an ambulance, and anyone on the property who can give first aid. Hurry, please hurry; this is really bad." The dispatcher asked for more precise information. She asked the following questions: "What happened? Where did it happen? How many victims are there?" All of this was done professionally and with reassurance that she would keep the channel open.

> **Record everything that is unusual and take credit for the care you provided.**

A 40-year-old man was at a construction site and had fallen about 30 feet, landing on a cement gymnasium floor. The man was unconscious, motionless, and silent. I was the first responder to arrive on the scene, along with a K-9 officer. Luckily, we were both already on the property, so we arrived within minutes of receiving the call. True to Murphy's Law, there was a complication. The patient's head was partially impaled on the metal flange on the I-beam. His vital signs indicated that he had sustained a serious injury. To our surprise, the patient regained consciousness, but he was not making sense, so I asked the K-9 officer to start documenting the incident while I began providing care.

Fifteen minutes passed before the ambulance arrived. During that time, the patient lapsed into and out of consciousness several times. After he initially regained consciousness, he lapsed into unconsciousness for several minutes. When he awoke, he started yelling very loudly, "Mamma! Mamma! Mamma!" Then he mumbled and was unconscious again for several minutes. The patient woke for a third time and began to moan and talk irrationally for about a minute. The entire time, we were observing the patient and documenting the incident.

The ambulance arrived and called the hospital with the information from our documentation. Because we were within minutes of the hospital, the emergency department surgeon and nurse met us at the scene. By this time, there were many responders to offer help and support on the scene. As the first responders on the scene, the K-9 officer and I gave our report to the EMTs and then to the surgeon. Our concise notes were taken to the emergency department with the patient for the neurosurgeon who would operate on him. Early that evening, the neurosurgeon contacted me to tell me that my concise and descriptive notes had helped him to quickly order tests and scans.

This call occurred early in my EMS career. I tell this story to every class of new EMS providers that I teach to remind them to always give concise and complete radio transmissions and to keep accurate patient information. It is important to always record all changes in patient behavior and levels of consciousness and follow up your oral report with written documentation of the run. Record everything that is unusual and take credit for the care you provided. It is a rule in EMS that if you didn't document it, it didn't happen.

Major Raymond W. Burton
Plymouth Regional Police Academy
Plymouth, Massachusetts

Tell the Truth

It is important to tell patients the truth. Telling the truth helps build trust with a patient. If you fail to tell the truth, the patient will not believe what you say in the future. There may be times when you do not need to tell the patient all the details in response to a question—and there will be times when you do not know the answer to a patient's question. In these cases, "I don't know" is an acceptable answer.

Allow Time for the Patient to Respond

Rushing a patient often hampers communication and delays the exchange of critical information. Because emergency situations can be hectic, you should bring a calm approach to the situation. Patients who are sick or injured may be confused and not thinking clearly. They will need time to answer even simple questions. Ask one question at a time and allow adequate time for the patient to respond to each question.

Limit the Number of People Talking With the Patient

Designate one provider to talk with the patient. This allows the patient to focus on the questions from one person. It avoids the confusion that results when multiple people are trying to question the patient at the same time. If other providers need to ask the patient questions, these questions can be addressed to the provider designated to talk with the patient.

Be Aware of Your Body Language

Your body language is a type of nonverbal communication. Do not talk down to a patient. If a patient is sitting or lying on the ground, kneel down to get close to the same level as the patient's face. Get close enough to the patient for comfortable conversation Figure 8-6 ▶. However, avoid getting so close that you invade the comfort zone of an agitated patient. Watch your stance. Crossing your arms in front of you may be interpreted as communicating an uncaring attitude.

Act and Speak in a Calm, Confident Manner

Emergency scenes can be noisy, confusing, and scary for patients. Remember that although it is not an emergency for you, this situation is an emergency for the patient. Your role is to render

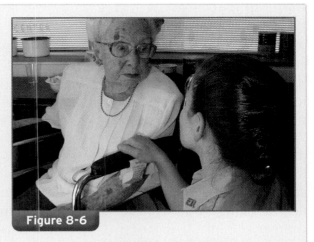

Figure 8-6

Use good body language. Get close enough to the patient to allow for comfortable conversation.

medical care that helps bring the emergency phase of this situation to an end. First responders need to convey a calm, caring, confident manner to the people present at the scene. Try to make the patient physically comfortable and relaxed.

Treat All Patients as if They Were Members of Your Family

Treat every patient the way you would like a member of your family to be treated. Remember that every patient you treat is someone's mother, father, sister, brother, daughter, or son. This guideline will facilitate effective communication with patients of all ages.

Communicating With Special Patients

Communicating with special types of patients requires additional considerations. Special patients include hearing-impaired patients, visually impaired patients, older patients, children, developmentally disabled patients, and persons displaying disruptive behavior.

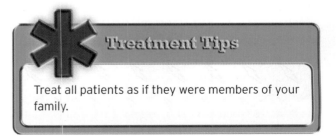

Treatment Tips

Treat all patients as if they were members of your family.

Communicating With Hearing-Impaired Patients

A major challenge faced by first responders is communicating with a deaf person. Most people have few skills for dealing with deaf persons and feel uncomfortable when asked to do so. A patient of any age may be unable to hear you for a variety of reasons: hereditary deafness; long-term deafness caused by illness, ear infections, or injury; or temporary deafness caused by an explosion or other loud noise. A patient who has been deaf for a long time usually develops skills to help compensate for the deafness. A patient who is temporarily deaf (such as from an explosion) does not have such skills.

In either case, your job is to address the medical needs of the patient. Ask, "Can you hear me?" A patient who is used to being deaf will probably respond by pointing at his or her ear and shaking his or her head to indicate deafness. The temporarily deaf person may feel anxious and panicky because he or she suddenly cannot hear. Help him or her focus on the problem by pointing at your ear and shaking your head to indicate deafness, or write out the question, "Can you hear?" on a piece of paper and show it to the patient.

After you determine that the patient is deaf, do not continue to rely on verbal communication; use other methods. It is difficult to read lips, and someone who is temporarily deaf will not have that skill anyway. A patient with long-term deafness may attempt to communicate with you by signing (using the hands and fingers to communicate). If you cannot sign, rely on writing and gestures to communicate.

As you examine the patient for injury or pain, use your own body to show the patient how to indicate whether there is pain in a particular location. Touch a place on your body and make a face to indicate pain. Then look at the patient and repeat the procedure on the patient's body. Most people will understand what you are trying to do. Do a complete patient assessment on every patient, whether or not he or she can communicate with you.

Keep the patient informed by making gestures to indicate that certain things are happening (for example, when the ambulance is arriving). Touch-

ing is an important part of communication and reassurance for both deaf and hearing patients. Hold the patient's hand so that he or she knows you are there to help.

When working with deaf patients:

- Identify yourself by showing the patient your patch or badge.
- Touch the patient; a deaf patient needs human contact just as much as a hearing patient.
- Face the patient when you speak so he or she can see your lips and facial expressions.
- Speak slowly and distinctly; do not shout.
- Watch the patient's face for expressions of understanding or uncertainty.
- Repeat or rephrase your comments in clear, simple language.
- If all this fails, write down your questions and offer paper and pencil to the patient to respond.
- Some people are both deaf and blind. This double loss may make these patients difficult to treat. Take your time, be patient, and use touch as a way of communicating.

If the patient is a hearing child of deaf parents, be sure to communicate with the parents about the child's condition and your actions. Like all other parents in similar circumstances, deaf parents must give their consent for you to treat their child. They have a right to know what is being done and are probably just as upset as hearing parents would be. If the patient is a deaf child of hearing parents, you need to involve the parents even more than usual. They can assist you in communicating with the child.

If the patient is a deaf parent with a hearing child, resist the urge to use the child as an interpreter unless the child is obviously mature and capable. Young children cannot understand medical terminology, and misinterpretation can have

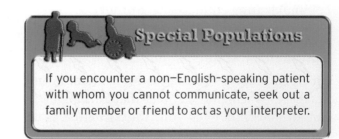

Special Populations

If you encounter a non–English-speaking patient with whom you cannot communicate, seek out a family member or friend to act as your interpreter.

very serious results. Communicate directly with the deaf patient, using whatever methods you can.

Communicating With Visually Impaired Patients

During your initial overview of the scene, look for signs that indicate the patient may be visually impaired. These may include the presence of eye glasses, a white cane, or a service dog. As you approach, introduce yourself to the patient. If you think the patient is blind, ask, "Can you see?"

A visually impaired patient may feel vulnerable, especially during the chaos of an accident scene. The patient may have learned to use other senses such as hearing, touch, and smell, to compensate for the loss of sight. The sounds and smells of an accident may be disorienting. The patient may rely on you to make sense of everything. Tell the patient what is happening, identify noises, and describe the situation and surroundings, particularly if you must move the patient.

Find out what the patient's name is and use it throughout your examination and treatment, just as you would with a sighted patient. Touch the patient to provide psychological support. If the patient has a service dog, he or she may initially be more concerned about the dog than about his or her own injuries. Recognize that the dog and the patient are a unique team who depend on each other. Let the patient direct the dog or tell you how to handle the dog. Use the techniques of restatement and redirection to focus the patient's attention on the problem at hand. Remember that service dogs are usually not aggressive and try to keep the patient and the dog together. If a blind patient must be moved and can walk, ask the patient to hold onto your elbow and stand slightly to your side and rear. Tell the patient about obstructions, steps, and curbs as you lead the way.

Many people make the mistake of talking louder when communicating with visually impaired patients. Remember that visual impairment and hearing impairment are not related. When dealing with a visually impaired patient, it may be helpful to maintain contact with them to let them know that you are still there. Emergencies are especially scary when a person is unable to see. Try to explain what you are doing for the patient. Tell them when they will feel move-

ment or noise and explain any treatments that they require.

Communicating With Non–English-Speaking Patients

In many areas of the country and in many urban areas, there are communities where English is not the first or even the most common language. If your patient speaks a language other than English and you cannot understand each other, you must find ways to communicate so that you can meet your responsibility as a first responder to provide the appropriate standard of care. You may be able to adapt some of the techniques recommended for communicating with a deaf patient. Determine how much English the patient speaks. Seek out a family member or friend to be your interpreter.

Supplement your questions with hand gestures, finger-pointing, and facial expressions. If your jurisdiction has a large non–English-speaking population, you should make a serious attempt to learn common phrases and questions so that you can use them when treating these patients.

Communicating With Older Patients

Older people tend to use emergency medical services more frequently than younger people. As people age, they are more likely to experience decreased vision and diminished hearing. When dealing with older people who suffer hearing or visual impairment, use the same communication skills you would for any other patients with similar conditions. Do not assume that all older patients have physical or mental impairments. Some older people are remarkably alert and healthy. Others suffer from a variety of physical and mental impairments. Assess all patients carefully and give them time to respond to your questions. Be aware of how older patients respond to you; it may give you clues as to how best to communicate with them.

Communicating With Pediatric Patients

Caring for ill or injured children is a stress-producing situation for most medical care providers. Children are often frightened, anxious, and unable to communicate the problem clearly; their parents are usually frightened and anxious

as well. Familiar objects and faces can help reduce this fright for children. Let a child keep a
favorite doll, toy, or blanket to give the child some
sense of comfort. Because children often take cues
from their parents, use the parents as allies in reassuring and calming the child. Talk to both the
parents and the child as much as possible and tell
them what is happening. Ask a parent to hold the
child if the illness or injury permits.

Speak to the child in a professional yet
friendly manner; tell the child your first name
and explain what you are doing. A child should
feel reassured that you are there to help in every
possible way. Do not stand over the child. Squat,
kneel, or sit down and establish eye contact
 Figure 8-7 ▾ . Ask the child simple questions
about the pain and to help you by pointing to
painful areas. Be honest. The level of understanding you can receive from an ill or injured
child is often remarkable.

Communicating With Developmentally Disabled Patients

You may find it difficult to communicate with developmentally disabled patients. Ask the family
about the patient's typical level of communication. Speak slowly, using short sentences and simple words. You may need to repeat statements
several times, or to rephrase them until the patient
understands what you want.

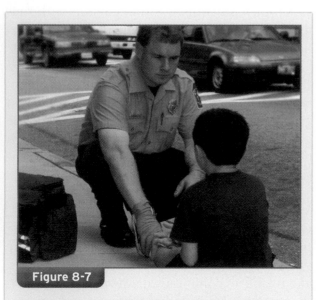

Figure 8-7

Squat, kneel, or sit when treating a pediatric patient.

Again, offer support by taking time to touch
your patients. Because the commotion surrounding an accident may confuse these patients
or make them afraid, use extra care in dealing
with developmentally disabled patients. You may
be able to adapt many of the techniques that you
use when treating children to your work with developmentally disabled patients.

Persons Displaying Disruptive Behavior

Disruptive behavior can present a danger to the
patient or others, and can cause delays in treatment. At some time in your career, you will encounter a person who challenges your patience
and communication skills.

In managing any patient who is exhibiting
disruptive behavior, take the following steps:
1. Assess the situation. Try to determine the
   cause of the patient's disruptive behavior.
2. Protect the patient and yourself.
3. Do not take your eyes off the patient or turn
   your back.
4. If the patient has a weapon, stay clear and wait
   for law enforcement personnel—no matter
   how badly injured the patient seems to be.
5. As soon as your personal safety is assured,
   carry out the appropriate emergency medical
   care.

There may be times when you are unable to
approach a patient; the person will not allow anyone to come near, despite all efforts to help. Sometimes family or friends of the disruptive patient
may insist that you take the person to the hospital, but you cannot take the patient to the hospital against his or her wishes (unless you are a
law enforcement officer). Frightened, agitated,
drugged, or disruptive patients can cause serious
injury to the first responder, bystanders, or themselves. It is best to wait for additional assistance
in these cases.

Documentation

Documentation constitutes the second major type
of communication. Documentation is a process
for verifying your actions using written records
 Figure 8-8 ▸ or computer-based records. By
recording the actions you took at an emergency
incident, you provide a record for others and a

Figure 8-8

A paper-based run form.

document you can refer to in the future if necessary. Documentation is helpful to you because you will not be able to remember all the details of every call. It also provides a legal record for the actions you took. It is often said that if you did not document it, it was not done. Documentation also provides a basis to evaluate the quality of care given. Remember that the call is not over until the paperwork is completed.

Proper documentation includes the following:
- The age and sex of the patient
- The history of the incident
- The condition of the patient when found
- The patient's description of the injury or illness
- The patient's chief complaint
- The patient's level of responsiveness
- The status of initial and later vital signs: airway, breathing, and circulation (including severe bleeding)

- The results of the physical examination
- Pertinent medical conditions using the SAMPLE format
- The treatment you gave the patient
- The agency and personnel who took over treatment of the patient
- Any other helpful facts
- Any reportable conditions present
- Any infectious disease exposure
- Anything unusual about the case

These topics include all the information in your hand-off report. Complete your run report as soon as possible after each call. Your documentation should be clear, concise, and accurate. Follow the standards of your organization for documentation. Some agencies use a paper-based reporting system, while others use a computer-based system. Either type of system can work well provided that you complete the reports accurately. If you make a mistake on the form, document and correct it.

Your organization may rely on run reports for documenting reportable events. Remember that reportable events include certain crimes and infectious diseases. Reportable crimes include knife wounds, gunshot wounds, motor vehicle collisions, suspected child abuse, domestic violence, elder abuse, dog bites, and rape. As a first responder, you need to learn which crimes are reportable in your area and your agency's procedures on reporting these crimes. Certain infectious diseases are also reportable. It is important that you learn how this process is handled in your agency and what you are required to do.

You are the Provider

SUMMARY

Review the *You are the Provider* case study provided at the beginning of the chapter.

Just as you are finishing your lunch, you hear the alert tones on your mobile radio. Your dispatcher announces, "Unit 403, respond to a vehicle collision with injuries at the corner of Main Street and University Drive. Your time out is thirteen forty-seven. Your run number is three-two-six-five."

1. How do the functions of the radio communications system change during different phases of an emergency medical call?

The functions of radio communications change throughout different phases of a call. The function of dispatch is to relay information about the location and type of call to responding units. Responding units then verify that they are en route. Upon arrival at the scene, the responding units notify the dispatcher that they are on the scene and transmit additional information about the call to the dispatcher. They may also update other responding units. EMS transport units use radio communications to give the receiving hospital a patient report. In addition, units notify the dispatcher when they are done with a call and ready for service.

2. Why is it important to have protocols for the use of a radio communications system?

Radio protocols are important because they improve the efficiency of radio communications and reduce the time each unit needs to spend on the air. Protocols also provide a standard format that reduces miscommunications.

3. Why is it important to document your observations, assessments, and treatments for each call?

Documenting observations, assessments, and treatments for each call is important because this information can be relayed to other members of the emergency medical services team and to hospital personnel. Written documentation is also important in the event of a court case because it will refresh your memory about the details of the incident.

Prep Kit

Ready for Review

The Ready for Review thoroughly summarizes this chapter.

- Communications systems allow you to relay information from one location to another when it is impossible to communicate face to face. Excellent communication skills are crucial during every phase of a call.

- It is important for you as a first responder to have a basic idea of how your department's communications system works.

- You must be familiar with two-way radio communications and have a working knowledge of mobile and hand-held portable radios. You must know when to use them and what type of information you can transmit.

- Throughout the difference phases of an EMS call, communication systems are used for different functions. The phases of an EMS call include dispatch, response to the scene, arrival at the scene, updating the responding EMS units, transferring care of the patient to other personnel, and postrun activities.

- The protocols for communicating with others during each phase of an EMS call may vary from one system to another. It is important that you learn and follow the standard procedures and protocols of your department.

- In addition to radio and oral communications, first responders must have excellent person-to-person communication skills. You should be able to interact with the patient and any family members, friends, or bystanders.

- It is important for you to remember that people who are sick or injured may not understand what you are doing or saying. Therefore, your body language and attitude are very important in gaining the trust of both the patient and family. You must also take special care of individuals such as children, geriatric patients, hearing-impaired and visually impaired patients, non–English-speaking patients, developmentally disabled patients, and persons displayed disruptive behavior.

- Along with your radio report and oral report, you must also complete a formal hand-off report to other EMS professionals at the scene. Documentation provides a legal record for the actions you took and provides a basis to evaluate the quality of care given. Remember that the call is not over until the paperwork is completed.

Technology

- Interactivities
- Vocabulary Explorer
- Anatomy Review
- Web Links
- Online Review Manual

Vital Vocabulary

The Vital Vocabulary are the key terms for this chapter.

base station A powerful two-way radio that is permanently mounted in a communications center.

fax machine A device used to send or receive printed text documents or images over a telephone or radio system.

mobile data terminal (MDT) A computer terminal mounted in a vehicle that sends and receives data through a radio communication system.

mobile radio A two-way radio that is permanently mounted in a vehicle such as a police car or fire truck.

paging systems Communications systems used to send voice or text messages over a radio system to specially designed radio receivers.

portable radio A hand-held, battery-operated, two-way radio.

repeater A radio system that automatically retransmits a radio signal on a different frequency.

telemetry A process in which electronic signals are transmitted and received by radio or telephone; commonly used for sending EKG tracings.

Assessment in Action

Assessment in Action presents a fictitious scenario to help you review what you learned in this chapter.

You are dispatched to 124 Ann Street for a 68-year-old female who is experiencing pain in the right side of her abdomen.

1. As you use your radio during this call, the agency that has responsibility for regulating your radio communications is:

   A. The Department of Homeland Security
   B. Your department
   C. The Federal Communications Commission
   D. Your state EMS agency

2. Which of the following is NOT a guideline for increasing effective communication with patients?

   A. Ask the patient's name and use it.
   B. Tell the truth.
   C. Allow a limited time for the patient to respond.
   D. Limit the number of people talking with the patient.

3. The husband of your patient on this call is hearing impaired. Which of the following actions is incorrect?

   A. Ask him if he can hear you.
   B. Stand in a position where he can see your lips while you talk to him.
   C. Write your questions on a sheet of paper and show them to him.
   D. Talk louder and louder until he can hear you.

4. The EMS transport unit arrives and is prepared to take over the care of this patient. Which of the following information should be included in your hand-off report?

   1. The history of the incident
   2. The patient's level of responsiveness
   3. The results of your physical exam
   4. The interventions you provided
      A. 1, 2, 3
      B. 1, 3, 4
      C. All of the above
      D. 1 and 3

5. Your documentation of this call should include:

   1. All information given in your hand-off report
   2. Pertinent medical conditions
   3. The agency and personnel who took over the care of this patient
   4. Anything unusual about this case
      A. None of the above should be included
      B. 1-3
      C. 1, 3, 4
      D. All of the above

Circulation

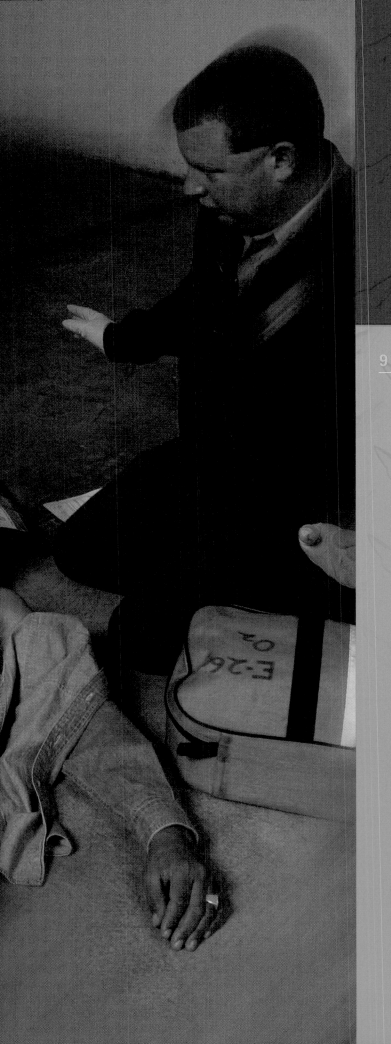

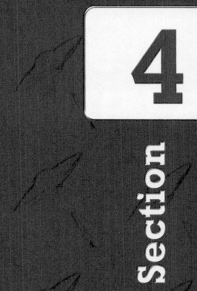

Professional Rescuer CPR

You are the Provider

You just started your morning shift and are in the middle of checking your equipment when you hear the click of the PA system that precedes an alarm. You stop what you are doing so you can hear the dispatcher. "Unit 433 respond to 10711 Mathews Court for a 74-year-old male experiencing shortness of breath. Time out is 0733."

You arrive on the scene 4 minutes later. As you and your partner enter the front door of the residence, a woman excitedly tells you that her husband slumped over in his chair just as you were pulling into the driveway.

1. What are the first steps you need to take?
2. What is the chance for a successful outcome on this call?
3. Your department has just placed automated external defibrillators on all units. How does this change your treatment of this patient?

Introduction

The purpose of this chapter is to teach you the remaining skills to perform cardiopulmonary resuscitation (CPR). CPR consists of three major skills: the A (airway) skills, the B (breathing) skills, and the C (circulation) skills. In Chapter 6, you learned the airway and breathing skills. These airway and breathing steps may be lifesaving procedures for a patient who has stopped breathing and whose heart is still beating. In most cases, however, by the time you arrive on the scene, the patient has not only stopped breathing, but the heart has stopped beating as well. If the patient is not breathing and has no heartbeat, rescue breathing alone will not save the patient's life. Forcing air into the lungs is useless unless the circulatory system can carry the oxygen in the lungs to all parts of the body.

In this chapter, you will learn the C (circulation) skills. If the patient's heart has stopped, you can maintain or restore circulation manually through the use of chest compressions (closed-chest cardiac massage). To maintain both breathing and heartbeat, rescue breathing and chest compressions must be done together. By combining the airway, breathing, and circulation skills, you will be able to perform CPR. Because about

70% of the patients who suffer cardiac arrest are in a state of ventricular fibrillation (V-fib)—a condition in which the heart muscle is "quivering" and not effectively pumping blood—this chapter covers the theory and steps needed to use an automated defibrillator to defibrillate these patients.

Anatomy and Function of the Circulatory System

The circulatory system is similar to a city water system because both consist of a pump (the heart), a network of pipes (the blood vessels), and fluid (blood). After blood picks up oxygen in the lungs, it goes to the heart, which pumps the oxygenated blood to the rest of the body.

In Chapter 4, you learned how the heart functions as a pump. The heart, which is about the size of your fist, is located in the chest between the lungs. The cells of the body absorb oxygen and nutrients from the blood and produce waste products (including carbon dioxide) that the blood carries back to the lungs. In the lungs, the blood exchanges the carbon dioxide for more oxygen. Blood then returns to the heart to be pumped out again.

The human heart consists of four chambers, two on the patient's right side and two on the patient's left side. Each upper chamber is called an atrium. The right atrium receives blood from the veins of the body; the left atrium receives highly oxygenated blood from the lungs. The bottom chambers are the ventricles. The right ventricle pumps deoxygenated blood to the lungs; the left ventricle pumps highly oxygenated blood throughout the body. The most muscular chamber of the heart is the left ventricle, which needs the most power because it must force blood to all parts of the body. Together the four chambers of the heart work in a well-ordered sequence to pump blood to the lungs and to the rest of the body Figure 9-1 ▶ .

One-way valves in the heart and veins allow the blood to flow only one direction through the circulatory system. The arteries carry blood away from the heart at high pressure and are therefore thick walled. The main artery carrying blood away

Technology

- Interactivities
- Vocabulary Explorer
- Anatomy Review
- Web Links
- Online Review Manual

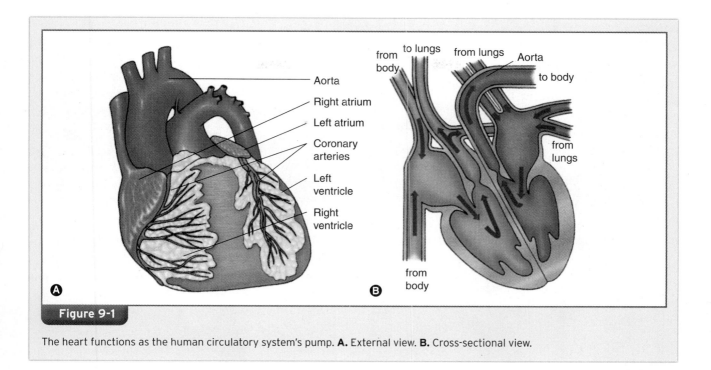

Figure 9-1

The heart functions as the human circulatory system's pump. **A.** External view. **B.** Cross-sectional view.

from the heart is quite large (about 1 inch in diameter) but arteries become smaller farther away from the heart.

The four major arteries are located in the neck, or (carotid) arteries; the wrist (radial) artery; the arm (brachial) artery; and the groin (femoral) artery. The locations of these arteries are shown in **Figure 9-2**. Because these arteries lie between a bony structure and the skin, they can be used to measure the patient's **pulse**. A pulse is generated when the heart contracts and sends a pressure wave through the artery. The capillaries are the smallest pipes in the circulatory system. Some capillaries are so small that only one blood cell at a time can go through them. At the capillary level, oxygen passes from the blood cells into the cells of body tissues, and carbon dioxide and other waste products pass from the tissue cells to the blood cells, which then return to the lungs. Veins are the thin-walled pipes of the circulatory system that carry blood back to the heart.

Blood has several components: **plasma** (a clear, straw-colored fluid), red blood cells, white blood cells, and **platelets** **Figure 9-3**. The red blood cells give blood its red color. Red blood cells carry oxygen from the lungs to the body and bring car-

bon dioxide back to the lungs. The white blood cells are called infection fighters because they devour bacteria and other disease-causing organisms. Platelets start the blood-clotting process.

Cardiac Arrest

<u>Cardiac arrest</u> occurs when the heart stops contracting, and no blood is pumped through the blood vessels. Without a supply of blood, the cells of the body will die because they cannot get any oxygen and nutrients and they cannot eliminate waste products. As the cells die, organ damage occurs. Some organs are more sensitive to low oxygen levels than others. Brain damage begins within 4 to 6 minutes after the patient has suffered cardiac arrest. Within 8 to 10 minutes, the damage to the brain may become irreversible. Cardiac arrest may have many different causes:

1. Heart and blood vessel diseases such as heart attack and stroke
2. Respiratory arrest, if untreated
3. Medical emergencies such as epilepsy, diabetes, allergic reactions, electrical shock, and poisoning
4. Drowning

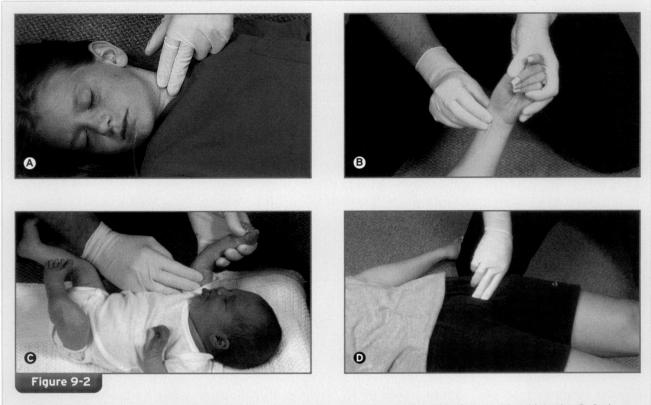

Figure 9-2

Locations for assessing the patient's pulse. **A.** Neck or carotid pulse. **B.** Wrist or radial pulse. **C.** Arm or brachial pulse. **D.** Groin or femoral pulse.

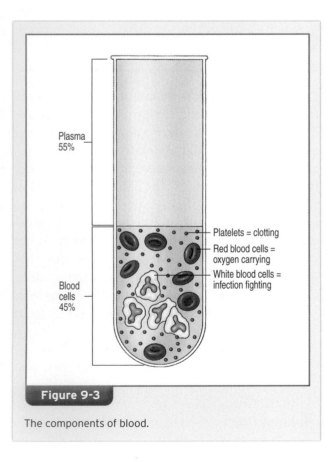

Figure 9-3

The components of blood.

Plasma 55%

Platelets = clotting

Red blood cells = oxygen carrying

White blood cells = infection fighting

Blood cells 45%

5. Suffocation
6. Trauma and shock caused by massive blood loss

A patient who has suffered cardiac arrest is unconscious and is not breathing. You cannot feel a pulse and the patient looks dead. Regardless of the cause of cardiac arrest, the initial treatment is the same: CPR.

Components of CPR

The technique of cardiopulmonary resuscitation requires three types of skills: the A (airway) skills, the B (breathing) skills, and the C (circulation) skills. In Chapter 6, you learned the airway and breathing skills. You learned how to check patients to determine if the airway is open and to correct a blocked airway by using the head tilt–chin lift or jaw-thrust maneuvers. You learned how to check patients to determine if they are breathing by using the look, listen, and feel technique. You learned to correct the absence of breathing by performing rescue breathing.

To perform CPR, you must combine the airway and breathing skills with circulation skills. You begin by checking the patient for a pulse. If there is no pulse, you must correct the patient's circulation by performing external chest compressions. The airway and breathing skills you know will push oxygen into the patient's lungs. External chest compressions move the oxygenated blood throughout the body. By compressing the patient's sternum (breastbone), you change the pressure in the patient's chest and force enough blood through the system to sustain life for a short period of time.

CPR by itself cannot sustain life indefinitely. However, it should be started as soon as possible to give the patient the best chance for survival. By performing all three parts of the CPR sequence, you can keep the patient alive until more advanced medical care can be administered. In many cases, the patient will need defibrillation and medication in order to be successfully resuscitated from cardiac arrest.

In the Field

Patients who are experiencing cardiac events—as well as their family members and friends—will usually be fearful and anxious about the episode. It is important for first responders to demonstrate a caring attitude and acknowledge those feelings. Although your primary goal is to ensure that the patient receives appropriate and timely care, you should also be sure to communicate with compassion during cardiac events.

The Cardiac Chain of Survival

In most cases of cardiac arrest, CPR alone is not sufficient to save lives, but it is the first treatment in the American Heart Association's Chain of Survival. The links in the chain include:
1. Early recognition of cardiac arrest and activation of the 9-1-1 system
2. Early bystander CPR
3. Early defibrillation by first responders or other EMS personnel
4. Early advanced care by paramedics and hospital personnel

As a first responder, you can help the patient by providing early CPR and by making sure that the EMS system has been activated. Some first responders may also be trained in the use of automated defibrillators. By keeping these links of the chain strong, you will help keep the patient alive until early advanced care can be administered by paramedics and hospital personnel. Just as an actual chain is only as strong as its weakest link, the Chain of Survival is only as good as its weakest link. Your actions in performing early CPR are vital to giving cardiac arrest patients their best chance for survival Figure 9-4 ▸ .

When to Start CPR

CPR should be started on all nonbreathing, pulseless patients, unless they are obviously dead or unless they have a do not resuscitate (DNR) order that is valid in your jurisdiction. (DNR orders are discussed more fully in this chapter under legal implications of CPR.) Few reliable criteria exist to determine death immediately.

The following criteria are reliable signs of death and indicate that CPR should not be started.
1. **Decapitation.** Decapitation occurs when the head is separated from the rest of the body. When this occurs, there is obviously no chance of saving the patient.
2. **Rigor mortis.** This is the temporary stiffening of muscles that occurs several hours after death. Rigor mortis indicates the patient has been dead for a prolonged period of time and cannot be resuscitated.
3. **Evidence of tissue decomposition.** Tissue decomposition or actual flesh decay occurs only after a person has been dead for more than a day.
4. **Dependent lividity.** Dependent lividity is the red or purple color that appears on the parts of the patient's body that are closest to the ground. It is caused by blood seeping into the tissues on the dependent, or lower, part of the person's body. Dependent lividity occurs after a person has been dead for several hours.

If any of the preceding signs of death is present in a pulseless, nonbreathing person, do not begin CPR. If none of these signs is present, you should activate the EMS system and then begin CPR. It is far better to start CPR on a person who is later de-

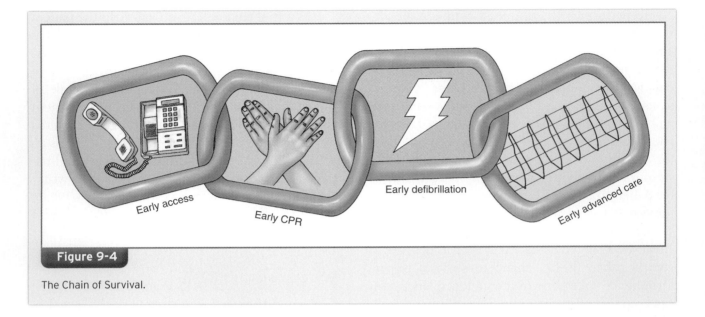

Figure 9-4

The Chain of Survival.

clared dead by a physician than to withhold CPR from a patient whose life might have been saved.

When to Stop CPR

You should discontinue CPR only when:
1. Effective spontaneous circulation and ventilation is restored.
2. Resuscitation efforts are transferred to another trained person who continues CPR.
3. A physician orders you to stop.
4. The patient is transferred to properly trained EMS personnel.
5. Reliable criteria for death (as previously listed) are recognized.
6. You are too exhausted to continue resuscitation, environmental hazards endanger your safety, or continued resuscitation would place the lives of others at risk.

The Technique of External Cardiac Compression in an Adult

A patient in cardiac arrest is unconscious and is not breathing. You cannot feel a pulse and the patient looks dead. If you suspect that the patient has suffered cardiac arrest, first check and correct the airway, then check and correct the breathing,

and finally check for circulation. Check for circulation by feeling the carotid pulse and looking for signs of coughing or movement. To check the carotid pulse, place your index and middle fingers on the larynx (Adam's apple). Now slide your fingers into the groove between the larynx and the muscles at the side of the neck Figure 9-5 ▾. Keep your fingers there for at least 5 seconds but no more than 10 seconds to be sure the pulse is absent and not just slow. As you check the pulse, look for signs of coughing or movement that may indicate circulation is present.

If there is no carotid pulse in an unresponsive patient, you must begin chest compressions. For chest compressions to be effective, the patient must be lying on a firm, horizontal surface. If the

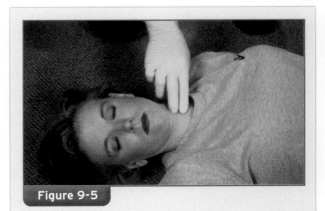

Figure 9-5

Check the patient's carotid pulse.

Safety Tips

Practice good body substance isolation (BSI) when doing CPR.

Treatment Tips

Do not let your fingers touch the chest wall; your fingers could dig into the patient, causing injury. Interlocking your fingers will help avoid this.

patient is on a soft surface, such as a bed, it is impossible to compress the chest. Immediately place all patients needing CPR on a firm, level surface.

To perform chest compressions effectively, stand or kneel beside the patient's chest and face the patient. Place the heel of one hand in the center of the patient's chest, in between the nipples. Place the heel of the other hand on top of the hand on the chest, and interlock your fingers **Skill Drill 9-1 ▶** .

SKILL DRILL 9-1

1. Locate the top and bottom of the sternum **Step 1** .
2. Place the heel of your hand in the center of the chest, in between the nipples **Step 2** .
3. Place your other hand on top of your first hand and interlock your fingers **Step 3** .

It is important to locate and maintain the proper hand position while applying chest compressions. If your hands are too high, the force you apply will not produce adequate chest compressions. If your hands are too low, the force you apply may damage the liver. If your hands slip sideways off the sternum and onto the ribs, the compressions will not be effective and you may damage the ribs and lungs.

After you have both hands in the proper position, compress the chest of an adult $1\frac{1}{2}$ to 2 inches straight down. For compressions to be effective, stay close to the patient's side and lean forward so that your arms are directly over the patient. Keep your back straight and your elbows stiff so you can apply the force of your whole body to each compression, not just your arm muscles. Between compressions, keep the heel of your hand on the patient's chest but allow the

chest to completely recoil. Compressions must be rhythmic and continuous. Each compression cycle consists of one downward push followed by a rest so that the heart can refill with blood. Push hard and push fast. Compressions should be at the rate of 100 compressions per minute in all patients—adults, children, and infants. After every 30 chest compressions, give two rescue breaths (1 second per breath). Practice on a manikin until you can compress the chest smoothly and rhythmically.

External Chest Compressions on an Infant

Infants (children under 1 year of age) who have suffered cardiac arrest will be unconscious and not breathing. They will have no pulse. To check for cardiac arrest, first check and correct the airway. Remember not to tilt the head back too far because this may occlude the infant's airway. Next check for breathing by using the look, listen, and feel technique. Correct the absence of breathing by giving mouth-to-mouth-and-nose rescue breathing.

To check an infant's circulation, feel for the brachial pulse on the inside of the upper arm **Figure 9-6 ▶** . Use two fingers of one hand to feel for the pulse and use the other hand to maintain the head tilt. If there is no pulse, begin chest compressions. Draw an imaginary horizontal line between the two nipples, and place your index finger just below the imaginary line in the center of the chest. Place your middle and ring fingers next to your index finger. Use your middle and ring fingers to compress the sternum approximately one half to one third the depth of the chest. Compress the sternum at a rate of 100 times per minute. If you are the only rescuer, give

Skill DRILL 9-1

Performing Chest Compressions

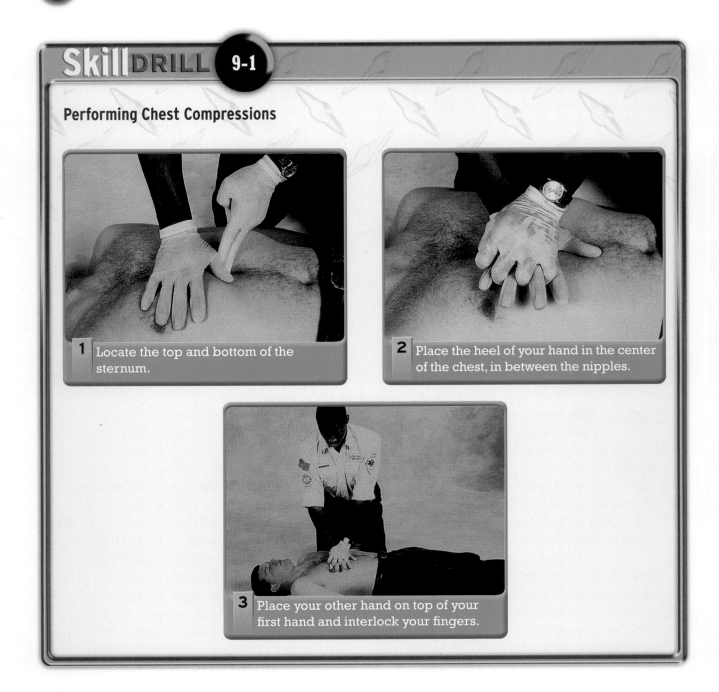

1 Locate the top and bottom of the sternum.

2 Place the heel of your hand in the center of the chest, in between the nipples.

3 Place your other hand on top of your first hand and interlock your fingers.

two rescue breaths (1 second per breath) after every 30 chest compressions. If two rescuers are present, give two rescue breaths after every 15 chest compressions.

Place the infant on a solid surface such as a table or cradle the infant in your arm, as shown in Figure 9-7 ▶ , when doing chest compressions. You will not need to use much force to achieve adequate compressions on infants be-

cause they are so small and their chests are so pliable.

External Chest Compressions on a Child

The signs of cardiac arrest in a **child** (from 1 year of age to the onset of puberty [12 to 14 years of age]) are the same as those for an adult

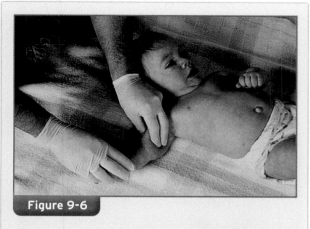

Figure 9-6

Check the brachial pulse on the inside of the infant's arm.

and for an infant. If you suspect that a child is in cardiac arrest, first check and correct the child's airway, then check and correct the child's breathing, and finally check for circulation. Check the carotid pulse by placing two or three fingers on the larynx. Slide your fingers into the groove between the Adam's apple and the muscle. Feel for the carotid pulse with one hand and maintain the head-tilt position with the other hand.

To perform chest compressions on a small child, place the heel of one hand in the center of the chest, in between the nipples. In larger children, perform chest compressions with two hands,

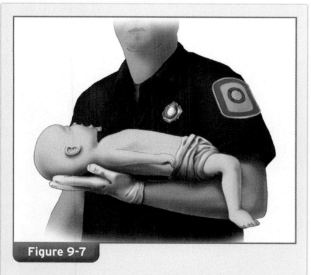

Figure 9-7

Positioning the infant patient for proper CPR.

as with the adult. Compress the sternum approximately one half to one third the depth of the chest. Compress the chest at a rate of 100 times per minute. If you are the only rescuer present, give two rescue breaths after every 30 chest compressions. If two rescuers are present, give two rescue breaths after every 15 compressions.

One-Rescuer Adult CPR

CPR consists of three skill sets: checking and correcting the airway, checking and correcting the breathing, and checking and correcting the circulation. In Chapter 6, you learned to perform the airway and breathing skill sets. Now that you have learned how to check for circulation and do chest compressions, you are ready to put all your skills together to perform CPR. If you are the only trained person at the scene, you must perform <u>one-rescuer CPR</u>. Follow the steps in **Skill Drill 9-2 ▶**:

SKILL DRILL 9-2

1. Establish the patient's level of consciousness **Step 1**. Ask the patient, "Are you okay?" Gently shake the patient's shoulder. If there is no response, call for additional help by activating the EMS system. (Even if you are alone, phone 9-1-1 before you begin CPR.)
2. Turn the patient on his or her back, supporting the head and neck as you do.
3. Open the airway **Step 2**. Use the head tilt–chin lift maneuver or, if the patient is injured, use the jaw-thrust maneuver. If the jaw-thrust maneuver does not adequately open the airway, carefully perform the head tilt–chin lift maneuver. Maintain the open airway.
4. Check for breathing **Step 3**. Place the side of your face and your ear close to the nose and mouth of the patient. Look, listen, and feel for the movement of air: Look for movement of the chest, listen

Skill DRILL 9-2

One-Rescuer Adult CPR

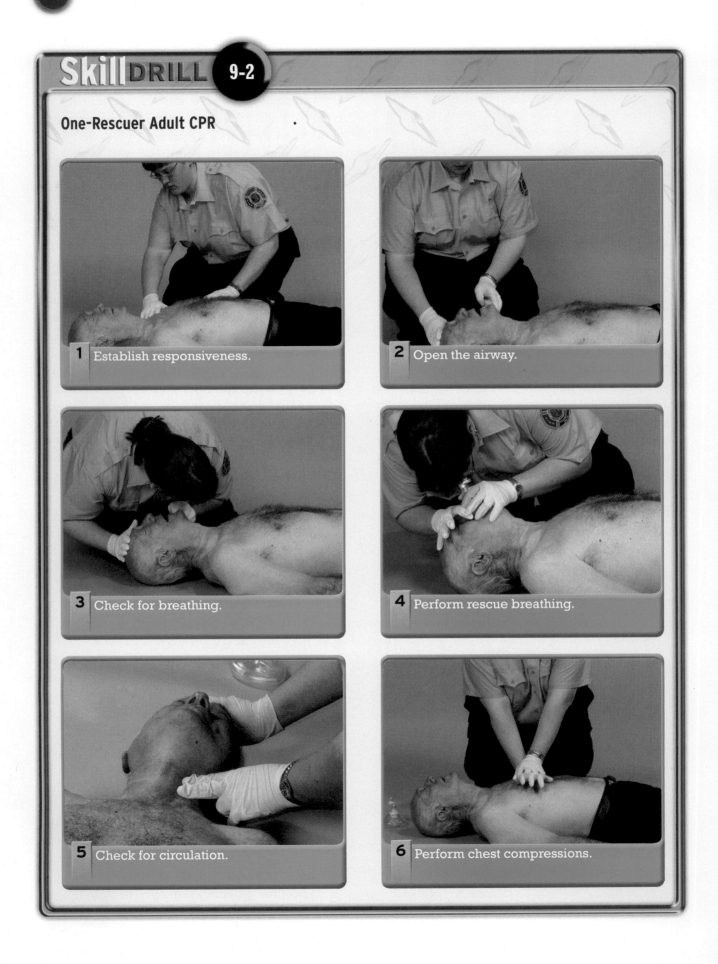

1. Establish responsiveness.

2. Open the airway.

3. Check for breathing.

4. Perform rescue breathing.

5. Check for circulation.

6. Perform chest compressions.

In the Field

If you do not have help, do not wait for another rescuer to arrive. Call 9-1-1 to activate EMS and then begin one-rescuer CPR immediately!

for sounds of air exchange, and feel for air movement on the side of your face. Your breathing check should last at least 5 seconds but no longer than 10 seconds. If there are no signs of breathing, begin rescue breathing. Use a mouth-to-mask ventilation device, if one is available, or place your mouth over the patient's mouth, seal the patient's nose with your thumb and index finger, and begin mouth-to-mouth rescue breathing.

5. Give two breaths `Step 4`. Blow slowly for 1 second using just enough force to make the chest visibly rise. Allow the lungs to deflate between breaths.

6. Check for signs of circulation by checking the carotid pulse and looking for signs of coughing or movement `Step 5`. Find the carotid pulse by locating the patient's larynx with your index and middle fingers, then sliding your fingers into the groove between the larynx and the muscles at the side of the neck. Check for at least 5 seconds but no more than 10 seconds. If the pulse is absent, proceed to the next step. If the pulse is present, continue rescue breathing every 5 to 6 seconds (10 to 12 breaths per minute).

7. Begin chest compressions `Step 6`. Place the heel of one hand in the center of the patient's chest, in between the nipples. Place the other hand on top of the first, so the hands are parallel. Now press down to compress the chest about 1½ to 2 inches. Apply 30 compressions at the rate of 100 compressions per minute. Count the compressions out loud: "One and two and three and."

8. After 30 chest compressions, give two rescue breaths.

9. Continue alternating compressions and **ventilations**. Deliver a sequence of 30 compressions followed by two ventilations.

10. After five cycles of CPR (about 2 minutes), check the carotid pulse.

11. If there is no pulse, continue CPR and recheck the patient in 2 minutes.

When performing one-rescuer CPR—whether the patient is an adult, child, or infant—you must deliver chest compressions and rescue breathing at a ratio of 30 compressions to two breaths. Immediately give two rescue breaths after each set of 30 chest compressions. Because you must interrupt chest compressions to ventilate, you should perform each series of 30 chest compressions in about 20 seconds (a rate of 100 compressions per minute).

A skill performance sheet titled One-Rescuer Adult CPR is shown in `Figure 9-8 ▸` for your review and practice.

Although one-rescuer CPR can keep the patient alive, two-rescuer CPR is preferable because it is less exhausting for the rescuers. Whenever possible, CPR for an adult should be performed by two rescuers.

Two-Rescuer Adult CPR

In many cases, a second trained person will be on the scene to help you perform CPR. Two-rescuer CPR is more effective than one-rescuer CPR. One rescuer can deliver chest compressions while the other performs rescue breathing. Chest compressions and ventilations can be given more regularly and without interruption. Two-rescuer CPR is also less tiring for the rescuers. However, to avoid rescuer fatigue—which may result in less effective chest compressions—two rescuers should switch roles after every five cycles of CPR (about every 2 minutes). Two rescuers should be able to switch roles quickly, interrupting CPR for 5 seconds or less. In any circumstance, CPR should not be interrupted for longer than 10 seconds.

In **two-rescuer CPR**, one rescuer delivers ventilations (mouth-to-mouth or mouth-to-mask

One-Rescuer Adult CPR

Steps	Adequately Performed
1. Establish unresponsiveness. Activate the EMS system.	
2. Open airway using head tilt–chin lift maneuver. (If trauma is present, use jaw-thrust maneuver.) Check for breathing (look, listen, and feel).*	
3. Give two slow breaths at 1 second per breath. If chest does not rise, reposition head and try to ventilate again. Watch for chest rise; allow for exhalation between breaths.	
4. Check for signs of circulation. Check carotid pulse and look for signs of coughing and movement. If breathing is absent but pulse is present, provide rescue breathing (one breath every 5 to 6 seconds [10 to 12 breaths per minute]).	
5. If no pulse, give cycles of 30 chest compressions (100 compressions per minute) followed by two slow breaths.	
6. After five cycles of 30 to 2 (about 2 minutes), check pulse.* If no pulse, continue CPR and recheck the patient in 2 minutes.	

*If victim is unresponsive but breathing, place in the recovery position.
Source: Based on the 2005 CPR and ECC guidelines.

Figure 9-8

Skill performance sheet.

breathing) and the other gives chest compressions. If possible, position yourselves on opposite sides of the patient—one near the head and the other near the chest. The sequence of steps is the same as for one-rescuer CPR, but the tasks are divided **Skill Drill 9-3** ▸:

Skill DRILL 9-3

1. Rescuer One (at the patient's head) determines the patient's level of consciousness by asking, "Are you okay?" If there is no response, the rescuer gently shakes the person's shoulder **Step 1**.
2. Call 9-1-1 to activate the EMS system if the patient is unconscious. If other people are present, ask them to call for EMS. If two rescuers are present, but no

bystanders are present, one rescuer should call 9-1-1 as the other continues to assess the patient.
3. Turn the patient on his or her back. Turn the patient as a unit, supporting the head and neck to protect the spine.
4. Rescuer One opens the airway using the head tilt–chin lift or jaw-thrust maneuver **Step 2**. If the jaw-thrust maneuver does not adequately open the airway, carefully perform a head tilt–chin lift.
5. Rescuer One checks for breathing by placing the side of his or her face close to the mouth and nose of the patient to look for chest movements, listen for breathing sounds, and feel for air movement for at least 5 seconds but no more than 10 seconds **Step 3**. If there

Skill DRILL 9-3

Two-Rescuer Adult CPR

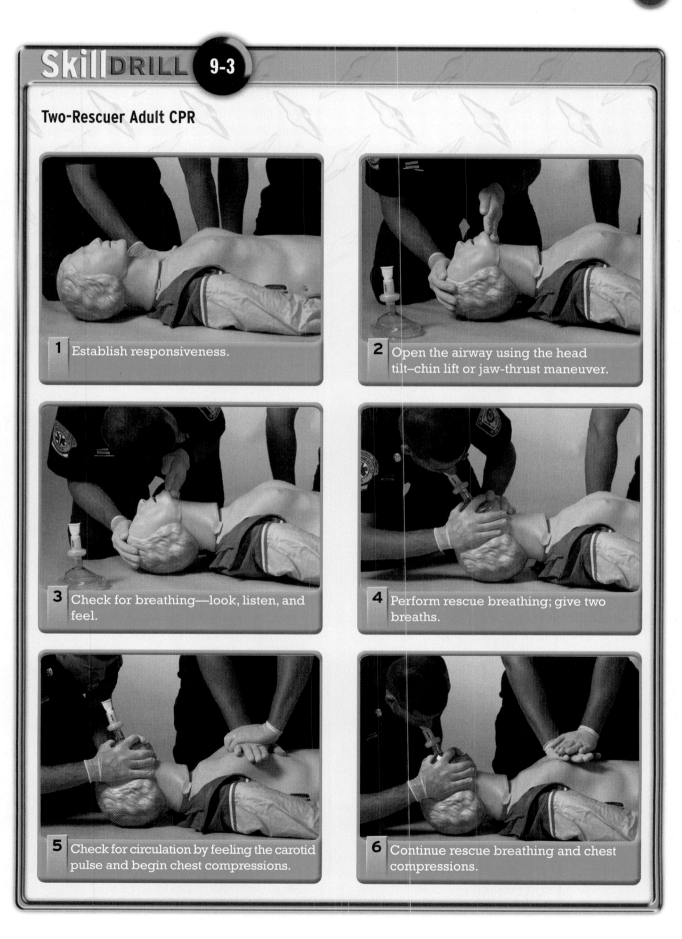

1 Establish responsiveness.

2 Open the airway using the head tilt–chin lift or jaw-thrust maneuver.

3 Check for breathing—look, listen, and feel.

4 Perform rescue breathing; give two breaths.

5 Check for circulation by feeling the carotid pulse and begin chest compressions.

6 Continue rescue breathing and chest compressions.

are no signs of breathing, proceed to the next step.

6. Rescuer One gives two breaths (1 second per breath). Allow time for complete deflation of the lungs between breaths `Step 4`.

7. Rescuer One checks for signs of circulation by checking for the presence of a carotid pulse and looking for signs of coughing and movement. Check the pulse for at least 5 seconds but no more than 10 seconds. If there is no carotid pulse, proceed to the following step.

8. Rescuer Two performs 30 chest compressions at a rate of 100 compressions per minute `Step 5`. Count "one and two and three" to maintain the proper rate of compressions and to let Rescuer One know when to ventilate.

9. After Rescuer Two completes 30 chest compressions, Rescuer One gives two ventilations. Rescuer Two should pause just long enough for Rescuer One to ventilate twice `Step 6`.

10. Periodically, Rescuer One should place his or her fingers on the carotid pulse of the patient as Rescuer Two continues the compressions. If the compressions are being done correctly, Rescuer One should feel a pulse with each compression. This confirms that the CPR is adequate.

11. After five cycles of CPR (about 2 minutes), Rescuer One should ask Rescuer Two to stop compressions as he or she rechecks the patient's pulse. If the patient's heart starts beating on its own, Rescuer One will continue to feel a pulse. In this case, Rescuer Two can stop doing compressions. Rescue breathing should be continued at a rate of 10 to 12 breaths per minute (one breath every 5 to 6 seconds) until spontaneous breathing resumes. If there is no pulse, CPR should be resumed.

Compressions and ventilations should remain rhythmic and uninterrupted. By counting out loud, Rescuer Two can continue to deliver compressions at the rate of 100 per minute, briefly pausing as Rescuer One delivers two rescue breaths. Once you and your partner establish a smooth pattern of CPR, you should limit interruptions in CPR to 10 seconds or less, such as when checking for a pulse or moving the patient. A skill performance sheet titled Two-Rescuer Adult CPR is shown in `Figure 9-9 ▸` for your review and practice.

FYI

Switching CPR Positions

If you and your partner must continue to perform two-rescuer CPR for an extended period of time, the person performing chest compressions will get tired. Once a rescuer gets tired, the effectiveness of chest compressions decreases. Because of this, rescuers should switch positions after every five cycles of CPR (about every 2 minutes). This will improve the quality of chest compressions and give the patient the best chance for survival.

A switch allows the person giving compressions (Rescuer Two) to rest his or her arms. Switching positions should be accomplished as smoothly and quickly (5 seconds or less) as possible to minimize the break in rate and regularity of compressions and ventilations. There are many orderly ways to switch positions. Learn the method practiced in your EMS system. One method is as follows:

1. As Rescuer Two tires, he or she says the following out loud (instead of counting): "We—will—switch—this—time." One word is spoken as each compression is done. These words replace the counting sequence for the first five compressions.

2. After 25 more chest compressions (a total of 30 compressions), Rescuer One completes two ventilations and moves to the chest to perform compressions.

3. Rescuer Two moves to the head of the patient to maintain the airway and ventilation and immediately checks the carotid pulse for at least 5 seconds but no more than 10 seconds. If the carotid pulse is absent, Rescuer Two says "No pulse; continue CPR."

Two-Rescuer Adult CPR

Steps	Adequately Performed
RESCUER ONE	
1. Establish unresponsiveness. If unresponsive, have someone activate the EMS system if not already done.	
2. Open airway using head tilt–chin lift maneuver. (If trauma is present, use jaw-thrust maneuver.) Check breathing (look, listen, and feel); try to ventilate; if the chest does not rise, reposition head and try to ventilate again.	
3. Give two slow breaths (1 second per breath), watch for chest rise, and allow for deflation between breaths.	
4. Check for circulation. Check carotid pulse and look for signs of coughing and movement.	
RESCUER TWO	
5. If no pulse, give cycles of 30 chest compressions (100 compressions per minute) followed by two slow breaths by Rescuer One.	
RESCUER ONE	
6. After five cycles of CPR (about 2 minutes), check pulse.* If no pulse, continue CPR and recheck the patient in 2 minutes.	

*If victim is unresponsive but breathing, place in the recovery position.
Source: Based on the 2005 CPR and ECC guidelines.

Figure 9-9

Skill performance sheet.

FYI cont.

4. Rescuer One then begins chest compressions. You should practice switching until you can do it smoothly and quickly. Switching is much easier if the rescuers work on opposite sides of the patient.

One-Rescuer Infant CPR

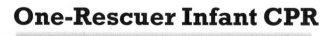

An infant is defined as anyone under 1 year of age. The principles of CPR are the same for adults and infants. In actual practice, however, you must use slightly different techniques for an infant. The steps for one-rescuer infant CPR are as follows:

1. Position the infant on a firm surface.
2. Establish the infant's level of responsiveness. An unresponsive infant is limp. Gently shake or tap the infant to determine whether he or she is unconscious. Call for additional help if the patient is unconscious. Activate the EMS system.
3. Open the airway. This is best done by the head tilt–chin lift maneuver. Be careful as you tilt the infant's head back because tilting it too far

can obstruct the airway. Continue holding the head with one hand.

4. Check for breathing. Place the side of your face close to the mouth and nose of the infant as you would for an adult. Look, listen, and feel for at least 5 seconds but no more than 10 seconds.

5. Give two breaths, each lasting 1 second. To breathe for an infant, place your mouth over the infant's mouth and nose. Because an infant has very small lungs, you should give only very small puffs of air, just enough to make the chest rise. Do not use large or forceful breaths **Figure 9-10 ▾**.

6. Check for circulation. Check the **brachial pulse** rather than the carotid pulse. The brachial pulse is on the inside of the arm **Figure 9-11 ▸**. You can feel it by placing your index and middle fingers on the inside of the infant's arm halfway between the shoulder and the elbow. Check for at least 5 seconds but no more than 10 seconds.

7. Begin chest compressions. An infant's heart is located relatively higher in the chest than an adult's heart. Imagine a horizontal line drawn between the infant's nipples. Place your index finger below that line in the middle of the chest. Place your middle and ring fingers next to your index finger. Use the middle and ring fingers to compress the ster-

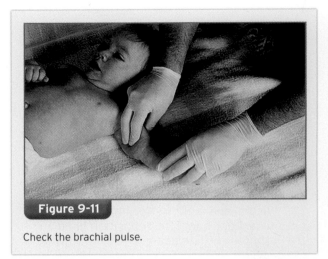
Figure 9-11

Check the brachial pulse.

num **Figure 9-12 ▾**. Because the chest of an infant is smaller and more pliable than the chest of an adult, use only two fingers to compress the chest. Compress the sternum approximately one half to one third the depth of the chest (about $\frac{1}{2}$ to 1 inch). To perform effective compressions, the infant must be lying on a firm surface. Deliver compressions at the rate of 100 per minute. The ratio of compressions to ventilations for one-rescuer infant CPR is 30 to 2.

8. Continue compressions and ventilations. Give two ventilations after each set of 30 compressions.

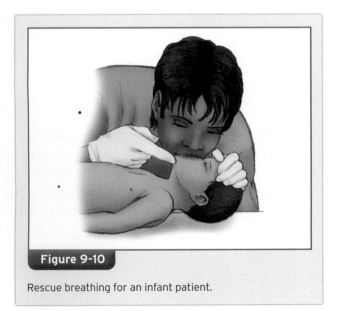
Figure 9-10

Rescue breathing for an infant patient.

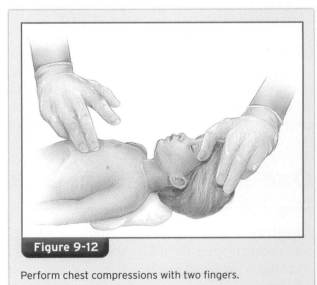
Figure 9-12

Perform chest compressions with two fingers.

One-Rescuer Infant CPR

Steps	Adequately Performed
1. Establish unresponsiveness. If a second rescuer is available, have him or her activate the EMS system.	
2. Open airway using the head tilt–chin lift maneuver. (If trauma is present, use jaw-thrust maneuver). Check breathing (look, listen, and feel).*	
3. Give two effective breaths (1 second per breath); if the chest does not rise, reposition head and try to ventilate again. Watch for chest rise; allow for exhalation between breaths.	
4. Check for signs of circulation. Check brachial pulse and look for signs of coughing or movement. If breathing is absent but pulse is present, provide rescue breathing (1 breath every 3 to 5 seconds [12 to 20 breaths per minute]).	
5. If no pulse, give 30 chest compressions (rate of 100 compressions per minute), followed by two slow breaths.	
6. After five cycles of CPR (about 2 minutes), check pulse.* If rescuer is alone, activate the EMS system and return to the patient. If no pulse, continue CPR.	

*If victim is unresponsive but breathing, place in the recovery position.
Source: Based on the 2005 CPR and ECC guidelines.

Figure 9-13

Skill performance sheet.

9. Reassess the patient after five cycles of compressions and ventilations (about 2 minutes) and every 2 minutes thereafter.

A skill performance sheet titled One-Rescuer Infant CPR is shown in 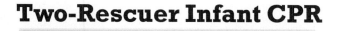 **Figure 9-13** ▲ for your review and practice.

Two-Rescuer Infant CPR

If you are performing two-rescuer infant CPR, use the two-thumb/encircling hands technique for chest compressions. This technique is done by placing both thumbs side-by-side over the lower half of the infant's sternum and encircling the infant's chest with your hands. Compress the sternum at a rate of 100 compressions per minute. When you are performing two-rescuer infant CPR, perform a compression-to-ventilation ratio of 15 to 2. As with any two-rescuer CPR technique, rescuers should switch roles after five cycles of CPR (about 2 minutes) to minimize rescuer fatigue.

One-Rescuer Child CPR

A child is defined as a person between 1 year of age and the onset of puberty (12 to 14 years of age). The steps for child CPR are essentially the same as for an adult; however, some steps may require modification for a child. These variations are:

- Use less force to ventilate the child. Ventilate only until the child's chest rises.
- In small children, use only one hand to depress the sternum one half to one third the depth of the chest; use two hands in larger children.
- Use less force to compress the child's chest.

Follow these steps to administer CPR to a child:

1. Establish the child's level of responsiveness. Tap and gently shake the shoulder and shout, "Are you okay?" If a second rescuer is available, have him or her activate the EMS system.
2. Turn the child on his or her back, as you support the head and neck.
3. Open the airway. Use the head tilt–chin lift maneuver or, if the child is injured, use the jaw-thrust maneuver. If the jaw-thrust maneuver does not adequately open the airway, carefully perform a head tilt–chin lift maneuver. Maintain the open airway.
4. Check for breathing. Place the side of your face and your ear close to the nose and mouth of the child. Look, listen, and feel for the movement of air: Look for movement of the chest, listen for sounds of air exchange, and feel for air movement on the side of your face. Check

for breathing for at least 5 seconds but no more than 10 seconds. If breathing is absent, place your mouth over the child's mouth, seal the child's nose with your thumb and index finger, and begin mouth-to-mouth rescue breathing. A mouth-to-mask ventilation device may be used.

5. Give two effective breaths. Blow slowly for 1 second, using just enough force to make the chest visibly rise. Allow the lungs to deflate between breaths.
6. Check for circulation. Locate the larynx with your index and middle fingers. Slide your fingers into the groove between the larynx and the muscles at the side of the neck to feel for the carotid pulse. Check for at least 5 seconds but no more than 10 seconds. If the pulse is absent, proceed to the following step. If the pulse is present, continue rescue breathing at a rate of 12 to 20 breaths per minute (one breath every 3 to 5 seconds).
7. Begin chest compressions. Place the heel of one hand in the center of the chest, in between the nipples Figure 9-14 ▾ . Compress the sternum approximately one half to one third the depth of the chest. Perform 30 compressions, using the heel of one hand (two hands in larger children). Compress the chest at the rate of 100 compressions per minute. Count the compressions out loud: "One and two and three and."

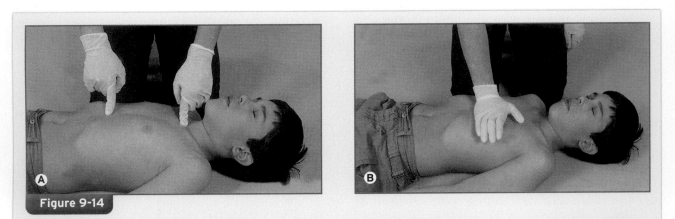

Figure 9-14

Performing chest compressions on a child. **A.** Locate the top and bottom of the sternum. **B.** Place the heel of your hand in the center of the chest, in between the nipples.

One-Rescuer Child CPR

Steps	Adequately Performed
1. Establish unresponsiveness. If a second rescuer is available, have him or her activate the EMS system.	
2. Open airway using head tilt–chin lift maneuver. (If trauma is present, use jaw-thrust maneuver.) Check breathing (look, listen, and feel).*	
3. Give two effective breaths (1 second per breath); if chest does not rise, reposition head and try to ventilate again. Watch for chest rise; allow for exhalation between breaths.	
4. Check for signs of circulation. Check carotid pulse and look for signs of coughing or movement. If breathing is absent but pulse is present, provide rescue breathing (one breath every 3 to 5 seconds, [12 to 20 breaths per minute]).	
5. If no pulse, perform 30 chest compressions (rate 100 compressions per minute) followed by two slow breaths.	
6. After five cycles of CPR (about 2 minutes), check pulse.* If rescuer is alone, activate the EMS system and return to the patient. If no pulse, continue CPR.	

*If victim is unresponsive but breathing, place in the recovery position.
Source: Based on the 2005 CPR and ECC guidelines.

Figure 9-15

Skill performance sheet.

8. After 30 chest compressions, deliver two effective rescuer breaths.
9. Continue compressions and ventilations. Continue a sequence of 30 compressions followed by two ventilations.
10. Check for a pulse after five cycles of CPR (about 2 minutes) and every 2 minutes thereafter.

A skill performance sheet titled One-Rescuer Child CPR is shown in **Figure 9-15** for your review and practice. In large children, you may need to use two hands to achieve an adequate depth of compression. When you are performing two-rescuer child CPR, administer 15 compressions followed by two rescue breaths.

Signs of Effective CPR

It is important to know the signs of effective CPR so you can assess your efforts to resuscitate the patient. The signs of effective CPR are:
1. A second rescuer feels a carotid pulse while you are compressing the chest.
2. The patient's skin color improves (from blue to pink).
3. The chest visibly rises during ventilations.

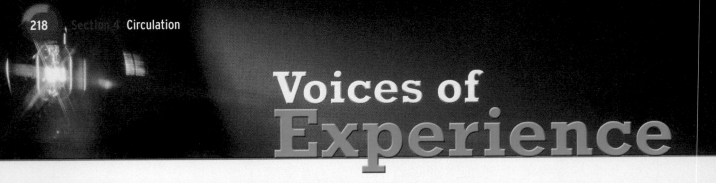

Voices of Experience

Teamwork in the Chain of Survival

It was a cool summer morning when a man saw his neighbor collapse in his backyard. He immediately jumped the fence separating the two properties to find his elderly male neighbor not breathing and without a pulse. He loudly yelled for help as he began CPR. The collapsed man's wife, who was inside the house at the time, heard her neighbor's scream. She looked out the window to see her husband lying on the ground and her neighbor administering CPR. Without hesitation, she dialed 9-1-1. Moments later, a law enforcement officer arrived with his automated external defibrillator (AED). He attached the AED, and after analyzing the rhythm, it stated, "No shock advised." Remaining calm, the neighbor and the police officer continued to perform CPR until the paramedics arrived.

> **We all play a role in responding to and caring for the victim of sudden cardiac arrest.**

Despite this early advanced care, we thought we may have passed a point of no return, but suddenly, we were able to regain a palpable pulse and blood pressure. We quickly transported this patient, and although we were unsure as to his ultimate outcome, we felt that everyone in the team had done an outstanding job.

Two weeks later, I received a copy of a thank-you note that had been given to everyone involved in the call. It was from the patient! He recovered and, showing no signs of mental or physical deficit, left the hospital on his own two feet.

When everyone works together to recognize emergencies; quickly accesses the emergency response system; and provides early CPR, early defibrillation, and early advanced care, the survival rates for sudden cardiac arrest (SCA) patients increases from 5% to 49%. When public access defibrillation is instituted in an area, survival rates are seen as high as 70%. Considering that around 250,000 people lose their lives every year as a result of SCA and that the chance of survival decreases by 10% per minute, this story exemplifies the importance of teamwork and how we all play a role in responding to and caring for the victim of SCA. I fully believe that the outcome of the incident hinged upon the swift, correct actions of a few individuals in the first moments of the emergency. Without effective first responders, a call like this one might not have had such a positive outcome.

Julie Chase, BS, NREMT-P
Emergency Medical Training and Consulting LLC
Austin, Texas

4. Compressions and ventilations are delivered at the appropriate rate and depth.

If some of these signs are not present, evaluate your technique to see if it can be improved.

Complications of CPR

A discussion of CPR would not be complete without mention of its complications, but they can be minimized by using the proper technique.

Broken Ribs

If your hands slip to the side of the sternum during chest compressions or if your fingers rest on the ribs, you may break ribs while delivering a compression. To prevent this, use proper hand position and do not let your fingers come in contact with the ribs. If you hear a cracking sound while performing CPR, check and correct your hand position but continue CPR. Sometimes you may break bones or cartilage even with proper CPR technique.

Gastric Distention

Bloating of the stomach is called **gastric distention** and is caused by too much air blown too fast and too forcefully into the stomach. A partially obstructed airway, which allows some of the air you breathe into the patient's airway to go into the stomach rather than into the lungs, can also cause gastric distention.

Gastric distention causes the abdomen to increase in size. A distended abdomen pushes on the diaphragm and prevents the lungs from inflating fully. Gastric distention also often causes regurgitation. If regurgitation occurs, quickly turn the patient to the side, wipe out the mouth with your gloved fingers, and then return the patient to a supine position.

Gastric distention is mentioned here so you will work hard to prevent it. Make sure you have opened the airway completely. Do not blow excessive amounts of air into the patient (deliver each breath over a period of 1 second). Be especially careful if you are a large person with a large lung capacity and the patient is smaller than you. If gastric distention is making it difficult for you to ventilate the patient, turn the patient's entire body to one side and press on the upper abdomen. This technique usually relieves the distention, but it is also likely to make the patient regurgitate stomach contents.

Regurgitation

Regurgitation (passive vomiting) is common during CPR, so you must be prepared to deal with it. You can minimize the risk of regurgitation by minimizing the amount of air that enters the patient's stomach. Regurgitation commonly occurs if the patient has suffered cardiac arrest. When cardiac arrest occurs, the muscle that keeps food in the stomach relaxes. If there is any food in the stomach, it backs up, causing the patient to vomit.

If the patient regurgitates as you are performing CPR, immediately turn the patient onto his or her side to allow the vomitus to drain from the mouth. Clear the patient's mouth of remaining vomitus, first with your fingers and then with a clean cloth (if one is handy). Use suction if it is available.

The patient may experience frequent episodes of regurgitation, so you must be prepared to take these actions repeatedly. EMS units carry a suction machine that can clear the patient's mouth. As a first responder, however, you cannot wait until the suction machine arrives before beginning or resuming CPR. You must simply deal with the regurgitation as it occurs.

Do your best to clear any vomitus from the patient's airway. If the airway is not cleared, three problems may arise:

1. The patient may breathe in (aspirate) the vomitus into the lungs.
2. You may force vomitus into the lungs with the next artificial ventilation.
3. It takes a strong stomach and the realization that you are trying to save the patient's life to continue with resuscitation after the patient has regurgitated—but you *must* continue. Remove the vomitus with a towel, the patient's shirt, your gloved fingers, or a suc-

tion unit if available. As soon as you have cleared away the vomitus, continue rescue breathing.

Creating Sufficient Space for CPR

As a first responder, you will frequently find yourself alone with a patient in cardiac arrest. One of the first things you must do is to create or find a space where you can perform CPR. Ask yourself, "Is there enough room in this location to perform effective CPR?" To perform CPR effectively, you need 3 to 4 feet of space on all sides of the patient. This will give enough space so that rescuers can change places, advanced life support procedures can be implemented, and an ambulance stretcher can be brought in. If there is not enough space around the patient, you have two options:

1. Quickly rearrange the furniture in the room to make space.
2. Quickly drag the patient into an area that has more room; for instance, out of the bathroom and into the living room—but not into a hallway Figure 9-16 ▾ .

Space is essential to a smooth rescue operation for a cardiac arrest patient. It takes a minimal amount of time to either clear a space

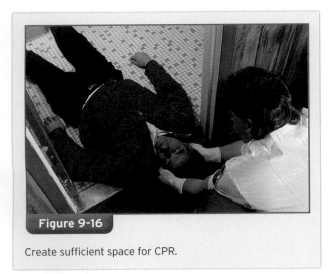

Figure 9-16

Create sufficient space for CPR.

around the patient or move the patient into a larger area.

Early Defibrillation by First Responders

Each year in the United States about 250,000 people die of coronary heart disease in an out-of-hospital setting. More than 70% of all out-of-hospital cardiac arrest patients have an irregular heart electrical rhythm called <u>ventricular fibrillation</u>. This condition, often referred to as V-fib, is the rapid, disorganized, and ineffective vibration of the heart. An electric shock applied to the heart will defibrillate it and reorganize the vibrations into effective heartbeats. A patient in cardiac arrest stands the greatest chance for survival when early defibrillation is available.

A first responder is often the first emergency care provider to reach a patient who has collapsed in cardiac arrest. A first responder who performs effective CPR helps to keep the patient's brain and heart supplied with oxygen until a defibrillator and advanced life support can arrive on the scene.

To get defibrillators to cardiac arrest patients more quickly, increasing numbers of EMS systems are equipping first responders with <u>automated external defibrillators (AEDs)</u> Figure 9-17 ▸ . These machines accurately identify ventricular fibrillation and advise you to deliver a shock if needed. Such equipment allows the first responder to combine effective CPR with early defibrillation to restore an organized heartbeat.

AEDs may be appropriate for your community if you work to strengthen all links of the cardiac Chain of Survival. The links of the Chain of Survival include:

- Early recognition of cardiac arrest and activation of the 9-1-1 system
- Early CPR: Early bystander CPR
- Early defibrillation by first responders or other EMS personnel
- Early advanced care by paramedics and hospital personnel

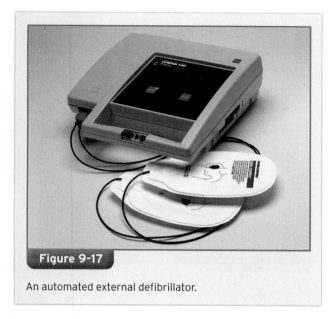

Figure 9-17

An automated external defibrillator.

Performing Automated External Defibrillation

The steps for using an AED are listed in **Skill Drill 9-4 ▶** :

SKILL DRILL 9-4

1. If you arrive on the scene before an AED is available, check the patient for responsiveness, airway, breathing, and circulation **Step 1**. If the patient is unresponsive, is not breathing, and has no pulse, you should begin CPR **Step 2**.
2. If you arrive with an AED and have been trained in its use, first check the patient for responsiveness, airway, breathing, and circulation. If the patient's cardiac arrest was not witnessed, perform five cycles of CPR (about 2 minutes) before beginning the AED procedure. If the cardiac arrest was witnessed, apply the AED as soon as possible.
3. Once the AED is brought to the scene, quickly attach the adhesive electrode pads to the patient **Step 3**. Minimize interruptions in performing CPR.
4. Stop CPR and remove your hands from the patient before you turn on the

defibrillator. No one should touch the patient once the machine has been turned on and is analyzing the heart rhythm.
5. Allow the defibrillator to analyze for a shockable rhythm. If a shockable rhythm is found, the machine quickly recommends defibrillation. You should first say, "Clear the patient" and ensure that no one is touching the patient before you press the "shock" button on the defibrillator **Step 4**.
6. After one shock is delivered, immediately resume CPR. Perform five cycles of CPR (about 2 minutes) starting with chest compressions **Step 5**. Stop CPR and remove your hands from the patient. Press the defibrillator to analyze the heart rhythm. If another shock is recommended, "clear" the patient, and administer another shock. Continue the sequence of five cycles of CPR, analyze, and shock until the defibrillator recommends no further shocks.
7. Check the patient's pulse. If a pulse is present, check breathing and support ventilations if necessary.
8. If no pulse, resume five cycles of CPR (about 2 minutes) starting with chest compressions. Check rhythm every five cycles. Continue until ALS providers take over or the patient starts to move **Step 6**.

If, after five cycles (about 2 minutes) of CPR, the defibrillator advises no shock, check the patient's pulse for at least 5 seconds but no more than 10 seconds. If the pulse is absent, resume CPR. If the pulse is present, check the breathing. Support ventilations if necessary. When advanced life support personnel arrive at the scene, they will assume control and responsibility for the patient's care.

AEDs vary in their operation so learn how to use your specific AED. You must have the training required by your medical director in order to practice this procedure. Practice until you can perform the procedure quickly and safely. Because the recommended guidelines for performing AED change, always follow the most current Emergency Cardiac Care (ECC) guidelines.

Skill DRILL 9-4

Procedure for Automated External Defibrillation

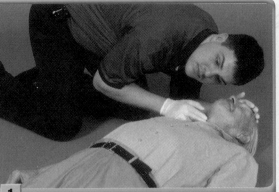

1 Check ABCs—look, listen, feel.

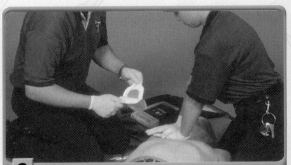

2 If patient is pulseless and not breathing, perform CPR for five cycles (about 2 minutes). If arrest is witnessed, proceed to step 3.

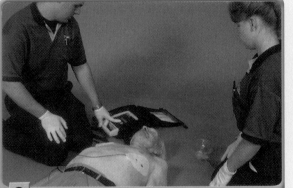

3 Apply adhesive electrode pads and connect to defibrillator.

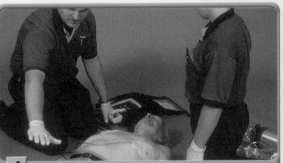

4 Turn AED on and allow machine to analyze rhythm. Determine if shock is indicated by the defibrillator. If shock is indicated, defibrillate the patient.

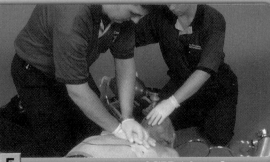

5 Perform five cycles of CPR (about 2 minutes) starting with chest compressions. Repeat Steps 4 and 5 until defibrillator no longer recommends a shock.

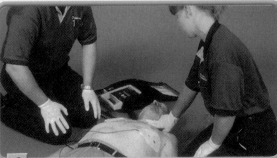

6 When no shock is recommended, check the pulse. If no pulse is present, resume five cycles of CPR starting with chest compressions.

CPR Training

As a first responder, you should successfully complete a CPR course through a recognized agency such as the Emergency Care and Safety Institute (ECSI). You should also regularly update your skills by successfully completing a recognized recertification course. You cannot achieve proficiency in CPR unless you have adequate practice on adult, child, and infant manikins. Your department should schedule periodic reviews of CPR theory and practice for all people who are trained as first responders.

Legal Implications of CPR

Living wills, advance directives, and DNR orders are legal documents that specify the patient's wishes regarding specified medical procedures.

These documents are explained in Chapter 3. First responders sometimes wonder if they should start CPR on a person who has a living will or an advance directive. Because you are not in a position to determine if the living will or advance directive is valid, CPR should be started on all patients unless signs of obvious death are present (such as rigor mortis or decapitation). If a patient has a living will or advance directive, the physician at the hospital will determine whether you should stop CPR. Follow your department's protocols regarding advance directives, living wills, and DNR orders.

Do not hesitate to begin CPR on a pulseless, nonbreathing patient. Without your help, the patient will certainly die. You may have legal problems if you begin CPR on a patient who does not need it and this action harms the patient. However, the chances of this happening are minimal if you assess the patient carefully before beginning CPR.

Another potential legal pitfall is abandonment—the discontinuation of CPR without the order of a licensed physician or without turning the patient over to someone who is at least as qualified as you are. If you avoid these pitfalls, you need not be overly concerned about the legal implications of performing CPR. Your most important protection against a possible legal suit is to become thoroughly proficient in the theory and practice of CPR.

You are the Provider

SUMMARY

Review the *You are the Provider* case study provided at the beginning of this chapter.

You just started your morning shift and are in the middle of checking your equipment when you hear the click of the PA system that precedes an alarm. You stop what you are doing so you can hear the dispatcher. "Unit 433 respond to 10711 Mathews Court for a 74-year-old male experiencing shortness of breath. Time out is 0733."

You arrive on the scene 4 minutes later. As you and your partner enter the front door of the residence, a woman excitedly tells you that her husband slumped over in his chair just as you were pulling into the driveway.

1. What are the first steps you need to take?

The information you get from your dispatcher may change by the time you arrive at the scene of the patient. In this case, the initial call was received for a patient who was short of breath. This condition changed to an unresponsive patient by the time the rescuers arrived. Always remain aware of the fact that the patient's condition can deteriorate between the time the call to 9-1-1 is placed and when you arrive at the scene.

The first step you need to take after determining that the scene is safe is to check responsiveness of the patient. If the patient is unresponsive, check and correct the patient's airway, breathing, and circulation. If the patient is not breathing, perform rescue breathing. If the carotid pulse is absent, proceed with chest compressions. One rescuer can begin CPR while the second rescuer notifies dispatch of the patient's condition. This will help to get additional EMS providers on the scene as soon as possible.

2. What is the chance for a successful outcome on this call?

This call has an increased chance for a positive outcome because the patient has been in cardiac arrest for a short time. The sooner CPR is started, the greater the chance for a successful outcome. The other major factor influencing the outcome is the amount of time it takes to defibrillate the patient.

3. Your department has just placed automated external defibrillators on all units. How does this change your treatment of this patient?

Having an automated external defibrillator would greatly increase the chance that you could successfully resuscitate this patient. If you have an AED available, you should apply it as soon as possible (because the duration of the patient's cardiac arrest is short) and then follow the steps for defibrillation. Avoid interruptions in chest compressions as much as possible.

Prep Kit

Ready for Review

The Ready for Review thoroughly summarizes the chapter.

- The circulatory system transports oxygenated blood from the lungs to the rest of the body. Each beat of the heart produces a pulse, which can be felt at various sites such as the inside of the wrist (radial), the neck (carotid), the inside of the upper arm (brachial), and the groin (femoral).

- Cardiac arrest occurs when the heart stops contracting and no blood is pumped through the blood vessels. Brain damage begins within 4 to 6 minutes after the patient has suffered cardiac arrest. Within 8 to 10 minutes, the damage to the brain may become irreversible.

- The Chain of Survival—early access to care, early CPR, early defibrillation, and early advanced cardiac life support (ACLS)—includes steps essential to successful emergency cardiac care.

- When you arrive at an emergency scene, you must first assess the area for potential safety hazards. If the scene is unsafe, make it as safe as possible for yourself and the patient. As you approach the patient, look for possible causes of illness or injury. Next, assess the patient by checking responsiveness and ABCs:

  - Airway

  - Breathing

  - Circulation

- Open the airway and look, listen, and feel for breathing. If the patient is not breathing, you must breathe for him or her. Check for a pulse. If it is absent, begin CPR.

- Basic life support for adults and children follows the same general steps: Check responsiveness, airway, breathing, and circulation. Intervene at any point where the patient's airway is obstructed, the patient is not breathing, or the patient has no circulation.

- Use the jaw-thrust maneuver to open the airway if you suspect a spinal injury, and the head tilt–chin lift maneuver if you do not suspect a spinal injury.

- Rescue breathing for adults should be performed at a rate of one breath every 5 to 6 seconds (10 to 12 breaths per minute) and one breath every 3 to 5 seconds (12 to 20 breaths per minute) for children.

- Chest compressions should be performed at a rate of 100 compressions per minute for adults and children. Perform 30 compressions and two breaths for adults and for all one-rescuer CPR. Perform 15 compressions and two breaths for two-rescuer child CPR.

- Basic life support for infants is similar to that provided for adults and children. The techniques may vary somewhat, but the same general steps apply: check responsiveness, airway, breathing, and circulation. Intervene at any point if the infant's airway is obstructed, if the infant is not breathing.

- Open the infant's airway by using the head tilt–chin lift maneuver if you do not suspect a spinal injury. Be careful not to hyperextend the neck; this could obstruct the airway. If the infant is not breathing, provide two initial breaths. If these breaths produce visible chest rise, check for a brachial pulse.

- If there is no pulse, or if the pulse rate is less than 60 beats per minute with poor perfusion, begin CPR. If you are alone, use two fingers to compress the chest 30 times, at a rate of 100 compressions per minute, to a depth equal to one half to one third the depth of the chest. After 30 compressions, give two breaths. If two rescuers are present, use the two-thumb technique with the hands encircling the chest and provide 15 compressions to two breaths. Continue CPR for 5 cycles (about 2 minutes) and then recheck the pulse. If the pulse is still absent, or less than 60 beats per minute with poor perfusion, continue CPR. If the pulse returns (or increases above 60 beats per minute), but the infant is still not breathing, provide rescue breathing.

- The single most important cardiac arrest survival factor is early defibrillation. The indications for using an automated external defibrillator (AED) are

Technology

- Interactivities
- Vocabulary Explorer
- Anatomy Review
- Web Links
- Online Review Manual

that the patient is unresponsive, not breathing, and pulseless. If the patient's cardiac arrest was witnessed by you, begin CPR and apply the AED as soon as possible. However, if the cardiac arrest was not witnessed by you, perform five cycles (about 2 minutes) of CPR before applying the AED.

- Once turned on and attached to the patient's bare chest, the AED will analyze the heart rhythm and advise whether or not a shock is indicated. If a shock is advised, ensure that nobody is touching the patient, deliver the shock, and immediately perform CPR for 2 minutes before reanalyzing the patient's rhythm. If no shock is advised, but the patient is pulseless, perform CPR for 2 minutes and then reanalyze the patient's rhythm. Continue CPR and rhythm analysis until advanced life support personnel arrive.

Vital Vocabulary

The Vital Vocabulary are the key terms for this chapter.

automated external defibrillators (AEDs) Portable battery-powered devices that recognize ventricular fibrillation and advise when a countershock is indicated. The AED delivers an electric shock to patients with ventricular fibrillation.

brachial pulse The pulse on the inside of the upper arm.

cardiac arrest Ceasing of breathing and a heartbeat.

chest compression Manual chest-pressing method that mimics the squeezing and relaxation cycles a normal heart goes through; administered to a person in cardiac arrest; also called external chest compression and closed-chest cardiac massage.

child Anyone between 1 year of age and the onset of puberty (12 to 14 years of age).

circulatory system The heart and blood vessels, which together are responsible for the continuous flow of blood throughout the body.

gastric distention Inflation of the stomach caused when excessive pressures are used during artificial ventilation and air is directed into the stomach rather than the lungs.

infant Anyone under 1 year of age.

one-rescuer CPR Cardiopulmonary resuscitation performed by one rescuer.

plasma The fluid part of the blood that carries blood cells, transports nutrients, and removes cellular waste materials.

platelets Microscopic disc-shaped elements in the blood that are essential to the process of blood clot formation, the mechanism that stops bleeding.

pulse The wave of pressure created by the heart as it contracts and forces blood out into the major arteries.

two-rescuer CPR Cardiopulmonary resuscitation performed by two rescuers.

ventilations The movement of air in and out of the lungs.

ventricular fibrillation An uncoordinated muscular quivering of the heart; the most common abnormal rhythm causing cardiac arrest.

Assessment in Action

Assessment in Action presents a fictitious scenario to help you review what you learned in this chapter.

You are dispatched to the Kruep Recreation Center for a man complaining of chest pain. Upon arrival, you find a 58-year-old man unconscious and unresponsive on the floor in the main lobby. Bystanders tell you that the man came to the front desk complaining of a pain in the center of his chest. Minutes later, he fell to the floor. He does not appear to be breathing.

1. What is your first step in providing care for this patient?

   A. Check for a pulse.
   B. Check for breathing.
   C. Perform chest compressions.
   D. Determine if he is unconscious.

2. Which of the following would indicate that CPR is needed?

   A. Shallow breathing
   B. Dilated pupils
   C. Absence of breathing and pulse
   D. Shortness of breath

3. All of the following are criteria that would negate performing CPR, EXCEPT:

   A. Evidence of tissue decomposition
   B. Rigor mortis
   C. Decapitation
   D. Dilated pupils

4. What is the appropriate depth of compressions for this patient?

   A. 1 to 1½ inches
   B. 1½ to 2 inches
   C. ½ to 1 inch
   D. 2 to 2½ inches

5. When performing CPR on this patient, what is the correct ratio of chest compressions to rescue breaths?

   A. 5 to 1
   B. 15 to 2
   C. 30 to 2
   D. 50 to 2

6. When performing rescue breathing on this patient, each breath should be given over a period of:

   A. 1 second
   B. 1½ seconds
   C. 2 seconds
   D. 2½ seconds

Illness and Injury

Section

5

Medical Emergencies

Chapter Objectives*

Knowledge and Attitude Objectives

1. Describe the general approach to a medical patient. (p 234)
2. Explain the causes, symptoms, and treatment of a patient with altered mental status. (p 235)
3. Explain the causes, symptoms, and treatment of a patient with seizures. (p 235-237)
4. Describe the treatment of a patient who shows signs and symptoms of exposure to heat. (p 238-239)
5. Describe the treatment of a patient who shows signs and symptoms of exposure to cold. (p 239-241)
6. Explain the causes of angina pectoris. (p 241-242)
7. Describe the signs, symptoms, and initial treatment of a patient with angina pectoris. (p 242)
8. Explain the major cause of a heart attack. (p 242)
9. Describe the signs, symptoms, and initial treatment of a patient with a heart attack. (p 242-243)
10. Explain the cause of congestive heart failure. (p 244)
11. Describe the signs, symptoms, and initial treatment of a patient with congestive heart failure. (p 244)
12. Describe the causes of dyspnea. (p 244)
13. Explain the signs, symptoms, and initial treatment of a patient with dyspnea. (p 244-245)
14. Describe the causes of asthma. (p 245)
15. Explain the signs, symptoms, and initial treatment of a patient suffering an asthma attack. (p 245-246)
16. Describe the major cause of a stroke. (p 246)
17. Explain the signs, symptoms, and initial treatment of a patient with a stroke. (p 246-247)
18. Describe the signs and symptoms of insulin shock. (p 247)
19. Describe the initial treatment of a patient in insulin shock. (p 248)
20. Describe the signs and symptoms of a patient in a diabetic coma. (p 248)
21. Describe the initial treatment of a patient in a diabetic coma. (p 249)
22. Describe the signs and symptoms of an abdominal problem. (p 249)
23. Describe the initial treatment of a patient with abdominal pain. (p 250)

Skill Objectives

1. Perform a patient assessment on a medical patient. (p 234)
2. Place an unconscious patient in the recovery position. (p 236)
3. Protect a patient who is seizing from sustaining further harm. (p 236)
4. Cool a patient who has suffered exposure to heat. (p 238-239)
5. Treat a patient who has suffered exposure to cold. (p 239-240)
6. Position a patient who has congestive heart failure. (p 244)
7. Administer fluids or oral glucose to a patient who is in insulin shock. (p 248)

*These are chapter learning objectives.

Medical Emergencies

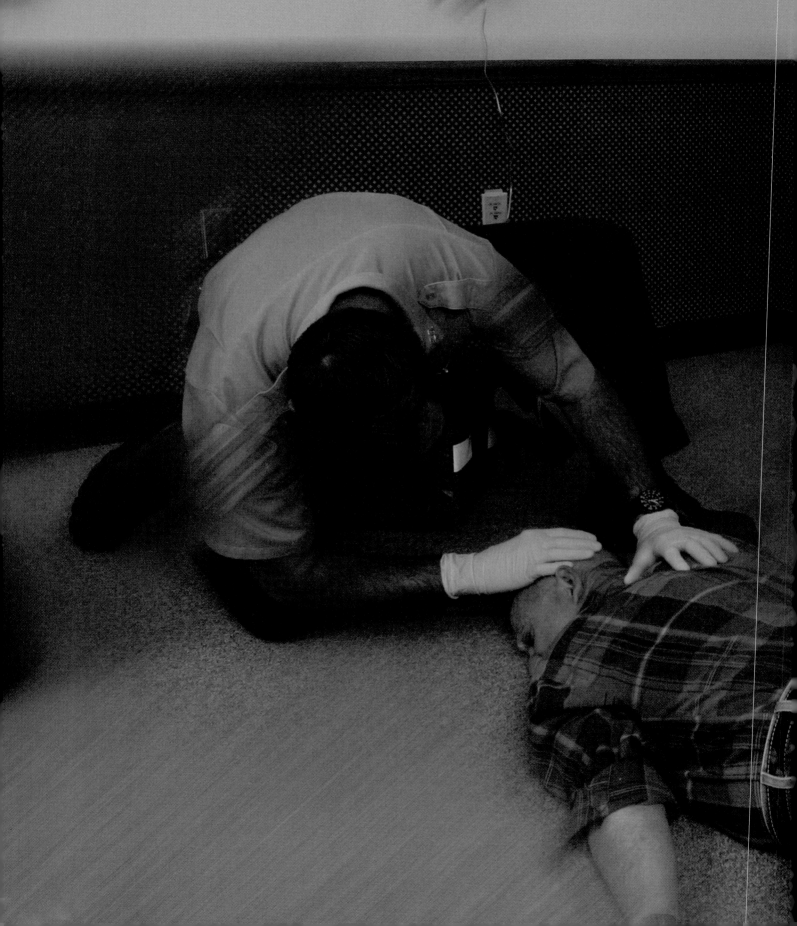

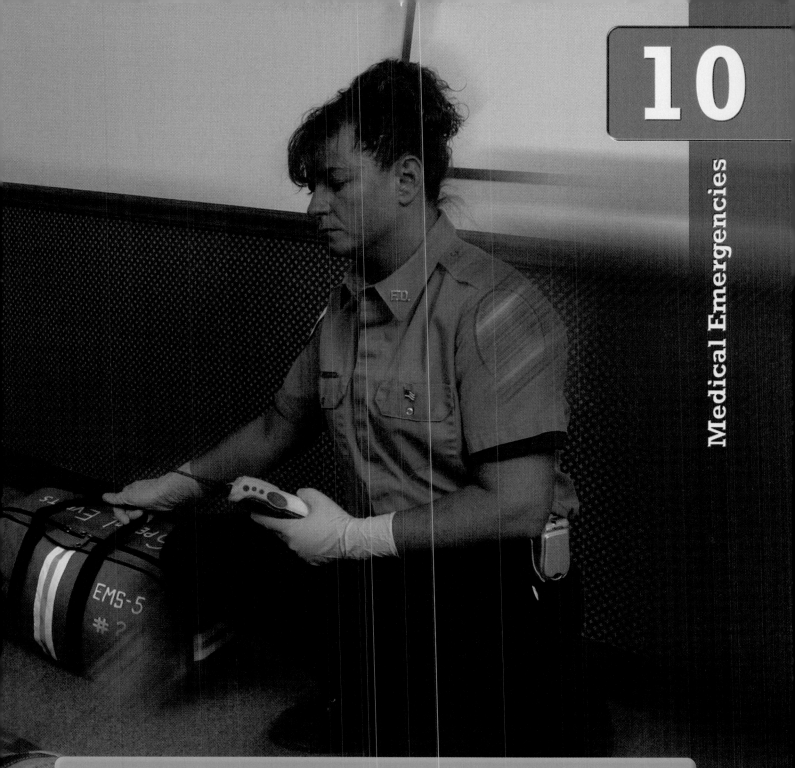

You are the Provider

You are dispatched to a private residence to assist a patient who is experiencing difficulty breathing. En route to the scene, you review what you have learned about patients who are short of breath.

1. Why is it important to obtain a thorough medical history on a patient like this?
2. Diseases of which two body systems are most likely to cause a patient to become short of breath?
3. Describe why a calm approach and a reassuring attitude benefit a patient who is short of breath.

Introduction

This chapter on medical conditions has two parts. The first part covers general medical complaints, including altered mental status and seizures. General medical complaints may result from a wide variety of medical conditions. You will learn the signs, symptoms, and common treatment steps for patients with these general medical complaints. The second part addresses some specific medical conditions you will encounter, including generalized heat emergencies, generalized cold emergencies, angina pectoris, heart attack, congestive heart failure, dyspnea, asthma, stroke, insulin shock, diabetic coma, and abdominal pain. You will learn the signs, symptoms, and treatment of patients with these specific medical conditions.

Treating patients with medical conditions can be some of the most challenging work you perform as a first responder. By carefully studying these conditions, you will be prepared to provide reassuring and sometimes life-saving care to patients suffering from medical emergencies.

General Medical Conditions

General medical conditions may have different causes, but they result in similar signs and symptoms. By learning to recognize the signs and symptoms of these conditions as well as general treatment guidelines, you will be able to provide immediate care for patients even if you cannot determine the exact cause of the problems. This initial treatment can stabilize the patient and allow other EMS and hospital personnel to diagnose and further treat the problem.

General Approaches to a Medical Patient

Your approach to a patient who has a general medical complaint should follow the systematic approach outlined in the patient assessment sequence in Chapter 7. Review your dispatch information for an idea of the possible problem. Carefully check the scene to assess your safety and that of the patient. As you perform the initial patient assessment, first try to get an impression of the patient's problem. Then determine the patient's responsiveness, introduce yourself, check the patient's ABCs, and acknowledge the patient's chief complaint.

Usually, it is best to collect a medical history on the patient experiencing a medical problem before you perform a physical examination. The medical history should be complete and include all factors that may relate to the patient's current illness.

The SAMPLE history format will help you secure the information you need:

S Signs/symptoms.
A Allergies.
M Medications.
P Pertinent past history.
L Last oral intake.
E Events associated with or leading to the illness or injury.

Although the physical examination should focus on the areas related to the patient's current illness, you should also realize that the patient may not always be aware of all facets of his or her

Technology

- Interactivities
- Vocabulary Explorer
- Anatomy Review
- Web Links
- Online Review Manual

problem. It is better to perform a complete physical examination and find all the problems than to perform a partial examination and miss an underlying problem. Determine the patient's vital signs and do not forget to perform ongoing assessment if additional EMS personnel are delayed.

As you perform the patient assessment, remember to reassure the patient. Any call for emergency medical care is a frightening experience for the patient. Many medical conditions are aggravated by stress: If you can reduce the patient's stress, you will go a long way toward making the patient more comfortable.

Altered Mental Status

Altered mental status is a sudden or gradual decrease in the patient's level of responsiveness. This change may range from a decrease in the level of understanding to unresponsiveness. Any patient who is unresponsive has suffered a severe change in mental status.

In assessing altered mental status, remember the AVPU scale:

A **Alert.** An alert patient will answer simple questions accurately and appropriately.

V **Verbal.** A patient who is responsive to verbal stimuli will react to loud voices.

P **Pain.** A patient who is responsive to a painful stimulus will react to the pain by moving or crying out.

U **Unresponsive.** An unresponsive patient will not respond to either verbal or painful stimuli.

When assessing the patient's mental status, you should consider two factors: the patient's initial level of consciousness and any change in that level of consciousness. A patient who is initially alert but later responds only to verbal stimuli has suffered a decrease in level of consciousness.

Many different conditions may cause an altered level of consciousness, including:

- Head injury
- Shock
- Decreased level of oxygen to the brain
- Stroke
- Slow heart rate
- High fever

Treatment Tips

The Patient Assessment Sequence

1. Scene size-up.
2. Perform an initial assessment.
   A. Form a general impression of the patient.
   B. Assess responsiveness—stabilize the spine if trauma.
   C. Check the patient's airway.
   D. Check the patient's breathing.
   E. Check the patient's circulation (including severe bleeding).
   F. Acknowledge the patient's primary complaint.
   G. Update responding EMS units.
3. Examine the patient from head to toe.
4. Obtain the patient's medical history (SAMPLE).
5. Perform an ongoing assessment.

Note: For medical patients, reverse steps 3 and 4.

- Infection
- Poisoning, including drugs and alcohol
- Low level of blood sugar (diabetic emergencies)
- Insulin reaction
- Psychiatric condition

Some of the specific conditions that cause altered mental status are explained in the second part of this chapter. Even if you cannot determine what is causing the patient's altered level of consciousness, you can help by treating the symptoms of the problem.

You should complete the patient assessment sequence to ensure scene safety and proper assessment. Initial treatment is to maintain the patient's ABCs and normal body temperature and to keep the patient from additional harm. If the patient is unconscious and has not suffered trauma, place the patient in the recovery position or use an airway adjunct to help maintain an open airway. Be prepared to suction if there is a chance that the patient may vomit or not be able to handle secretions.

Seizures

Seizures are caused by sudden episodes of uncontrolled electrical impulses in the brain. Seizures that produce shaking movements and involve the entire body are called <u>generalized seizures</u> or grand mal seizures. These seizures usually last less than 5 minutes, although prolonged seizures may continue for more than 5 minutes. Patients are usually unconscious during generalized seizures and do not remember them afterwards. Although seizures are rarely life threatening, they are a serious medical emergency and may be the sign of a life-threatening condition. When seizures occur, the patient may need help to maintain an open airway. The patient may lose bowel or bladder control, soiling his or her clothing.

One cause of generalized seizures is a sudden high fever. These seizures are called febrile seizures. Febrile seizures are most common in infants and young children. Febrile seizures are discussed in the chapter on pediatric emergencies.

Some seizures result in only a brief lapse of consciousness. These seizures are called <u>absence seizures</u> or petit mal seizures. Patients experiencing absence seizures may blink their eyes, stare vacantly, or jerk one part of their body. Because these seizures are of brief duration and severity, the family or bystanders of the patient do not usually call EMS. A physician should examine patients exhibiting signs and symptoms of an absence seizure.

Many times you will not be able to determine the cause of the patient's seizure. After a seizure, the patient may be sleepy, confused, upset, hostile, or out of touch with reality for up to an hour. You must monitor the patient's ABCs and arrange for **transport** to an appropriate medical facility.

Usually, the seizure will be over by the time you arrive at the scene. If it has not ended, your treatment should focus on protecting the patient from injury. Do not restrain the patient's movements. If you attempt to restrain the patient, you may cause further injury. If a patient suffers a seizure while on a hard surface, control the patient's arms by grasping them at the wrists. Allow the patient's arms to move but prevent the elbows from hitting the hard surface. To prevent the patient's head from hitting a hard surface, quickly slide the toes of your shoes under the patient's head. The patient should be moved only if he or she is in a dangerous location, such as in a busy street or close to something hard, hot, or sharp.

During a seizure, the patient generally does not breathe and may turn blue. You cannot do anything about the patient's airway during the seizure, but once the seizure has stopped, it is essential that you ensure an open airway. This is usually best accomplished with the head tilt–chin lift technique. Observe the seizure activity and report your observations and assessment findings to other EMS providers. They may be important in determining the cause of the seizure.

After you have opened the airway, place the patient in the recovery position to help keep the airway open and to allow any secretions (saliva or blood from a bitten tongue) to drain out **Figure 10-1 ▼**. Patients who have suffered a seizure may have excess oral secretions.

In the Field

There are many different types of seizures and they can be caused by many factors, including:

- Epilepsy
- Trauma
- Head injury
- Stroke
- Shock
- Decreased level of oxygen to the brain
- High fever
- Infection
- Poisoning, including drugs and alcohol
- Brain tumor
- Diabetic emergencies
- Complication of pregnancy
- Unknown causes

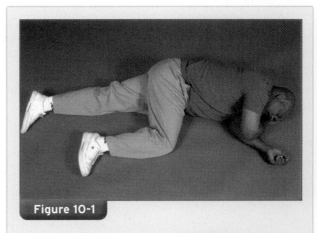

Figure 10-1

Recovery position for an unconscious patient.

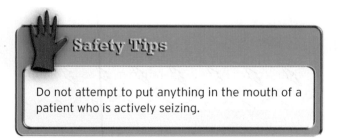

Treatment Tips

Treatment for Seizures

- Stay calm. You cannot stop a seizure once it has started.
- Do not restrain the patient.
- Protect the patient from contact with hard, sharp, or hot objects.
- Do not force anything between the patient's teeth.
- Do not be concerned if the patient stops breathing temporarily during the seizure.
- After the seizure, turn the patient on his or her side and make sure breathing is not obstructed.
- If the patient does not begin breathing after a seizure, start rescue breathing.

Treatment Tips

Although there is a strong tendency to quickly categorize patients as "medical patients" or as "trauma patients," it is important to realize that many of the patients you encounter may have both a medical condition and a traumatic injury. For example, the altered level of consciousness experienced by a diabetic in insulin shock may contribute to a motor vehicle crash. As you study this chapter, try to imagine how you can use your knowledge to treat patients with a single problem or a variety of problems. Remember to carefully assess each patient and treat the problems that you identify.

Most patients start to breathe soon after the seizure ends. If the patient does not resume breathing after a seizure or if the seizure is prolonged, begin mouth-to-mask or mouth-to-mouth breathing (see Chapter 6). Supplemental oxygen should be administered as soon as it is available.

Many patients may be confused after a seizure and may become anxious, hostile, or belligerent. At this point, the patient needs privacy. Because the person is probably embarrassed about what happened or where it happened (perhaps in a public place such as a restaurant or shopping mall), move the patient to a more comfortable, private place if other EMS personnel are delayed. The state of confusion after a seizure may last for 30 to 45 minutes. Do not leave the patient. First responders should encourage any patient who suffers a seizure to go to a medical facility for examination and treatment. The best treatment you can provide for a seizure patient is to protect him or her from self-injury. After the seizure,

you should ensure that the airway is open, the patient is breathing adequately, and secretions and blood in the mouth are cleared. (See the Treatment for Seizures tip box.)

Specific Medical Conditions

In the first part of this chapter, you learned how to assess general medical complaints and treat patients based on their signs and symptoms. This should be the foundation for your assessment and treatment of patients who present with medical conditions. You will find it helpful, however, to know about some of the more specific medical conditions you may encounter as a first responder, particularly those covered in this second part of the chapter.

Sometimes the patient or the patient's family will tell you that the patient has a certain medical condition. At other times, your careful assessment of the patient will reveal information that

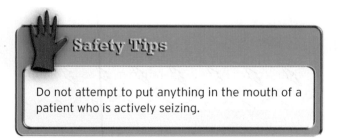

Safety Tips

Do not attempt to put anything in the mouth of a patient who is actively seizing.

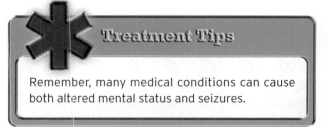

Treatment Tips

Remember, many medical conditions can cause both altered mental status and seizures.

leads you to suspect a particular condition. Your determination may help you take specific steps to help the patient. The added knowledge you gain from the second part of this chapter will help you assess, treat, and communicate more effectively with patients who have medical conditions.

Exposure to Heat and Cold

As a first responder, you will encounter patients who have been exposed to heat and to cold. When you assess these patients, you should follow the steps of the patient assessment sequence. The signs and symptoms exhibited by the patient will guide you in your treatment. To help you recognize and treat these patients, the signs, symptoms, and treatment for heat exhaustion, heatstroke, frostbite, and hypothermia are presented.

Heat Exhaustion

<u>Heat exhaustion</u> can occur when a person is exposed to temperatures above 80°F (26°C), usually in combination with high humidity. A person suffering from heat exhaustion sweats profusely and becomes lightheaded, dizzy, and nauseated.

Predisposing factors may make some people more susceptible to heat-related illnesses. The very young, older people, and people who have preexisting medical conditions or who are taking certain medications are more likely to suffer from heat-related illness. High ambient temperatures reduce the body's ability to cool itself by radiation. High humidity reduces the body's ability to lose heat through evaporation. Exercise results in greater production of sweat.

The patient's blood pressure drops (causing a weak pulse), and the patient frequently complains of feeling weak. Body temperature is usually normal. The signs and symptoms of heat exhaustion are similar to the early signs of shock and its treatment is similar as well.

When you encounter a patient suffering from heat exhaustion, complete a scene size-up and initial patient assessment. Patients experiencing heat exhaustion sweat heavily and are in mild shock from fluid loss. To treat heat exhaustion, move the patient to a cooler place (for example, from a baseball diamond to a shady spot under a tree) and treat him or her for shock. Unless the patient is unconscious, nauseated, or vomiting, give fluids by mouth to replace the fluids lost through sweating. Drinking cool water is excellent treatment for cases of heat exhaustion. Monitor ABCs and arrange for **transport** to a medical facility.

Heatstroke

<u>Heatstroke</u> results when a person has been in a hot environment for a long period of time, overwhelming the body's sweating mechanism. The patient's body temperature rises until it reaches a level at which brain damage occurs. Without prompt and proper treatment, a patient with heatstroke will die.

The patient usually has flushed, dry skin that feels hot to the touch. A person who is suffering from heatstroke may be semiconscious; unconsciousness may develop rapidly. Such patients may have temperatures as high as 106°F (41.1°C).

Maintain the patient's ABCs. Move the patient from the heat and into a cool place as soon

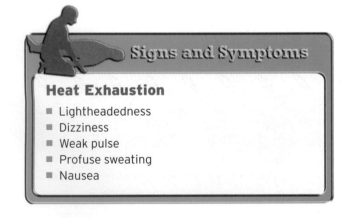

Signs and Symptoms

Heat Exhaustion

- Lightheadedness
- Dizziness
- Weak pulse
- Profuse sweating
- Nausea

Treatment Tips

Heatstroke is an emergency that requires immediate action. Body temperature must be lowered quickly!

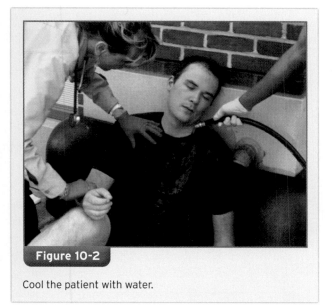

Figure 10-2

Cool the patient with water.

as possible. Remove the patient's clothes, down to the underwear. Soak the patient with water **Figure 10-2 ▲**. You can cool the patient with water from a garden hose, a shower in the home or factory, or a low-pressure hose from a fire truck. Ice packs can be placed on the groin. If the patient is conscious and not nauseated, administer small amounts of cool water. Arrange for **rapid transport** to an appropriate medical facility for further treatment. **Table 10-1 ▼** compares the signs and symptoms of heat exhaustion with those of heatstroke.

Frostbite

<u>Frostbite</u> can result when exposed parts of the body are in a cold environment. It can occur on a winter day, in a walk-in food freezer, or in a cold-

storage warehouse in the middle of the summer. Exposed body parts actually freeze. The body parts most susceptible to frostbite are the face, ears, fingers, and toes. Depending on the temperature and wind velocity, frostbite can occur in even a short period of time.

Increases in wind speed have the same effect as decreases in temperature. Imagine holding your hand outside an automobile traveling at 55 mph on a cold winter day! The combination of wind speed and low temperature produces a wind-chill factor **Figure 10-3 ▶**. When the temperature is relatively mild, 35°F (2°C), an accompanying 20-mph wind will produce a wind chill equivalent to an actual temperature of 12°F (−11°C). If there is a combination of low temperature and high wind, protect yourself and your patient from the dangers of wind chill.

People weakened by old age, medical conditions, exhaustion, or hunger are the most susceptible to frostbite. In superficial frostbite, sometimes called frostnip, the affected body part first becomes numb and then acquires a bright red color. Eventually the area loses its color and changes to pale white. There may be a loss of feeling and sensation in the injured area. If the area is rewarmed, the patient may experience a tingling feeling.

Warming a frostbitten part must be done quickly and carefully. Usually, putting the fingers, toes, or ears next to a warm body part is sufficient. For example, place frostbitten fingers in the armpits. Do not try to warm a frostbitten area by rubbing it with your hands or a blanket and never rub snow or ice onto a suspected frostbitten area. Doing so will only make the problem worse. Treat the frostbitten patient for shock.

TABLE 10-1	Comparing Heat Exhaustion and Heatstroke	
Heat Exhaustion	**Heatstroke**
Normal body temperature	High body temperature
Sweating	Dry skin (usually)
Cool and clammy skin	Hot and red skin
Dizziness and nausea	Semiconscious (or unconscious)

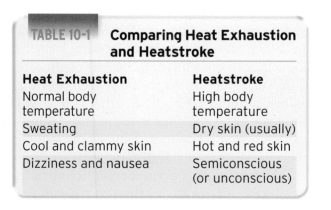

Safety Tips

Prevention is the only effective means of combating frostbite. If you are going outside in freezing weather, dress warmly and make sure the vulnerable parts of the body are well covered or protected.

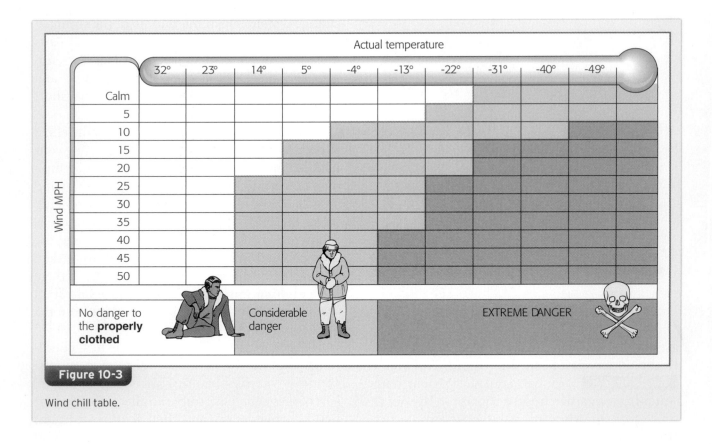

Figure 10-3

Wind chill table.

A frostbitten patient who has been outside for an extended period of time may suffer deep frostbite. In this case, the skin will be white and waxy. The skin may be firm or frozen. Swelling and blisters may be present. If the skin has thawed, it may appear flushed with areas of purple and white or may be mottled and cyanotic. Follow the usual sequence of scene size-up, initial patient assessment, and physical exam. Remove any jewelry the patient is wearing and cover the extremity with dry clothing or dry dressings. Do not break blisters, rub the injured area, apply heat, or allow the patient to walk on an affected lower extremity. Patients with deep frostbite should receive **prompt transport** to a medical facility so they can be warmed under carefully controlled conditions.

Hypothermia

When the body temperature falls into the subnormal area (below about 95°F or 35°C), the condition is called **hypothermia** ("low temperature"). Hypothermia occurs when a person's body is not able to produce enough energy to keep the internal (core) body temperature at a satisfactory level.

Hypothermia is not only a winter problem; it can occur in temperatures as high as 50°F (10°C). People who become cold because of inadequate or wet clothing are susceptible to hypothermia, especially if they are weakened by illness. The initial signs of hypothermia include feelings of being cold, shivering, decreasing level of consciousness, and sleepiness. Shivering is the body's attempt to produce more heat. As hypothermia progresses, shivering stops. A patient who is so cold that he or she cannot even shiver cools down even faster than before. Signs of increasing hypothermia include a lack of coordination, mental confusion, and slowed reactions. As the body's temperature goes below about 90°F (32°C), the patient will lose consciousness. Without treatment and warming to reverse the downward spiral, the patient will eventually die. See **Table 10-2 ▶**.

If you suspect that a patient is suffering from hypothermia, move the patient to a warm (or warmer) location. Remove wet clothing and place warm blankets over and under the patient. Doing this helps retain body heat and begins the warming process. If the patient is conscious, give warm fluids to drink.

If you are outdoors and cannot easily take the patient inside a building, move the patient into a heated vehicle as soon as possible. If you cannot move the patient to a warmer environment, keep the patient dry and place as many blankets and insulating materials as possible around the patient. Sometimes you can use your own body heat to warm the patient. Wrap blankets around yourself and the patient or get into a sleeping bag with the patient to use your body heat to start the warming process even during transport. Handle the patient gently. Any patient suffering from hypothermia must be examined by a physician.

FYI

The remaining material in this chapter is supplemental to The First Responder DOT curriculum.

Cardiac Arrest and Hypothermia

If the patient's temperature falls below 83°F (or 28°C), the heart may stop and you will need to begin CPR. Strange as it may seem, hypothermia may actually protect patients from death in some cases. Therefore, always start CPR on hypothermic patients even if you believe they have been "dead" for several hours. Hypothermic patients should never be considered dead until they have been warmed in an appropriate medical facility.

Treatment Tips

A special example of hypothermia protecting a patient from death is an apparent drowning in water colder than 70°F (21°C). Many children who fell in cold water and apparently drowned have been resuscitated successfully. Always start CPR on apparent drowning victims pulled from cold water.

Heart Conditions

The heart must receive a constant supply of oxygen or it will die. The heart receives its oxygen through a complex system of coronary (heart) arteries. As long as these arteries continue to supply the heart with an adequate amount of oxygen, the heart can continue to function properly.

As the body ages, however, the coronary arteries may narrow as a result of a disease process called **atherosclerosis**. Atherosclerosis causes layers of fat to coat the inner walls of the arteries. Progressive atherosclerosis can cause angina pectoris, heart attack, and even **cardiac arrest**.

Angina Pectoris

As atherosclerosis progresses, it can reduce the blood (oxygen) supply to the heart enough to cause pain or pressure in the chest. This pain is known as **angina pectoris** or simply angina. The heart simply needs more oxygen than the narrowed coronary arteries can deliver.

TABLE 10-2 Characteristics of Systemic Hypothermia

Core Temperature	93° to 95°F (34° to 35°C)	89° to 92°F (32° to 33°C)	80° to 88°F (27° to 31°C)	< 80°F (< 27°C)
Signs and Symptoms	Shivering, foot stamping	Loss of coordination, muscle stiffness	Coma	Apparent death
Cardiorespiratory Response	Constricted blood vessels, rapid breathing	Slowing respirations, slow pulse	Weak pulse, arrhythmias, very slow respirations	Cardiac arrest
Level of Consciousness	Withdrawn	Confused, lethargic, sleepy	Unresponsive	Unresponsive

When a patient has chest pain, you should first ask the person to describe the pain. Angina is often described as pressure or heavy discomfort. The patient may say something like, "It feels like an elephant is sitting on my chest." Angina attacks are usually brought on by exertion, emotion, or eating. Crushing pain may be felt in the chest and may radiate to either or both arms, the neck, jaw, or any combination of these sites. The patient is often short of breath and sweating, is extremely frightened, and has a sense of doom.

Ask whether the patient is already being treated for a diagnosed heart condition. If the answer is "yes," ask if the patient has a pill or spray to take for angina pain. A patient who has suffered previous bouts of angina usually has medication that can be taken (placed or sprayed under the tongue) to relieve the pain. The most common medication of this type is <u>nitroglycerin</u>, and the patient may have already taken a dose by the time you arrive on the scene Figure 10-4 ▾ .

If the patient has nitroglycerin but has not taken it during the past 5 minutes, help place one of the tiny pills under the patient's tongue or help the patient administer the aerosol spray. You should follow your local protocols regarding the administration of nitroglycerin. Nitroglycerin usually relieves angina pain within 5 minutes. If the pain has not diminished after 5 minutes, help the patient take a second dose. If the pain still has not lessened 5 minutes after the second dose, assume the patient is having a heart attack. Before you assist with the administration of nitroglycerin, you need to receive training and have permission from your medical director.

Heart Attack

A heart attack (myocardial infarction) results when one or more of the coronary arteries is completely blocked. The two primary causes of coronary artery blockage are severe atherosclerosis and a blood clot from somewhere else in the circulatory system that has broken free and become lodged in the artery. If one of the coronary arteries becomes blocked, the part of the heart muscle served by that artery is deprived of oxygen and dies Figure 10-5 ▶ .

Blockage of a coronary artery causes the patient to suffer immediate and severe pain. The pain of angina pectoris and heart attack may be similar at first. Most heart attack patients describe the pain as crushing. The pain may radiate from the chest to the left arm or to the jaw Figure 10-6 ▶ . The patient is usually short of breath, weak, sweating, nauseated, and may vomit. The pain of a heart attack is not relieved by nitroglycerin pills, and it will persist, unlike the pain of angina that rarely lasts more than 5 minutes.

If the area of heart muscle supplied by the blocked artery is either critical or large, the heart may stop completely. Complete cessation of heartbeat is called cardiac arrest. CPR is your first emergency treatment for cardiac arrest (see Chapters

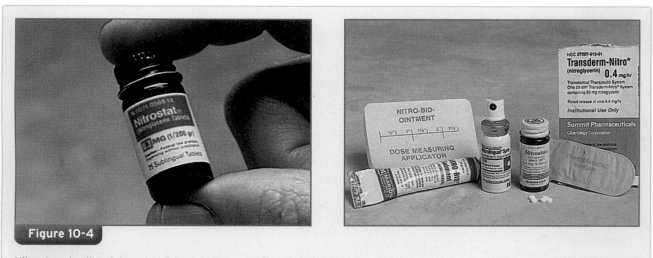

Figure 10-4

Nitroglycerin pills, ointment, patch, and spray used for relief of chest pain.

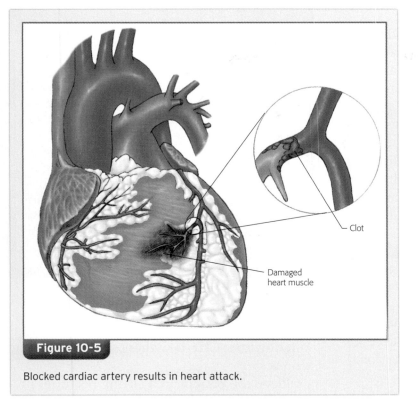

Figure 10-5

Blocked cardiac artery results in heart attack.

Clot

Damaged
heart muscle

6 and 9). Most heart attack patients do not experience immediate cardiac arrest. To support the patient and reduce the probability of cardiac arrest, you can take the following actions:

- Summon additional help.
- Talk to the patient to relieve his or her anxiety.
- Touch the patient to establish a bond. Hold the person's hand.
- Reassure the patient that you are there to help. The person is afraid that death is close and fear can create tension and make the pain worse.
- Move the patient as little as possible and do not allow the person to move! If the patient must be moved, you and other bystanders must move the patient.
- Place the patient in the position he or she finds most comfortable. This is usually a semireclining or sitting position.
- If oxygen is available and you are trained to use it, administer it to the patient. Supplemental oxygen increases the amount of oxygen the blood can carry. The increase in oxygen reduces pain and anxiety. It also eases the minds of the patient's family and friends to see that something is being done to relieve the patient's physical distress. Because you do not have extensive equipment available to help the heart attack patient, your primary role is to provide psychological support and arrange for **prompt transport** to an appropriate medical facility. Because the patient's emotional state can affect his or her physical condition, psychological support is valuable. It can prevent cardiac arrest.

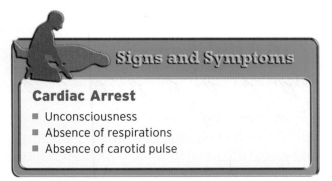

Signs and Symptoms

Cardiac Arrest

- Unconsciousness
- Absence of respirations
- Absence of carotid pulse

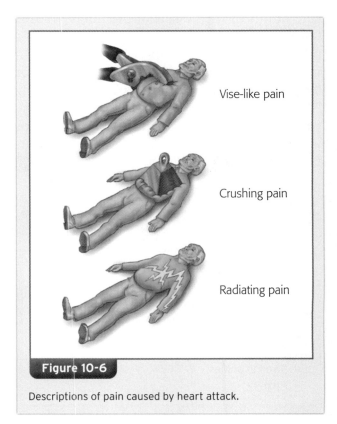

Vise-like pain

Crushing pain

Radiating pain

Figure 10-6

Descriptions of pain caused by heart attack.

Congestive Heart Failure

Congestive heart failure (CHF) is not directly caused by narrow or blocked coronary arteries, but by failure of the heart to pump adequately. As explained in Chapters 4 and 9, the heart has two sides. The right side receives "used" blood from the body and sends it to the lungs; the left side receives "fresh" oxygenated blood from the lungs and pumps it to the body. If one side of the heart becomes weak and cannot pump as well as the other side, the circulatory system becomes unbalanced, resulting in circulatory congestion. In CHF, the failure is in the heart muscle, but the congestion is in the blood vessels. **Figure 10-7 ▶** shows what happens if CHF occurs on the left side of the heart, which sends blood to the body. Because the left side cannot send blood to the body as efficiently as the right side can send blood to the lungs, more blood goes to the lungs than to the body. This results in congestion (overload) in the blood vessels of the lungs.

The major symptom of CHF is breathing difficulty, not chest pain. If you are called to assist a patient who has respiratory problems but no signs of injury or airway obstruction are present, look for the signs and symptoms of CHF. As blood pressure builds in the vessels of the lungs, fluid is forced into lung tissue, causing it to swell. The patient may make a gurgling sound when breathing and start spitting up a white or pink froth or foamy fluid. At this point, the patient is actually "drowning" in his or her own body fluids. The patient is very anxious but is usually in little or no pain (unless he or she is suffering a heart attack coupled with CHF).

Signs and Symptoms

Congestive Heart Failure

- Shortness of breath
- Rapid, shallow breathing
- Moist or gurgling respirations
- Profuse sweating
- Enlarged neck veins
- Swollen ankles
- Anxiety

Treatment Tips

Within the last 15 years, the use of "clot-buster" drugs has been an important advance in treating heart attack patients. Clot-buster drugs can often open the blocked coronary vessels and prevent the need for costly and painful operations.

Because clot busters must be administered by a specially trained physician within a few hours of the start of a heart attack to be effective, your prompt response and thoughtful care of a heart attack patient may be the first step in returning that patient to a comfortable, healthy, and productive life.

As soon as you determine that the patient is suffering from CHF, take these simple, lifesaving actions:

1. Place the patient in a sitting position, preferably on a bed or chair. Having the legs hang down over the edge of the bed or chair helps drain some of the fluid back into the lower parts of the body and may improve breathing.
2. Administer oxygen (if it is available and you are trained to give it) in large quantities and at a high flow rate.
3. Summon additional help.
4. Arrange for **prompt transport** to an appropriate medical facility.

The most important action is to place the patient in a sitting position with the legs down. This position helps relieve CHF symptoms until more highly trained EMS personnel arrive.

Dyspnea

Dyspnea means shortness of breath or difficulty breathing. Although healthy people may experience shortness of breath during intense physical exertion or at high altitudes, this condition is usually associated with serious heart or lung disease. Heart-related causes of dyspnea include angina pectoris, heart attack, and CHF. These conditions have already been discussed. Pulmonary (lung) diseases such as **chronic obstructive pulmonary disease (COPD)**, emphysema, chronic **bronchitis**, pneumonia, and asthma can also cause dyspnea.

Chronic obstructive pulmonary disease and emphysema are caused by damage to the small air sacs (alveoli) in the lungs. This damage decreases the amount of working lung capacity, resulting in shortness of breath. Chronic bronchitis is caused by an inflammation of the airways in the lungs. Pneumonia is caused by an infection in the lungs. Asthma is discussed in the next section.

As a first responder, you will not always be able to determine what is causing a patient to be short of breath. Do not spend too much time trying to determine the specific cause, but focus on treating the symptoms of dyspnea.

General treatment for patients with dyspnea consists of the following steps:

1. Check the patient's airway to be sure it is not obstructed.
2. Check the rate and depth of the patient's breathing. If the rate is below eight breaths per minute or above 40 breaths per minute, be prepared to assist with mouth-to-mask or mouth-to-barrier-device rescue breathing.
3. Place the patient in a comfortable position. A conscious patient is usually most comfortable when sitting.
4. Provide reassurance.
5. Loosen any tight clothing.
6. Administer oxygen, if it is available and you are trained to do so.

Asthma

One common cause of dyspnea is asthma. Asthma is an acute clamping down or spasm of the smaller air passages. It is associated with excess mucus production and swelling of the small airways and is caused by a type of allergic reaction. Asthma is a common condition that affects 6 million people in the United States. It is a serious disease that kills 4,000 to 5,000 people each year.

Patients experiencing an asthma attack have great difficulty exhaling through partially obstructed air passages. A wheezing sound will be heard during exhalation. If there is a limited

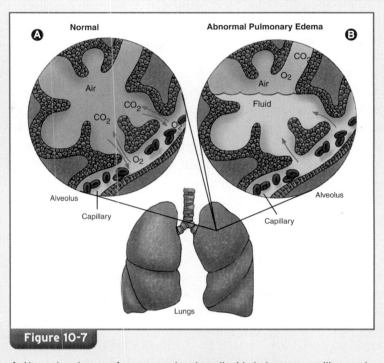

Figure 10-7

A. Normal exchange of oxygen and carbon dioxide between a capillary and an alveolus. **B.** Pulmonary edema: Congestive heart failure causes fluid to leak from the capillary and build in the alveolus, impeding oxygen and carbon dioxide exchange.

In the Field

The major symptom of heart attack is chest pain; the major symptom of CHF is difficulty breathing.

Treatment Tips

Patients who are short of breath or receiving oxygen should have their breathing and pulse monitored at least every 5 minutes. Underlying illness or trauma may cause certain patients to stop breathing and require you to begin rescue breathing.

amount of air moving through the small air passages, wheezing may be absent. Fatigued patients may be so short of breath that they are unable to talk. Many asthmatic patients will have taken medications before your arrival.

Patients can die during asthma attacks. It is important that you follow the steps just listed for treating dyspnea. In addition to these steps, you can instruct the patient to perform pursed-lip breathing. Ask the patient to purse his or her lips as if blowing up a balloon when exhaling. Tell the patient to blow out with force. Pursed-lip breathing relieves some of the internal lung pressures that cause the asthma attack. Treatment by paramedics or in the hospital includes medications that help to relax the constricted air passages. If advanced life support is not available, arrange for **prompt transport** to an appropriate medical facility.

Stroke

Strokes are a leading cause of brain injury and disability in adults. Each year millions of adults suffer strokes. Nearly a quarter of them die. Most strokes (70%) are caused by a blood clot that lodges in an artery of the brain. The clot blocks the blood supply to part of the brain. Without treatment, that part of the brain will be damaged or die. Think of a stroke as a "brain attack," similar to a heart attack. People with high blood pressure have an increased risk of having a stroke.

The signs and symptoms of stroke vary depending on which portion of the brain is affected. A stroke patient may be alert, confused, or unresponsive. Responsive patients may not be aware that they have signs of a stroke. Some stroke patients are unable to speak; others are unable to move one side of their body. The patient may have a headache and may describe it as "the worst headache of my life." Some stroke patients suffer seizures. The signs and symptoms of a stroke may be similar to the signs and symptoms of a head injury, insulin shock, or seizures.

The Cincinnati Prehospital Stroke Scale is an easy to administer and accurate tool used to determine if a patient might have suffered a stroke. It requires no tools to administer. It assesses facial muscles by having the patient smile, arm drift by having the patient hold their arms in front of them, and speech by having the patient repeat a simple phrase. If the patient is not able to complete one or more of these tasks, you should suspect they may be suffering from a stroke. Table 10-3 ▼ describes the specific steps for administering the Cincinnati Prehospital Stroke Scale.

Your first priority is to maintain an open airway. Administer oxygen (if available and you are trained to use it) using a nonrebreathing face mask. If the patient is having convulsions, try to prevent further injury from occurring. Be prepared to administer rescue breathing if the patient stops breathing. Place unresponsive patients in the recovery position to help them maintain an open airway (see Figure 10-1, page 236). This is especially important because some stroke patients are unable to swallow. Give psychological support by talking to and touching the patient. Be especially careful if you must move a patient

---

TABLE 10-3   The Cincinnati Prehospital Stroke Scale

The Cincinnati Prehospital Stroke Scale is a tool you can use to tell if there is a high probability that a patient has suffered a stroke. This scale requires you to quickly assess three things: Facial Droop, Arm Drift, and Abnormal Speech.

Facial Droop	**Have patient show teeth or smile.**
Normal	Both sides of the face move equally.
Abnormal	One side of the face does not move as well as the other side.
Arm Drift	**Patient closes eyes and holds both arms straight out for 10 seconds.**
Normal	Both arms move the same or both arms do not move the same.
Abnormal	One arm does not move or one arm drifts down compared to the other.
Abnormal Speech	**Have patient say, "You can't teach an old dog new tricks."**
Normal	Patient uses correct words with no slurring.
Abnormal	Patient slurs words, uses the wrong words, or is unable to speak.

Note: If any of these three signs is abnormal, the probability of a stroke is 72%.

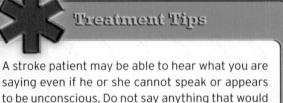

Signs and Symptoms

Stroke

- Headache
- Numbness or paralysis on one side of the body
- Dizziness
- Confusion
- Drooling
- Inability to speak
- Difficulty seeing
- Unequal pupil size
- Unconsciousness
- Convulsions
- Respiratory arrest
- Incontinence

Treatment Tips

A stroke patient may be able to hear what you are saying even if he or she cannot speak or appears to be unconscious. Do not say anything that would increase the patient's anxiety.

because some patients may not be able to feel one side of their body.

Some stroke patients can be treated with special drugs to dissolve the blood clot in their brain. These "clot-buster" drugs must be given in the hospital within the first few hours after the stroke. For this reason, it important for you to determine the time the stroke began from the patient, family, or bystanders. If the patient has signs or symptoms of a stroke, it is important for you to arrange for **prompt transport** of the patient to a medical facility that is equipped to treat stroke patients.

Diabetes

Diabetes is caused by the body's inability to process and use the type of sugar that is carried by the bloodstream to the body's cells. Sugar is an essential nutrient. The body's cells need both oxygen and sugar to survive. The body produces a hormone (chemical) called insulin that enables sugar carried by the blood to move into individual cells, where it is used as fuel.

If the body does not produce enough insulin, the cells become "starved" for sugar. This condition is called diabetes. Many diabetics (people with diabetes) must take supplemental insulin injections to bring their insulin levels up to normal. Mild diabetes can sometimes be treated by oral medicine rather than insulin.

Diabetes is a serious medical condition. Therefore, all diabetic patients who are sick must be evaluated and treated in an appropriate medical facility. Two specific things can go wrong in the management of diabetes: insulin shock and diabetic coma. Both are medical emergencies that you must deal with as a first responder.

Insulin Shock

Insulin shock occurs if the body has enough insulin but not enough blood sugar. A diabetic may take insulin in the morning and then alter his or her usual routine by not eating or by exercising vigorously. In either case, the level of blood sugar drops and the patient suffers insulin shock.

The signs and symptoms of insulin shock are similar to those of other types of shock. Suspect insulin shock if a patient has a history of diabetes or is wearing medical emergency information, such as a medical alert tag necklace or bracelet.

Insulin shock is a serious medical emergency that can occur quickly, often within a few minutes. If insulin shock is not diagnosed and corrected by the administration of sugar in some form, the patient may die.

A person experiencing insulin shock may appear to be drunk. You must keep this fact in mind. Mistakes have been and will continue to be made by first responders and others who misinterpret insulin shock as intoxication. If you suspect that a patient is suffering from insulin shock, try to get answers to the following questions:

- Are you a diabetic?
- Did you take your insulin today?
- Have you eaten today?

If the patient is diabetic and has taken insulin that day, but has not yet eaten, you should suspect that the patient is going into insulin shock. If the patient is able to swallow, attempt to get the pa-

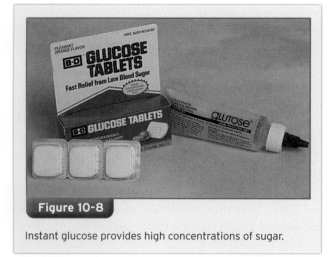

Figure 10-8

Instant glucose provides high concentrations of sugar.

TABLE 10-4	Comparing Insulin Shock and Diabetic Coma	
Insulin Shock		**Diabetic Coma**
Pale, moist, cool skin		Warm, dry skin
Rapid, weak pulse		Rapid pulse
Normal breathing		Deep, rapid breathing
Dizziness or headache		–
Confusion or unconsciousness		Unresponsiveness or unconsciousness
Rapid onset of symptoms (minutes)		Slow onset of symptoms (days)

In the Field

Progression into insulin shock is rapid and may be fatal; progression into diabetic coma usually takes several days.

Signs and Symptoms

Insulin Shock

- Pale, moist, cool skin
- Rapid, weak pulse
- Dizziness or headache
- Confusion or unconsciousness
- Rapid onset of symptoms (within minutes)

tient to eat or drink something sweet. For example, you could use a drink that has a high sugar concentration such as a cola or orange juice; honey is another possibility. Do not give a diet beverage to these patients. Diet beverages do not contain the necessary sugar.

If the patient is unconscious, do not try to administer fluids by mouth because the patient may choke and aspirate the fluid into the lungs. Summon help immediately. Open the patient's airway and assist breathing and circulation, if necessary. The patient must have sugar administered intravenously as soon as possible. This can be done by a paramedic or a physician. Some first responders carry a tube of oral glucose that can be placed inside the cheek **Figure 10-8 ▲**. This can be administered to unconscious patients and may be effective in providing the patient with the needed sugar. Even though the patient's body may absorb only a small amount of sugar as a result of your efforts, it may be enough to prolong consciousness until the patient receives further medical treatment.

Diabetic Coma

Diabetic coma occurs when the body has too much blood sugar and not enough insulin. A person with diabetes may fail to take insulin for several days. Blood sugar builds to higher and higher levels, but there is no insulin to process it for use by body cells.

The patient may be unresponsive or unconscious. A patient suffering from diabetic coma may appear to have the flu (influenza) or a severe cold. As with insulin shock, misdiagnosis is common. It is not always easy to tell the difference between insulin shock and diabetic coma **Table 10-4 ▲**.

If the patient is conscious or partly conscious, if you cannot get definite answers to your questions, or if you are not sure whether the patient is suffering from insulin shock or diabetic coma,

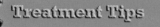

Treatment Tips

During your initial examination of every patient, look for an emergency medical alerting device to find out whether the patient has a preexisting medical condition, such as diabetes.

Signs and Symptoms

Diabetic Coma

- History of diabetes
- Warm, dry skin
- Rapid, pulse
- Deep, rapid breathing
- Fruity odor on the patient's breath
- Slow onset of symptoms (days)

you can do no harm by administering a liquid sugar substance. Sugar may improve the condition of a patient suffering from insulin shock and will not raise blood sugar levels enough to do further harm to the patient entering a diabetic coma. In general, give conscious diabetic patients sugar by mouth and arrange for **prompt transport** to an appropriate medical facility.

If the diabetic patient is unconscious, arrange for **prompt transport** to an appropriate medical facility and administer oral glucose only if approved by your medical director. Every sick diabetic patient must be transported by ambulance to an appropriate medical facility for further treatment and examination.

Abdominal Pain

Separated from the chest by the diaphragm, the abdomen is a crossroads for several body systems, including the circulatory, skeletal, nervous, digestive, and genitourinary systems. For example, the aorta carries blood from the heart through

the abdomen to the lower parts of the body while a large vein, the vena cava, carries blood back to the heart. The spine, with its large trunks of nerves, runs through this area, and parts of the rib cage surround the abdominal cavity. Most of the digestive system including the stomach, small intestine, large intestine, liver, gallbladder, and pancreas are in the abdomen. The kidneys and ureters are located in the abdominal area as well as parts of the male and female reproductive systems.

The contents of the abdomen are divided into hollow and solid structures. Hollow structures, such as the small intestine, are really tubes through which contents pass. Solid structures, such as the pancreas and the liver, produce substances. The structures in the abdomen are sometimes identified by quadrant, according to their location. As a first responder, you do not have to learn the names, types, and locations of all the abdominal structures.

The abdomen occupies a large part of the body and abdominal pain is a common complaint. Because of the number of body systems and organs located in the abdomen, even physicians may have a difficult time identifying the cause of abdominal pain. As a first responder, you need to be able to recognize that a patient has an abdominal problem. You are not expected to determine the cause of the abdominal pain.

One condition you may encounter is called an **acute abdomen**. An acute abdomen is caused by irritation of the abdominal wall. This irritation may be due to infection or to the presence of blood in the abdominal cavity as the result of disease or trauma. A patient with an acute abdomen

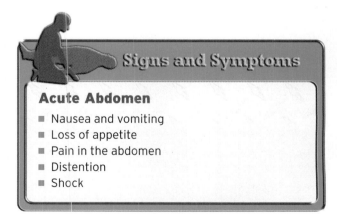

Signs and Symptoms

Acute Abdomen

- Nausea and vomiting
- Loss of appetite
- Pain in the abdomen
- Distention
- Shock

may have referred pain in other parts of the body such as the shoulder. The abdomen may feel as hard as a board.

If a patient has abdominal pain, monitor vital signs, treat symptoms of shock, keep the patient comfortable, and arrange for **transport** to an appropriate medical facility. It is important for these patients to be examined by a physician.

One cause of an acute abdomen is an **abdominal aortic aneurysm (AAA)**. An abdominal aortic aneurysm occurs when one or more layers of the aorta become weakened and separate from other layers of the aorta. Patients who have diabetes, high blood pressure, or atherosclerosis as well as heavy smokers are at high risk for developing an AAA. The weakening of the aorta causes a ballooning of the vessel, much like a weak spot on thin rubber tubing. If this weak spot or aneurysm ruptures, the patient will rapidly lose huge quantities of blood into his or her abdomen. This massive internal blood loss will cause profound shock.

Patients with an AAA may complain of pain in the abdomen. Some patients describe this pain as a tearing sensation. They may have pain referred to the shoulder. If an AAA ruptures, the patient will experience severe pain and profound shock from the blood spilling into the abdomen.

Any patient who experiences these signs and symptoms should be placed in a comfortable position. This is often sidelying with the legs drawn up. Treat the patient for shock. Handle these patients gently and arrange for **prompt transport** to an appropriate medical facility. The sooner these patients receive medical care the better their chance of survival will be.

You are the Provider SUMMARY

Review the *You are the Provider* case study provided at the beginning of the chapter.

You are dispatched to a private residence to assist a patient who is experiencing difficulty breathing. En route to the scene you review what you have learned about patients who are short of breath.

1. **Why is it important to obtain a thorough medical history on a patient like this?**

   By obtaining a thorough medical history, you will learn the signs and symptoms associated with the patient's shortness of breath, allergies, medications the patient is taking, past medical history, and events leading to this present illness. This medical history will help you to put the pieces of the illness "puzzle" together.

2. **Diseases of which two body systems are most likely to cause a patient to become short of breath?**

   The two body systems most likely to cause a patient to be short of breath are the cardiovascular system and the respiratory system. Although you will not be expected to be able to identify the patient's exact problem, reviewing the common causes of these symptoms may help you to assist the patient.

3. **Describe why a calm approach and a reassuring attitude benefit a patient who is short of breath.**

   By maintaining a calm approach and helping the patient to remain calm, you can help to reduce the amount of oxygen the patient needs and help the patient to be less anxious during this frightening time.

Many emergency calls are for patients who are suffering shortness of breath. These calls can be challenging for you as a first responder.

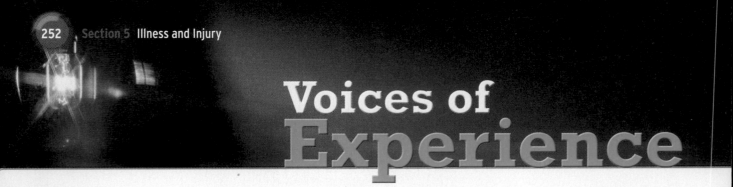

Voices of Experience

Things Are Not Always How They Seem

The call came in on a Sunday morning for a "man down." When my partner and I arrived at the patient's residence, an older woman, who was obviously dressed for church, waved us inside the house.

As soon as I walked into the house, I heard a blood-curdling scream and looked around the corner to find the patient rolling around on the floor, obviously in pain. The patient kept saying, "My back is killing me." His wife was upset. She was yelling at him to stop faking, saying that she knew he was doing this in an attempt to stay home from church and watch fishing on TV.

> " You can't let the attitudes of other people on the scene influence your diagnosis. "

While my partner got the vital signs, I spoke to the patient's wife. She told me that he was 68 years old, pretty healthy, and that his only significant medical history was for high blood pressure. At about this time, my patience for the patient's screaming complaint was really beginning to wear thin. My partner looked up and stated, "I can't get a blood pressure."

Well, I knew he had to have a blood pressure, so I decided to take it myself. I pumped up the blood pressure cuff and noted that the patient was still complaining of pain. I began to deflate the cuff, waiting and waiting to hear the familiar ticking, and I continued to wait and wait. After inflating the cuff another time without any success, I figured I would just get a palpable blood pressure. I reached down to palpate the patient's radial pulse, and that's when it hit me, he didn't have one.

All that training and I was missing something really big. I thought for a quick second, then went back to the ABCs. What could cause severe back pain and shock? I quickly unbuckled the patient's belt and trousers and attempted to palpate a femoral pulse. Not only could I not get a femoral pulse, but I noticed that both of the patient's legs were blue—and I mean blue!

We quickly placed the patient in a Reeves stretcher and began a rapid code 3 response to the hospital. I called into the emergency department at the hospital and advised the physician that I had a patient who had a leaking or ruptured abdominal aortic aneurysm and who was extremely hypotensive. On arrival, we were met by the emergency room physician and the surgeon, and the patient was taken directly to the operating room.

A few weeks after the incident, the surgeon told me that the only thing that had saved the patient was our rapid diagnosis and transport. I didn't have the fortitude to tell him that I had originally thought the patient was faking, but I did learn an important lesson. As a responder, you can't let the attitudes of other people on the scene influence your diagnosis. The wife was convinced that her husband was faking, and as a result, I became convinced as well. Even though the patient appeared to be healthy, as responders, our eyes are trained to see beyond appearances. We must exhaust every option because sometimes things aren't how they appear to be. In this case, my ability to quickly realize that I was missing something saved this patient's life.

Matthew Zavarella, MS, RN, NREMT-P, CFRN, CCRN, CEN

Flight Nurse/Clinical Education
Life Flight–St. Vincent Mercy Medical Center
Medical University of Ohio
Toledo, Ohio

Prep Kit

Ready for Review

The Ready for Review thoroughly summarizes the chapter.

- General medical conditions may have different causes, but they result in similar signs and symptoms. By learning to recognize the signs and symptoms of these conditions as well as general treatment guidelines, you will be able to provide immediate care for patients even if you cannot determine the exact cause of the problems.

- Your approach to a patient who has a general medical complaint should follow the systematic patient assessment sequence. Usually, it is best to collect a medical history on the patient experiencing a medical problem before you perform a physical examination. The SAMPLE history format will help you secure the information you need.

- Altered mental status is a sudden or gradual decrease in the patient's level of responsiveness. In assessing altered mental status, remember the AVPU scale. You should complete the patient assessment sequence to ensure scene safety and proper assessment. Initial treatment is to maintain the patient's ABCs and normal body temperature and to keep the patient from additional harm. If the patient is unconscious and has not suffered trauma, place the patient in the recovery position or use an airway adjunct to help maintain an open airway.

- Seizures are caused by sudden episodes of uncontrolled electrical impulses in the brain. Usually, the seizure will be over by the time you arrive at the scene. If it has not ended, your treatment should focus on protecting the patient from injury. Do not restrain the patient's movements. You cannot do anything about the patient's airway during the seizure, but once the seizure has stopped, it is essential that you ensure an open airway. After you have opened the airway, place the patient in the recovery position and arrange for transport to an appropriate medical facility.

- A person suffering from heat exhaustion sweats profusely and becomes lightheaded, dizzy, and nauseated. To treat heat exhaustion, move the patient to a cooler place and treat him or her for shock. Unless the patient is unconscious, nauseated, or vomiting, give fluids by mouth to replace the fluids lost through sweating.

- A person suffering from heatstroke may be semi-conscious; unconsciousness may develop rapidly. Such patients may have temperatures as high as 106°F. Maintain the patient's ABCs. Move the patient from the heat and into a cool place as soon as possible. Remove the patient's clothes and soak the patient with water. Arrange for rapid transport.

- The body parts most susceptible to frostbite are the face, ears, fingers, and toes. Warming the frostbitten part must be done quickly and carefully. Usually, putting the fingers, toes, or ears next to a warm body part is sufficient.

- The initial signs of hypothermia include feeling of being cold, shivering, decreasing level of consciousness, and sleepiness. Signs of increasing hypothermia include a lack of coordination, mental confusion, and slowed reactions. If you suspect hypothermia, move the patient to a warm location, remove wet clothing, and place warm blankets over and under the patient.

- The second part of this chapter covers some specific medical conditions. By learning about the causes and knowing the signs and symptoms of these conditions, you may be able to provide more specific care for the patient. Although these conditions must be diagnosed and treated by a physician, you can greatly improve the patient's chances of survival by taking the simple actions described here until more highly trained EMS personnel arrive on the scene to assist you.

Technology

- Interactivities
- Vocabulary Explorer
- Anatomy Review
- Web Links
- Online Review Manual

www.FirstResponder.EMSzone.com

Vital Vocabulary

The Vital Vocabulary are the key terms for this chapter.

abdominal aortic aneurysm (AAA) A condition in which the layers of the aorta in the abdomen weaken. This causes blood to leak between the layers of the artery, causing it to bulge and sometimes rupture.

absence seizures Seizures that are characterized by a brief lapse of attention. The patient may stare and not respond. Also known as petit mal seizures.

acute abdomen The sudden onset of abdominal pain caused by disease or trauma which irritates the lining of the abdominal cavity and requires immediate medical or surgical treatment.

angina pectoris Chest pain with squeezing or tightness in the chest caused by an inadequate flow of blood to the heart muscle.

atherosclerosis A disease characterized by a thickening and destruction of the arterial walls and caused by fatty deposits within them; the arteries lose the ability to dilate and carry blood.

bronchitis Inflammation of the airways in the lungs.

cardiac arrest Sudden cessation of heart function.

chronic obstructive pulmonary disease (COPD) A slow process of destruction of the airways, alveoli, and pulmonary blood vessels caused by chronic bronchial obstruction (emphysema).

diabetes A disease in which the body is unable to use sugar normally because of a deficiency or total lack of insulin.

diabetic coma A state of unconsciousness that occurs when the body has too much sugar and not enough insulin.

dyspnea Difficulty or pain with breathing.

frostbite Partial or complete freezing of the skin and deeper tissues caused by exposure to the cold.

generalized seizures Seizures characterized by contraction of all the body's muscle groups. May last for several minutes. Also known as grand mal seizures.

heat exhaustion A form of shock that occurs when the body loses too much water and too many electrolytes through very heavy sweating after exposure to heat.

heatstroke A condition of rapidly rising internal body temperature that occurs when the body's mechanisms for the release of heat are overwhelmed. Untreated heatstroke can result in death.

hypothermia A condition in which the internal body temperature falls below 95ºF after prolonged exposure to cool or freezing temperatures.

insulin shock Condition that occurs in a diabetic who has taken too much insulin or has not eaten enough food.

nitroglycerin A medication used to treat angina pectoris; it increases blood flow and oxygen supply to the heart muscle and reduces or eliminates the pain of angina pectoris.

Assessment in Action

Assessment in Action presents a fictitious scenario to help you review what you learned in this chapter.

You are dispatched to a restaurant for the report of an ill patron. As you are responding, your dispatcher reports that the patient is experiencing chest pain. When you arrive on scene, you find a 68-year-old man who is pale, sweating, and holding his hand to his chest.

1. Describe the factors you need to assess in this scenario when performing a scene size-up.

2. What information related to the general impression of the patient can you gain as you approach this patient?

3. The next step in the initial assessment is:
   A. Patient's medical history
   B. Determining the patient's ABCs
   C. Physical examination
   D. Ongoing assessment

4. Obtaining a medical history will give you all but which of the following:
   A. Allergies
   B. Medications
   C. Signs and symptoms
   D. Name of his illness

5. Your patient becomes confused and starts to seize. You should:
   A. Insert an oral airway
   B. Insert a nasal airway
   C. Protect the patient from further harm
   D. Open the patient's airway

6. If the patient is not able to answer your questions, you could obtain a medical history by:
   A. Calling the patient's physician
   B. Asking the wait staff if they know the patient
   C. Questioning family members or friends
   D. Looking for medical bracelets or necklaces

Poisoning and Substance Abuse

Chapter Objectives*

Knowledge and Attitude Objectives

1. Understand what a poison is. (p 258)
2. Describe the signs and symptoms of ingested poisons. (p 259)
3. Describe how to treat a patient who has ingested a poison. (p 259-260)
4. Describe the signs and symptoms of inhaled poisons. (p 261, 263)
5. Describe how to treat a patient who has inhaled a poison. (p 261)
6. Describe the signs and symptoms of injected poisons. (p 263)
7. Describe how to treat a patient who has injected a poison. (p 263-264)
8. Describe the signs and symptoms of absorbed poisons. (p 264-265)

9. Describe how to treat a patient who has absorbed a poison. (p 264-265)
10. Describe the signs and symptoms of a drug overdose caused by uppers, downers, hallucinogens, and abused inhalants. (p 267)
11. Describe the general treatment for a patient who has suffered a drug overdose. (p 267-268)

Skill Objectives

1. Use water to flush a patient who has come in contact with liquid poison. (p 264-265)
2. Brush a dry chemical off the patient and then flush with water. (p 264-265)

*These are chapter learning objectives.

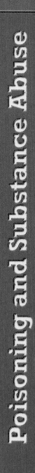
You are the Provider

It is late afternoon and so far you have had a quiet tour of duty. You are dispatched to a residence for a patient suffering from an overdose. En route you call back to your dispatcher to determine the age of the patient. The dispatcher indicates that the age of the patient is not known. As you continue to respond, you mentally prepare yourself for the types of situations you might encounter on this call.

What types of overdoses would you most likely encounter if this patient were:
1. A young child?
2. A young adult?
3. A geriatric patient?

Introduction

A **poison** is a substance that causes illness or death when eaten, drunk, inhaled, injected, or absorbed in relatively small quantities. This chapter covers signs, symptoms, emergency care, and treatment of patients suffering from accidental or intentional poisoning, bites, stings, or alcohol or substance abuse. You can save a patient's life by quickly recognizing and promptly treating a serious poisoning.

FYI

All material in this chapter is supplemental to the First Responder DOT curriculum.

General Considerations

As a first responder, you need to be a good detective when dealing with patients who have come in contact with poisons. Poisoning can be classified according to the way the poison enters the body.

Poisons can enter the body by four primary routes:

1. *Ingestion* occurs when a poison enters the body through the mouth and is absorbed by the digestive system.
2. *Inhalation* occurs when a poison enters the body through the mouth or nose and is absorbed by the mucous membranes lining the respiratory system.
3. *Injection* occurs when a poison enters the body through a small opening in the skin and spreads through the circulatory system. Injection can occur as a result of an insect sting, a snake bite, or the intentional use of a hypodermic needle to inject a poisonous substance into the body.
4. *Absorption* occurs when a poison enters the body through intact skin and spreads through the circulatory system.

Even though poisons can be introduced into the body by different routes, some of the effects of the poison on the body may be very similar. In general, to assess and treat patients who have been poisoned, begin with a thorough assessment that follows the patient assessment sequence. If you suspect

Technology

Interactivities

Vocabulary Explorer

Anatomy Review

Web Links

Online Review Manual

Special Populations

Accidental poisonings can occur in people of all ages. In the past, the rate of deaths from accidental poisonings was highest in children between birth and 4 years of age. The advent of childproof caps and other safety containers has significantly decreased poisoning deaths among children. Today, deaths from accidental poisonings are highest in adults between 25 and 44 years of age, primarily because of the increase in the use of illegal drugs **Figure 11-1 ▾** .

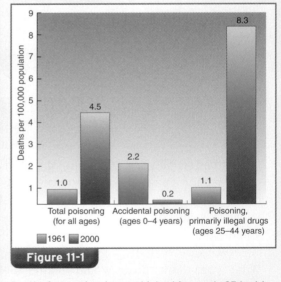

Figure 11-1

Deaths from poisoning are highest in people 25 to 44 years of age.

Safety Tips

Be especially careful when performing an overview of the scene to determine if it is safe to enter. Be alert for odors. Look for containers close to the patient. If you believe the scene is unsafe, stay a safe distance away and call for specialized assistance.

TABLE 11-1	General Signs and Symptoms of Poisoning
History	History of ingesting, inhaling, injecting, or absorbing a poison
Respiratory	Difficulty breathing or decreased respirations
Digestive	Nausea and vomiting
Abdominal pain
Diarrhea
Central Nervous System	Unconsciousness or altered mental status
Dilation or constriction of the pupils
Convulsions
Other	Excess salivation
Sweating
Cyanosis
Empty containers

poisoning, obtain a thorough history from the patient or from bystanders. A good history of the incident will help guide you in your patient assessment.

Be alert for any visual clues that may indicate the patient has been in contact with a poison. These include traces of the substance on the patient's face and mouth (ingested poisons), traces of the substance on the skin (absorbed poisons), needle pricks or sting marks (injected poisons), and respiratory distress (inhaled poisons).

Much of the emergency care you give will be based on the patient's symptoms. A patient with a poisonous substance on the skin needs to have the substance removed. A patient who is showing signs of respiratory distress needs to receive respiratory support. A patient who is exhibiting signs of digestive distress needs to receive support for

that problem. Sometimes the patient's signs and symptoms will be less specific, and you will have to base your treatment on general signs and symptoms. The general signs and symptoms of poisoning are shown in Table 11-1.

Ingested Poisons

An ingested poison is taken by mouth. More than 80% of all poisoning cases are caused by ingestion. Often, there are chemical burns, odors, or stains around the mouth. The person may also be suffering from nausea, vomiting, abdominal pain, or diarrhea. Later symptoms may include abnormal or decreased respirations, unconsciousness, or seizures.

Treatment for Ingested Poisons

To treat a person who has ingested a poison:
- Identify the poison.
- Call the poison control center for instructions and follow instructions (800-222-1222). If you are unable to contact the poison control center, dilute the poison by giving water.
- Arrange for **prompt transport** to a hospital.

Treatment Tips

Place an unconscious patient in the recovery position to help keep the airway open and to facilitate the drainage of mucus and vomitus from the mouth and nose Figure 11-2.

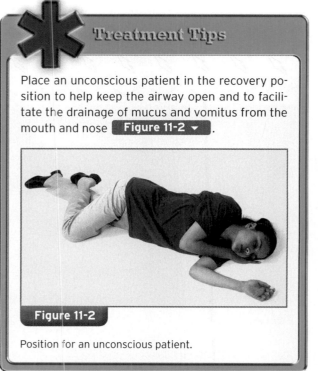
Figure 11-2
Position for an unconscious patient.

Before treating a person who has ingested a poison, attempt to identify the substance that has been ingested. Question the patient's family or bystanders and look for empty containers such as empty pill bottles that may indicate what the patient ate or drank. If there will be a delay in transporting the patient, contact the poison control center in your community. You should have the number of your local poison control center accessible in your first responder life support kit Figure 11-3 ▾ . The poison control center can tell you if you should start any treatment before the patient is transported to the hospital.

Dilution

Most poisons can be diluted by giving the patient large quantities of water, providing the patient is conscious and able to swallow.

Activated Charcoal

Administering activated charcoal is another method of treating ingested poisons Figure 11-4 ▸ . Activated charcoal is a finely ground powder that is mixed with water to make it easier to swallow. It works by binding to the poison, thereby preventing the poison from being absorbed in the patient's digestive tract.

Activated charcoal may be used by some first responder systems to treat poisonings if the nearest medical facility is a long distance away. However, you should give activated charcoal only if

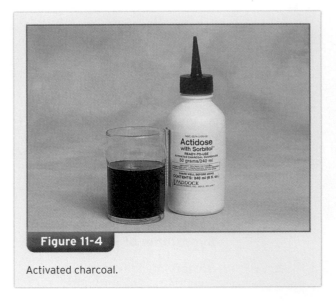

Figure 11-4

Activated charcoal.

you are trained in its use and have approval from your medical director or your poison control center. Do not give it if the patient has ingested an **acid** (a chemical substance with a pH of less than 7.0 that can cause severe burns) or an alkali, such as liquid drain cleaner, or if the patient is unconscious. The usual dose for an adult patient is 25 to 50 grams. The usual dose for a pediatric patient is 12.5 to 25 grams. Because the mixture looks like mud, you can serve the mixture in a covered cup and give the patient a straw. This may make it easier for the patient to drink.

Vomiting

In the past, syrup of ipecac was used to cause vomiting, but today it is recommended in only a few situations in which the risk of losing consciousness is clearly ruled out. Because syrup of

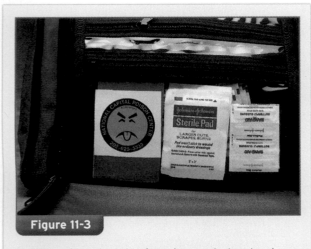

Figure 11-3

Post the universal number for poison control centers in your first responder life support kit: 800-222-1222.

Signs and Symptoms

Ingested Poisons

- Unusual breath odors
- Discoloration or burning around the mouth
- Nausea and vomiting
- Abdominal pain
- Diarrhea
- Any of the other signs and symptoms of poisoning listed in Table 11-1.

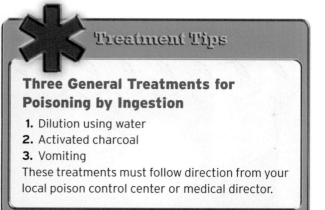

Treatment Tips

Three General Treatments for Poisoning by Ingestion

1. Dilution using water
2. Activated charcoal
3. Vomiting

These treatments must follow direction from your local poison control center or medical director.

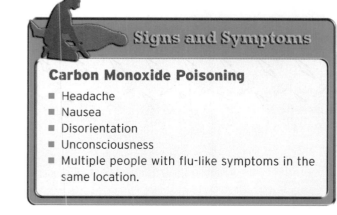

Signs and Symptoms

Carbon Monoxide Poisoning

- Headache
- Nausea
- Disorientation
- Unconsciousness
- Multiple people with flu-like symptoms in the same location.

ipecac induces vomiting, individuals who have ingested substances that may cause diminished alertness over time may vomit and inhale the vomit into the lungs as they lose consciousness. Activated charcoal is considered more effective and safer that syrup of ipecac.

Inhaled Poisons

Poisoning by inhalation occurs if a **toxic** substance is breathed in and absorbed through the lungs. Some toxic substances such as carbon monoxide are very poisonous but are not irritating. **Carbon monoxide (CO)** is an odorless, colorless, tasteless gas that cannot be detected by your normal senses. Other toxic gases such as chlorine gas and ammonia are very irritating and will cause coughing and severe respiratory distress. These gases can be classified as irritants.

Carbon Monoxide

One of the most common causes of carbon monoxide poisoning is an improperly vented heating appliance. Carbon monoxide also is present in smoke. People caught in building fires often suffer carbon monoxide poisoning. Inhaling relatively small quantities of carbon monoxide gas can result in severe poisoning because carbon monoxide combines with red blood cells about 200 times more readily than oxygen. Therefore, a small quantity of carbon monoxide can "monopolize" the red blood cells and prevent them from transporting oxygen to all parts of the body.

Safety Tips

Residential carbon monoxide detectors are being installed in many homes. These detectors are designed to sound an alarm before the residents of the house show signs and symptoms of carbon monoxide poisoning. Once the residential carbon monoxide detector is activated, specially trained and equipped personnel must be summoned to investigate the source of the carbon monoxide.

The signs and symptoms of carbon monoxide poisoning include headache, nausea, disorientation, and unconsciousness. Low levels of carbon monoxide poisoning have signs and symptoms that are just like the flu. If you find several patients together who all have these symptoms (especially in winter), suspect carbon monoxide poisoning and remove everyone from the structure or vehicle.

Irritants

Many gases irritate the respiratory tract. Two of the more frequently encountered gases are:

1. **Ammonia.** Inhalation of ammonia usually occurs in agricultural settings where it is used as a fertilizer Figure 11-5 ▶. It has a strong, irritating odor that is highly toxic. Inhaling large amounts of ammonia gas deadens the sense of smell and severely irritates the lungs and upper respiratory tract, causing violent cough-

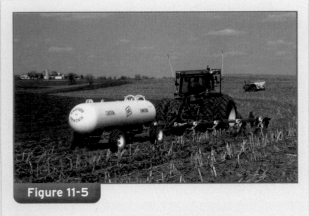

Figure 11-5

Fertilizer trucks on farms often carry ammonia.

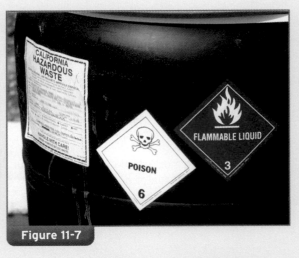

Figure 11-7

Placards used to identify the presence of hazardous materials.

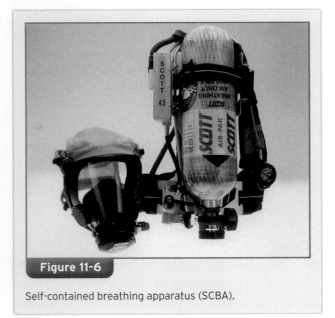

Figure 11-6

Self-contained breathing apparatus (SCBA).

ing. Ammonia can also severely burn the skin. Anyone who enters an environment containing ammonia must wear a proper encapsulating suit with a **self-contained breathing apparatus (SCBA)** Figure 11-6 ▲ . This apparatus contains a mask, regulator, and air supply and delivers air to rescuers when they enter contaminated areas.

2. **Chlorine.** Chlorine gas is commonly found in large quantities around swimming pools and water treatment plants. The odor of chlorine is familiar to anyone who has used chlorine bleach or been in a swimming pool or hot tub. Chlorine can severely irritate the lungs and the upper respiratory tract, causing violent coughing. Chlorine gas can also cause skin burns. Anyone who enters an environment containing chlorine must wear a proper encapsulating suit with a SCBA.

The presence of hazardous materials that are toxic (poisonous) and those in which there is danger of fire or explosion should be indicated by the appropriate hazardous materials warning placard Figure 11-7 ▲ .

Treatment for Inhaled Poisons

The first step in treating a patient who has inhaled any poison gas is to remove him or her from the source of the gas. If the patient is not breathing, begin mouth-to-mask breathing. If the patient is breathing, administer large quantities of oxygen (if available). Any patient who has inhaled a poisonous gas should be **transported promptly** to a medical facility for further examination because there may be a delayed reaction to the poison.

In some situations, your first response is to evacuate people. If you are called to the scene of a large poison gas leak (or other hazardous material leak), you may have to evacuate large numbers of people to prevent further injuries.

Signs and Symptoms

Inhaled Poisons

- Respiratory distress
- Dizziness
- Cough
- Headache
- Hoarseness
- Confusion
- Chest pain
- Any other signs and symptoms of poisoning listed in Table 11-1.

Safety Tips

Do not venture into areas where poisonous gases might be present. Call an agency (such as the fire department) that is equipped with SCBA. You should be especially aware of the hidden dangers found in tanks, confined spaces, farm silos, sewers, and other below-ground structures. Every year, rescuers lose their lives by venturing into a silo, sewer, or pit to save a person who may already be dead.

Once this has been done, begin to treat the evacuees as necessary.

Injected Poisons

The two major causes of poisoning by injection are (1) animal bites and stings and (2) toxic injection. This section covers animal bites and stings; toxic injection will be discussed later, as part of substance abuse. The signs and symptoms of poisonous stings and bites are shown in the box below. If a person has received a large amount of poison (for example, multiple bee stings) or if a person is especially sensitive to this poison (has an anaphylactic reaction), he or she may collapse and become unconscious.

Treatment for Insect Stings and Bites

A person who has been bitten or stung by an insect should be kept quiet and still. This will help slow the spread of the poison throughout the body. A light constricting band (*not* a tourniquet) may be used if there is severe swelling. Apply the band between the sting or bite and the patient's heart. It should be snug, but not so snug that it cuts off circulation. (Check for a distal pulse after application.) Ice packs may help reduce local swelling and pain.

Some people suffer an extreme allergic reaction to stings and bites and may go into anaphylactic shock (see Chapter 13). The signs and symptoms of **anaphylactic shock** include itching; **hives** (patches of swelling, redness, and intense itching on the skin); swelling; generalized weakness; unconsciousness; rapid, weak pulse; and rapid, shallow breathing. The patient's blood pressure drops, and the patient may even suffer cardiac arrest.

Elevating the patient's legs (shock treatment) may help in some cases. If the patient's condition progresses to the point of respiratory or cardiac arrest, begin mouth-to-mask breathing or CPR.

If a patient appears to be going into anaphylactic shock, immediately arrange for **rapid transport** to a medical facility where the patient can

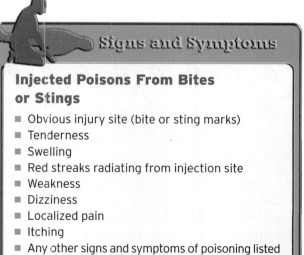

Signs and Symptoms

Injected Poisons From Bites or Stings

- Obvious injury site (bite or sting marks)
- Tenderness
- Swelling
- Red streaks radiating from injection site
- Weakness
- Dizziness
- Localized pain
- Itching
- Any other signs and symptoms of poisoning listed in Table 11-1.

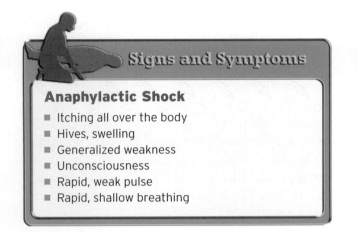

Signs and Symptoms

Anaphylactic Shock

- Itching all over the body
- Hives, swelling
- Generalized weakness
- Unconsciousness
- Rapid, weak pulse
- Rapid, shallow breathing

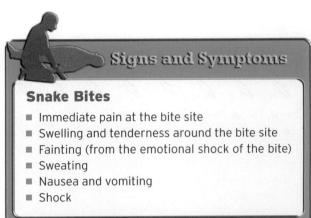

Signs and Symptoms

Snake Bites

- Immediate pain at the bite site
- Swelling and tenderness around the bite site
- Fainting (from the emotional shock of the bite)
- Sweating
- Nausea and vomiting
- Shock

receive treatment with specific medications. Medication may also be started by a paramedic who is working under the direction of a physician.

Snake Bites

There are four kinds of poisonous snakes in the United States: rattlesnake, cottonmouth, copperhead, and coral snake. The snake injects its poison into the skin and muscles with its fangs. This poison can cause local injury to the skin and muscle and may even involve the entire extremity. Signs and symptoms may affect the entire body (see the accompanying Signs and Symptoms box). A bite from a poisonous snake is rarely fatal; although nearly 7,000 people are bitten by snakes each year in the United States, fewer than 20 will die from the bite. However, permanent injury can sometimes result. The bite of the coral snake delivers a slightly different poison that may cause these additional problems:

- Respiratory difficulties
- Slurred speech
- Paralysis
- <u>Coma</u> (state of unconsciousness from which the patient cannot be aroused)
- Seizures

Treatment for Snake Bites

The field treatment for poisonous snake bite is basically the same as the treatment for shock (see Chapter 13). Keep the patient calm and quiet; have the patient lie down and try to relax. Gently wash the bite area with soap and water. If the bite occurred on the arm or leg, splint the affected

extremity to decrease movement. Place the splinted extremity below the level of the heart to decrease the absorption of the poison. Treat the patient carefully and arrange for **prompt transport** to the hospital or medical facility. The only effective treatment for poisonous snake bites is the administration of antivenin in the hospital.

Absorbed Poisons

Poisoning by absorption occurs when a poisonous substance enters the body through the skin. Insecticides and toxic industrial chemicals are two common poisons absorbed through the skin. A person suffering from absorption poisoning may have both localized and systemic signs and symptoms, as shown in the Signs and Symptoms box.

Treatment for Absorbed Poisons

The first step in treating a patient who has absorbed a poisonous substance is to ensure that the patient is no longer in contact with the toxic substance. You may have to ask the patient to remove all clothing. Then brush—do not wash—any dry chemical off the patient. Contact with water may activate the dry chemical and result in a burning or caustic reaction.

After removing all the dry chemical, wash the patient completely for at least 20 minutes. Use any water source that is available: an industrial shower, a home shower, a garden hose, or even a fire engine's booster hose. Do not forget to wash

Signs and Symptoms

Absorbed Poisons

- Traces of powder or liquid on the skin
- Inflammation or redness of the skin
- Chemical burns
- Skin rash
- Burning
- Itching
- Nausea and vomiting
- Dizziness
- Shock
- Any other signs and symptoms of poisoning listed in Table 11-1.

Treatment Tips

When in doubt in absorbed-poison situations, have the patient remove all clothing so that he or she is no longer in contact with the toxic substance.

out the patient's eyes if they have been in contact with the poison. If additional EMS personnel are delayed, contact the poison control center or your medical director for additional treatment information.

If the patient is suffering from shock, have the patient lie down and elevate the legs. If the patient is having difficulty breathing, administer oxygen if it is available and you are trained to use it.

Substance Abuse

Alcohol

Alcohol is the most commonly abused drug in U.S. society today. Alcohol intoxication may be seen in people of any age, including children and teenagers. Alcohol usage is involved in more than one half of all traffic fatalities, more than one half of all murders, and more than one third of all suicides. Deaths as a result of alcohol abuse are two and one half times as numerous as deaths from motor vehicle crashes. However, because the symptoms of alcohol intoxication are similar to those of other medical illnesses or severe injuries, you should never assume that an apparently intoxicated person is "just another drunk."

In addition, people who have been drinking can be injured or suddenly develop a serious illness. You cannot assume that the symptoms (including the smell of alcohol on someone's breath) are caused by drunkenness. If you are unsure about whether a patient who appears to be intoxicated has a serious injury or illness, be extra careful with your examination. You should arrange for **prompt transport** to an appropriate medical facility, where a physician can make a complete assessment.

Alcohol is an addictive, depressant drug. A person who is physically dependent on alcohol and then is suddenly deprived of it may develop withdrawal symptoms, such as convulsions or seizures. The most severe withdrawal symptoms are called <u>**delirium tremens (DTs)**</u>. The signs and symptoms of DTs include shaking, restlessness, confusion, hallucinations, gastrointestinal distress, chest pain, and fever. These signs and symptoms usually appear 3 to 4 days after the person stops drinking. **Transport** a person suffering from DTs to an appropriate medical facility. DTs are a serious medical emergency and can be fatal.

Drugs

In today's society, people of all ages abuse many different prescription and street drugs. Drugs may be ingested, inhaled, or injected into the body. As a first responder, you may not be able to identify the type of drug used, although this information will be helpful to medical providers. When you do your scene assessment, look for clues that can indicate what type of drug was used and how it was administered. Today, the most popular drugs fall into four categories: uppers, downers, hallucinogens, and inhalants **Figure 11-8 ▼** .

Voices of Experience

Recognizing the Accidental Overdose

My partner and I had just begun our shift on a paramedic transport unit when a call came in for a 43-year-old woman, possibly in cardiac arrest. A first responder engine company was also dispatched to assist. When the engine arrived, they found the patient in respiratory arrest and cyanotic. They began ventilating with a bag-mask device and high-flow oxygen, which improved the patient's color and oxygen saturation. They updated us on the patient's status, and we used this information to mentally prepare for the call.

> **Our EMS training can only take us so far, and working in the field is an extension of our classroom learning.**

When my partner and I arrived, the engine crew was maintaining the patient's airway and ventilating. The patient's daughter handed me several bottles of medications and a box containing a narcotic patch for pain management. The patient's unresponsiveness, respiratory impairment, and pinpoint pupils indicated to me that the patient was overdosing from the narcotic patch. My partner and I located a patch on the patient's left upper chest, removed it, and wiped away any remaining medication. We were able to reverse the immediate effects of the narcotic, and within minutes she began breathing on her own. Her mental status improved, but she remained confused.

We transferred her to the truck and began to transport. Throughout the ride, she remained awake but was slow to respond to questions. She also tried to vomit several times without bringing up anything. We did not realize at the time that she was continuing to overdose from the narcotics.

When we arrived at the emergency department and transferred care, the nurses removed all of the patient's clothing and found three additional narcotic patches. Once these were removed, the patient began to stabilize and recover. Although the outcome was favorable, we had omitted exposing the patient as part of the initial exam. If we had, we would have located the remaining narcotic patches and would have been able to stabilize her quicker.

I learned two important lessons from this call. First, patients who are prescribed a medication may not be educated properly in its use. Our patient was prescribed the narcotic patch the day before the call, and she continued applying patches in an attempt to relieve her pain, which resulted in an overdose. Second, it is important to expose all unresponsive patients as part of the initial assessment. Items such as medication patches and medical alert tags may be found, which give clues about the patient's condition and can help you figure out how best to treat the patient.

Not all EMS responses can be executed perfectly. Our EMS training can only take us so far, and working in the field is an extension of our classroom learning. When something goes wrong on a call, take the lessons you learned to improve your performance as an EMS provider. On this call, we were very fortunate to have a positive outcome. Our decision to transport quickly may have saved this patient's life. At any level of the EMS, it is important not to dwell on mistakes, but to learn from them and use them to the benefit of future patients.

Robert Shields, NREMT-P
Lieutenant, Cumberland Rescue Service
Cumberland, Rhode Island

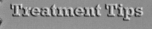

Treatment Tips

A person who appears intoxicated may be suffering instead from any one of a number of serious illnesses or injuries. Insulin shock, diabetic coma, head injury, traumatic shock, and drug reactions may all display the same symptoms as alcohol intoxication.

Uppers

Uppers are drugs that stimulate the **central nervous system (CNS)** (the brain and spinal cord). They include **amphetamines** (speed, ice, or crystal) and **cocaine** (coke). People using these substances show signs of restlessness, irritability, and talkativeness. They may need to be kept from harming themselves and should be taken to a facility where they can be monitored until the effects of the drug wear off.

Downers

Like alcohol, **downers** are depressants. Downers include **barbiturates** (drugs that depress the nervous system), tranquilizers, opiates, and marijuana. An overdose of one of these drugs can result in respiratory depression or arrest. A person who has overdosed on downers may be breathing shallowly or not at all. If the person is not breathing, begin mouth-to-mask resuscitation. If cardiac arrest occurs, begin CPR immediately.

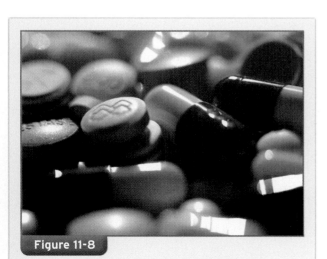

Figure 11-8

Types of drugs that are commonly abused.

Hallucinogens

Hallucinogens include PCP, LSD, peyote, mescaline, and some types of mushrooms. **Hallucinogens** are chemicals that cause people to see things that are not there. A patient who is hallucinating may become frightened and unable to distinguish between reality and fantasy. One hallucinogen, PCP, also blocks the body's pain receptors. People on PCP may feel no pain and may seriously injure themselves or others. Large doses of PCP can produce convulsions, coma, heart and lung failure, or stroke.

Abused Inhalants

Recently the intentional inhalation of volatile chemicals has increased, especially among teenagers who are seeking an alcohol-like high. Many of these substances can be bought in hardware stores and include gasoline, paint thinners, cleaning compounds, lacquers, and a wide variety of substances used as aerosol propellants. Users put the chemical in a plastic bag and inhale from the bag. The combination of a lack of oxygen and the effects of the poisonous substance inhaled can lead to unconsciousness and death. Some abused inhalants cause drowsiness or unresponsiveness. Some cause seizures. Others overstimulate the heart and produce sudden cardiac death from ventricular fibrillation.

Treat these patients carefully. Try to keep them from struggling. Support their airway, breathing, and circulation. Give high-flow oxygen as soon as it is available. Carefully monitor their vital signs and arrange for **prompt transport** to an appropriate medical facility.

Treatment for a Drug Overdose

Once you have determined that a patient is suffering from a drug overdose, the job of the first responder is to:

- Provide basic life support (clear the airway and perform mouth-to-mask breathing or CPR, as necessary).
- Keep the patient from hurting him- or herself and others.
- Provide reassurance and psychological support.
- Arrange for **prompt transport** to a medical facility for treatment.

The effects of some drugs can only be counteracted by other drugs administered by a paramedic or a physician. If a patient is acting out, speak to him or her in a calm, reassuring tone of voice and try to keep the patient from harming anyone. If a person reports seeing things that are not there, say, "I believe you are seeing those things; however, I do not see them myself." This statement lets the patient know that you understand his or her experience, but that in reality, the perceived object is not present.

Patients who are suffering adverse reactions from a drug overdose require specialized treatment. You and other EMS personnel should be aware of local facilities equipped to deal with such cases. Keep in mind that a person suffering from a drug overdose may also have other injuries or medical conditions that require medical treatment. Try to avoid classifying or judging the patient.

Toxic Injection From Drugs

Drugs that are injected into the bloodstream can result in toxic injection. The patient's reaction depends on the quantity and type of drug injected. Because street drugs may be diluted (*cut*) with sugar or other substances that should not be injected into the bloodstream, the patient may be unaware of exactly what has been injected. After a toxic injection, the patient may complain of weakness, dizziness, fever, or chills. This type of emergency requires you to support the patient, treat the symp-

Safety Tips

People who use intravenous drugs have a high incidence of bloodborne diseases such as hepatitis B and AIDS. Use body substance isolation (BSI) techniques to reduce your chances of coming in contact with bloodborne pathogens.

toms, and provide transport to an appropriate medical facility. You should also check the injection site for redness, swelling, and increased skin temperature. The presence of any of these signs may indicate an infection that will require medical care.

Intentional Poisoning

Intentional self-poisoning is attempted suicide and may involve ingested poisons (or drugs) or inhaled poisons (such as carbon monoxide). Regardless of whether the poisoning was accidental or intentional, medical treatment is the same. A patient who has attempted suicide needs both medical and psychological support. The patient may not want your help and may be difficult to treat. Nevertheless you and all other EMS personnel must make every effort to preserve life and offer reassurance.

You are the Provider SUMMARY

Review the *You are the Provider* case study provided at the beginning of the chapter.

It is late afternoon and so far you have had a quiet tour of duty. You are dispatched to a residence for a patient suffering from an overdose. En route you call back to your dispatcher to determine the age of the patient. The dispatcher indicates that the age of the patient is not known. As you continue to respond, you mentally prepare yourself for the types of situations you might encounter on this call.

1. What types of overdoses would you most likely encounter if this patient were a young child?

Young children tend to put objects in their mouths. Medications that are left within the reach of unsupervised children may result in overdoses. Likewise, young children may ingest cleaning supplies or other poisonous substances.

2. What types of overdoses would you most likely encounter if this patient were a young adult?

Overdoses that occur in young adults are most frequently the result of an attempted suicide or the result of an accidental overdose of recreational drugs.

3. What types of overdoses would you most likely encounter if this patient were a geriatric patient?

Many geriatric patients take a wide variety of medications for a multitude of ailments. Taking large numbers of medications coupled with confusion often leads to unintentional overdoses of prescribed medications.

The most likely pattern of overdoses changes with the age of the patient. Recognizing these patterns may help you to gain a better picture of a given incident.

Prep Kit

Ready for Review

The Ready for Review thoroughly summarizes the chapter.

- This chapter discusses the signs, symptoms, and treatment of patients who have suffered accidental or intentional poisoning.

- The four primary routes by which poisons enter the body are ingestion, inhalation, injection, and absorption.

- An ingested poison is taken by mouth. Often, there are chemical burns, odors, or stains around the mouth. The person may also be suffering from nausea, vomiting, abdominal pain, or diarrhea.

- An inhaled poison is breathed in and absorbed through the lungs. Some toxic substances such as carbon monoxide are very poisonous but are not irritating. Other toxic gases such as chlorine gas and ammonia are very irritating and will cause coughing and severe respiratory distress.

- The two major causes of poisoning by injection are (1) animal bites and stings and (2) toxic injection.

- Poisoning by absorption occurs when a poisonous substance enters the body through the skin. A person suffering from absorption poisoning may have both localized and systemic signs and symptoms.

- It is important to pay special attention to scene safety and not enter a hazardous environment without the proper training and equipment.

Technology

- Interactivities
- Vocabulary Explorer
- Anatomy Review
- Web Links
- Online Review Manual

Vital Vocabulary

The Vital Vocabulary are the key terms for this chapter.

acid A chemical substance with a pH of less than 7.0 that can cause severe burns.

amphetamines Stimulants that produce a general mood elevation, improve task performance, suppress appetite, or prevent sleepiness.

anaphylactic shock Severe shock caused by an allergic reaction to food, medicine, or insect stings.

barbiturates Drugs that depress the nervous system; they can alter the state of consciousness so that the individual may appear drowsy or peaceful.

carbon monoxide (CO) A colorless, odorless, poisonous gas formed by incomplete combustion, such as in a fire.

central nervous system (CNS) The brain and spinal cord.

cocaine A powerful stimulant that induces an extreme state of euphoria. Legitimately, it is a potent local anesthetic. On the street, it is commonly known as coke. Synthetic cocaine is known as crack.

coma A state of unconsciousness from which the patient cannot be aroused.

delirium tremens (DTs) A severe, often fatal, complication of alcohol withdrawal that can occur from 1 to 7 days after withdrawal. It is characterized by restlessness, fever, sweating, confusion, disorientation, agitation, hallucinations, and convulsions.

downers Depressants; barbiturates.

hallucinogens Chemicals that cause a person to see visions or hear sounds that are not real.

hives An allergic skin disorder marked by patches of swelling, redness, and intense itching.

poison Any substance that may cause injury or death if relatively small amounts are ingested, inhaled, or absorbed, or applied to, or injected into the body.

self-contained breathing apparatus (SCBA) A complete unit for delivery of air to a rescuer who enters a contaminated area; contains a mask, regulator, and air supply.

toxic Poisonous.

uppers Drugs that stimulate the central nervous system. These include amphetamines and cocaine.

Assessment in Action

Assessment in Action presents a fictitious scenario to help you review what you learned in this chapter.

On a night when temperatures are reported to be near freezing, you and your first responder partner are en route to 512 Maple Lane for a sick person. Upon arrival, as you enter the residence, you find a homemade gas heater to be the primary heat source for the home. You find four patients, all complaining of flu-like symptoms.

1. With the information given, which of the following is the most likely cause of the illness?

   A. Carbon monoxide poisoning
   B. Chlorine gas poisoning
   C. The bird flu
   D. None of the above

2. What is your first step in treating these patients?

3. Which is NOT a sign or symptom of carbon monoxide poisoning?

   A. Headache
   B. Vomiting
   C. Itching
   D. Disorientation

4. Carbon monoxide attaches to the red blood cells affecting the transportation of oxygen to the body.

   A. True
   B. False

5. All of these patients should receive prompt transport to the hospital for further observation.

   A. True
   B. False

Behavioral Emergencies

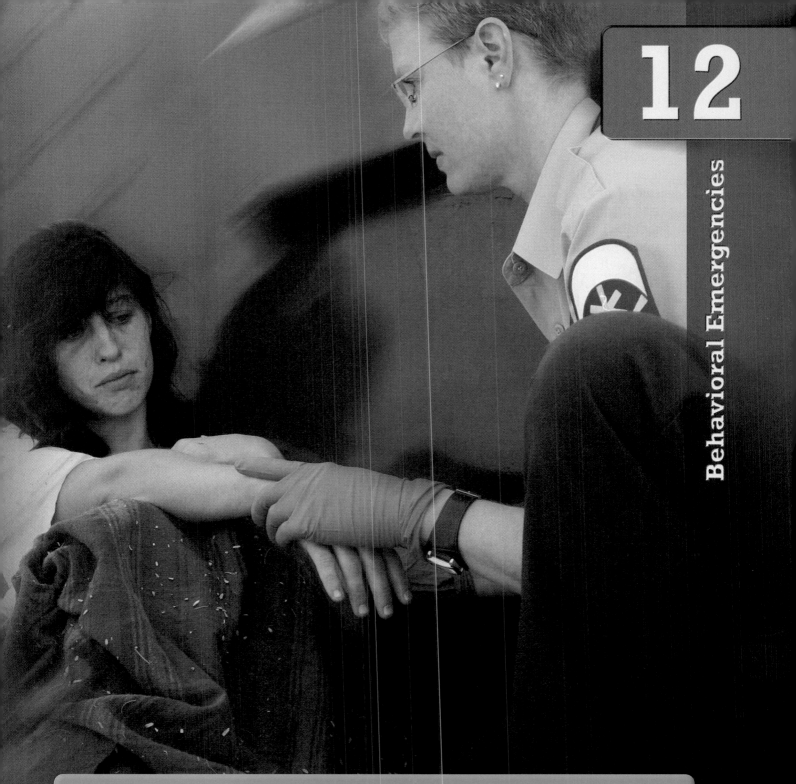

You are the Provider

You are dispatched to a residence located about 7 minutes from your station for a report of a "disturbed patient." This neighborhood is a middle-class suburban part of town with modest single-family homes. As you respond, you mentally review the types of situations you might encounter on this call.

1. What types of conditions could be included in the dispatcher's label of "disturbed patient"?
2. What factors should you consider and evaluate as you approach this patient?
3. What types of skills and interventions might be appropriate in dealing with this patient?

Introduction

Every emergency situation, whether it is an illness or an injury, has emotional and psychological effects on everyone involved—you, the patient, the patient's family and friends, and even bystanders. As a first responder to a behavioral emergency, you will need to give psychological support as well as necessary emergency medical care. This chapter explains the five major factors that cause behavioral crises: medical conditions, physical trauma conditions, psychiatric illnesses, mind-altering substances, and situational stresses.

The simple intervention techniques addressed in this chapter will help prepare you to deal with patients and their families during the stressful experience of a medical emergency. You will also be better able to identify and understand the reactions to the grief that you observe.

Many patients experience high anxiety, denial, anger, remorse, and grief during a situational crisis. Three skills that are useful when communicating with patients in crisis are restatement, redirection, and empathy. This chapter also provides information on how to deal with crowd control, domestic violence, violent patients, armed patients, suicide crisis, sexual assault, and death and dying. Medical and legal considerations and the role of critical incident stress debriefings are also covered.

Behavioral Crises

As a first responder, you will encounter situations in which patients exhibit abnormal behavior. Sometimes this abnormal behavior is the primary reason that you are called and sometimes it is a secondary reaction to another situation such as an accident or illness. **Behavioral emergencies** are defined as situations in which a person exhibits abnormal, unacceptable behavior that cannot be tolerated by the patients themselves or by family, friends, or the community. Some behavioral emergencies involve your patient, and others involve the patient's family or friends.

Five main factors contribute to behavioral changes. They are:

1. *Medical conditions* such as uncontrolled diabetes that causes low blood sugar, respiratory conditions that prevent the patient's brain from receiving enough oxygen, high fevers, and excess cold
2. *Physical trauma conditions* such as head injuries and injuries that result in shock and an inadequate blood supply to the brain
3. *Psychiatric illnesses* such as depression, panic, or **psychotic behavior** (behavior characterized by defective or lost contact with reality)
4. *Mind-altering substances* such as alcohol and a wide variety of chemical substances
5. *Situational stresses* from a variety of emotional traumas such as death or serious injury to a loved one

To better understand a behavioral crisis, you need to look at the stages a person passes through when experiencing a situational crisis.

What Is a Situational Crisis?

Simply put, a **situational crisis** is a state of emotional upset or turmoil. It is caused by a sudden and disruptive event such as a physical illness, a traumatic injury, or the death of a loved one. Every

Technology

- Interactivities
- Vocabulary Explorer
- Anatomy Review
- Web Links
- Online Review Manual

emergency creates some form of situational crisis for the patient and those persons close to the patient. You will often encounter this type of crisis as a first responder. Some of the concepts covered here are similar to the concepts covered in Chapter 2.

Most situational crises are sudden and unexpected (such as an automobile crash), cannot be handled by the person's usual coping mechanisms, last only a short time, and can cause socially unacceptable, self-destructive, or dangerous behavior.

Phases of a Situational Crisis

There are four emotional phases to each situational crisis. Although a person may not experience every phase during a crisis, he or she will certainly experience one or more. If you understand what these phases are and why they occur, you can better understand how to help people who are experiencing an emotional crisis.

High Anxiety or Emotional Shock

In the first phase of a situational crisis, a person exhibits high anxiety or emotional shock. High anxiety is characterized by rather obvious signs and symptoms: flushed (red) face, rapid breathing, rapid speech, increased activity, loud or screaming voice, and general agitation. **Emotional shock** is often the result of sudden illness, accident, or sudden death of a loved one. Like most other types of shock, emotional shock is characterized by cool, clammy skin; a rapid, weak pulse; vomiting and nausea; and general inactivity and weakness.

Denial

The next phase of a situational crisis may be denial or a refusal to accept the fact that an event has occurred. For example, a child who has just lost a parent may refuse to accept the death by telling everyone that the parent is sleeping or has gone away.

Allow the patient to express denial. Do not argue with the patient, but try to understand the emotional and psychological trauma that he or she is experiencing.

Anger

Anger is a normal human response to emotional overload or frustration. Anger may follow denial or, in some cases, may occur instead of denial. For example, the spouse of a patient may, for no apparent reason, begin screaming at you, calling you incompetent, or using foul language or racial slurs. Although it may be difficult, you should remain calm and not respond angrily as well.

In crisis situations, it is often easier to vent angry feelings on an unknown person (the first responder) or an authority figure (a law enforcement officer) than on a friend or family member. Anger is perhaps the most difficult emotion to deal with objectively because the angry person seems to be directing his or her anger at you. Do not take the person's anger personally, but acknowledge that it is a reaction to stress.

Frustration and a sense of helplessness can often build to anger. If these emotions are not released, the anger may be expressed by aggressive physical behavior. For example, in a serious crash involving a school bus, you may have to demonstrate to bystanders that you and other rescue personnel are indeed removing children from the crashed bus. If little activity is apparent to the bystanders, they may become angry, hostile, and even violent. In such situations,

---

In the Field

Emotional Phases of a Situational Crisis

- High anxiety or emotional shock
- Denial
- Anger
- Remorse and grief

Treatment Tips

Virtually every emergency call requires some degree of psychological intervention.

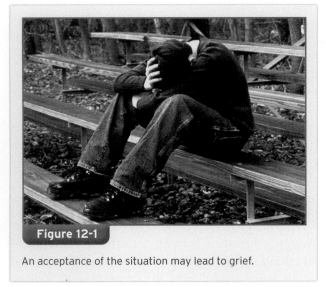

Figure 12-1

An acceptance of the situation may lead to grief.

show confidence. Demonstrate that you are making progress. Be professional and do not react to anger by becoming angry yourself. Remain calm and unhurried to prevent escalation of violence. If necessary, a member of the EMS team may have to explain the situation—what is being done and why it appears to be taking so long. Acknowledge anger by saying something like, "What's the matter? Can you tell me what I can do to help?" Then allow the person to express his or her anger.

Remorse or Grief

An acceptance of the situation may lead to remorse or grief **Figure 12-1 ▲**. People may feel guilty or apologetic about their behavior or actions during an incident. They may also express grief about the incident itself.

Crisis Management

As a first responder, you should consider how you can deal with the patient's emotional concerns or crises. You need to approach patients who are experiencing behavioral or situational crises using the same general framework for patient assessment that applies to other types of patients.

In this section, you will learn about some additional skills that you can use for patients who are exhibiting behavioral crises or emotional stress.

Role of the First Responder

As a first responder, your approach to a patient who may be exhibiting abnormal behavior is to follow the steps of your patient assessment sequence:

1. Perform a scene size-up.
2. Perform an initial patient assessment.
3. Perform a physical examination—examine the patient from head to toe.
4. Obtain the patient's medical history (SAMPLE).
5. Provide ongoing assessment.

After you have completed the initial patient assessment, you may need to perform a physical examination or obtain the patient's medical history, depending on the needs of that individual patient. As you perform these steps, it is important that you remain calm and reassuring to the patient.

Your most important assessment skill may be your ability to communicate with the patient. Your communication skills will help you obtain needed information from the patient as you calm and reassure the patient.

Communicating With the Patient

The first and most important step in crisis management is to talk with the person. Talking lets the person know that someone cares. Ask the patient his or her name, tell them yours, and ask what you can do to help. When communicating with the patient, be honest, warm, caring, and empathetic.

When you begin talking with the patient, your body language is as important as your words. Try to position yourself so you are at the patient's eye level **Figure 12-2 ▶**. If the person is lying down,

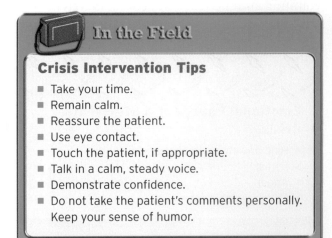

In the Field

Crisis Intervention Tips

- Take your time.
- Remain calm.
- Reassure the patient.
- Use eye contact.
- Touch the patient, if appropriate.
- Talk in a calm, steady voice.
- Demonstrate confidence.
- Do not take the patient's comments personally. Keep your sense of humor.

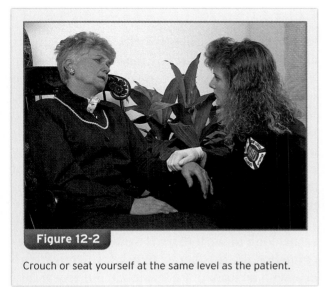

Figure 12-2

Crouch or seat yourself at the same level as the patient.

In the Field

Body language is very important.

person and provide honest reassurance. Avoid making false statements or giving false assurances. The patient does not want to be told that everything is all right when it obviously is not.

Try not to let negative personal feelings about the person or about the person's behavior interfere with your attempt to assist. Your function is to help the person deal with the events that caused the crisis. You should remain neutral and avoid taking sides in any situation or argument.

Sometimes a simple act, such as offering a tissue or a warm blanket, defuses the person's immediate crisis reaction. Simple acts of kindness can comfort and reassure the person that you are there to help.

Restatement

To show the person that you understand what he or she is saying, you can use a technique known as **restatement**. This means rephrasing a person's own words and thoughts and repeating them back to the person. Here is one example of restatement:

> Patient with broken arm: "I can't take any more of this pain!"
>
> First responder: "The pain seems unbearable to you now, but it will ease up when we finish applying this splint."

It is not usually helpful simply to say, "I know what you mean," or "I know how you feel." You do not know exactly how the patient is feeling, even though you may have been through a similar experience. Be honest and give the patient hope, but do not give false hope.

Redirection

Sometimes, a patient may be embarrassed about being the center of attention or may be concerned about others involved in the situation. **Redirection** helps focus a patient's attention on the immediate situation or crisis. This is an attempt to alleviate the patient's expressed concerns and draw his

kneel beside him or her. If the person is sitting, move down to his or her level. Do not stand above the person with your hands on your hips. This is a threatening position and communicates an uncaring attitude and indifference to the patient's problem **Figure 12-3 ▾** .

Establish eye contact. This assures the person that you are, indeed, interested in helping. Use a calm, steady voice when you talk to the

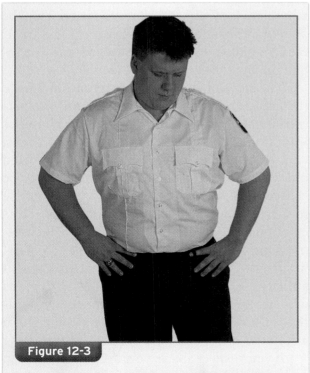

Figure 12-3

This body language communicates an uncaring attitude.

or her attention back to the immediate situation. An example of redirection follows:

> Patient involved in a motor vehicle crash: "Oh my God! Where are my children? What's wrong with my children?"

> First responder: "Your children are being taken care of by my partner; they are in good hands. Now, we must take care of you."

If the patient is in a public place such as on a sidewalk or in the lobby of a building, move the patient to a location that is quieter and more private, if the injury or illness permits.

Empathy

The ability to empathize involves imagining yourself in another person's situation, sharing their feelings or ideas. <u>Empathy</u> helps you understand the emotional or psychological trauma the patient is experiencing. Ask yourself, "How would I feel if I were lying on the sidewalk with my clothes all torn and bloody and strangers looking down at me?" Empathy is one of the most helpful concepts you can use in dealing with patients in crisis situations.

Communication Skills

By using these various communication skills, you will be able to deal more effectively with the patient's problems. Practice these skills with another person until you are able to use them comfortably. Some principles you can use when assessing patients with a behavioral problem are listed here.

1. Identify yourself and let the patient know you are there to help.
2. Inform the patient of what you are doing.
3. Ask questions in a calm, reassuring voice.
4. Allow the patient to tell what happened. Do not be judgmental.
5. Show you are listening by using restatement and redirection.
6. Acknowledge the patient's feelings.
7. Assess the patient's mental status:
   A. Appearance
   B. Activity
   C. Speech
   D. Orientation to person, place, and time

FYI

Crowd Control

Simple crowd control may help reduce a patient's anxiety when there are too many people around. Encourage bystanders to leave. Sometimes too many emergency personnel have been dispatched to the scene. The presence of many uniformed personnel in a small apartment, for instance, is overwhelming or threatening to some people. Any emergency personnel who are not needed right away should leave the room or immediate vicinity until the patient calms down.

During your initial overview of the emergency scene, look to see if there is a crowd that may become hostile. It is better to ask for help early to deal with an unhappy crowd than it is to wait until the situation is unsafe for you and your patient.

Domestic Violence

Domestic violence is a common occurrence in today's society. Its different forms include elder abuse, child abuse, and spouse and domestic partner abuse. As a first responder, you need to be able to recognize the signs and symptoms of abuse and to understand the three phases in the cycle of abuse. When you respond to a situation involving domestic violence, you will have to maintain safety for yourself and for the patient and be able to perform effective assessment and treatment. Finally, you need to understand the requirements for reporting abuse in your state.

The signs of abuse include physical injuries, the emotional state of the victim, and the personality indicators of the abuser. Physical injuries from domestic violence include broken bones, cuts, head injuries, bruises, burns, and scars from old injuries. Internal injuries may also be caused by abuse. In some cases, injuries will be in varying stages of healing. The abused person's emotional scars and symptoms may include depression, suicide attempts, and abuse of alcohol or drugs. The patient may have feelings of anxiety, distress, and hopelessness. Persons who are abusers may be paranoid, overly sensitive, obsessive, or threatening. They often abuse alcohol or drugs and have access to weapons.

If you suspect abuse, your responsibility is to maintain safety for yourself and for the patient.

Dealing with a violent person is covered later. To diffuse a tense situation, try to separate the patient from the person who may have been the abuser. This will create a safe place for the patient, give you a chance to gather needed information, and allow you to treat the patient's injuries. As you question the patient, express your concern. Ask the patient if she or he is all right. Try to keep from judging the patient. If the patient refuses to be transported, some agencies provide information about domestic abuse shelters. In some cases, the presence of law enforcement personnel will be helpful. Finally, learn the requirements for reporting cases of suspected abuse in your state.

Cycles of Abuse

Abuse has been described as a three-part cycle. In the tension phase, the abuser becomes angry and often blames the victim. If the victim has been in the relationship for some time, he or she may recognize the tension build up and react by trying to placate the abuser. The victim may also try to minimize or deny the abuse. The tension phase is usually the longest part of the abuse cycle.

The second stage is the explosive phase, when the batterer becomes enraged and loses control as well as the ability to think clearly. Most injuries to the victim occur during this stage. The third phase is the make-up phase. During this stage, the abuser may make all sorts of promises, which are seldom kept. This phase helps keep the abused person in the relationship with the abuser. As a first responder, you may enter a domestic scene anywhere in this cycle. Understanding this cycle will help you to anticipate the actions of both abuser and victim.

Violent Patient

If you must treat an unarmed patient who is or may become violent, immediately attempt to establish verbal and eye contact with the patient. This begins the process of establishing rapport with the patient and is important for communicating with a potentially violent person.

If family members or friends are present, check with them about the patient's past history of violence. A patient with a past history of violence is

Most violent patients calm down as time passes. The longer you can keep the patient talking, the better your chances are of resolving the situation without violence. Time is on your side.

more likely to become violent again. Listen to the patient for yelling or verbal threatening. Loud, obscene, or bizarre speech indicates emotional instability. Assess the patient's posture to determine if he or she shows threatening behavior **Figure 12-4 ▾**. A person who is pacing, cannot sit still, or tries to protect personal space is more likely to become violent. Patients who have been abusing alcohol or drugs are also at high risk for developing violent behavior. Do not force the patient into a corner, and do not allow yourself to be cut off from a route of retreat.

In situations like this, it is usually best to have only one person talk with the patient. Having

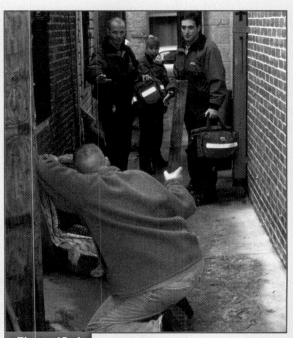

Figure 12-4

A patient's posture will indicate the potential for violent behavior.

FYI
cont.

more than one rescuer attempt conversation is often very threatening. The communicator should be the rescuer with whom the patient seems to have the best initial rapport.

If all other means of approach and intervention fail, it may be necessary to summon law enforcement personnel to control a violent patient.

Violence Against First Responders

According to the National Institute for Occupational Safety and Health, the following factors increase the risk of violence in the workplace:

- Working alone or in small numbers
- Working late at night or early in the morning hours
- Working in high-crime areas
- Working in community settings

All of those factors describe your job as a first responder. You come in contact with all kinds of people at all hours of the day and night. You work in the community and may be called to high-crime areas. You should be alert when you respond to a call that has an increased chance for violence. These include crime scenes, incidents involving gangs, large gatherings of hostile or potentially hostile people, and domestic disputes (previously discussed). However, even though you are more likely to be involved in potentially violent situations than the average citizen, there are steps you can take to minimize the chance of injury to you and to patients.

Prevention

Prevention is the best way to avoid violence. It is far better to avoid or prevent an incident of violence than to have to deal with actual violence. You may have several different opportunities for preventing violence. Can you learn anything from the dispatch information? As you arrive at the

FYI
cont.

scene use your personal "antenna" to pick up any signs that you may be approaching a violent situation. (Review the section on scene safety in Chapter 2.) Be sure you have an escape route in mind as you approach any suspicious scene.

Your ability to use good interpersonal communication skills will help prevent many situations from becoming violent. Empathy can defuse tense situations. Practice the communication skills reviewed in this chapter. If you think you need backup or law enforcement personnel, request it early. If you are unable to handle a situation by yourself, remember your escape route. Learn your local protocols for violent situations and avail yourself of additional training for handling this type of situation.

The Armed Patient

You may encounter a person who is armed with a gun, knife, or other weapon. It is not your role to handle this situation unless you are a law enforcement officer. Be alert for potentially threatening situations and summon assistance if you think the person is armed. Do not proceed into an area where there may be an armed person without assistance from law enforcement personnel. If you must wait for the arrival of law enforcement personnel, stay with your vehicle in a safe location. If, despite caution, you are confronted by an armed person, immediately attempt to withdraw. Your best defense is to avoid confronting a person who is armed!

Medical and Legal Considerations

To protect the rights of the patient and to protect yourself from any possible legal action, you must understand the laws of your state and community

Safety Tips

If you have any doubts about your safety at a scene, wait at a safe distance and request help from law enforcement officials.

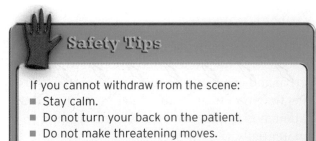

Safety Tips

If you cannot withdraw from the scene:
- Stay calm.
- Do not turn your back on the patient.
- Do not make threatening moves.
- Try to talk with the person and explain that you are there to give emergency medical assistance.

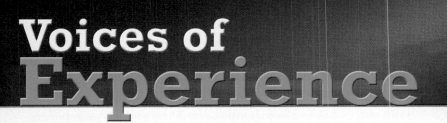

Voices of Experience

Perception is Reality

It has been said that a person's perception of the world is his or her reality. This statement held quite true during a call I responded to for a man who was threatening to kill himself with a knife. The man was a Vietnam War veteran who had a history of post-traumatic stress disorder and behavioral problems. He had threatened to harm himself in the past. On this particular day, the man was found sitting on his bed holding a large knife to his throat. He was keeping first responders from entering the apartment by telling them that he would kill himself if they came into the room. He also claimed that his floor, a large checkerboard pattern of green and white tiles, was full of land mines.

I took my time and allowed the man to maintain his space. I did not fully enter the room, as he had requested. In a calm voice, I asked him to explain to us how he thought we could help him. After several minutes of conversation he revealed that he did not want to hurt us, but he didn't want us to come into his room because the green tiles on his floor were land mines and we would be risking our lives by stepping on them. It occurred to me to ask the man about the white tiles: "If the green tiles are land mines, why can't we just walk on the white tiles?" The man's face lit up with a surprised look that said, "Now why didn't I think of that!" He quickly agreed to walk over to us on the white tiles. He set the knife down and carefully stepped on only the "non–land mine" tiles and made his way over to us. He was grateful for our help.

> " The first responder should resist the urge to become complacent or callous when dealing with people who are experiencing behavioral problems. "

This particular call could have been potentially dangerous for the patient and ourselves had we not taken time to establish a rapport with the patient and help him through his crisis.

Few calls tax the first responder's patience, knowledge base, and communication skills the way behavioral emergency calls often do. I have found myself in several situations with patients who were threatening to harm themselves or others. Other times, I have been called to behavioral emergencies that take on a much more mundane tone. The first responder should resist the urge to become complacent or callous when dealing with people who are experiencing behavioral problems.

The best single piece of advice I could pass on to new first responders is to make sure they take their time on behavioral emergency calls. You may feel you don't have a significant amount of time to spare; however, whenever possible, behavioral emergency patients should be approached in a calm, cool, collected manner. When patients feel rushed or threatened, they are less likely to respond positively to your aid.

Sherm Syverson, BS, NREMT-P
Education Manager
Emergency Medical Education Center at F-M Ambulance Service
Fargo, North Dakota

that relate to dealing with emotionally disturbed patients. If an emotionally disturbed patient agrees to be treated, there should be few legal issues. However, if a patient who appears to be disturbed refuses to accept treatment, it may be necessary to provide care against the patient's will. To do this, you must have a reasonable belief that the patient would harm him- or herself or others. Usually, if patients are a threat to themselves or to others, it is possible to treat and transport them without their consent. As a first responder, you will usually not be responsible for transporting the patient, but you should know what the laws permit you to do. This direction should come from your medical director and from legal counsel.

There may be times when it is necessary for you to apply reasonable force to keep patients from injuring themselves or others. If you are required to restrain a patient, you should consider the following factors: the patient's size and apparent strength, the sex of the patient, the type of abnormal behavior, the mental state of the patient, and the method of restraint. Whenever possible, you should avoid acts of physical force that may injure the patient. You may, however, use reasonable force to defend yourself against an attack by an emotionally disturbed patient.

To prevent problems if you must restrain a patient, seek assistance from law enforcement officials or from your medical director. It is also important to document the conditions present in cases where you must restrain or subdue a patient. To prevent accusations of sexual misconduct by emotionally disturbed patients, a caregiver of the same sex should take primary responsibility for the care of the patient, whenever possible.

FYI
Other Types of Emotional Crises

Three other types of emotional crises—attempted suicide, sexual assault, and death and dying—also require good communication skills from the first responder. Each of these is difficult for the patient and for the first responder.

Attempted Suicide

Each year, thousands of people, from teenagers to the elderly, attempt **suicide** (self-inflicted death). People attempt suicide by ingesting poi-

sons, jumping from heights or in front of cars or trains, cutting their wrists or neck, and shooting or hanging themselves. Not all suicide attempts result in death, and many patients who fail at first will attempt suicide again. Most people who attempt suicide have a serious psychiatric illness, such as depression or alcohol or substance abuse. Many people attempt suicide while under the influence of alcohol or drugs. The underlying psychiatric disease is usually treatable, however, and with proper treatment the patient will no longer be suicidal. However, until that treatment is carried out, the patient must at all times be considered suicidal. All suicide attempts should be taken seriously.

Management of an attempted suicide consists of the following steps:

1. Get a complete history of the incident.
2. Determine if the patient still has a weapon or drugs on them.
3. Support the patient's ABCs, as needed.
4. Dress open wounds.
5. Treat the patient for spinal injuries, if indicated.
6. Do not judge the patient. Treat him or her for the injuries or conditions you discover.
7. Provide emotional support for the patient and family.

Talk with the patient during treatment. Remember that many suicide attempts are cries for help Figure 12-5 ▾ . In addition to treating the patient, you should provide emotional support for the patient's family. Help the family under-

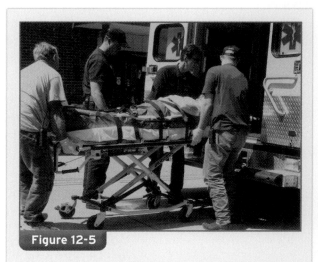

Figure 12-5

Many suicide attempts are cries for help.

FYI cont.

stand that a suicide attempt usually indicates an underlying psychiatric illness and that it is not the fault of the family or friends. It is not your role as a first responder to pass judgment on a patient; it is your role to provide a caring attitude and good medical care.

Sexual Assault

Special consideration should be given to any victim of sexual assault. Such victims may be male or female, old or young. Because sexual assault creates an emotional crisis, the psychological aspects of treatment are important. The patient may have a hard time dealing with a rescuer who is the same sex as the person who has committed the assault. You may have to delay all but the most essential treatment until a rescuer of the same sex as the victim arrives. Your first priority is the medical well-being of the patient, so you will need to treat any injuries the person may have (knife wounds, gunshot wounds, and so forth). However, because sexual assault is a crime, you should not remove clothing except to give medical care. Try to convince the victim not to bathe or use the toilet. Keep the scene and any evidence as undisturbed and intact as possible and avoid aggressively questioning the patient as to what happened.

In addition to giving medical care, treat the patient with empathy. Maintain the patient's privacy by covering her or him with a sheet or blanket and do not leave the patient alone. Contact your local law enforcement agency and rape crisis center, if one is available in your community.

Death and Dying

As a first responder, you will encounter death and dying from natural, accidental, and intentional causes. How well you can help the dying patient

FYI cont.

and the person's family or relatives largely depends on your own feelings about death. The material presented here expands on the material introduced in Chapter 2.

In some situations, there is nothing you can do and the patient dies. In other situations, the patient dies despite everyone's best efforts. In yet other situations, the patient's death is completely unexpected. In every case, you must do whatever you can to meet the patient's medical needs. Your attempts to save or give comfort to the patient help everyone (the patient, the family, and you) to deal emotionally with the patient's death.

Most human beings are afraid of dying. Witnessing the death of another human being brings that fear to the forefront, if only for a brief time. You must work through your personal feelings about death so you can confront it in the field. Although you may be somewhat uncomfortable bringing up the subject, it helps to discuss it with others in the emergency care field. If you are uncomfortable talking with your peers, talk to a member of your hospital's emergency department staff.

Once you have done everything you can to treat a patient medically, consider the psychological needs of the patient and his or her family. Being there as an empathetic caregiver is helpful. Do not be afraid to touch. Putting an arm around a shoulder or holding the hand of the patient or a member of the family helps everyone, including you **Figure 12-6 ▶**. Do not make false statements about the situation, but it is just as important not to destroy hope. Even if, in your judgment, the situation is hopeless, try to give comfort by making such positive statements as, "We're here to help you, and we are doing everything we can. The ambulance is on its way, and you will be at the hospital as soon as possible."

Dealing with the deaths of others is a routine aspect of your job as a first responder. You must, therefore, constantly be on guard to prevent any callousness from entering into your interactions with patients and their families.

One specific type of death, sudden infant death syndrome (SIDS), is discussed in Chapter 16.

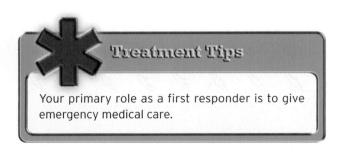

Treatment Tips

Your primary role as a first responder is to give emergency medical care.

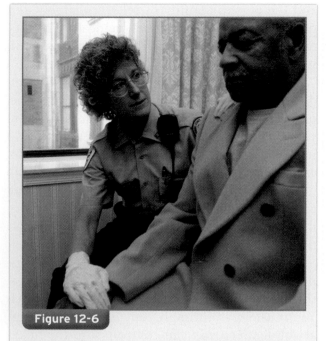

Figure 12-6

Do not be afraid to show empathy to patients and family members.

Critical Incident Stress Debriefing

Providing emergency care is stressful for you as well as for the patient. As a first responder, you will deal with patients experiencing high levels of stress and anxiety. In emergency situations, you may not always be able to help patients. Some types of situations, such as rescue missions involving children or mass-casualty incidents, tend to produce more stress than others. You may need counseling to deal with these stresses.

If you let stress build up without releasing it in healthy ways, it can begin to have negative effects on you and your performance. Signs and symptoms of extreme stress include depression, inability to sleep, weight change, increased alcohol consumption, inability to get along with family and coworkers, and lack of interest in food or sex.

To help prevent excess stress and to relieve stress caused by critical incidents, psychologists have developed a process called **critical incident stress debriefing (CISD)**. CISD brings rescuers and a trained person together to talk about the rescuers' feelings. CISD may help rescuers understand the signs and symptoms of stress and receive reassurance from the group leader. It also allows people to obtain more help from trained professionals, if needed. Some public safety agencies have set up CISD teams to handle stressful events. These teams may be helpful to rescuers who have been through an overwhelming or stressful event. Additional information about critical incident stress debriefing is presented in Chapter 2. Check with your agency to see what types of counseling and CISD resources are available **Figure 12-7 ▼**.

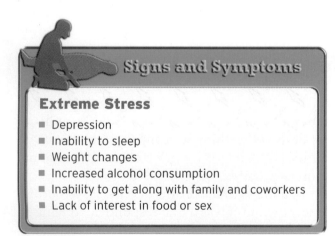

Signs and Symptoms

Extreme Stress

- Depression
- Inability to sleep
- Weight changes
- Increased alcohol consumption
- Inability to get along with family and coworkers
- Lack of interest in food or sex

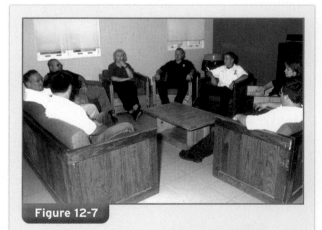

Figure 12-7

A critical incident stress debriefing session.

You are the Provider   SUMMARY

Review the *You are the Provider* case study provided at the beginning of this chapter.

You are dispatched to a residence located about 7 minutes from your station for a report of a "disturbed patient." This neighborhood is a middle-class suburban part of town with modest single-family homes. As you respond, you mentally review the types of situations you might encounter on this call.

1. What types of conditions could be included in the dispatcher's label of "disturbed patient"?

Many conditions can cause patients to be labeled as "disturbed." These include:

- Medical conditions such as uncontrolled diabetes, low blood sugar, and conditions that prevent the patient's brain from receiving enough oxygen
- Physical trauma such as head injuries and shock
- Psychiatric illnesses such as depression, panic disorders, and psychotic behaviors
- Mind-altering substances
- Situational stressors such as serious injury or death of a loved one

2. What factors should you consider and evaluate as you approach this patient?

As you approach the patient, assess the patient's mental status by evaluating the patient's appearance, activity, speech patterns, and orientation to persons, place, and time.

3. What types of skills and interventions might be appropriate in dealing with this patient?

When dealing with patients during a behavioral crisis, consider the use of the following skills and interventions:

- Ensure the safety of yourself, your partner, and bystanders.
- Follow the patient assessment sequence.
- Use good communication tools such as restatement, redirection, and empathy.
- Remain calm.
- Take your time.
- Use good eye contact.
- Touch the patient, if appropriate.
- Talk in a calm, steady voice.
- Demonstrate confidence.
- Do not take the patient's comments personally.
- Keep your sense of humor.

Prep Kit

Ready for Review

The Ready for Review thoroughly summarizes the chapter.

- Only a small percentage of the patients you treat are severely mentally disturbed, but almost every patient you deal with is experiencing some degree of mental and emotional crisis. No matter what the incident or crisis, your response must be to help the patient.

- Behavioral emergencies are situations in which a person exhibits abnormal, unacceptable behavior that cannot be tolerated by the patients themselves or by family, friends, or the community.

- This chapter explains the five major factors that cause behavioral crises: medical conditions, physical trauma conditions, psychiatric illnesses, mind-altering substances, and situational stresses.

- The four emotional phases to each crisis include high anxiety or emotional shock, denial, anger, and remorse or grief. Although a person may not experience every phase during a crisis, he or she will certainly experience one or more.

- Your role as a first responder consists of assessing the patient and providing physical and emotional care. Your most important assessment skill may be your ability to communicate with the patient.

- You must understand the laws of your state and community that relate to dealing with emotionally disturbed patients. If an emotionally disturbed patient agrees to be treated, there should be few legal issues. However, if a patient who appears to be disturbed refuses to accept treatment, it may be necessary to provide care against the patient's will.

To do this, you must have a reasonable belief that the patient would harm him- or herself or others. Usually, if patients are a threat to themselves or to others, it is possible to treat and transport them without their consent.

- Even with these tools for managing behavioral crises, it is important to remember that sometimes the best approach is to ask yourself, "How would I like to be treated if I were in this situation?"

Vital Vocabulary

The Vital Vocabulary are the key terms for this chapter.

behavioral emergencies Situations in which a person exhibits abnormal behavior that is unacceptable or cannot be tolerated by the patients themselves or by family, friends, or the community.

critical incident stress debriefing (CISD) A system of psychological support designed to reduce stress on emergency personnel.

emotional shock A state of shock caused by sudden illness, accident, or death of a loved one.

empathy The ability to participate in another person's feelings or ideas.

psychotic behavior Mental disturbance characterized by defective or lost contact with reality.

redirection A means of focusing the patient's attention on the immediate situation or crisis.

restatement Rephrasing a patient's own statement to show that he or she is being heard and understood by the rescuer.

situational crisis A state of emotional upset or turmoil caused by a sudden and disruptive event.

suicide Self-inflicted death.

Technology

- Interactivities
- Vocabulary Explorer
- Anatomy Review
- Web Links
- Online Review Manual

Assessment in Action

Assessment in Action presents a fictitious scenario to help you review what you learned in this chapter.

You and your partner are dispatched to John Glenn Middle School for a sick person. Upon arrival, you are met by the school nurse who explains that two students found your 13-year-old patient Hailey in the bathroom bleeding from both wrists. The nurse has stopped the bleeding and dressed the wounds. The school has attempted to reach the student's parents but have been unable to do so. Hailey explains that she has been fighting with her mom a lot lately and can't handle it any more. She wants to give up.

1. What type of consent do you have in order to treat this patient?

   A. Expressed
   B. Implied
   C. Informed
   D. You cannot treat this patient because she is a minor.

2. Which of the following would NOT be part of management of an attempted suicide?

   A. Dress open wounds.
   B. Support the patient's ABCs, as needed.
   C. Get a complete history of the incident.
   D. Judge the patient for his or her actions.

3. When interacting with this patient, you should:

   A. Take your time.
   B. Provide emotional support for the patient and family.
   C. Talk in a calm, steady voice.
   D. All of the above.

4. When documenting this call, you should:

   A. Only include the information given to you by the school nurse.
   B. Document all statements made by the patient referring to her desire to kill herself.
   C. Document what the witnesses saw in the bathroom.
   D. Document every aspect of the call.

5. Describe the condition under which you could take a disturbed patient to a medical facility against his or her will.

6. Explain how restatement might be used to improve your communication with this patient.

Bleeding, Shock, and Soft-Tissue Injuries

11. Describe the signs, symptoms, and possible complications associated with each of the following types of burns:
    - Thermal (p 318)
    - Respiratory (p 319)
    - Chemical (p 319)
    - Electrical (p 320)
12. Explain the emergency treatment for each of the following types of burns:
    - Thermal (p 318)
    - Respiratory (p 319)
    - Chemical (p 319)
    - Electrical (p 320)
13. List and explain four types of soft-tissue injuries. (p 304-305)
14. Describe the principles of treatment for soft-tissue injuries. (p 306)
15. Explain the functions of dressings and bandages. (p 306)
16. Discuss the emergency medical care for patients with the following injuries:
    - Face wounds (p 309)
    - Nosebleeds (p 310)
    - Eye injuries (p 310)
    - Neck wounds (p 311)
    - Chest and back wounds (p 313)
    - Impaled objects (p 313)
    - Closed abdominal wounds (p 313)
    - Open abdominal wounds (p 314-315)
    - Genital wounds (p 315)
    - Extremity wounds (p 315-316)
    - Gunshot wounds (p 316)
    - Bites (p 316)
    - Avulsions and amputations (p 305-306)

Skill Objectives

1. Perform body substance isolation procedures for patients with wounds. (p 302)
2. Perform emergency medical care for patients suffering the following types of burns:
   - Thermal (p 318)
   - Respiratory (p 319)
   - Chemical (p 319)
   - Electrical (p 319)

*These are chapter learning objectives.

Bleeding, Shock, and Soft-Tissue Injuries

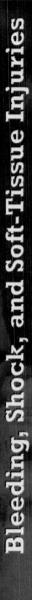

You are the Provider

It is a warm summer day, and you are dispatched for the report of an injured party in a suburban part of town. As you are responding, you receive further dispatch information that the patient's leg has been cut by a power lawn mower.

1. What safety considerations should you keep in mind as you approach this situation?
2. What equipment and supplies do you want to take with you?
3. What are the treatment goals for this type of incident?

3

...uction

...r presents the skills you need to rec-
...care for patients who are suffering from
sho...eding, or soft-tissue injuries. Because
most soft-tissue injuries result in bleeding, maintaining good body substance isolation (BSI) is important when you are caring for these injuries. The
chapter describes four types of wounds: abrasions,
lacerations, punctures, and avulsions. Techniques
for controlling external bleeding are stressed. It is
important that you learn the techniques for dressing and bandaging wounds presented here.

Damage to internal soft tissues and organs
can cause life-threatening problems. Internal
bleeding causes the patient to lose blood in the circulatory system and results in shock. <u>Shock</u> is a
state of collapse of the cardiovascular system that
results in inadequate delivery of blood to the organs. More trauma patients die from shock than
from any other reason. Your ability to recognize
the signs and symptoms of shock and to take simple measures to aid shock patients will give them
the best chance for survival. This chapter explains
the causes and types of shock using an analogy of
a pump, pipes, and fluid. You will learn how the
failure of any part of the system can cause shock.

Burns are another type of soft-tissue injury.
Burns may be caused by heat, chemicals, or
electricity. They may damage any part of the

Technology

- Interactivities
- Vocabulary Explorer
- Anatomy Review
- Web Links
- Online Review Manual

Safety Tips

Most soft-tissue injuries involve some degree of
bleeding. Any time you approach a patient with a
potential soft-tissue injury, you need to consider
your BSI strategy.

body and are especially harmful if they occur
inside the respiratory tract. This chapter examines the extent, depth, and cause of burns.

As you study this chapter, keep in mind the
importance of maintaining good BSI techniques to
prevent the spread of disease-carrying organisms.

Body Substance Isolation and Soft-Tissue Injuries

The BSI concept assumes that all body fluids are
potentially dangerous. Therefore, you must take
appropriate measures to prevent contact with the
patient's body fluids. When dealing with patients
who have soft-tissue injuries, wear gloves to prevent contact with the patient's blood. At times,
you may also need to wear a surgical mask and eye
protection if there is danger of blood splatter from
a massive wound or if the patient is coughing or
vomiting bloody material.

FYI

Review of the Parts and Function of the Circulatory System

The three parts of the circulatory system are
the pump (heart), the pipes (arteries, veins, and
capillaries), and the fluid (blood cells and other
blood components). **Figure 13-1 ▶** presents a
schematic illustration of the circulatory system.

The Pump

The heart functions as the human circulatory
system's pump. The heart consists of four separate chambers, two on top and two on the bottom. The lower chambers are the left and right

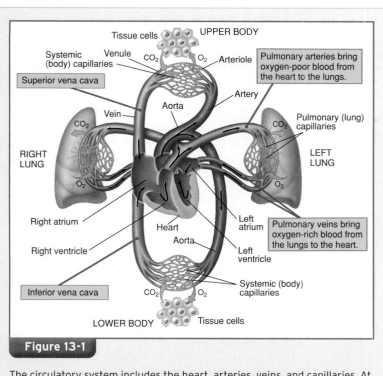

Figure 13-1

The circulatory system includes the heart, arteries, veins, and capillaries. At the center of the system is the heart, which pumps the blood.

FYI cont.

ventricles and the upper chambers are the left and right atria (a single chamber is called an **atrium**). The ventricles are the larger chambers and do most of the actual pumping. The atria are somewhat less muscular and serve more as reservoirs for blood flowing into the heart from the body and the lungs **Figure 13-2 ▸** .

The Pipes

The human body has three main types of blood vessels: arteries, capillaries, and veins. The arteries (big-flow, heavy-duty, high-pressure pipes) carry blood away from the heart. The capillaries (distribution pipes), the smallest of the blood vessels, form a network that distributes blood to all parts of the body. The smallest capillaries are so narrow that blood cells have to flow through them "single file." The veins return the blood from the capillaries to the heart, where it is pumped to the lungs. There, the blood gives off carbon dioxide and absorbs oxygen.

FYI cont.

The Fluid

Fluid consists of blood cells and other blood components, each with a specific function. The liquid part of the blood is known as plasma. Plasma serves as the transporting medium for the "solid" parts of the blood, which are the red blood cells, white blood cells, and platelets. Red blood cells carry oxygen and carbon dioxide **Figure 13-3 ▸** . White blood cells have a "search-and-destroy" function. They consume bacteria and viruses to combat infections in the body. Platelets interact with each other and with other substances in the blood to form clots that help stop bleeding.

Pulse

A pulse is the pressure wave generated by the pumping action of the heart. The beat you feel is caused by the surge of blood from the left ventricle as it contracts and pushes blood out into the main arteries of the body. In counting the number of pulsations per minute, you also count heartbeats per minute. In other words, the pulse rate reflects the heart rate.

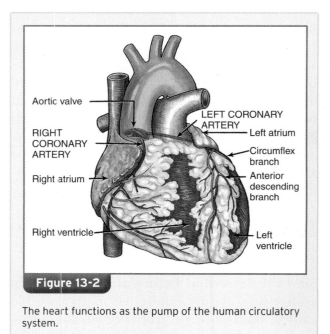

Figure 13-2

The heart functions as the pump of the human circulatory system.

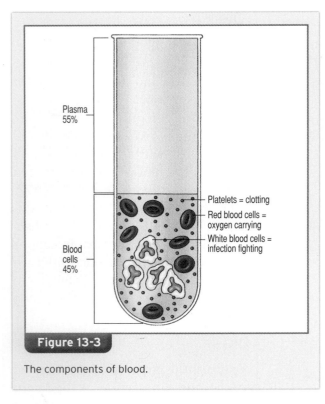

Figure 13-3

The components of blood.

Plasma 55%

Blood cells 45%

Platelets = clotting
Red blood cells = oxygen carrying
White blood cells = infection fighting

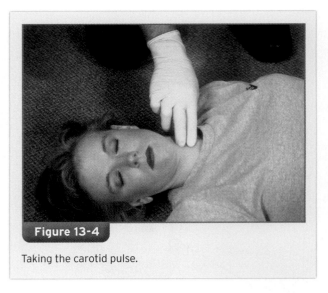

Figure 13-4

Taking the carotid pulse.

FYI cont.

Usually you can feel a patient's radial and carotid pulses. In a conscious patient, you can easily find the radial (wrist) pulse at the base of the thumb. If the patient is unconscious, suffering from shock, or both, it may be impossible for you to feel a radial pulse. Therefore, it is vital that you know how to locate the carotid (neck) pulse. If the patient appears to be in shock or is unconscious, attempt to locate the carotid pulse first. You locate the carotid pulse by placing two fingers lightly on the larynx and sliding the fingers off to one side until you feel a slight notch. You should be able to feel the carotid pulse at this spot **Figure 13-4 ▶**. Practice locating the carotid pulse of another person in a dark room. You should be able to locate the pulse within 3 seconds of touching the person's larynx.

Shock

Shock is defined as failure of the circulatory system. Circulatory failure has many possible causes, but the three primary causes are discussed here.

Pump Failure

Cardiogenic shock occurs if the heart cannot pump enough blood to supply the needs of the body. Pump failure can result if the heart has been weakened by a heart attack. Inadequate pumping of the heart can cause blood to back up in the vessels of the lungs, resulting in a condition known as **congestive heart failure (CHF)**.

Pipe Failure

Pipe failure is caused by the expansion (dilation) of the capillaries to as much as three or four times their normal size. This causes blood to pool in the capillaries, instead of circulating throughout the system. When blood pools in the capillaries, the rest of the body, including the heart and other vital organs, is deprived of blood. Blood pressure falls and shock results. **Blood pressure** is the pressure of the circulating blood against the walls of the arteries.

In shock caused by sudden expansion of the capillaries, blood pressure may drop so rapidly that you are unable to feel either a radial or a carotid pulse.

Special Populations

In an infant, you should check the brachial (upper arm) pulse instead of the carotid pulse.

Three types of shock caused by capillary expansion are:
1. Shock induced by fainting
2. Anaphylactic shock
3. Spinal shock

The least serious type of shock caused by pipe failure is fainting. Fainting (**psychogenic shock**) is the body's response to a major psychological or emotional stress. The capillaries suddenly expand to three or four times their normal size. Fainting is a short-term condition that corrects itself once the patient is placed in a horizontal position.

Anaphylactic shock is caused by an extreme allergic reaction to a foreign substance, such as venom from bee stings (see Chapter 11), penicillin, or certain foods. Shock develops very quickly following exposure. The patient may suddenly start to itch, a rash or hives may appear, the face and tongue may swell very quickly, and a blue color may appear around the mouth. The patient appears flushed (reddish) and breathing may quickly become difficult, with wheezing sounds coming from the chest. Blood pressure drops rapidly as the blood pools in the expanded capillaries. The pulse may be so weak that you cannot feel it. Pipe failure has occurred and death will result if prompt action to counteract the toxin is not taken.

Spinal shock may occur in patients who have suffered a spinal cord injury. The injury to the spinal cord allows the capillaries to expand and blood pools in the lower extremities. The brain, heart, lungs, and other vital organs are deprived of blood, resulting in shock.

Fluid Loss

The third general type of shock is caused by fluid loss. Fluid loss caused by excessive bleeding (**hemorrhage**) is the most common cause of shock. Blood escapes from the normally closed circulatory system through an internal or external wound, and the system's total fluid level (blood volume) drops until the pump cannot operate efficiently. To compensate for fluid loss, the heart begins to pump faster to maintain pressure in the pipes.

However, as the fluid continues to drain out, the pump eventually stops pumping altogether.

External bleeding is not difficult to detect because you can see blood escaping from the circulatory system to the outside. With internal bleeding, blood escapes from the system, but you cannot see it. Even though the escaped blood remains inside the body, it cannot reenter the circulatory system and is not available to be pumped by the heart. Whether external or internal, unchecked bleeding causes shock, eventual pump failure, and death.

An average adult has about 12 pints of blood circulating in the system. Losing a single pint of blood will not produce shock in a healthy adult. In fact, 1 pint per donor is the amount that blood banks collect. However, the loss of 2 or more pints of blood can produce shock. This amount of blood can be lost as a result of injuries such as a fractured femur. **Figure 13-5 ▾** shows the amount of blood that can be lost as a result of various injuries.

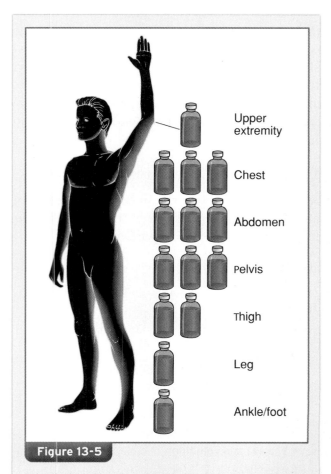

Upper extremity

Chest

Abdomen

Pelvis

Thigh

Leg

Ankle/foot

Figure 13-5

Potential blood loss from injuries in various parts of the body. Each bottle equals 1 pint.

Signs and Symptoms of Shock

Shock deprives the body of sufficient blood to function normally. As shock progresses, the body alters some of its functions in an attempt to maintain sufficient blood supply to its vital parts. A patient who is suffering from shock may exhibit some or all of the signs and symptoms shown in the box below. Initially, the patient's breathing may be rapid and deep, but as shock progresses in severity, breathing becomes rapid and shallow.

Changes in mental status may be the first signs of shock, so monitoring the overall mental status of a patient can help you detect shock. Any change in mental status may be significant. In severe cases, the patient loses consciousness. If a trauma patient who has been quiet suddenly becomes agitated, restless, and vocal, you should suspect shock. If a trauma patient who has been loud, vocal, and belligerent becomes quiet, you should also suspect shock and begin treatment. If the patient has dark skin, you may not be able to use skin color changes to help you detect shock. Therefore, you must be especially alert for other signs of shock. The capillary refill test and the condition of the skin (cool and clammy) will help you recognize shock in patients who have dark skin.

General Treatment for Shock

As a first responder, you can combat shock from any cause and keep it from getting worse by taking several simple but important steps.

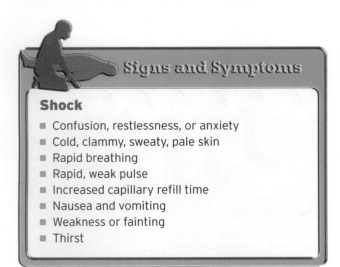

Signs and Symptoms

Shock

- Confusion, restlessness, or anxiety
- Cold, clammy, sweaty, pale skin
- Rapid breathing
- Rapid, weak pulse
- Increased capillary refill time
- Nausea and vomiting
- Weakness or fainting
- Thirst

Treatment Tips

General Treatment for Shock

1. Position the patient correctly.
2. Maintain the patient's ABCs.
3. Treat the cause of shock, if possible.
4. Maintain the patient's body temperature by placing blankets under and over the patient.
5. Make sure the patient does not eat or drink anything.
6. Assist with other treatments (such as administering oxygen, if available).
7. Arrange for immediate and **prompt transport** to an appropriate medical facility.

Position the Patient Correctly

If there is no head injury, extreme discomfort, or difficulty breathing, lay the patient flat on the back on a horizontal surface. Place the patient on a blanket, if available. Elevate the patient's legs 6 to 12 inches off the floor or ground Figure 13-6 ▾ . This enables some blood to drain from the legs back into the circulatory system. If the patient has a head injury, do not elevate the legs. If the patient is having chest pain or difficulty breathing (which is likely to occur in cases of heart attack and emphysema), and no spinal injury is suspected, place the patient in a sitting or semireclining position.

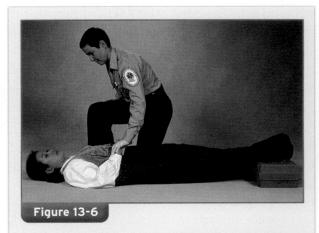

Figure 13-6

Position for treatment of shock if there is no head injury. Note the elevated legs. If the patient is experiencing difficulty breathing and no spinal injury is suspected, place the patient in a sitting or semireclining position.

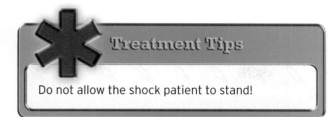

Maintain the Patient's ABCs

Check the patient's airway, breathing, and circulation at least every 5 minutes. If necessary, open the airway, perform rescue breathing, or begin CPR.

Treat the Cause of Shock, if Possible

Most causes of shock must be treated in the hospital. Often this treatment consists of surgery by specially trained physicians. However, you will be able to treat one common cause of shock—external bleeding. By controlling external bleeding with direct pressure, elevation, or **pressure points**, you will be able to temporarily treat this cause of shock until the patient can be transported to an appropriate medical facility for more advanced treatment.

Maintain the Patient's Body Temperature

Attempt to keep the patient comfortably warm. A patient with cold, clammy skin should be covered. It is as important to place blankets under the patient to keep body heat from escaping into the ground as it is to cover the patient with blankets.

Make Sure the Patient Does Not Eat or Drink Anything

Even though a patient in shock is very thirsty, do not give liquids by mouth. There are two reasons for this:

1. A patient in shock may be nauseated and eating or drinking may cause vomiting.

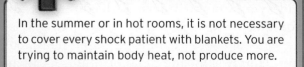

2. A patient in shock may need emergency surgery. Patients should not have anything in their stomachs before surgery.

If you are working in an area where ambulance response time is more than 20 minutes, you may give patients a clean cloth or gauze pad that has been soaked in water to suck. This relieves dryness of the mouth but does not quench thirst. No matter how thirsty patients are, do not permit them to drink anything.

FYI

Assist With Other Treatments

When a basic life support (BLS) or advanced life support (ALS) unit arrives on the scene, be ready to assist unit personnel with further treatment. Patients may be given oxygen or IV solutions. If you are trained in the administration of oxygen and have it available, give it to shock patients. Oxygen benefits such patients by ensuring that the reduced number of red blood cells are as oxygen saturated as they can be.

EMTs or paramedics can administer **intravenous (IV) fluids**. Adding fluid to the body combats the loss of blood volume. Some EMS personnel use **pneumatic antishock garments (PASGs)** in the field to treat pelvic fractures and to treat shock. PASGs are placed around the patient's legs and abdomen and inflated with air. As the PASG inflates, it exerts pressure around the legs and abdomen. Although you, as a first responder, will not use these devices yourself, you should know their purpose and function. It is also important to understand that PASGs must not be removed in the field. Removing PASGs must be done in a hospital and under the direct supervision of a physician.

Arrange for Transport

As soon as you realize that you have a patient who is suffering from shock, you should make sure that an ambulance has been dispatched. When the ambulance arrives, give the EMS personnel a concise hand-off report emphasizing the signs and symptoms of shock that you noted. The EMTs or paramedics should make sure that the patient is quickly prepared for **prompt transport** to an appropriate medical facility that can handle a patient with these severe problems. The cure for shock is usually surgical repair, and the sooner the patient gets to the hospital, the better the chance of survival will be.

Treatment for Shock Caused by Pump Failure

Patients suffering from pump failure may be confused, restless, anxious, or unconscious. Their pulse is usually rapid and weak; their skin is cold and clammy, sweaty, and pale. Their respirations are often rapid and shallow. Pump failure is a serious condition. Your proper treatment and prompt transport by ambulance to a medical center will give these patients their best chance for survival.

Treatment for Shock Caused by Pipe Failure

Patients who have fainted, who are suffering from anaphylactic shock, or who have suffered a severe spinal cord injury will have pipe failure. The size of their capillaries may increase three or four times, causing signs and symptoms of shock.

Treatment for Anaphylactic Shock

The initial treatment for anaphylactic shock is similar to the treatment for any other type of shock. Anaphylactic shock is an extreme emergency and the patient must be transported as soon as possible. Paramedics, nurses, and doctors can give medications that may reverse the allergic reaction. Some patients who have severe allergies may carry an epinephrine auto-injector. If the patient has a prescribed auto-injector, help the patient use it. Support the patient's thigh and place the tip of the auto-injector lightly against the outer thigh. Using a quick motion, push the auto-injector firmly against the thigh and hold it in place for several seconds. This will inject the medication.

Treatment for Shock Caused by Fluid Loss

Shock may be caused by internal blood loss (blood that escapes from damaged blood vessels and stays inside the body) or by external blood loss (blood

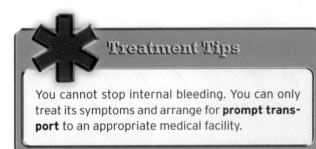

Signs and Symptoms

Internal Bleeding

- Coughing or vomiting of blood
- Abdominal tenderness, rigidity, or distention
- Rectal bleeding
- Vaginal bleeding in women
- Classic signs of shock

Treatment Tips

You cannot stop internal bleeding. You can only treat its symptoms and arrange for **prompt transport** to an appropriate medical facility.

that escapes from the body). Excessive bleeding is the most common cause of shock.

Shock Caused by Internal Blood Loss

Patients die quickly and quietly from internal bleeding following abdominal injuries that rupture the spleen, liver, or large blood vessels. You must be alert to catch the earliest signs and symptoms of internal bleeding and to begin treatment for shock. If you are treating several injured patients, those with internal bleeding should be **transported promptly** to the medical facility first, because immediate surgery may be needed. (Chapter 18 discusses how to decide which patients should receive care first.)

Bleeding from stomach ulcers, ruptured blood vessels, or tumors can all cause internal bleeding and shock. This bleeding can be spontaneous, massive, and rapid, often leading to the loss of large quantities of blood by vomiting or bloody diarrhea.

It is important that you recognize the signs and symptoms of internal bleeding and take prompt corrective action. In addition to the classic signs of shock (confusion, rapid pulse, cold and clammy skin, and rapid breathing), patients with internal bleeding may show some of the signs and symptoms depicted in the box on this page.

Bleeding

Controlling External Blood Loss

There are three types of external blood loss: capillary, venous, and arterial **Figure 13-7 ▸**. The most common type of external blood loss is **capillary bleeding**. In capillary bleeding, the blood oozes out (such as from a cut finger). You can control capillary bleeding simply by applying direct pressure to the site.

The next most common type of bleeding is **venous bleeding**. This bleeding has a steady flow. Bleeding from a large vein may be profuse and life

---

Treatment Tips

Treatment for Shock Caused by Pump Failure

1. Keep the patient lying down unless breathing is better in a sitting position.
2. Maintain the patient's ABCs. Be prepared to do CPR, if necessary.
3. Conserve the patient's normal body temperature.
4. Make sure the patient does not eat or drink anything.
5. Keep the patient quiet and do any necessary moving for him or her.
6. Provide reassurance.
7. Arrange for **prompt transport** by ambulance to an appropriate medical facility.
8. Provide high-flow oxygen as soon as it is available.

Treatment for Shock Caused by Pipe Failure

Fainting

1. Examine the patient to make sure there is no injury.
2. Keep the patient lying down with legs elevated 6 to 12 inches off the floor or ground. This enables the blood to drain from the legs back into the central circulatory system.
3. Maintain the ABCs.
4. Maintain the patient's normal body temperature.
5. Provide reassurance.

Anaphylactic Shock

1. Keep the patient lying down. Elevate the legs 6 to 12 inches off the floor or ground.
2. If the patient has an epinephrine auto-injector, help the patient use it.
3. Maintain the patient's ABCs. Anaphylactic shock may cause airway swelling. In severe reactions, the patient may require mouth-to-mask breathing or full CPR.
4. Maintain the patient's normal body temperature.
5. Provide reassurance.
6. Arrange for **rapid transport** by ambulance to an appropriate medical facility.

Spinal Shock

1. Place the patient on his or her back. Because the spine may be injured, keep the patient's head and neck stabilized to protect the spinal cord (Chapter 14). Do not elevate the patient's feet because this will make breathing more difficult.
2. Maintain the patient's ABCs.
3. Maintain the patient's body temperature.
4. Make sure the patient does not eat or drink anything.
5. Assist with other treatments. Help other medical providers place the patient on a backboard.

Treatment for Shock Caused by Fluid Loss

Internal Blood Loss

1. Keep the patient lying down. Elevate the legs 6 to 12 inches off the floor or ground.
2. Maintain the patient's ABCs.
3. Maintain the patient's normal body temperature.
4. Make sure the patient does not eat or drink anything.
5. Provide reassurance.
6. Keep the patient quiet and do any necessary moving for him or her.
7. Provide high-flow oxygen as soon as it is available.
8. Monitor the patient's vital signs at least every 5 minutes.
9. Arrange for **prompt transport** by ambulance to an appropriate medical facility.

External Blood Loss

1. Control bleeding by applying direct pressure on the wound, elevating the injured part, and using pressure points (compressing a major artery against the bone). This is the most important step. Maintain BSI precautions.
2. Make sure the patient is lying down. Elevate the legs 6 to 12 inches off the floor or ground.
3. Maintain the patient's ABCs.
4. Maintain the patient's body temperature.
5. Make sure the patient does not eat or drink anything.
6. Provide reassurance.
7. Provide high-flow oxygen as soon as it is available.
8. Arrange for **prompt transport** by ambulance to an appropriate medical facility.

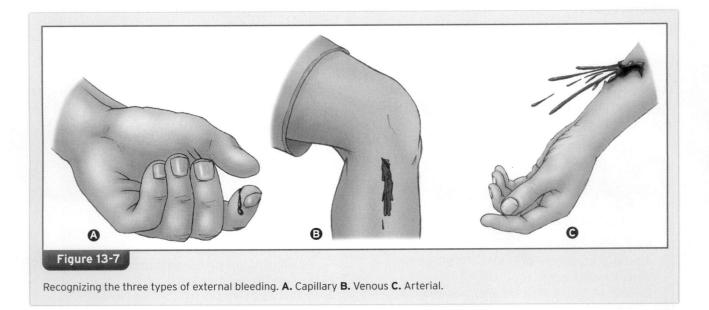

Figure 13-7

Recognizing the three types of external bleeding. **A.** Capillary **B.** Venous **C.** Arterial.

threatening. To control venous bleeding, apply direct pressure for at least 5 minutes.

The most serious type of bleeding is __arterial bleeding__. Arterial blood spurts or surges from the laceration or wound with each heartbeat. Blood pressure in arteries is higher than in capillaries or veins, and unchecked arterial bleeding can result in death from loss of blood in a short time. To control arterial bleeding, exert direct pressure and, if necessary, apply pressure to a pressure point. This is done by compressing a major artery against the underlying bone, as explained later. Maintain pressure until EMS arrives.

Because many injured patients actually die from shock caused by blood loss, it is vitally important that you control external bleeding quickly.

Direct Pressure

Most external bleeding can be controlled by applying direct pressure to the wound. Place a dry, sterile __dressing__ directly on the wound and press on it with your gloved hand Figure 13-8 ▶ . Wear the gloves from your first responder life

support kit. If you do not have a sterile dressing or gauze bandage, use the cleanest cloth available. To maintain direct pressure on the wound, wrap the dressing and wound snugly with a roller gauze bandage. Do not remove a dressing after you have applied it, even if it becomes blood soaked. Place another dressing on top of the first and keep them both in place. According to the American Medical Association, it is extremely unlikely that you—as a first responder providing emergency care—will contract AIDS or hepatitis from a patient who is bleeding if you follow BSI precautions. For more information, call the Centers for Disease Control and Prevention National AIDS Hotline at 800-342-AIDS.

Safety Tips

It is extremely unlikely that you will contract AIDS or hepatitis from a patient who is bleeding if you follow BSI precautions.

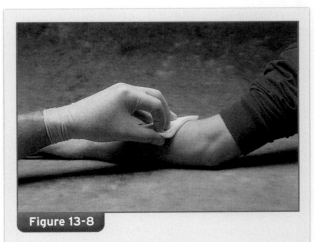

Figure 13-8

Applying direct pressure to a wound.

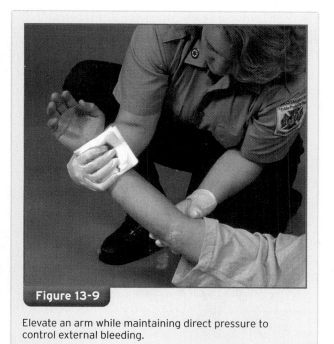

Figure 13-9

Elevate an arm while maintaining direct pressure to control external bleeding.

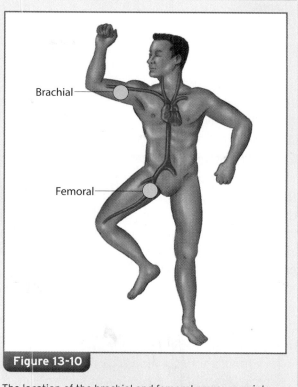

Figure 13-10

The location of the brachial and femoral pressure points.

Elevation

If direct pressure does not stop external bleeding from an extremity, elevate the injured arm or leg as you maintain direct pressure. Elevation, in conjunction with direct pressure, will usually stop severe bleeding **Figure 13-9 ▲** .

Pressure Points

If the combination of direct pressure and elevation does not control bleeding from an arm or leg wound, you must try to control it indirectly by preventing blood from flowing into the limb. This is accomplished by compressing a major artery against the bone at a pressure point.

Compressing the artery at a pressure point stops blood flow in much the same way that stepping on a garden hose stops the flow of water. Although there are several pressure points in the body, the <u>brachial artery pressure point</u> (in the upper arm) and the <u>femoral artery pressure</u> <u>point</u> (in the groin) are the most important **Figure 13-10 ▲** .

In applying pressure to the brachial artery, you should remember the words "slap, slide, and squeeze." Proceed as follows:

1. Position the patient's arm so the elbow is bent at a right angle (90°) and hold the upper arm away from the patient's body.
2. Gently "slap" the inside of the biceps with your fingers halfway between the shoulder and the elbow to push the biceps out of the way.
3. "Slide" your fingers up to push the biceps away.
4. "Squeeze" (press) your hand down on the humerus (upper arm bone). You should be able to feel the pulse as you press down.

If the patient is sitting down, squeeze by placing your fingers halfway between the shoulder and

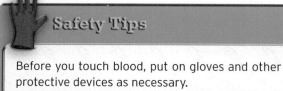

Safety Tips

Before you touch blood, put on gloves and other protective devices as necessary.

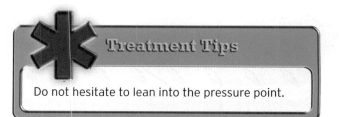

Treatment Tips

Do not hesitate to lean into the pressure point.

Treatment Tips

Three Methods of Controlling External Bleeding

1. Apply direct pressure.
2. Elevate the body part.
3. Apply pressure at a pressure point.

the elbow and your thumb on the opposite side of the patient's arm. If done properly, this technique (in combination with direct wound pressure and elevation) will quickly stop any bleeding below the point of application Figure 13-11.

Figure 13-11

Applying pressure to the brachial artery.

The femoral artery pressure point is more difficult to locate and squeeze. Proceed as follows:

1. Position the patient on his or her back and kneel next to the patient's hips, facing the patient's head. You should be on the side of the patient opposite the extremity that is bleeding.
2. Find the pelvis and place the little finger of your hand closest to the injured leg along the anterior crest on the injured side Figure 13-12A.
3. Rotate your hand down firmly into the groin area between the genitals and the pelvic bone. This compresses the femoral artery and usually stops the bleeding, when combined with elevation and direct pressure over the bleeding site Figure 13-12B.
4. If the bleeding does not slow immediately, reposition your hand and try again.

Body Substance Isolation and Bleeding Control

Certain communicable diseases such as hepatitis or AIDS can be spread by contact with blood from an infected person. This risk is greatly increased when the infected blood contacts a cut or an open sore on your skin. Although the risk of contracting hepatitis or AIDS through intact skin is small, you should minimize this risk as much as possible by wearing vinyl or latex gloves whenever you might come in contact with a patient's blood or bodily fluids Figure 13-13. Carry your gloves on top of your first respon-

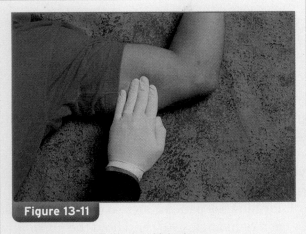

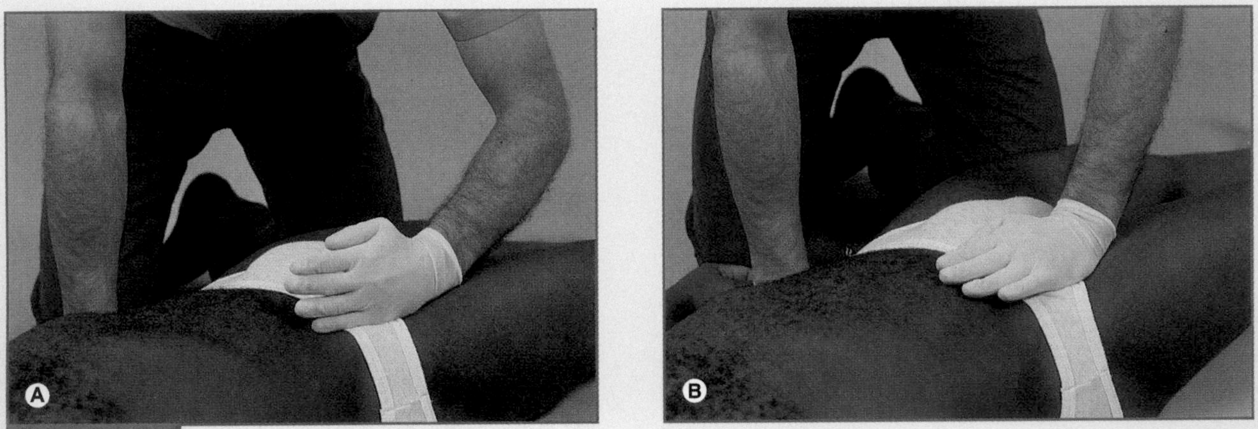

Figure 13-12

Locating and applying pressure to the femoral artery. **A.** Locate the femoral pressure point. **B.** Apply pressure to the femoral artery.

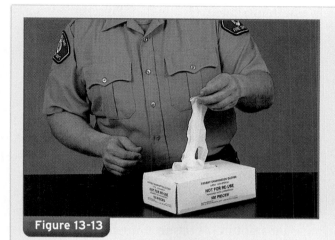
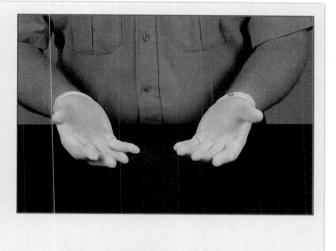

Figure 13-13

Wear gloves to minimize your risk of infection.

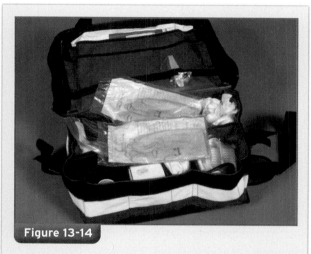

Figure 13-14

Keep your gloves on top in your first responder life support kit.

der life support kit or in a pouch on your belt for quick access **Figure 13-14 ▲**. If you do get blood on your hands, wash it off as soon as possible with soap and water. If you are in the field and cannot wash your hands, use a waterless hand-cleaning solution that contains an effective germ-killing agent.

Wounds

A wound is an injury caused by any physical means that leads to damage of a body part. Wounds are classified as closed or open. In a **closed wound**, the skin remains intact; in an **open wound**, the skin is disrupted.

Treatment Tips

A word about tourniquets: rarely! A tourniquet is made of a band of material placed around an arm or leg above a wound and tightened to control severe bleeding. Tourniquets can be difficult to make from improvised materials, difficult to tighten, and difficult to maintain at sufficient tension. Several tourniquets designed for military application are currently available commercially that alleviate some of these problems. Use of a tourniquet is only indicated in situations where bleeding cannot be controlled by other means, including elevation, direct pressure, and pressure point application. Such wounds are typically extensive—involving large portions of an arm or leg—as seen after injury from an explosive device. Tourniquet application is typically considered a last-ditch effort to save a life when all other means of bleeding control have failed.

Closed Wounds

The only closed wound is the **bruise** (contusion). A bruise is an injury of the soft-tissue beneath the skin. Because small blood vessels are broken, the injured area becomes discolored and swells. The severity of these closed soft-tissue injuries varies greatly. A simple bruise heals quickly.

In contrast, bruising and swelling following an injury may also be a sign of an underlying fracture that could take months to heal. Whenever you encounter a significant amount of swelling or bruising, suspect the possibility of an underlying fracture.

Open Wounds

Abrasion

Commonly called a scrape, <u>road rash</u>, or rug burn, an <u>abrasion</u> occurs when the skin is rubbed across a rough surface Figure 13-15 ▾ .

Puncture

<u>Puncture</u> wounds are caused by a sharp object that penetrates the skin Figure 13-16 ▾ . These wounds may cause a significant deep injury that is not immediately recognized. Puncture wounds do not bleed freely. If the object that caused the puncture wound remains sticking out of the skin, it is called an <u>impaled object</u>.

A <u>gunshot wound</u> is a special type of puncture wound. The amount of damage done by a gunshot depends on the type of gun used and the distance between the gun and the victim. A gunshot wound may appear as an insignificant hole but can do massive damage to internal organs. Some gunshot wounds are smaller than a dime, and some are large enough to destroy significant amounts of tissue. Gunshot wounds usually have both an <u>entrance wound</u> and an <u>exit wound</u>. The entrance wound is usually smaller

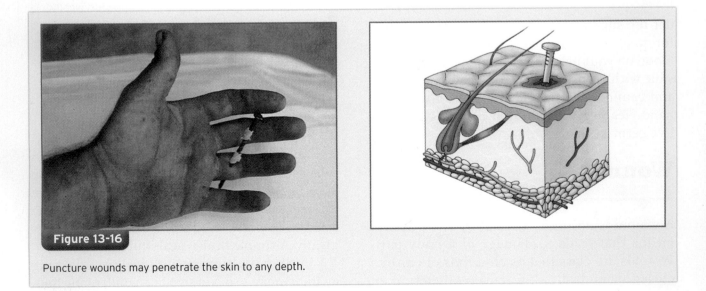

Figure 13-15

Abrasions involve variable depth of the skin; they are often called scrapes or road rashes.

Figure 13-16

Puncture wounds may penetrate the skin to any depth.

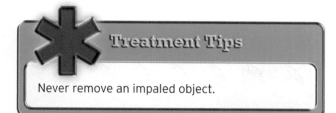

Treatment Tips

Never remove an impaled object.

than the exit wound. Most deaths from gunshot wounds result from internal blood loss caused by damage to internal organs and major blood vessels as the bullet passes through the body. There is often more than one gunshot wound. A thorough patient examination is important to be sure that you have discovered all of the entrance and exit wounds.

Laceration

The most common type of open wound is a **laceration** [Figure 13-17 ▾]. Lacerations are commonly called cuts. Minor lacerations may require little care, but large lacerations can cause extensive bleeding and even be life threatening.

Avulsions and Amputations

An **avulsion** is a tearing away of body tissue [Figure 13-18 ▾]. The avulsed part may be totally severed from the body or it may be attached by a flap of skin. Avulsions may involve small or large amounts of tissue. If an entire body part is torn away, the wound is called a traumatic amputation [Figure 13-19 ▸]. Any amputated body part

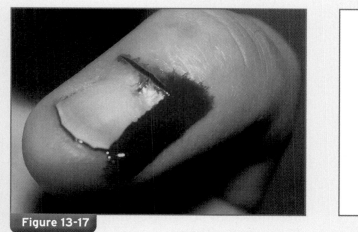

Figure 13-17

Lacerations are cuts produced by sharp objects.

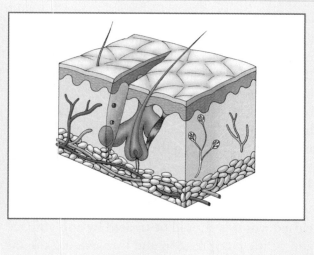

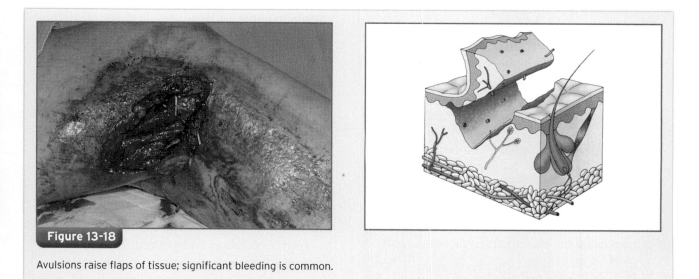

Figure 13-18

Avulsions raise flaps of tissue; significant bleeding is common.

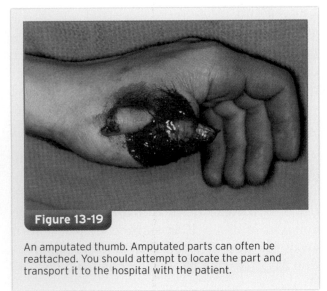

Figure 13-19

An amputated thumb. Amputated parts can often be reattached. You should attempt to locate the part and transport it to the hospital with the patient.

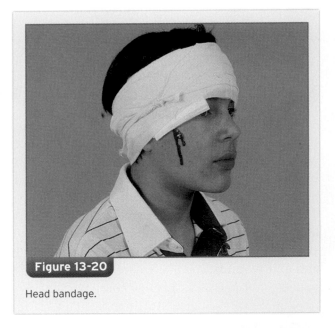

Figure 13-20

Head bandage.

should be located, placed in a clean plastic bag, kept cool, and taken with the patient to the hospital for possible reattachment (reimplantation). If the amputated part is small and a clean plastic bag is not available, you can use a surgical glove turned inside out. Cold packs or iced water can be used to keep the detached body parts cold. Do not allow ice to touch the body part directly.

Principles of Wound Treatment

Very minor bruises need no treatment. Other closed wounds should be treated by applying ice and gentle compression and by elevating the injured part. Because extensive bruising may indicate an underlying fracture, you should **splint** all contusions (see Chapter 14).

It is important to stop bleeding as quickly as possible using the cleanest dressing available. You can usually control bleeding by covering an

open wound with a dry, clean, or sterile dressing and applying pressure to the dressing with your hand. If the first dressing does not control the bleeding, reinforce it with a second layer. Additional ways to control bleeding include elevating an extremity and using pressure points.

A dressing should cover the entire wound to prevent further contamination. Do not attempt to clean the contaminated wound in the field, because cleaning will only cause more bleeding. A thorough cleaning will be done at the hospital. All dressings should be secured in place by a compression bandage.

Learning to dress and bandage wounds requires practice. As a trained first responder, you should be able to bandage all parts of the body quickly and competently **Figure 13-20 ▲**.

Dressing and Bandaging Wounds

Dressing and bandaging are done to:

- Control bleeding.
- Prevent further contamination.
- Immobilize the injured area.
- Prevent movement of impaled objects.

Dressings

A dressing is an object placed directly on a wound to control bleeding and prevent further contamination. Once a dressing is in place, apply firm, direct manual pressure on it to stop the bleeding. It is important to stop severe bleeding as quickly

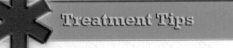

Treatment Tips

The major principles of open-wound treatment are to:

- Control bleeding.
- Prevent further contamination of the wound.
- **Immobilize** the injured part (reduce or prevent movement).
- Stabilize any impaled object.

as possible using the cleanest dressing available. If no equipment is available, you may have to apply direct pressure with your hand to a wound that is bleeding extensively, even though you should normally wear gloves.

Sterile dressings come packaged in many different sizes. Three of the most common sizes are 4-inch by 4-inch gauze squares (commonly known as 4 × 4s). Heavier pads measure 5 inches by 9 inches (5 × 9s). A trauma dressing is a thick sterile dressing that measures 10 inches by 30 inches. Use a trauma dressing to cover a large wound on the abdomen, neck, thigh, or scalp—or as padding for splints **Figure 13-21 ▾**.

When you open a package containing a sterile dressing, touch only one corner of the dressing **Figure 13-22 ▾**. Place it on the wound with-

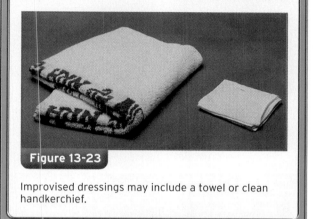

Treatment Tips

If commercially prepared dressings are not available, use the cleanest cloth object available, such as a clean handkerchief, wash cloth, disposable diaper, or article of clothing **Figure 13-23 ▾**.

Figure 13-23

Improvised dressings may include a towel or clean handkerchief.

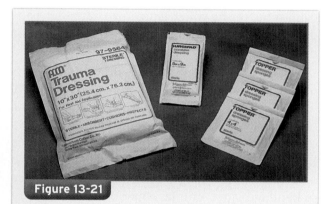

Figure 13-21

Common sizes of wound dressings are 10 inches × 30 inches, 5 inches × 9 inches, and 4 inches × 4 inches.

out touching the side of the dressing that will be next to the wound. If bleeding continues after you have applied a compression dressing to the wound, put additional gauze pads over the original dressing. Do not remove the original dressing because the blood-clotting process will have already started and should not be disrupted. When you are satisfied that the wound is sufficiently dressed, proceed to bandage.

Bandaging

A bandage is used to hold the dressing in place. Two types of bandages commonly used in the field are roller gauze and triangular bandages. The first type, conforming roller gauze, stretches slightly and is easy to wrap around the body part **Figure 13-24 ▸**. Triangular bandages are usually 36 inches across **Figure 13-25 ▸**. A triangular bandage can be folded and used as a wide **cravat** or it can be used without folding **Figure 13-26 ▸**. Roller gauze is easier to apply and stays in place better than a triangular bandage, but a triangular bandage is very useful for bandaging scalp lacerations and lacerations of the chest, back, or thigh.

You must follow certain principles if the bandage is to hold the dressing in place, control bleeding, and prevent further contamination. Before you apply a bandage, check to ensure that the dressing completely covers the wound

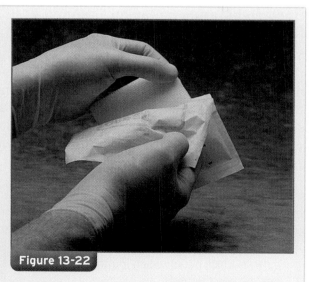

Figure 13-22

Open the package containing a sterile dressing carefully.

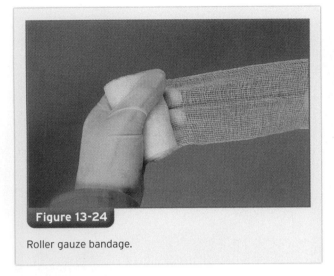

Figure 13-24

Roller gauze bandage.

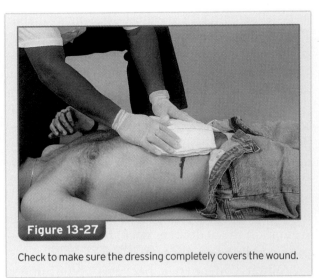

Figure 13-27

Check to make sure the dressing completely covers the wound.

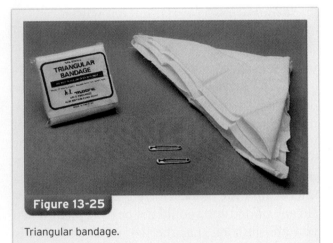

Figure 13-25

Triangular bandage.

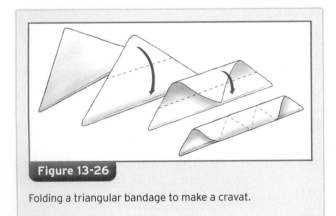

Figure 13-26

Folding a triangular bandage to make a cravat.

because swelling may make the bandage too tight. If this happens while the patient is under your care, remove the roller gauze or triangular bandage and reapply it, making sure that you do not disturb the dressing beneath.

Once bandaging is complete, secure the bandage so it cannot slip. Tape, tie, or tuck in any loose ends. Figures 13-29 through 13-37 show how to dress and bandage wounds of various parts of the body. Practice these bandaging techniques for several types of wounds using both roller gauze and triangular bandages. Although the principles of bandaging are simple, some parts of the body are difficult to bandage. It is important to practice bandaging different parts of the body to ensure competency in emergency situations.

Body Substance Isolation Techniques for the First Responder

Some infectious disease organisms, including the hepatitis and AIDS viruses, can be transmitted if blood from an infected person enters the bloodstream of a healthy person through a small cut or opening in the skin. Because you may have such a cut, it is important that you

and extends beyond all sides of the wound **Figure 13-27 ▶**. Wrap the bandage just tightly enough to control bleeding. Do not apply it too tightly because it may cut off all circulation. It is important to regularly check circulation at a point farther away from the heart than the injury itself

Safety Tips

Providing for your own safety and that of patients is always a high priority when you are examining and treating open wounds.

wear gloves to avoid contact with patients' blood **Figure 13-28 ▼**. Using gloves also protects wounds from being contaminated by dirt or infectious organisms you may have on your hands. Vinyl or latex medical gloves can be stored on the top of your first responder life support kit or in a pouch on your belt, where they will be readily available. (See Chapter 2 for more information on infectious diseases.)

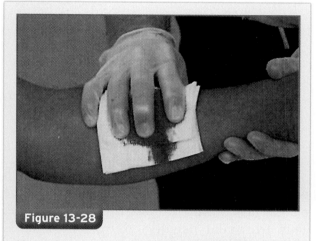

Figure 13-28

Always wear gloves when in contact with body fluids.

FYI

Specific Wound Treatment

Face and Scalp Wounds

The face and scalp have many blood vessels. Because of this generous blood supply, a relatively small laceration can result in a large amount of bleeding. Although face and scalp lacerations may not be life threatening, they are always bloody and cause much anxiety for the patient and first responder.

You can control almost all facial or scalp bleeding by applying direct manual pressure. Direct pressure is effective because the bones of the skull are so close to the skin. Direct pressure compresses the blood vessels against the skull and stops the bleeding. If bleeding continues, do not remove the dressing. Instead, reinforce it with a second layer and continue to apply manual pressure. After the bleeding stops, wrap the head with a bandage **Figure 13-29 ▼**.

For wounds inside the cheek, hold a gauze pad inside the cheek (in the mouth). If necessary, you can also apply a pad outside the cheek. Always keep the airway open. Severe scalp lacerations may be associated with skull fractures or even brain injury. If any brain tissue or bone

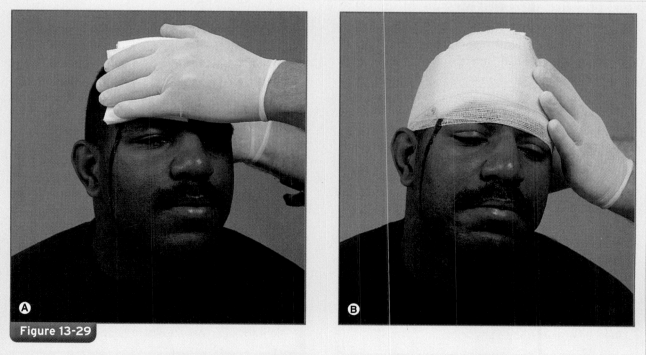

Ⓐ   Ⓑ

Figure 13-29

Bandaging a head wound. **A.** Apply direct pressure until bleeding stops. **B.** Wrap the head with a bandage.

In the Field

Remember that patients who have injuries or are bleeding will likely be worried. It is your job to assure them that you are doing everything you can to treat them. Don't forget to show your patients and their families that you care!

FYI cont.

fragments are visible, do not apply pressure to the wound. Instead, cover the wound loosely, being careful not to exert direct pressure on the brain or the bone fragments.

If the patient has a head injury, the neck and spine may also be injured. Move the head as little as possible and stabilize the neck. (Treatment of spinal injuries is discussed in Chapter 14.) In cases of head injury, always evaluate the patient's level of consciousness. Carefully monitor the patient's airway and breathing and protect the spine.

Nosebleeds

Nosebleeds can result from injury or high blood pressure. In some cases, there is no apparent cause. A nosebleed with no apparent cause is called a **spontaneous nosebleed**. In a patient with high blood pressure, increased pressure in the small blood vessels of the nose may cause one to rupture, resulting in bleeding. A patient with high blood pressure should be seen and treated by a physician.

Most nosebleeds can be controlled easily. Unless the patient is suffering from shock, seat the person and tilt the head slightly forward. This position keeps the blood from dripping down the throat. Swallowing blood may cause coughing or vomiting and make the nosebleed worse.

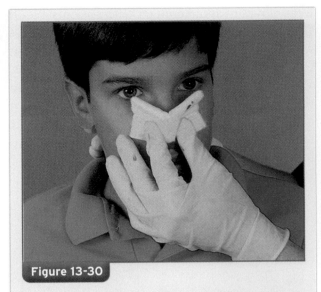
Figure 13-30

Pinch nostrils together to control a nosebleed.

FYI cont.

After the patient is seated correctly, pinch both nostrils together for at least 5 minutes. The patient may wish to do this without assistance. This treatment usually controls nosebleeds **Figure 13-30 ▲**. If a nosebleed persists or is very severe, arrange for **transport** to an appropriate medical facility. Instruct the patient to avoid blowing his or her nose because this will often cause additional bleeding.

Eye Injuries

All eye injuries are potentially serious and require medical evaluation. When an eye laceration is suspected, cover the entire eye with a dry gauze pad. Have the patient lie on his or her back and arrange for **transport** to an appropriate medical facility.

Occasionally an object will be impaled in the eye. Immediately place the patient on his

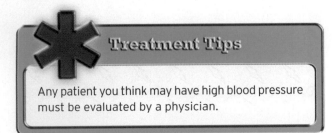
Treatment Tips

Any patient you think may have high blood pressure must be evaluated by a physician.

Treatment Tips

Whenever you must bandage both eyes, explain to the patient why you are doing so. Having both eyes covered can be very distressing. Stay with the patient to help reassure him or her.

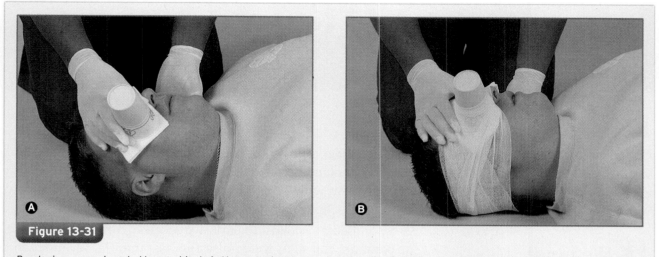

Figure 13-31

Bandaging an eye impaled by an object. **A.** Use a cup to cover an impaled object. **B.** Bandage both eyes to minimize eye movement.

FYI cont.

or her back and cover the injured eye with a dressing and a paper cup so the impaled object cannot move. Bandage both eyes. This is important because both eyes move together, and if the patient attempts to look at something with the uninjured eye, the injured eye will move also, aggravating the injury **Figure 13-31 ▲**. Arrange for **transport** of the patient to the hospital.

Neck Wounds

The neck contains many important structures: the trachea, the esophagus, large arteries, veins, muscles, vertebrae, and the spinal cord.

FYI cont.

Because an injury to any of these structures may be life threatening, all neck injuries are serious.

Use direct pressure to control bleeding neck wounds. Once bleeding is controlled, bandage the neck **Figure 13-32 ▼**. In rare cases, you may have to exert finger pressure above and below the injury site to prevent further neck bleeding.

Always keep in mind that major trauma to the neck may be associated with airway problems and with neck fracture or spinal cord injury. Therefore, maintain the patient's airway and stabilize the head and neck.

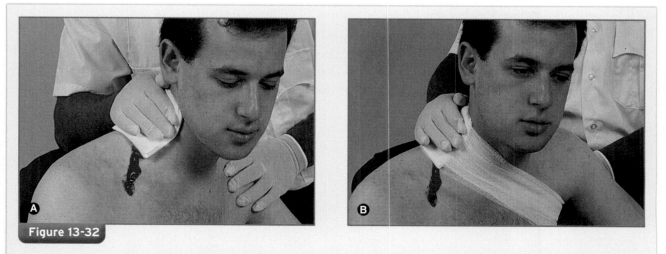

Figure 13-32

Bandaging a neck wound. **A.** Place dressing over wound. **B.** Place bandage over wound and under the arm on the opposite side.

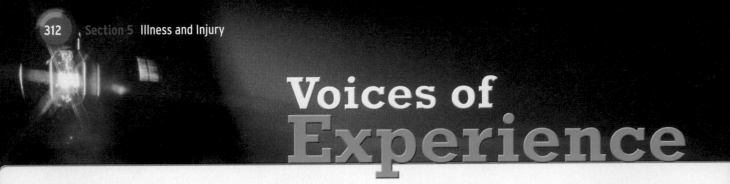

Voices of Experience

Back to Basics

Our pagers alerted us to a run: "LifeFlight 1, meet a private ambulance on Rt. 33 between 270 and Coonpath Road." The report was for a 26-year-old female who accidentally shot herself in the foot with a .22 handgun. Her condition was becoming worse, and they were concerned that she might die before we arrived.

> **We must remember that it is the basics that save lives.**

As we landed at a roadside park, we received a radio report that the patient's vital signs were pulse 146, respirations 32, and blood pressure 60/palp. At a small, local emergency department 90 miles to the southeast, the doctor advised that the patient be transported to a trauma center and a private ALS ambulance was called to transport. En route, the patient's wound kept bleeding through the pressure dressing, so the medic kept packing on more dressings in an attempt to protect the clot that was forming on the wound. Because she was becoming shocky, the ambulance crew stopped at a hospital along the way for help. At that hospital, the dressing was replaced with a new pressure dressing and the patient received a unit of O-negative blood. They placed her back in the ambulance and our helicopter was called to meet them en route. In preparation for meeting the ambulance, we were thinking that we would intubate her and place a turbo, 8.5F catheter in an existing IV so we could really "dump in" some fluids.

The squad arrived and we climbed in. I noticed a huge puddle of blood on the floor and a sizable blood-soaked dressing on the patient's right foot. As I intubated her, the nurse removed the dressing and found two small holes with moderate bleeding. He held direct pressure to the two bullet holes with 5 × 9 dressings, as we elected to load the patient into the helicopter and start back to the trauma center, which was 12 minutes away by helicopter. My partner Mel kept holding direct pressure and I maintained her airway and fluid administration. Mel was able to stop the bleeding with direct pressure in the 12 minutes it took to fly to the trauma center. I couldn't help but think that if someone had just taken that action earlier in her treatment, she might have been treated and released from the emergency department. As it turned out, she was discharged 2 months later with an anoxic brain injury, which left her with vision and short-term memory problems.

This single event left a deep impression on me and how I deal with bleeding and shocky patients. Each of us is taught early on in the educational process that direct pressure stops bleeding—PERIOD! As we learn more and receive additional education, we must remember that it is the basics that save lives.

Michael D. Smith, EMT-P, EMSI
Firefighter/Flight Paramedic
City of Grandview Heights, Division of Fire and
   MedFlight of Ohio
Columbus, Ohio

Chest Wounds and Back Wounds

The major organs affected by chest wounds and back wounds are the lungs, large blood vessels, and heart. Any wound involving these organs is a life-threatening injury. Place the patient with a chest injury in a comfortable position (usually sitting) (see Chapter 14).

If a lung is punctured, air can escape and the lung will collapse. The patient may cough up bright red blood. To help maintain air pressure in the lung, your first act should be to cover any open chest wound with airtight material, sealing it. This covering is called an **occlusive dressing**. Use a clear plastic cover from your medical supplies, aluminum foil, plastic wrap, or a special dressing that has been impregnated with petroleum jelly (Vaseline). Any material that will occlude (seal off) the wound is sufficient **Figure 13-33 ▾**.

Administering oxygen is important early treatment for an injured lung. It should be given by EMS personnel when they arrive or by first responders who are trained and have the equipment available.

Chest wounds may also damage the heart. Seal the wound in the manner described and monitor the patient's airway, breathing, and circulation. Treat the patient for shock and perform CPR, if necessary.

If the patient's breathing becomes more labored after you seal the chest wound, you may need to remove the seal briefly to allow excess air to escape and then reseal the wound.

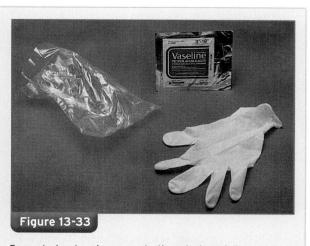

Figure 13-33

For occlusive dressings, use plastic, petroleum jelly, or gloves.

Impaled Objects

If an object is impaled in the patient, apply a stabilizing dressing and arrange for the patient's immediate and **prompt transport** to an appropriate medical facility. Sometimes an impaled object is too long to permit the patient to be removed from the accident scene and transported to an appropriate medical facility. In these cases, it may be necessary to stabilize the impaled object and carefully cut it close to the patient's body. If you encounter a situation like this, stabilize the impaled object as well as you can and immediately request a specialized rescue team that has the tools and training to handle such a situation.

If you find the patient with a knife or other object protruding from the abdomen, do not attempt to remove it. Instead, support the impaled object so it cannot move. Place a large roll of gauze or towels on either side of the object and secure the rolls with additional gauze wrapped around the body. It is important to stabilize the object so it will not move while the patient is being transported to the hospital **Figure 13-34 ▸**. Any movement of the object may cause further internal damage.

FYI

Closed Abdominal Wounds

Closed abdominal wounds commonly occur as the result of a direct blow from a blunt object. You should check for a closed abdominal wound whenever force has been applied to the abdomen. Look for bruises or other marks on the abdomen that indicate blunt injury.

Any time an injured patient is suffering from shock, you should remember that there may be internal abdominal injuries accompanied by bleeding. When there is internal bleeding, the abdomen may become swollen, rigid, or hard like a board. Treat patients with closed abdominal injuries and signs of shock by placing them on their backs and elevating their legs at least 6 inches (unless they are having difficulty breathing). Conserve their body heat.

If the patient is vomiting blood (ranging in color from bright red to dark brown), it may be an indication of bleeding from the esophagus or stomach. Monitor the patient's vital functions carefully because shock may result. Give the patient nothing by mouth. Arrange for **prompt transport** to an appropriate medical facility.

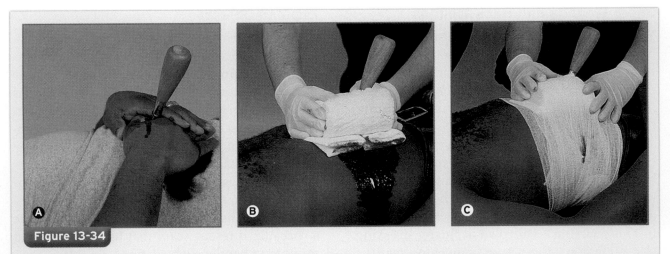

Figure 13-34

Bandaging an impaled object. **A.** Do not attempt to remove or move an impaled object. **B.** Stabilize the object in place with dressings. **C.** Place a bandage over the dressings.

Treatment Tips

To treat an open abdominal wound, follow these steps:

1. Apply a dry, sterile dressing to the wound.
2. Maintain the patient's body temperature.
3. Place the patient on his or her back with the legs elevated.
4. Place the patient who is having difficulty breathing in a semireclining position.
5. Administer oxygen, if it is available, and you are trained to use it.

Open Abdominal Wounds

Open abdominal wounds usually result from slashing with a knife or other sharp object and are always serious injuries.

If the intestines are protruding from the abdomen, place the patient on his or her back with the knees bent, to relax the abdominal muscles. Cover the injured area with a sterile dressing **Figure 13-35 ▾**. Do not attempt to replace the intestines inside the abdomen.

You can make a bandage from a large trauma pad (10 inches × 30 inches) and several cravats to cover protruding abdominal intestines. Position the trauma pad to cover the whole area of the wound. Tie two or three wide cravats loosely over

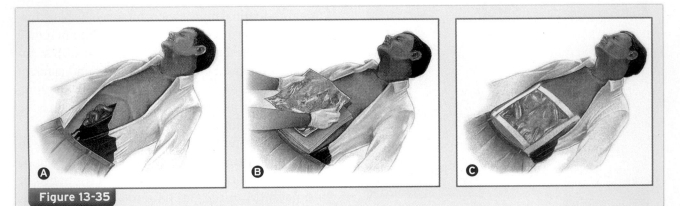

Figure 13-35

Bandaging an open abdominal wound. **A.** Open abdominal wounds are serious injuries. **B.** Cover with a moist, sterile dressing or occlusive dressing, depending on local protocol. **C.** Secure the dressing.

the trauma pad, just tightly enough to keep it firmly in place, but not tightly enough to push the intestines back into the abdomen.

EMTs and paramedics carry sterile <u>saline</u> (salt water), which can be poured on the dressing to keep the protruding organs moist so they do not dry out. Only sterile saline should be used.

FYI

Genital Wounds

Both male and female genitals have a rich blood supply. Injury to the genitals can often result in severe bleeding. Apply direct pressure to any genital wound with a dry, sterile dressing.

FYI cont.

Direct pressure usually stops the bleeding. Although it may be embarrassing to examine the patient's genital area to determine the severity of the injury, you must do so if you suspect such injuries. The patient can suffer a critical loss of blood if you do not find the injury and control the bleeding.

Extremity Wounds

To treat all open extremity wounds, apply a dry, sterile compression dressing and bandage it securely in place **Figure 13-36 ▼** and **Figure 13-37 ▼**. Elevating the injured part decreases bleeding and

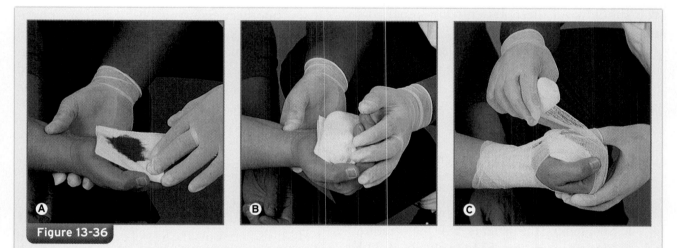

Figure 13-36

Bandaging a hand wound. **A.** Place a dressing over the wound. **B.** Place a gauze roll in the palm of the hand to apply pressure. **C.** Secure the dressing with a gauze roller bandage.

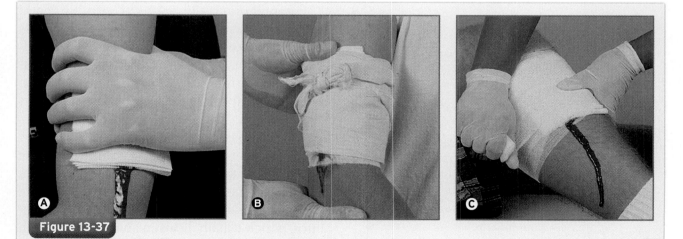

Figure 13-37

Bandaging an extremity wound. **A.** Place a dressing over the wound. **B.** Secure the dressing with a cravat. **C.** Secure the dressing with a roller gauze.

swelling. You should splint all injured extremities prior to transport because there may be an underlying fracture.

Gunshot Wounds

Some gunshot wounds are easy to miss unless you perform a thorough patient examination Figure 13-38 ▾ . Most deaths from gunshot wounds result from internal blood loss caused by damage to internal organs and major blood vessels. Because gunshot wounds are so serious, prompt and effective treatment is important. Gunshot wounds of the trunk and neck are a major cause of spinal cord injuries. Because you cannot see the bullet's path through the body, you should treat these patients for spinal cord injuries.

To treat a gunshot wound, follow these steps:

1. Open the airway and establish adequate ventilation and circulation.
2. Control any external bleeding by covering wounds with sterile dressings and applying pressure with your hand or a bandage.
3. Examine the patient thoroughly to be sure you have discovered all entrance and exit wounds.
4. Treat for symptoms of shock by:
   A. Maintaining the patient's body temperature.
   B. Placing the patient on his or her back with the legs elevated 6 inches.
   C. Placing a patient who is having difficulty breathing in a semireclining position.
   D. Administering oxygen, if available.

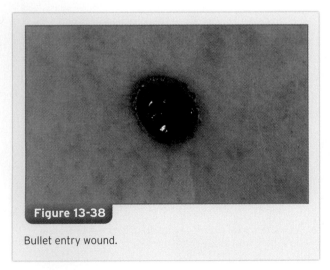

Figure 13-38

Bullet entry wound.

5. Arrange for **prompt transport** of the patient to an appropriate medical facility.
6. Perform CPR if the patient's heart stops as a result of loss of blood.

Bites

Bites from animals or humans may range from minor to severe. All bites have a high chance of causing infection. Bites from an unvaccinated animal may cause **rabies**. Minor bites can be washed with soap and water, if they are available. Major bite wounds should be treated by controlling the bleeding and applying a suitable dressing and bandage.

All patients who have been bitten by an animal or another person must be treated by a physician. In most states, EMS personnel are required to report animal bites to the local health department or a law enforcement agency. You should check the laws in your local area to determine requirements.

Burns

The skin serves as a barrier that prevents foreign substances, such as bacteria, from entering the body. It also prevents the loss of body fluids. When the skin is damaged, such as by a burn, it can no longer perform these essential functions.

Burn Depth

There are three classifications of burns by depth: superficial (first-degree) burns, partial-thickness (second-degree) burns, and full-thickness (third-degree) burns. Although it is not always possible to determine the exact degree of a burn injury, it is important for you to understand this concept.

Superficial burns (first-degree burns) are characterized by reddened and painful skin. The injury is confined to the outermost layers of skin, and the patient experiences minor to moderate pain. An example of a superficial burn is a sunburn, which usually heals in about a week, with or without treatment Figure 13-39 ▸ .

Partial-thickness burns (second-degree burns) are somewhat deeper but do not damage the deep-

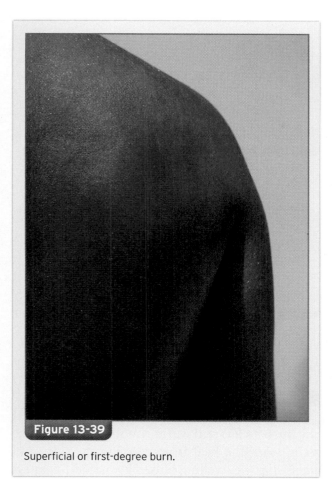

Figure 13-39

Superficial or first-degree burn.

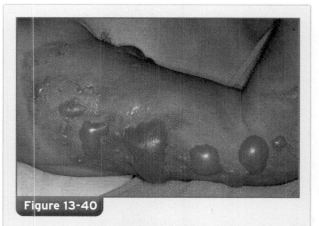

Figure 13-40

Partial-thickness or second-degree burn.

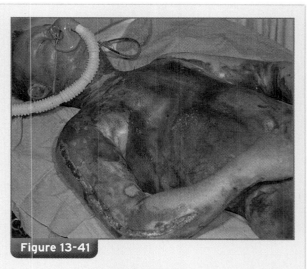

Figure 13-41

Full-thickness or third-degree burn.

est layers of the skin Figure 13-40 ▶ . Blistering is present, although blisters may not form for several hours in some cases. There may be some fluid loss and moderate to severe pain because the nerve endings are damaged. Partial-thickness burns require medical treatment. They usually heal within 2 to 3 weeks.

Full-thickness burns (third-degree burns) damage all layers of the skin. In some cases, the damage is deep enough to injure and destroy underlying muscles and other tissues Figure 13-41 ▶ . Pain is often absent because the nerve endings have been destroyed. Without the protection provided by the skin, patients with extensive full-thickness burns lose large quantities of body fluids and are susceptible to shock and infection.

FYI

Extent of Burns

The **Rule of Nines** is a method for determining what percentage of the body has been burned.

FYI cont.

Although this rule is most useful for EMTs and paramedics who report information to the hospital from the field, first responders should be able to roughly estimate the extent of a burn. Figure 13-42 ▶ shows how the Rule of Nines divides the body. In an adult, the head and arms each equal 9% of the total body surface. The front and back of the trunk and each leg are equal to 18% of the total body surface. For example, if one half of the back and all of the right arm of a patient are burned, the burn involves about 18% of the total body area. The Rule of Nines is slightly modified for young children, but the adult figures serve as an adequate guide.

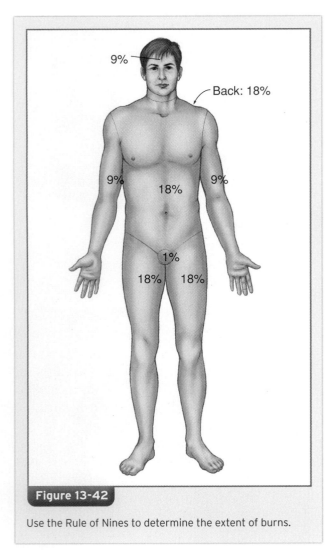

Figure 13-42

Use the Rule of Nines to determine the extent of burns.

Cause or Type of Burns

Burns are caused by exposure to the following elements:

- Heat (thermal burns)
- Chemicals
- Electricity

Thermal Burns

<u>Thermal burns</u> are caused by heat. The first step in treating thermal burns is to cool the skin by "putting out the fire." Superficial burns can be quite painful, but if there is clean, cold water available, you can place the burning area in cold water to help reduce the pain. You can also wet a clean towel with cold water and put it on superficial burns. After the burned area is cooled, cover it with a dry, sterile dress-

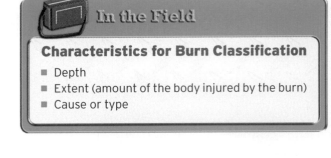

In the Field

Characteristics for Burn Classification

- Depth
- Extent (amount of the body injured by the burn)
- Cause or type

Treatment Tips

Do not apply burn ointments, butter, grease, or cream to any burn!

ing or the large sterile cloth called a burn sheet (found in your first responder life support kit) **Figure 13-43 ▼**.

Partial-thickness burns should be cooled if the burn area is still warm. Cooling helps reduce pain, stops the heat from cooking the skin, and helps stop the swelling caused by partial-thickness burns.

If blisters are present, be very careful not to break the blisters. Intact skin, even if blistered, provides an excellent barrier against infection. If the blisters break, the danger of infection increases. Cover partial-thickness burns with a dry, sterile dressing or burn sheet.

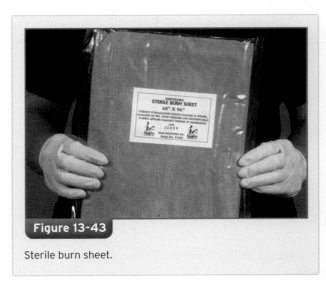

Figure 13-43

Sterile burn sheet.

Full-thickness burns, if still warm, should also be cooled with water to keep the heat from damaging more skin and tissue. Cut any clothing away from the burned area, but leave any clothing that is stuck to the burn. Cover full-thickness burns with a dry, sterile dressing or burn sheet **Figure 13-44 ▾**.

Patients with large superficial burns or any partial-thickness or full-thickness burns must be treated for shock and **transported** to a hospital.

FYI

Respiratory Burns

A burn to any part of the airway is a <u>respiratory burn</u>. If a patient has been burned around the head and face or while in a confined space (such as in a burning house), you should look for the signs and symptoms of respiratory burns, listed in the Signs and Symptoms box.

Watch the patient carefully. Breathing problems that result from this type of burn can develop rapidly or slowly over several hours. Administer oxygen as soon as it is available and be prepared to perform CPR. If you suspect that a patient has suffered respiratory burns, arrange for **prompt transport** to a medical facility.

If the patient has injuries in addition to the burn, treat the injuries before transporting the patient. For example, if a patient who has a partial-thickness burn of the arm has also fallen off a ladder and fractured both legs, splint the fractures and place the patient on a backboard, in addition to treating the burn injury.

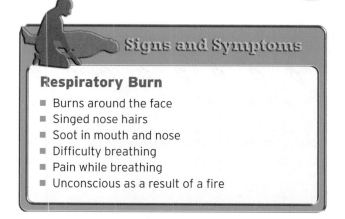

Signs and Symptoms

Respiratory Burn

- Burns around the face
- Singed nose hairs
- Soot in mouth and nose
- Difficulty breathing
- Pain while breathing
- Unconscious as a result of a fire

Chemical Burns

Many strong substances can cause <u>chemical burns</u> to the skin. These substances include strong acids such as battery acid or strong alkalis such as drain cleaners. Some chemicals cause damage even if they are on the skin or in the eyes for only a short period of time. The longer the chemical remains in contact with the skin, the more it damages the skin and underlying tissues. Chemicals are extremely dangerous to the eyes and can cause superficial, partial-thickness, or full-thickness burns to the skin.

The initial treatment for chemical burns is to remove as much of the chemical as possible from the patient's skin. Brush away any dry chemical on the patient's clothes or skin, being careful not to get any on yourself. You may have to ask the patient to remove all clothing.

After you have removed as much of the dry chemical as possible, flush the contaminated skin

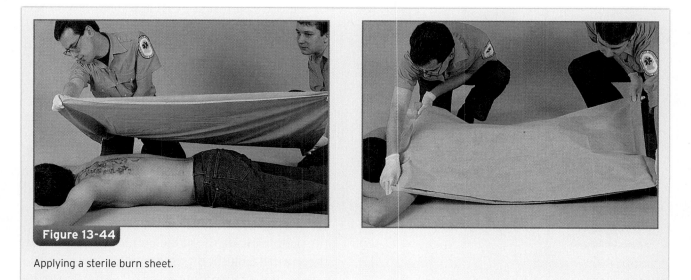

Figure 13-44

Applying a sterile burn sheet.

with abundant quantities of water. You can use water from a garden hose, a shower in the home or factory, or even the booster hose of a fire engine. It is essential that the chemical be washed off the skin quickly to avoid further injury. Flush the affected area of the body for at least 10 minutes, then cover the burned area with a dry, sterile dressing or a burn sheet and arrange for **prompt transport** to an appropriate medical facility.

Chemical burns to the eyes cause extreme pain and severe injury. Gently flush the affected eye or eyes with water for at least 20 minutes Figure 13-45 ▼. You must hold the eye open to allow water to flow over its entire surface. Direct the water from the inner corner of the eye to the outward edge of the eye. You may have to put the patient's face under a shower, garden hose, or faucet so that the water flows across the patient's entire face. Flushing the eyes can continue while the patient is being transported.

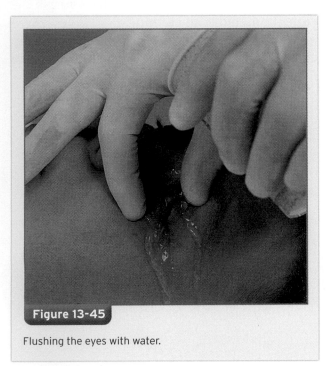

Figure 13-45

Flushing the eyes with water.

After flushing the eyes for 20 minutes, loosely cover the injured eye or eyes with gauze bandages and arrange for **prompt transport** to an appropriate medical facility. All chemical burns should be examined by a physician.

Electrical Burns

Electrical burns can cause severe injuries or even death, but they leave little evidence of injury on the outside of the body. These burns are caused by an electrical current that enters the body at one point (for example, the hand that touches the live electrical wire), travels through the body tissues and organs, and exits from the body at the point of ground contact Figure 13-46 ▶.

Electricity causes major internal damage, rather than external damage. A strong electrical current can actually "cook" muscles, nerves, blood vessels, and internal organs, resulting in major damage. Patients who have been subjected to a strong electrical current can also suffer irregularities of cardiac rhythm or even full cardiac arrest and death. Children often suffer electrical burns by chewing on an electrical cord or by pushing something into an outlet. Although the burn may not look serious at first, it is often quite severe because of underlying tissue injury.

Persons who have been hit or nearly hit by lightning frequently suffer electrical burns. Treat these patients as you would electrical burn patients. Evaluate them carefully because they may also suffer cardiac arrest. Arrange for **prompt transport** to an appropriate medical facility.

Before you touch or treat a person who has suffered an electrical burn, be certain that the patient is not still in contact with the electrical power source that caused the burn. If the patient is still in contact with the power source, anyone who touches him or her may be electrocuted. If the patient is touching a live power source, your first act must be to unplug, disconnect, or turn off the power Figure 13-47 ▶. If you cannot do this alone, call for assistance from the power company or from a qualified rescue squad or fire department.

If a power line falls on top of a motor vehicle, the people inside the vehicle must be told to stay there until qualified personnel can remove the power line or turn the power off. After ensuring

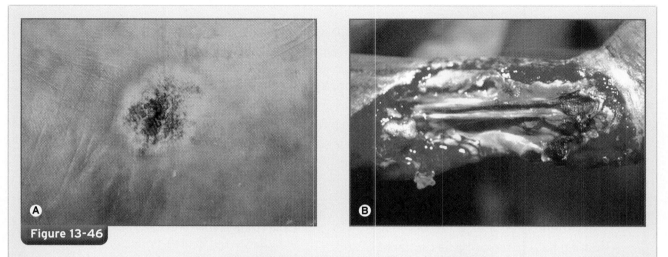

Figure 13-46

Electrical burns. **A.** An entrance wound is often small. **B.** An exit wound can be extensive and deep.

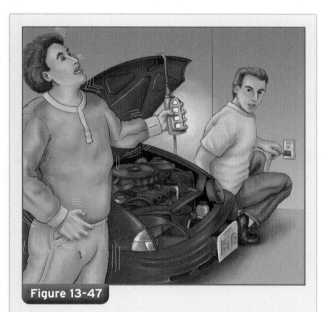

Figure 13-47

Do not touch the patient without unplugging, disconnecting, or turning off the power first.

Safety Tips

Avoid direct or indirect contact with live electrical wires. Direct contact occurs when you touch a live electrical wire. Indirect contact occurs when you touch a vehicle, a patient, a fence, a tree, or any other object that is in contact with a live electrical wire.

that the power has been disconnected, examine each electrical burn patient carefully, assess the ABCs, and treat the patient for visible, external burns. Cover these external burns with a dry, sterile dressing and arrange for **prompt transport** to an appropriate medical facility.

Monitor the airway, breathing, and circulation of electrical burn patients closely and arrange to have such patients transported promptly to an emergency department for further treatment.

You are the Provider   SUMMARY

Review the *You are the Provider* case study provided at the beginning of the chapter.

It is a warm summer day, and you are dispatched for the report of an injured party in a suburban part of town. As you are responding, you receive further dispatch information that the patient's leg has been cut by a power lawn mower.

1. **What safety considerations should you keep in mind as you approach this situation?**

   Caring for a person who has suffered a soft-tissue injury involves several safety considerations. Be certain the machinery has been turned off so it cannot cause further harm to the patient or to rescuers. BSI is a major concern any time external bleeding is present.

2. **What equipment and supplies do you want to take with you?**

   The equipment needed for treating soft-tissue injuries includes BSI equipment such as gloves to protect the rescuer, dressings and bandages to treat the soft-tissue injury, splinting materials to immobilize the injured body part, and blankets to conserve body heat.

3. **What are the treatment goals for this type of incident?**

   The goals of treating soft-tissue injuries are to ensure BSI, control external bleeding, prevent further contamination of the wound site, and immobilize the affected extremity. Meeting these objectives requires different actions to be taken in different situations.

Prep Kit

Ready for Review

The Ready for Review thoroughly summarizes the chapter.

- This chapter covers the knowledge and skills you need to treat patients suffering shock, bleeding, and soft-tissue injuries.

- You must take appropriate body substance isolation measures to prevent contact with the patient's body fluids.

- The three parts of the circulatory system are the pump (heart), the pipes (arteries, veins, and capillaries), and the fluid (blood cells and other blood components).

- Shock is a state of collapse of the cardiovascular system that results in inadequate delivery of blood to the organs. The three primary causes of shock are pump failure, pipe failure, and fluid loss. The general treatment for shock is positioning the patient correctly, maintaining the patient's ABCs, and treating the cause of shock, if possible.

- There are three types of external blood loss: capillary (blood oozes out), venous (bleeds at a steady flow), and arterial (blood spurts or surges). Most external bleeding can be controlled by applying direct pressure to the wound.

- A wound is an injury caused by any physical means that leads to damage of a body part. Wounds are classified as closed (skin remains intact) or open (skin is disrupted). Open wounds are classified as abrasions, punctures, lacerations, and avulsions or amputations.

- Control bleeding by covering an open wound with a dry, clean, or sterile dressing and apply pressure to the dressing with your hand. Additional ways to control bleeding include elevating an extremity and using pressure points.

- There are three classifications of burns by depth: superficial (first-degree) burns, partial-thickness (second-degree) burns, and full-thickness (third-degree) burns. Burns may be caused by heat, chemicals, or electricity.

- By learning to recognize and provide initial emergency treatment for patients suffering shock, bleeding, and soft-tissue injuries, you will be able to provide physical and emotional assistance to these patients in their time of need. At times, your prompt recognition and treatment will make a real difference.

Vital Vocabulary

The Vital Vocabulary are the key terms for this chapter.

abrasion Loss of skin as a result of a body part being rubbed or scraped across a rough or hard surface.

anaphylactic shock Severe shock caused by an allergic reaction to food, medicine, or insect stings.

arterial bleeding Serious bleeding from an artery in which blood frequently pulses or spurts from an open wound.

atrium Either of the two upper chambers of the heart.

avulsion An injury in which a piece of skin is either torn completely loose from all of its attachments or is left hanging as a flap.

blood pressure The pressure of the circulating blood against the walls of the arteries.

brachial artery pressure point Pressure point located in the arm between the elbow and the shoulder; also used in taking blood pressure and for checking the pulse in infants.

bruise Injury caused by a blunt object striking the body and crushing the tissue beneath the skin. Also called a contusion.

capillary bleeding Bleeding from the capillaries in which blood oozes from the open wound.

cardiogenic shock Shock resulting from inadequate functioning of the heart.

chemical burns Burns that occur when any toxic substance comes in contact with the skin. Most chemical burns are caused by strong acids or alkalis.

Technology

- Interactivities
- Vocabulary Explorer
- Anatomy Review
- Web Links
- Online Review Manual

closed wound Injury in which soft-tissue damage occurs beneath the skin but there is no break in the surface of the skin.

congestive heart failure (CHF) Heart disease characterized by breathlessness, fluid retention in the lungs, and generalized swelling of the body.

cravat A triangular swathe of cloth that is used to hold a body part splinted against the body.

dressing A bandage.

electrical burns Burns caused by contact with high- or low-voltage electricity. Electrical wounds have an entrance and an exit wound.

entrance wound Point where an injurious object such as a bullet enters the body.

exit wound Point where an injurious object such as a bullet passes out of the body.

femoral artery pressure point Pressure point located in the groin, where the femoral artery is close to the skin.

full-thickness burns Burns that extend through the skin and into or beyond the underlying tissues; the most serious class of burn.

gunshot wound A puncture wound caused by a bullet or shotgun pellet.

hemorrhage Excessive bleeding.

immobilize To reduce or prevent movement of a limb, usually by splinting.

impaled object An object such as a knife, splinter of wood, or glass that penetrates the skin and remains in the body.

intravenous (IV) fluids Fluids other than blood or blood products infused into the vascular system to maintain an adequate circulatory blood volume.

laceration An irregular cut or tear through the skin.

occlusive dressing An airtight dressing or bandage for a wound.

open wound Injury that breaks the skin or mucous membrane.

partial-thickness burns Burns in which the outer layers of skin are burned; these burns are characterized by blister formation.

pneumatic antishock garments (PASGs) Trouser-like devices placed around a shock victim's legs and abdomen and inflated with air.

pressure points Points where a blood vessel lies near a bone; pressure can be applied to these points to help control bleeding.

psychogenic shock Commonly known as fainting; caused by a temporary reduction in blood supply to the brain.

puncture A wound resulting from a bullet, knife, ice pick, splinter, or any other pointed object.

rabies An acute viral infection of the central nervous system transmitted by the bite of an infected animal.

respiratory burn Burn to the respiratory system resulting from inhaling superheated air.

road rash An abrasion caused by sliding on pavement. Usually seen after motorcycle or bicycle accidents.

Rule of Nines A way to calculate the amount of body surface burned; the body is divided into sections, each of which constitutes approximately 9% or 18% of the total body surface area.

saline Salt water.

shock A state of collapse of the cardiovascular system; the state of inadequate delivery of blood to the organs of the body.

splint A means of immobilizing an injured part by using a rigid or soft support.

spontaneous nosebleed A nosebleed with no apparent cause.

superficial burns Burns in which only the superficial part of the skin has been injured; an example is a sunburn.

thermal burns Burns caused by heat; the most common type of burn.

venous bleeding External bleeding from a vein, characterized by steady flow; the bleeding may be profuse and life threatening.

ventricles The two lower chambers of the heart.

Assessment in Action

Assessment in Action presents a fictitious scenario to help you review what you learned in this chapter.

You are dispatched to a local car repair shop for a traumatic injury. Upon arrival, you find a 27-year-old male holding a rag against his lower forearm. The rag is soaked with bright red blood. As you remove the rag to inspect the injury, you find a 4-inch full-thickness laceration that is spurting bright red blood.

1. What is your first step in the treatment of this patient?

   A. Irrigate the wound.
   B. Apply direct pressure.
   C. Apply a bandage and dressing.
   D. Elevate the extremity.

2. What type of body substance isolation should you as the first responder use when treating this patient?

   A. Gloves
   B. Eye protection
   C. Gown
   D. All of the above

3. What is the proper order of use for the following bleeding control measures?

   1. Elevation
   2. Pressure points
   3. Direct pressure
      A. 3, 1, 2
      B. 2, 3, 1
      C. 3, 2, 1

4. What type of bleeding is this patient presenting with?

   A. Venous
   B. Arterial
   C. Capillary
   D. None of the above

5. If using a pressure point to assist in bleeding control, what artery will you apply pressure to?

   A. Femoral artery
   B. Brachial artery
   C. Carotid artery
   D. Radial artery

Injuries to Muscles and Bones

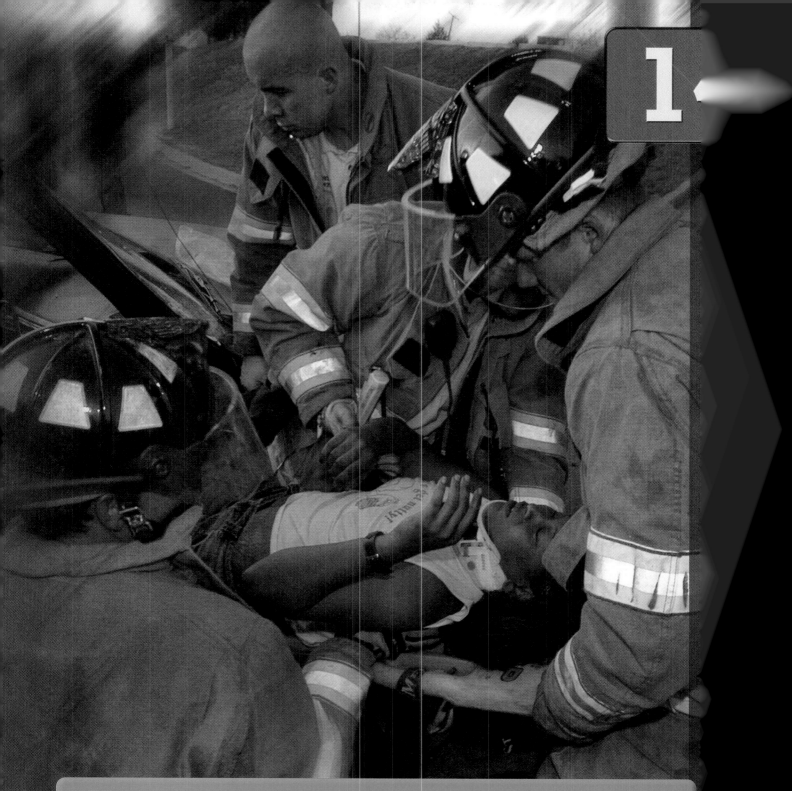

You are the Provider

It is a warm, sunny, spring day. You are dispatched to a residence for the report of a senior citizen who has fallen. When you arrive, you find a conscious and alert 74-year-old woman lying at the bottom of the four steps leading up to the front porch. The woman complains of pain in her right leg.

1. What are the body substance isolation considerations in this case?
2. What type of physical examination is needed for this patient?
3. Under what conditions would you move this patient?

Introduction

As a first responder, you will encounter many types of musculoskeletal injuries, including fractures, dislocations, sprains, strains, head injuries, spinal cord injuries, and chest injuries. You need to understand the anatomy and functioning of the musculoskeletal system and to study the causes or mechanisms of injury. This will give you a better understanding of the results of various injuries.

Before you can treat musculoskeletal injuries, you must be able to recognize their signs and symptoms and to differentiate between open and closed injuries. Giving proper care at the scene can prevent additional injury or disability. This chapter describes how to manage injuries to the upper and lower extremities, the head, the spinal cord, and the chest. It also provides information on body substance isolation techniques and their relation to musculoskeletal injuries.

The Anatomy and Function of the Musculoskeletal System

The musculoskeletal system has two parts: the skeletal system, which provides support and form for the body, and the muscular system, which provides both support and movement.

Technology

Interactivities

Vocabulary Explorer

Anatomy Review

Web Links

Online Review Manual

The Skeletal System

The skeletal system consists of 206 bones and is the supporting framework for the body. The four functions of the skeletal system are:

1. To support the body
2. To protect vital structures
3. To assist in body movement
4. To manufacture red blood cells

The skeletal system Figure 14-1 ▾ is divided into seven areas:

1. Head, skull, and face
2. Spinal column
3. Shoulder girdle
4. Upper extremities
5. Rib cage (thorax)
6. Pelvis
7. Lower extremities

The bones of the head include the skull and the lower jawbone. The skull is actually many bones fused together to form a hollow sphere that

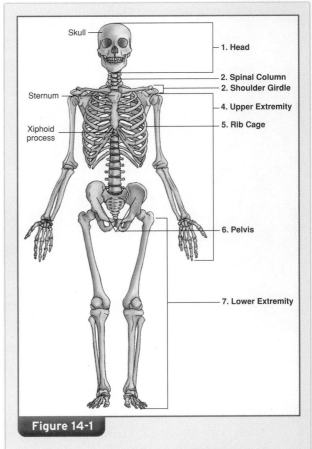

Figure 14-1

The seven major areas of the human skeleton.

contains and protects the brain. The jawbone is a movable bone attached to the skull that completes the structure of the face.

The spine consists of a series of separate bones called vertebrae. The spinal vertebrae are stacked on top of each other and are held together by muscles, tendons, disks, and ligaments. The spinal cord, a group of nerves that carry messages to and from the brain, passes through a hole in the center of each vertebra. In addition to protecting the spinal cord, the spine is the primary support structure for the entire body.

The spine has five sections Figure 14-2 ▾ :
1. Cervical spine (neck)
2. Thoracic spine (upper back)
3. Lumbar spine (lower back)
4. Sacrum
5. Coccyx (tailbone)

The shoulder girdles form the third area of the skeletal system. Each shoulder girdle supports an arm and consists of the collarbone (clavicle) and the shoulder blade (scapula). The fourth area of the skeletal system, the upper extremities, consists of three major bones as well as the wrist and hand. The arm has one bone (the humerus), and the forearm has two bones (the radius and the ulna). The radius is located on the thumb side of the arm; the ulna is located on the side of the little finger. There are several bones in the wrist and hand. However, you do not need to learn their names and you can consider them as one unit for the purposes of emergency treatment.

The fifth area of the skeletal system is the rib cage or chest (thorax). The 12 sets of ribs protect the heart, lungs, liver, and spleen. All of the ribs are attached to the spine Figure 14-3 ▾ . The upper five rib sets connect directly to the sternum (breastbone). A bridge of cartilage connects the ends of the 6th through 10th rib sets to each other and to the sternum. The 11th and 12th rib sets are called floating ribs because they are not attached to the sternum. The sternum is located in the front of the chest. The pointed structure at the bottom of the sternum is called the xiphoid process.

The sixth area of the skeletal system is the pelvis, which links the body and the lower extremities. The pelvis also protects the reproductive organs and the other organs located in the lower abdominal cavity.

The lower extremities (the thigh and the leg) form the seventh area of the skeletal system. The thigh bone (femur) is the longest and strongest

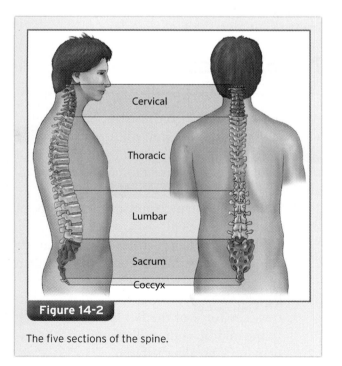

Figure 14-2

The five sections of the spine.

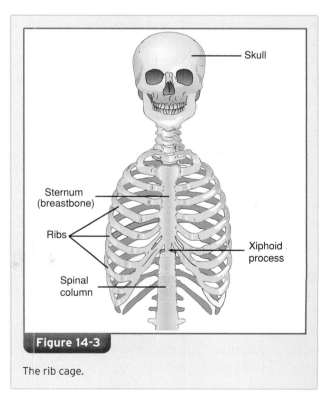

Figure 14-3

The rib cage.

bone in the entire body. The leg consists of two major bones, the tibia and fibula, as well as the ankle and foot. The kneecap (patella) is a small, relatively flat bone that protects the front of the knee **joint**. Like the wrist and hand, the ankle and foot contain a large number of smaller bones that can be considered as one unit.

A protective bony structure surrounds each of the body's essential organs. The skull protects the brain. The vertebrae protect the spinal cord. The ribs protect the heart and lungs. The pelvis protects the lower abdominal and reproductive organs. A vital but often overlooked function of the skeletal system is to produce red blood cells. Red blood cells are manufactured primarily within the spaces inside the bone called the marrow.

The Muscular System

The muscles of the body provide both support and movement. Muscles are attached to bones by tendons and cause movement by alternately contracting (shortening) and relaxing (lengthening). Muscles are usually paired in opposition: As one member of the pair contracts, the other relaxes. This mechanical opposition moves bones and enables you to open and close your hand, turn your head, and bend and straighten your knee or other joints. To straighten the elbow, for example, the biceps muscle relaxes, and an opposing muscle on the back of the arm contracts.

The musculoskeletal system gets its name from the coordination between the muscular system and the skeletal system to produce movement. Movement occurs at joints, where two bones come together. The bones are held together by ligaments, thick bands that arise from one bone, span the joint, and insert into the adjacent bone.

The body has three types of muscles: voluntary, involuntary, and cardiac. Voluntary, or skeletal, muscles are attached to bones and can be contracted and relaxed by a person at will. They are responsible for the movement of the body. Involuntary, or smooth, muscles are found on the inside of the digestive tract and other internal organs of the body. They are not under

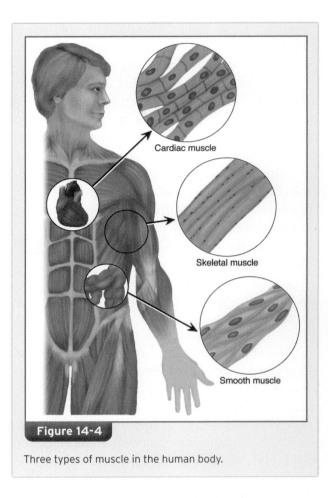

Figure 14-4

Three types of muscle in the human body.

Cardiac muscle
Skeletal muscle
Smooth muscle

conscious control and perform their functions automatically. Cardiac muscle is found only in the heart **Figure 14-4 ▲**. Most musculoskeltal injuries involve skeletal muscles.

Mechanism of Injury

As a first responder, you must understand the **mechanism of injury** or how injuries occur. Musculoskeletal injuries are caused by three types of mechanisms of injury: direct force, indirect force, and twisting force **Figure 14-5 ▶**.

Examples of each mechanism and the type of injury it causes are:

- **Direct force.** A car strikes a pedestrian on the leg. The pedestrian sustains a broken leg.
- **Indirect force.** A woman falls on her shoulder. The force of the fall transmits energy to the middle of the collarbone and the excess force breaks the bone.

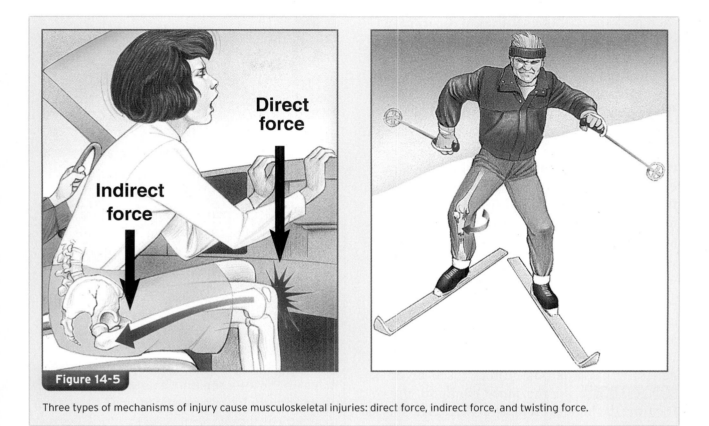

Figure 14-5

Three types of mechanisms of injury cause musculoskeletal injuries: direct force, indirect force, and twisting force.

- **Twisting force.** A football player is tackled as he is turning. He twists his leg, causing a severe injury to his knee. Injuries can be caused by direct force at the site of impact or can be caused by indirect force at an impact site removed from the site of the injury.

As a first responder, you will see many different types of traumatic injuries. Some of these will be the result of motor vehicle crashes or auto/pedestrian accidents; others will be the result of athletic activities, work-related accidents, falls, or violence. You will see injuries in people of all ages—from very young children to older people. Use the information provided by your dispatcher and gathered from your overview of the scene to identify the possible mechanisms of injury. You will gain additional information from examining and questioning the patient. By understanding the mechanism of injury (how the injury occurred), you will be better able to assess the patient and provide the needed treatment.

FYI

A Word About Terminology

There are different ways to describe a patient's injuries. You must rely on your senses of sight and touch to determine the type of injury the patient has experienced. You must also listen to the information that the patient can give you. However, keep in mind that, as a first responder, you do not have the training or tools to diagnose an injury as a physician can.

The next section defines fractures, dislocations, and sprains. Although you are not expected to diagnose these injuries, the patient's signs and symptoms will lead you to suspect that a certain injury is most probable. Some instructors and medical directors may choose to identify musculoskeletal injuries strictly in terms of the signs and symptoms present, such as a painful, swollen, deformed extremity. Others may choose to use terms such as suspected or possible fracture, dislocation, or sprain. To meet the needs of both groups of instructors and medical directors, this text uses "PSDE" (painful, swollen, deformed extremity) after

FYI cont.

each relevant term. Regardless of the terminology used, the most important part of the first responder's job is to provide the best assessment and treatment for the patient.

Types of Injuries

It is often difficult to distinguish one type of musculoskeletal extremity injury from another. All three types are serious, and all extremity injuries must be identified so they can receive appropriate medical treatment.

Fractures

A fracture is a broken bone. Fractures can be caused by a variety of mechanisms, but require a significant force, unless the bone is weakened by a disease such as osteoporosis. Fractures are generally classified as either closed or open **Figure 14-6 ▾**. In the more common **closed fracture**, the bone is broken but there is no break in the skin.

In an **open fracture**, the bone is broken and the overlying skin is lacerated. The open wound can be caused by a penetrating object, such as a bullet, or by the fractured bone end itself protruding through the skin. Open fractures are contaminated by dirt and bacteria that may lead to

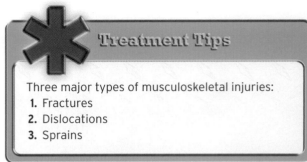

Treatment Tips

Three major types of musculoskeletal injuries:
1. Fractures
2. Dislocations
3. Sprains

FYI cont.

infection. Both open and closed fractures injure adjacent soft tissues, resulting in bleeding at the fracture site. Fractures can also injure nearby nerves and blood vessels, causing severe nerve injury and excessive bleeding.

Dislocations

A **dislocation** is a disruption that tears the supporting ligaments of the joint. The bone ends that make up the joint separate completely from each other and can lock in one position. Any attempt to move a dislocated joint is very painful. Because many nerves and blood vessels lie near joints, a dislocation can damage these structures as well.

Sprains and Strains

A **sprain** is a joint injury caused by excessive stretching of the supporting ligaments. It can be

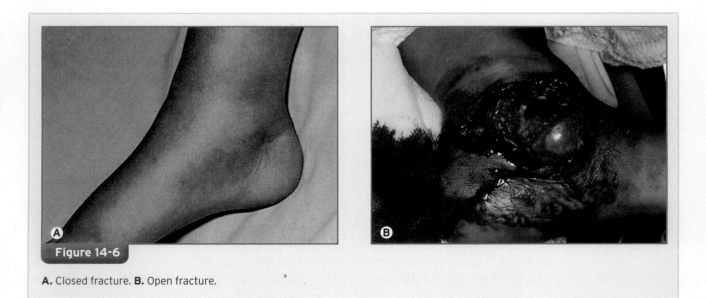

Figure 14-6

A. Closed fracture. **B.** Open fracture.

FYI cont.

thought of as a partial dislocation. Strains are caused by stretching or tearing of a muscle.

Body Substance Isolation and Musculoskeletal Injuries

As you examine and treat patients with musculoskeletal injuries, you need to practice BSI. These patients may have open wounds related to the musculoskeletal injury or to a separate, open soft-tissue injury. You should assume that trauma patients have open wounds that pose a threat of infection. Wear approved gloves. When responding to motor vehicle crashes or other situations that may present a hazard from broken glass or other sharp objects, it is wise to wear heavy rescue gloves that provide protection from sharp objects. Some first responders wear latex or vinyl gloves under the heavy rescue gloves for added BSI protection. If the patient has active bleeding that may splatter, you should have protection for your eyes, nose, and mouth as well.

Safety Tips

BSI is for *your* protection.

Signs and Symptoms

Extremity Injuries

- Pain at the injury site
- An open wound
- Swelling and discoloration (bruising)
- The patient's inability or unwillingness to move the extremity
- Deformity or angulation
- Tenderness at the injury site

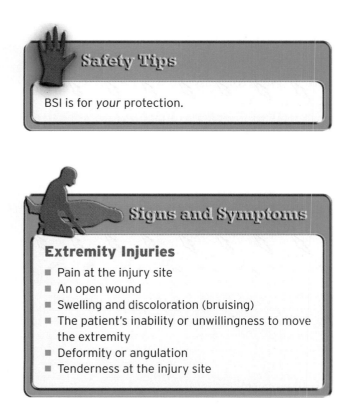

Examination of Musculoskeletal Injuries

There are three essential steps in examining a patient with a limb injury:

1. General assessment of the patient according to the patient assessment sequence
2. Examination of the injured part
3. Evaluation of the circulation and sensation in the injured limb

General Patient Assessment

A general, initial assessment of the injured patient must be carried out before focusing attention on any injured limb. All of the steps in the patient assessment must be followed. Once you have checked and stabilized the patient's airway, breathing, and circulation (ABCs), you can then direct your attention to the injured limb identified during the physical examination.

Limb injuries are not life threatening unless there is excessive bleeding from an open wound. Therefore, it is essential that you stabilize the airway, breathing, and circulation before you focus on the limb injury, regardless of the pain or deformity that may be present at that injury site.

As you examine and treat patients with musculoskeletal injuries, remember that this is a scary and painful experience for them. Explain what you are doing as you conduct your examination and stabilize the patient. Treat the patient with the same care and consideration that you would give to a close member of your own family.

Examining the Injured Limb

As a first responder, you should initially inspect the injured limb and compare it to the

In the Field

Listen to the patient. He or she is usually right about the location and type of injury.

opposite, uninjured limb. To do this, gently and carefully cut away any clothing covering the wound, if necessary. (Do not ever hesitate to cut clothing in order to uncover a suspected injury.)

When you examine the limb, you may find any one of the following:

- An open wound
- Deformity
- Swelling
- Bruising

After you have uncovered and looked at the injured limb, you should gently feel it for any points of tenderness. Tenderness is the best indicator of an underlying fracture, dislocation, or sprain (PSDE).

To detect limb injury, start at the top of each limb (where it connects to the body) and using both hands, squeeze the entire limb in a systematic, firm (yet gentle) manner, moving down the limb and away from the body **Figure 14-7 ▶**. Make sure you examine the entire extremity.

As you carry out your hands-on examination, it is important to ask the patient where it hurts most; the location of greatest pain is probably the injury site. Also ask if the patient feels tingling or numbness in the extremity because this may indicate nerve damage or lack of circulation.

Careful inspection and a gentle hands-on examination will identify most musculoskeletal injuries. After you have made a careful visual and hands-on examination, and if the patient shows no sign of injury, ask the patient to move the limb carefully. If there is an injury, the patient will complain of pain and refuse to move the limb.

Any of the signs or symptoms described earlier (deformity, swelling, bruising, tenderness, or

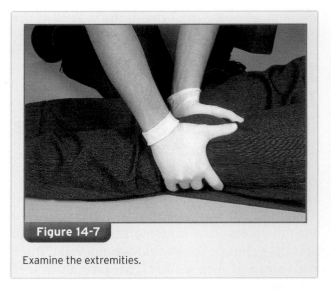

Figure 14-7

Examine the extremities.

pain with motion) indicate the presence of a limb injury (PSDE). Only one sign is necessary to indicate an injury to the limb. All limb injuries, regardless of type or severity, are managed in the same way.

Evaluation of Circulation, Sensation, and Movement

Once you suspect limb injury, you must evaluate the circulation and sensation in that limb. Many important blood vessels and nerves lie close to the bones, especially around major joints. Therefore, any injury may have associated blood vessel or nerve damage. It is also essential to check circulation and sensation after any movement of the limb (such as for splinting). Moving the limb during splinting

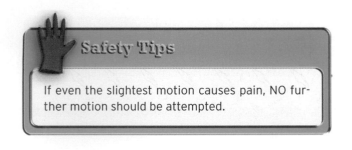

Safety Tips

If even the slightest motion causes pain, NO further motion should be attempted.

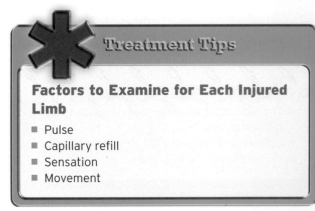

Treatment Tips

Factors to Examine for Each Injured Limb

- Pulse
- Capillary refill
- Sensation
- Movement

might have caused a bone fragment to press against or even cut a blood vessel or nerve **Skill Drill 14-1 ▸** :

SKILL DRILL 14-1

1. **Pulse.** Feel the pulse distal to the point of injury. If the patient has an upper extremity injury, check the radial (wrist) pulse **Step 1** . If the patient has a lower extremity injury, check the tibial (posterior ankle) pulse **Step 2** .
2. **Capillary refill.** Test the capillary refill in a finger or toe of any injured limb. Firm pressure on the tip of the nail causes the nail bed to turn white **Step 3** . Release the pressure and the normal pink color should return by the time it takes to say "capillary refill" **Step 4** . If the pink color does not return in this 2-second interval, it is considered to be delayed or absent and indicates a circulation problem in the limb. A cold environment will naturally delay capillary refill, so in that situation, do not use capillary refill to assess an injured limb. The absence of a pulse or capillary refill indicates that a limb is in immediate danger. Impaired circulation demands **prompt transportation** and prompt medical treatment at an appropriate medical facility.
3. **Sensation.** The patient's ability to feel your light touch on the fingers or toes is a good indication that the nerve supply is intact. In the hand, check sensation by touching lightly the tips of the index and little fingers. In the foot, the tip of the big toe and the top of the foot should be checked for sensation **Step 5** and **Step 6** .
4. **Movement.** If the hand or foot is injured, do not have the patient do this part of the test. When the injury is between the hand or foot and the body, have the patient open and close the fist or flex the foot of the injured limb **Step 7** and **Step 8** . These simple movements indicate that the nerves to these muscles are working. Sometimes any attempt at motion will produce pain. In this

case, do not ask the patient to move the limb any further. Any open wound, deformity, swelling, or bruising of a limb should be considered evidence of a possible limb injury and treated as such.

Treatment of Musculoskeletal Injuries

Regardless of their extent or severity, all limb injuries are treated in the same way in the field. For all open extremity wounds, first cover the entire wound with a dry, sterile dressing and then apply firm but gentle pressure to control bleeding, if necessary. The sterile compression dressing protects the wound and underlying tissues from further contamination. The injured limb should then be splinted.

General Principles of Splinting

All limb injuries (PSDE) should be splinted before a patient is moved, unless the environment prevents effective splinting or threatens the patient's life (or that of the rescuer). Splinting prevents the movement of broken bone ends, a dislocated joint, or damaged soft tissues and thereby reduces pain. With less pain, the patient relaxes and the trip to the medical facility is easier. Splinting also helps to control bleeding and decreases the risk of damage to the nearby nerves and vessels by sharp bone fragments. Splinting prevents closed fractures (PSDE) from becoming open fractures (PSDE) during movement or transportation.

All first responders should know the following general principles of splinting:

1. In most situations, remove clothing from the injured limb (PSDE) to inspect the limb for open wounds, deformity, swelling, bruising, and capillary refill.
2. Note and record the pulse, capillary refill, sensation, and movement distal to the point of injury, both before and after splinting.
3. Cover all open wounds with a dry, sterile dressing before applying the splint.

Skill DRILL 14-1

Checking Circulation, Sensation, and Movement in an Injured Extremity

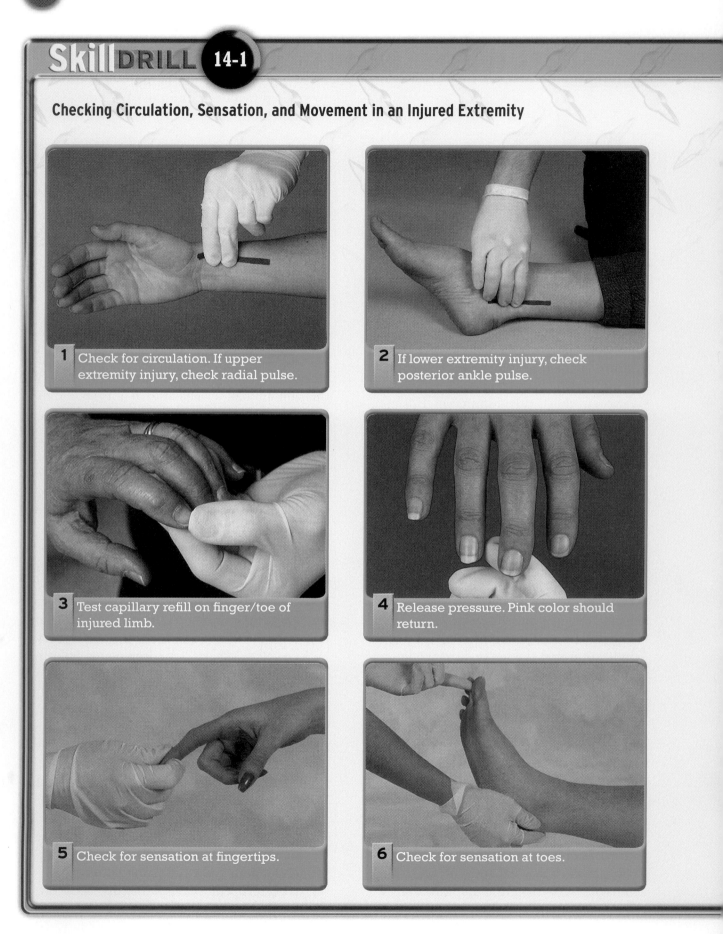

1 Check for circulation. If upper extremity injury, check radial pulse.

2 If lower extremity injury, check posterior ankle pulse.

3 Test capillary refill on finger/toe of injured limb.

4 Release pressure. Pink color should return.

5 Check for sensation at fingertips.

6 Check for sensation at toes.

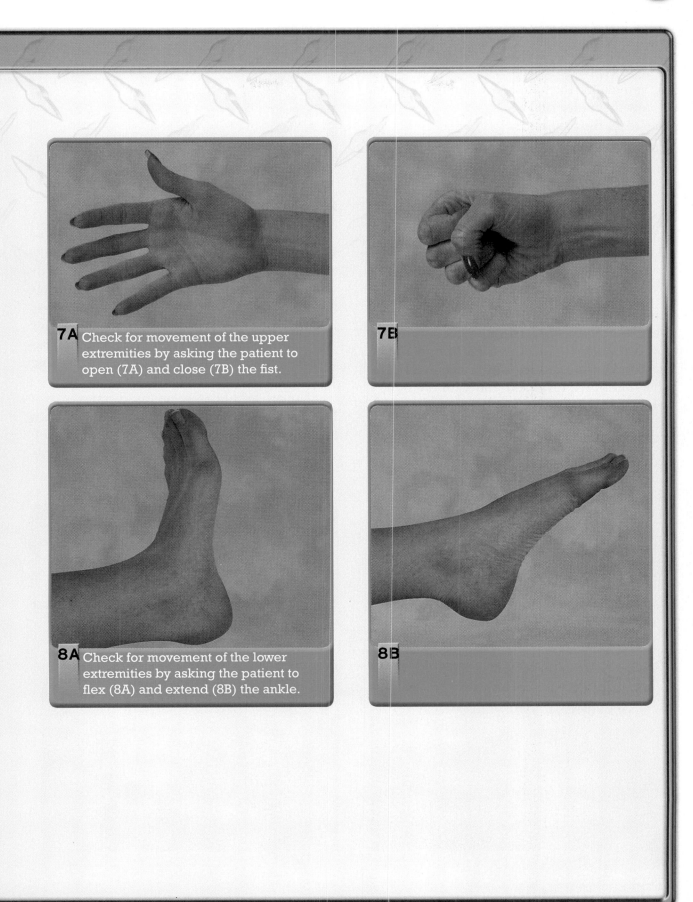

7A Check for movement of the upper extremities by asking the patient to open (7A) and close (7B) the fist.

7B

8A Check for movement of the lower extremities by asking the patient to flex (8A) and extend (8B) the ankle.

8B

4. Do not move the patient before splinting, unless there is an immediate danger to the patient or the first responder.

5. Immobilize the joint above and the joint below the injury site.

6. Pad all rigid splints.

7. When applying the splint, use your hands to support the injury site and minimize movement of the limb until splinting is completed.

8. Splint the limb in the position in which it is found.

9. When in doubt, splint.

Materials Used for Splinting

Many different materials can be used as splints, if necessary. Even when standard splints are not available, the arm can be bound to the chest and an injured leg can be secured to the other, uninjured lower extremity for temporary stability.

Rigid Splints

Rigid splints are made from firm material and are applied to the sides, front, or back of an injured extremity. Common types of rigid splints include padded board splints, molded plastic or aluminum splints, padded wire ladder splints, SAM splints, and folded cardboard splints Figure 14-8 ▾ . Padded wire ladder or SAM splints can be molded to the shape of the limb to splint it in the position found.

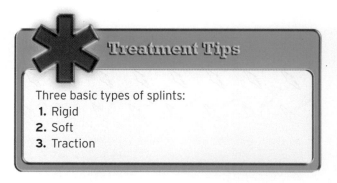

Three basic types of splints:
1. Rigid
2. Soft
3. Traction

Soft Splints

The most commonly used soft splint is the inflatable, clear plastic air splint. This splint is available in a variety of sizes and shapes, with or without a zipper, that runs the length of the splint Figure 14-9 ▸ . After it is applied, the splint is inflated by mouth—never by using a pump or air cylinder. The air splint is comfortable for the patient and provides uniform pressure to a bleeding wound.

The air splint has some disadvantages. If it must be used in cold, dirty areas, the zipper can stick, clog with dirt, or freeze. After it is inflated, the splint can be punctured by sharp fragments

Safety Tips

NEVER use anything but the air from your mouth to inflate air splints!

Figure 14-8

A. Rigid cardboard splints. **B.** SAM splint.

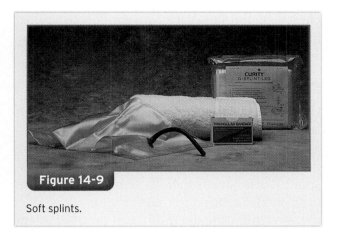

Figure 14-9

Soft splints.

Improvised splints can be made from rolled newspapers, magazines, towels, or belts **Figure 14-10 ▼**.

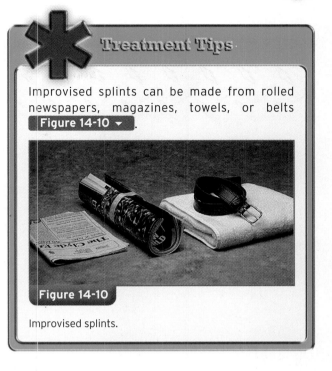

Figure 14-10

Improvised splints.

of glass or other objects. Temperature and altitude changes can increase or decrease the pressure in the air splint, so careful monitoring by emergency care personnel is required.

Traction Splints

A **traction splint** holds a lower extremity fracture (PSDE) in alignment by applying a constant, steady pull on the extremity. Properly applying a traction splint requires two well-trained EMTs working together; one person cannot do it alone. First responders do not learn the skills necessary to apply this type of splint. However, you may be asked to assist trained medical personnel in the placement of a traction splint, and you should be familiar with the general techniques, as shown later in Skill Drill 14-4.

FYI

Splinting Specific Injury Sites

The treatment techniques described here can be carried out by a person with a first-responder level of training and with materials readily available to you. Most splinting techniques are two-person operations. One person stabilizes and supports the injured limb, while the other person applies the splint.

Shoulder Girdle Injuries

The easiest way to splint most shoulder injuries is to apply a **sling** made of a triangular bandage and to secure the sling (and arm) to the body with swathes around the arm and chest. Apply the sling by tying a knot in the point of the triangular bandage, placing the elbow into the cup formed by

FYI cont.

the knot, and passing the two ends of the bandage up and around the patient's neck. Tie the sling so the wrist is slightly higher than the elbow **Figure 14-11 ▼**.

To keep the arm immobilized, fold another triangular bandage until you have a long swathe that is 3 to 4 inches wide **Figure 14-12 ▶**. Tie one or two swathes around the upper arm and chest of the patient. This easily applied splint adequately immobilizes fractures of the collarbone, most shoulder injuries, and fractures of the arm.

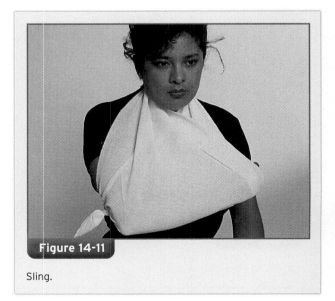

Figure 14-11

Sling.

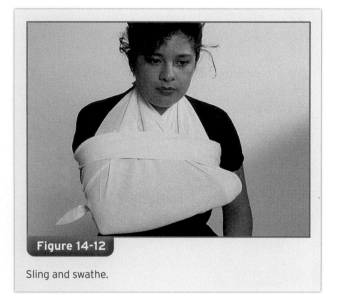

Figure 14-12

Sling and swathe.

Dislocation of the Shoulder

The dislocated shoulder is the only shoulder girdle injury that is difficult to immobilize with a sling and swathe. In a shoulder dislocation, there is often a space between the upper arm and the chest wall. Fill this space with a pillow or a rolled blanket and before applying a sling and swathe as for other shoulder injuries (see Figure 14-12).

Elbow Injuries

Do not move an injured elbow from the position in which you find it. The elbow must be splinted as it lies because any movement can cause nerve or blood vessel damage. If the elbow is straight, splint it straight. If the elbow is bent at an unusual angle, splint it in that position.

After splinting the injured elbow of a patient who does not have a significant shoulder injury (and only if it does not cause pain), gently move the splinted injury to the patient's side for comfort and ease of transport. An effective splint for an injured elbow is a pillow splint. Wrap the elbow in a pillow, add additional padding to keep the elbow in the position found, and secure the pillow as shown in **Figure 14-15 ▶**.

The patient is usually transported in a sitting position with the splinted elbow resting on his or her lap. A padded wire ladder or SAM splint is

In the Field

When triangular bandages are not available, loop a length of gauze (or even a belt) around the patient's wrist and suspend the limb from the neck **Figure 14-13 ▼**. Secure the arm gently, but firmly, to the chest wall with another length of gauze or belt.

If you haven't cut away the coat, you can also pin a coat sleeve to the front of the patient's coat as a temporary splint **Figure 14-14 ▼**. This technique is less secure than a sling and swathe, but it may be of use in cold weather areas.

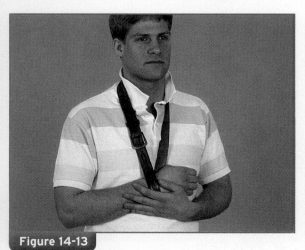

Figure 14-13

Improvised sling using a belt.

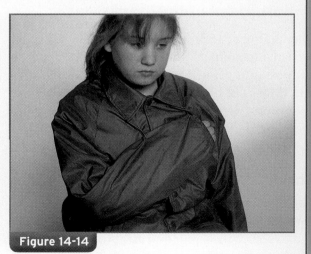

Figure 14-14

Improvised sling using safety pins.

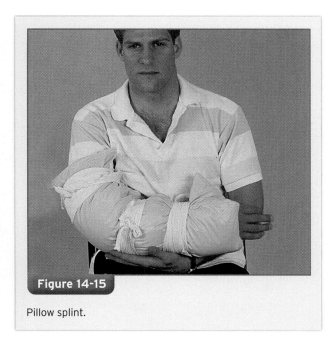

Figure 14-15

Pillow splint.

FYI cont.

also effective for splinting elbows that are found in severely deformed positions.

Injuries of the Forearm

Several splints can be used to stabilize the **forearm**: the air splint, the cardboard splint, the SAM splint **Skill Drill 14-2 ▶**, and even rolled newspapers and magazines. Be sure to pad all rigid splints adequately.

FYI cont.

SKILL DRILL 14-2

1. Support and stabilize the injured limb.
2. Form the SAM splint to the injured forearm **Step 1**.
3. Place the splint under the injured limb **Step 2**.
4. Secure the splint in place with gauze **Step 3**.
5. Recheck the pulse, capillary refill, and sensation of the injured forearm.

An air splint can be applied quickly and immobilizes the forearm quite well. Of the several types of air splints available, the one with a full-length zipper is easiest to use **Skill Drill 14-3 ▶**:

SKILL DRILL 14-3

1. Unzip the air splint completely, keeping the air intake valve on the outside of the splint. Stabilize the injured forearm and place the air splint over your arm **Step 1**.
2. Carefully support the injured forearm and slip the unzipped air splint under it. Slide the air splint over the injured arm **Step 2**.
3. After the air splint is positioned to correctly support the injured site, connect the zipper, zip it shut, and inflate it by mouth until the plastic can be depressed slightly when you exert firm pressure with your fingers **Step 3**.

Treatment Tips

If you have to improvise a splint for a forearm injury, **Figure 14-16 ▼** shows how to apply a splint made of magazines and newspapers.

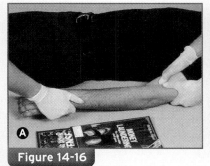

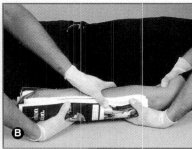

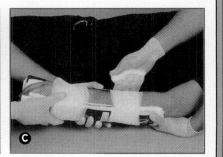

Figure 14-16

Applying an improvised splint using magazines. **A.** Stabilize injured limb. **B.** Place padded magazines under injured arm. **C.** Secure splint with gauze.

Skill DRILL 14-2

Applying a SAM Splint

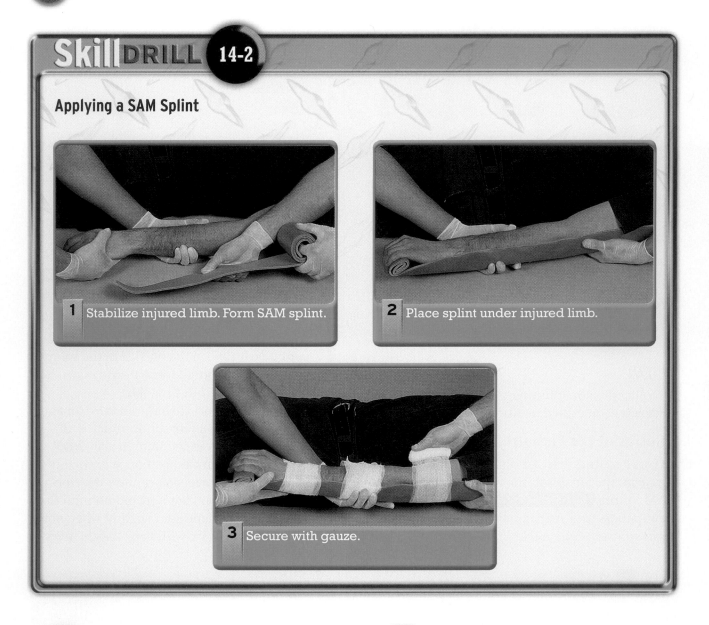

1 Stabilize injured limb. Form SAM splint.

2 Place splint under injured limb.

3 Secure with gauze.

To apply an air splint without a zipper, place the air splint over your hand and lower arm and grasp the patient's hand. Have a second person support the patient's elbow and upper arm to prevent movement. Apply slight pull in the long axis of the forearm. Slip the air splint off your arm and onto the patient's injured forearm. The air splint should extend over the patient's hand and wrist to prevent swelling. Inflate the splint, as described earlier.

Injuries of the Hand, Wrist, and Fingers

As a first responder, you will see a variety of hand injuries, all of which can be potentially serious. The functions of the fingers and hand are so com-

plex that any injury, if poorly or inadequately treated, may result in permanent deformity and disability. Treat even seemingly simple lacerations carefully. Send any amputated parts to the hospital with the patient. You can use a bulky hand dressing and a short splint to immobilize all injuries of the wrist, hand, and fingers.

First, cover all wounds with a dry, sterile dressing. Then place the injured hand and wrist into what is called the position of function **Figure 14-17 ▶**. Place one or two soft roller dressings into the palm of the patient's hand. Apply a splint to hold the wrist, hand, and fingers in the position of function and secure the splint with a soft roller bandage.

Skill DRILL 14-3

Applying an Air Splint

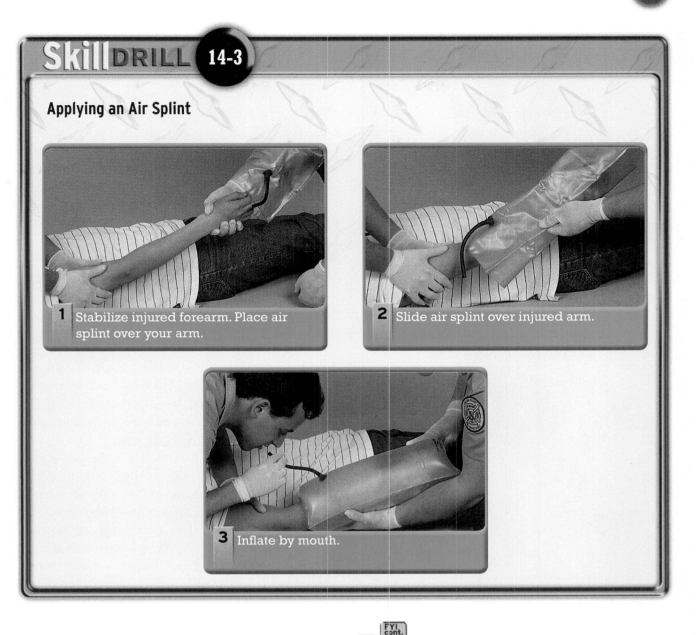

1 Stabilize injured forearm. Place air splint over your arm.

2 Slide air splint over injured arm.

3 Inflate by mouth.

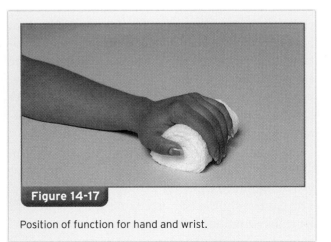

Figure 14-17

Position of function for hand and wrist.

FYI cont.

Pelvic Fractures

Fractures of the pelvis often involve severe blood loss because the broken bones can easily lacerate the large blood vessels that run directly beside the pelvis. These vessels can release a great deal of blood into the pelvic area. Pelvic fractures commonly cause shock. Therefore, the first responder must always treat the patient for shock. However, do not raise the patient's legs until he or she is secured on a backboard.

The surest sign of pelvic fracture is tenderness when both your hands firmly compress the patient's pelvis Figure 14-18 ▶ . Immobilize fractures of the pelvis with a long backboard, as illustrated in Figure 14–21. EMTs may apply a

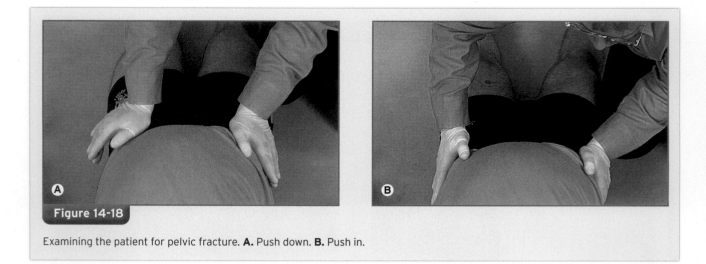

Figure 14-18

Examining the patient for pelvic fracture. **A.** Push down. **B.** Push in.

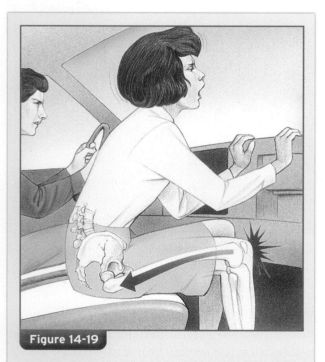

Figure 14-19

Posterior dislocation of the hip can occur as a result of the knee hitting the dashboard in an automobile collision.

FYI cont.

pneumatic antishock garment (PASG) to stabilize the fracture and treat shock.

Hip Injuries

Two types of hip injuries are commonly seen: dislocations and fractures. Both injuries may result from high-energy <u>trauma</u>. When an unbelted automobile passenger is thrown forward in an acci-

FYI cont.

dent and crashes against the dashboard, the impact of the knee against the dashboard is transmitted up the shaft of the thigh bone (femur), injuring the hip and often producing either a dislocation or a fracture, or both Figure 14-19 .

Hip fractures actually occur at the upper end of the femur, rather than in the hip joint itself. Hip fractures do not occur only as a result of high-energy trauma; they can occur in elderly people, especially women, after only minimal trauma (such as falling down). These fractures in the elderly occur because bone weakens and becomes more fragile with advancing age, a condition called <u>osteoporosis</u>. Patients with osteoporosis may suffer major fractures from minor falls.

A dislocated hip is extremely painful, especially when any movement is attempted. The joint is usually locked with the thigh flexed and rotated inward across the midline of the body. The knee joint is often flexed as well. Fractures of the hip region usually cause the injured limb to become shortened and externally (outwardly) rotated Figure 14-20 .

Treat all hip injuries by immobilizing the hip in the position found. Use several pillows and/or rolled blankets, especially under the flexed knee. The patient should be placed on a long backboard for transportation. The patient and the limb should be well stabilized to eliminate all motion in the hip region Figure 14-21 .

Because fractures of the upper end of the femur are so common in elderly patients, any

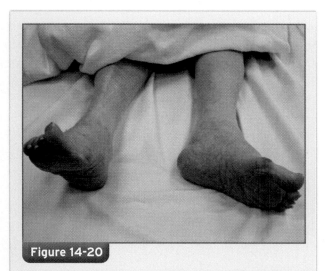

Figure 14-20

Signs of a hip fracture may include external rotation and shortening of the injured leg.

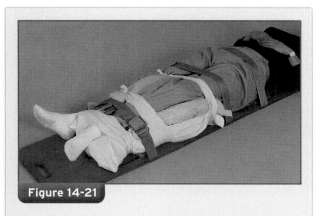

Figure 14-21

Immobilization of hip or pelvic injuries using a backboard.

FYI cont.

elderly person who has fallen and complains of pain in the hip, thigh, or knee—even if there is no deformity—should be splinted and transported to the hospital for X-ray evaluation.

Injuries of the Thigh

Trauma to the thigh can bruise the muscles or fracture the shaft of the femur. A fractured femur is very unstable and usually produces significant thigh deformity. There is much bleeding and swelling.

The treatment of femur fractures (PSDE) requires skill and proper equipment. As a first responder, you can treat for shock and help prevent further injury. Place the patient in as comfortable a position as possible, treat for shock, and call for additional personnel and equipment.

FYI cont.

However, after a motor vehicle crash, you may have to move the patient quickly, even before proper equipment and additional personnel arrive. You should learn and practice emergency temporary splinting for lower extremity injuries. Secure both legs together with several swathes, cravats, or bandages so that the two lower extremities are immobilized as one unit. This technique allows you to remove the patient from a dangerous environment quickly.

A traction splint is the most effective way to splint a unilateral fractured femur. Traction splints are designed specifically for this purpose. Although you may not have a traction splint in your first responder life support kit, you should know how it works so that you can assist other EMS personnel, as needed.

Before applying a traction splint, trained EMTs align deformed fractures (PSDE) by applying manual longitudinal traction. Once manual traction is applied, it must be maintained until the traction splint is fully in place **Figure 14-22 ▶**. Because many different types of traction splints are available, you should learn to use the one that your department uses. Most are applied basically using the same method. **Skill Drill 14-4 ▶** illustrates the steps for applying a Hare traction splint.

SKILL DRILL 14-4

1. Place the splint beside the patient's uninjured leg and adjust it to the proper length. Open and adjust the four support straps, which should be positioned at the midthigh, above the knee, below the knee, and above the ankle **Step 1**.
2. The first rescuer supports and stabilizes the injured limb while the second rescuer fastens the ankle hitch about the patient's ankle and foot **Step 2**.
3. The first rescuer supports the leg at the site of the suspected injury while the second rescuer manually applies gentle traction to the ankle hitch and foot. Use only enough force to reposition the limb so that will fit into the splint **Step 3**. The first rescuer slides the splint into position under the patient's injured limb **Step 4**.
4. Pad the groin area and gently apply the strap around the midthigh **Step 5**.

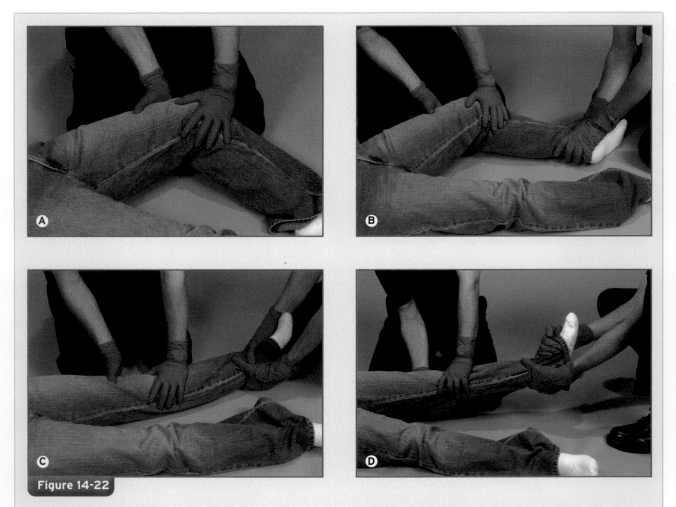

Figure 14-22

Straightening an injured leg for splinting. **A.** The first rescuer grasps the injured leg at the knee and applies traction in the long axis of the body. **B.** The second rescuer grasps the ankle. **C.** The second rescuer straightens the leg. **D.** The second rescuer maintains traction by leaning back.

FYI
cont.

5. The first rescuer connects the loops of the ankle hitch to the end of the splint while the second rescuer continues to maintain traction. Then apply gentle traction to the connecting strap between the ankle hitch and the splint, just strongly enough to maintain limb alignment.

6. Once the proper traction has been applied, fasten the support straps so that the limb is securely held in the splint. Check all support straps to make sure they are secure Step 6 .

FYI
cont.

To apply proper traction using this type of splint, it is essential that the foot end of the traction splint be elevated 6 to 8 inches off the ground. If the heel of the injured leg touches the ground, traction is lost and must be reapplied. Most traction splints include a foot stand that elevates the limb. Check and recheck pulse, capillary refill, and nerve function before and after a splint is applied Figure 14-23 ▸ . If your department uses a different type of traction splint, you will need to be instructed in how to properly apply it.

Skill DRILL 14-4

Applying a Traction Splint

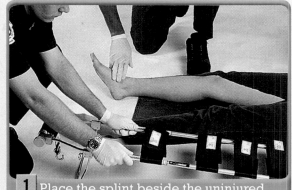

1 Place the splint beside the uninjured limb, adjust the splint to the proper length, and prepare the straps.

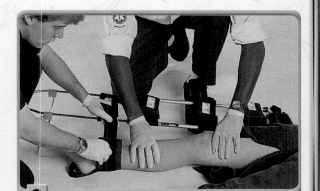

2 Support the injured limb as your partner fastens the ankle hitch about the foot and ankle.

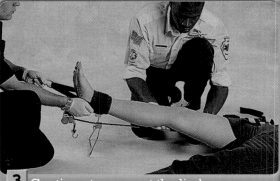

3 Continue to support the limb as your partner applies gentle traction to the ankle hitch and foot.

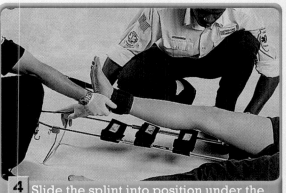

4 Slide the splint into position under the injured limb.

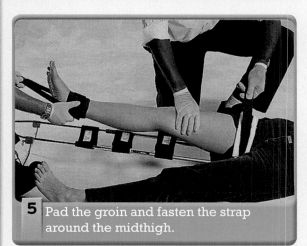

5 Pad the groin and fasten the strap around the midthigh.

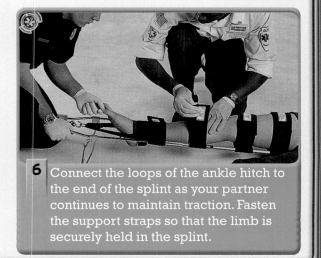

6 Connect the loops of the ankle hitch to the end of the splint as your partner continues to maintain traction. Fasten the support straps so that the limb is securely held in the splint.

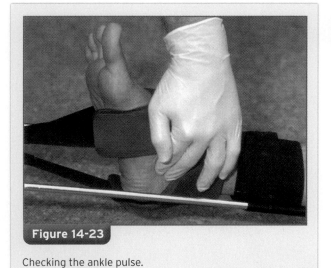

Figure 14-23

Checking the ankle pulse.

FYI cont.

Knee Injuries

Always immobilize an injured knee in the same position that you find it. If it is straight, use long, padded board splints or a long-leg air splint. If there is a significant deformity, place pillows, blankets, or clothing beneath the knee **Figure 14-24 ▾**, secure the splint materials to the leg with bandages, swathes, or cravats, and secure the injured leg to the uninjured leg. Then place the patient on a backboard.

Leg Injuries

Like fractures of the forearm, fractures of the leg can be splinted with air splints, cardboard splints, and even magazines and newspapers. **Skill Drill 14-5 ▸** shows how to apply an air splint

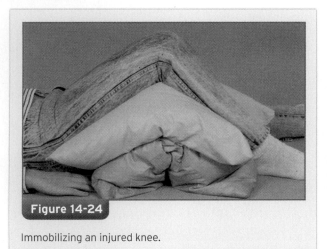

Figure 14-24

Immobilizing an injured knee.

Safety Tips

DO NOT elevate the injured leg when treating for shock.

FYI cont.

to the leg. It takes two trained people to splint an injured leg. One person supports the leg with both hands (above and below the injury site), while the other person applies the splint.

SKILL DRILL 14-5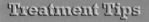

1. The first rescuer supports the injured limb.
2. The second rescuer slides the splint under the limb **Step 1**.
3. The second rescuer places the splint around limb **Step 2**.
4. The first rescuer slides his or her hands out of the splint while the second rescuer inflates the splint **Step 3**.
5. Either rescuer rechecks the pulse capillary refill and sensation of the injured leg.

Treatment Tips

Pad all rigid splints to provide the best stabilization and pain relief. Do not apply any splint too tightly. Recheck pulse, capillary refill, and sensation after the splint is applied to make sure that no damage has been done **Figure 14-25 ▾**.

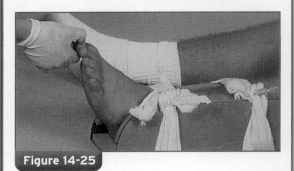

Figure 14-25

Checking capillary refill on splinted injured leg.

Skill DRILL 14-5

Applying an Air Splint to the Leg

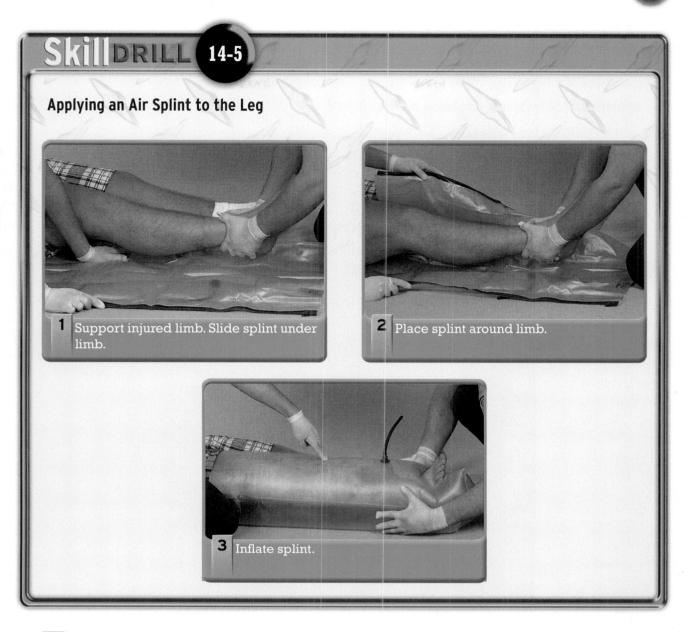

1 Support injured limb. Slide splint under limb.

2 Place splint around limb.

3 Inflate splint.

Injuries of the Ankle and Foot

Fractures of the ankle and foot can be splinted with either a pillow or an air splint. Place the pillow splint around the injured ankle and foot, and tie or pin it in place Skill Drill 14-6 ▶ :

Skill DRILL 14-6

1. Place a pillow under the injured limb Step 1 .
2. Mold the pillow around the foot and ankle.
3. Secure the pillow with cravats, swathes, or bandages Step 2 .
4. Recheck pulse, capillary refill, and sensation Step 3 .

Additional Considerations

Remember that extremity injuries are not, in themselves, life threatening unless excessive bleeding is present. You may not always have the equipment or help you need to manage all types of extremity injuries. You may not even have time to splint an injury before additional EMS personnel arrive. There will be times, however, when you are the only trained person at the scene of an accident. To prepare for such situations, practice splinting until you can apply the principles in any situation. Because you may find the patient in a variety of positions and locations, practice splinting both a sitting and a prone volunteer.

Skill DRILL 14-6

Applying a Pillow Splint for Ankle or Foot Injury

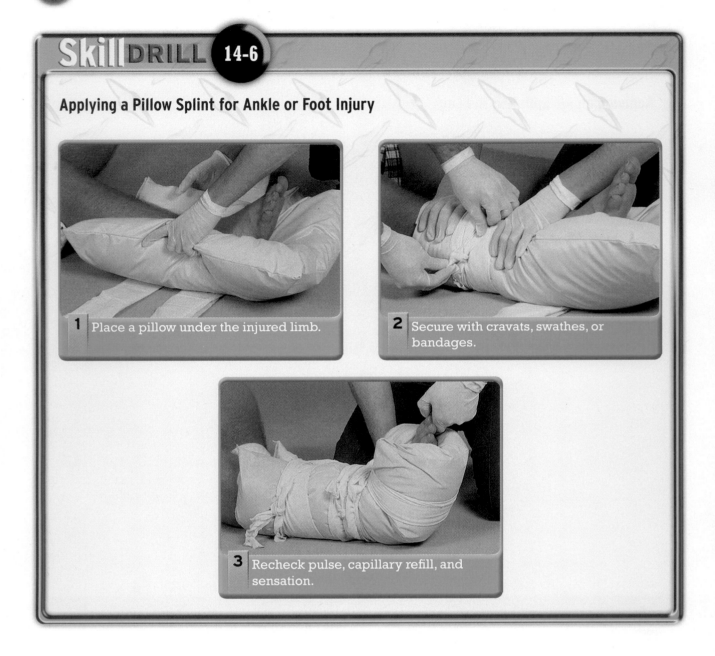

1 Place a pillow under the injured limb.

2 Secure with cravats, swathes, or bandages.

3 Recheck pulse, capillary refill, and sensation.

It takes two people to adequately splint most limb injuries: one to stabilize and support the extremity and one to apply the splint. Most of the principles and techniques of splinting covered in this chapter require that you work with another member of the EMS team. Learn how the team functions as a unit during stressful situations and be prepared to work with any member of the EMS team who arrives to assist you.

Injuries of the Head (Skull and Brain)

Severe head and spinal cord injuries can result from many different kinds of trauma. These injuries are common causes of death and can also lead to irreversible <u>paralysis</u> and permanent brain damage. Improperly handling a patient after an accident can cause further injury or death. Spinal

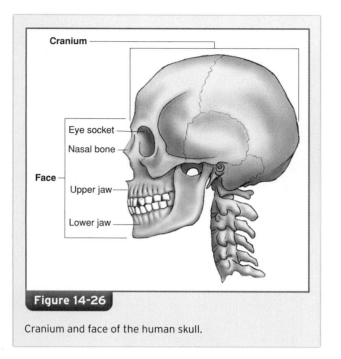

Figure 14-26

Cranium and face of the human skull.

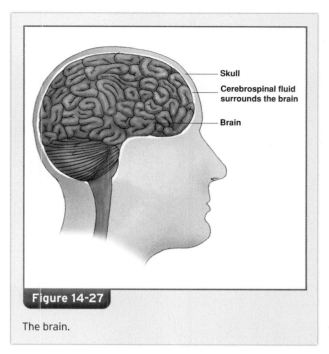

Figure 14-27

The brain.

injuries can be caused, for example, by well-intentioned citizens pulling a patient from a wrecked car or by poor treatment from inadequately trained emergency personnel. As a first responder, you must know what to do to provide prompt treatment and avoid errors that may make the injury worse.

The human skull has two primary parts **Figure 14-26 ▲**:

1. The cranium, a tough four-bone shell that protects the brain
2. The facial bones, which give form to the face and furnish frontal protection for the brain

Mechanisms of Injury

Head injuries are common with certain types of trauma. Of patients involved in automobile accidents, 70% suffer some degree of head injury. Imagine the cranium as a rigid bowl, containing the delicate brain **Figure 14-27 ▶**. Between the skull and brain, a fluid called <u>cerebrospinal fluid (CSF)</u> cushions the brain from direct blows. A direct force such as a hammer blow can injure the skull and the brain inside. Indirect forces can also cause injury, as in an automobile accident when the head strikes the windshield and causes the brain to bounce against the inside of the skull.

Spinal injury is often associated with head injury. The force of direct blows to the head is often transmitted to the spine, producing a fracture or dislocation. The injuries may damage the spinal cord or at least put it at risk for injury. Any time you suspect or identify an injury to the head or skull, you should also suspect injury to the neck and spinal cord. Therefore, all patients with head injuries must have the cervical spine splinted to protect the spinal cord.

Types of Head Injuries

Injuries of the head are classified as open or closed **Figure 14-28 ▶**. In a <u>closed head injury</u>, bleeding and swelling within the skull may increase pressure on the brain, leading to irreversible brain damage and death if it is not relieved. An open injury of the head usually bleeds profusely. Severe open head injuries are serious but not always fatal.

Examine the nose, eyes, and the wound itself to see if any blood or CSF is seeping out. The CSF is clear, watery, and straw-colored. In severe cases of open head injury, brain tissue or bone may be visible.

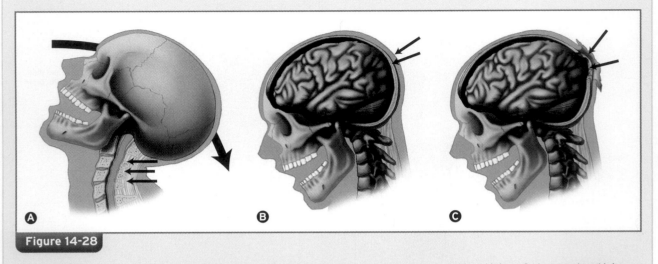

Figure 14-28

Open and closed head injuries. **A.** A head injury may cause a cervical spine injury. **B.** A closed head injury. **C.** An open head injury.

Signs and Symptoms of Head Injuries

A patient suffering from a head injury may exhibit some or all of the signs and symptoms shown in the Signs and Symptoms box below. A serious head injury may also produce raccoon eyes and Battle's sign. Raccoon eyes look like the black eyes that develop after a fistfight. Battle's sign appears as a bruise behind one or both ears Figure 14-29 ▸ .

Treatment of Head Injuries

When any one sign or symptom of head injury is present, proceed as follows:

1. Immobilize the head in a neutral position. Stabilize the patient's neck and prevent movement of the head. If returning the head to neutral is met with resistance, leave it in the position found.

2. Maintain an open airway. Use the jaw-thrust technique to open the airway (see Chapter 6). Be prepared to suction if the patient vomits. Avoid movement of the head and neck.

3. Support the patient's breathing. Be sure that the patient is breathing adequately on his or her own. If not, institute mouth-to-mask or mouth-to-barrier ventilation. As soon as oxygen becomes available, it should be administered to the patient. Oxygen is important to keep brain cells alive, particularly when brain swelling is present after serious head injury.

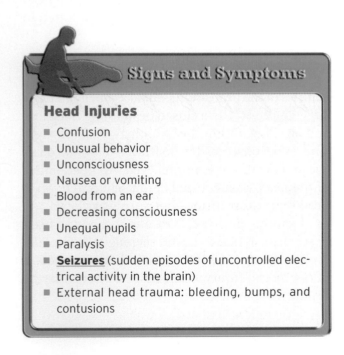

Signs and Symptoms

Head Injuries

- Confusion
- Unusual behavior
- Unconsciousness
- Nausea or vomiting
- Blood from an ear
- Decreasing consciousness
- Unequal pupils
- Paralysis
- **Seizures** (sudden episodes of uncontrolled electrical activity in the brain)
- External head trauma: bleeding, bumps, and contusions

Safety Tips

If a patient has a head injury, assume that an associated neck or spinal cord injury is also present. Do nothing that would cause undue movement of the head and spine. Always splint the entire spine before moving the patient.

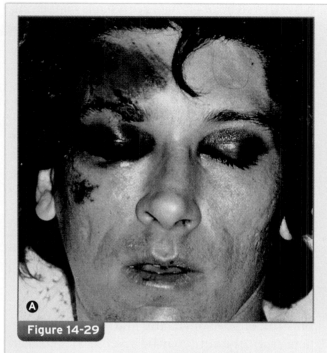
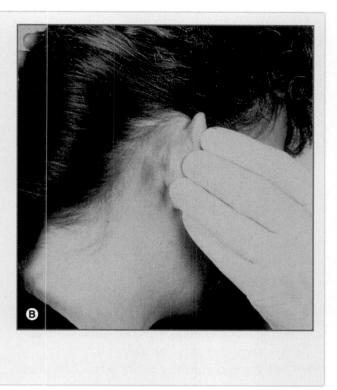

Figure 14-29

Signs of head injury. **A.** Raccoon eyes. **B.** Battle's sign.

4. Monitor circulation. Be prepared to support circulation by performing full CPR if the patient's heart stops.
5. Check to see if CSF or blood is seeping from a wound or from the nose or ears Figure 14-30 ▾. CSF is clear, watery, and straw-colored. Do not try to stop leakage of CSF from a wound or any other opening because leakage from inside the skull relieves internal pressure.

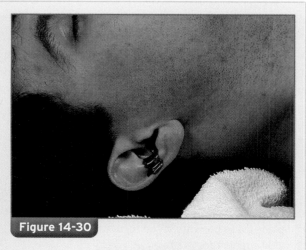

Figure 14-30

Blood or CSF from the ear indicates head injury.

6. Control bleeding from all head wounds with dry, sterile dressings. Use enough direct pressure to control the bleeding without disturbing the underlying tissue.
7. Examine and treat other serious injuries.
8. Arrange for **prompt transport** to an appropriate medical facility.

Injuries of the Face

Facial injuries commonly result from:
- Motor vehicle accidents in which the patient's face hits the steering wheel or windshield
- Assaults
- Falls

Airway obstruction is the primary danger in severe facial injuries. Severe damage to the face and facial bones can cause bleeding and the collapse of the facial bones, leading to airway problems. If the patient has facial injuries, you should also suspect a spinal injury. Although facial injuries may bleed considerably, they are rarely life threatening unless the airway is obstructed.

Treatment of Facial Injuries

When facial injuries are present, proceed as follows:

1. Immobilize the head in a neutral position. Stabilize it to prevent further movement of the neck.
2. Maintain an open airway. Use the jaw-thrust technique to open the airway. Clear any blood or vomitus from the patient's mouth with your gloved fingers.
3. Support breathing. Be prepared to ventilate the patient, if necessary.
4. Monitor circulation.
5. Control bleeding by covering any wound with a dry, sterile dressing and applying direct pressure. Be sure to check for wounds inside the mouth. Try to prevent the patient from swallowing blood because this can cause vomiting. Have suction ready for use.
6. Look for and stabilize other serious injuries.
7. Arrange for **prompt transport** to an appropriate medical facility.

If these measures do not keep the airway clear or if you are unable to control severe facial bleeding, log roll the patient onto his or her side, keeping the head and spine stable and rolling the whole body as a unit. Turn the head and body at the same time. The neck must not be allowed to twist **Figure 14-31 ▼** .

Bandage facial injuries as described in Chapter 13. If possible, leave the patient's eyes clear of bandages so he or she can see what is happening. Being able to see reduces the patient's tendency to panic.

Injuries of the Spine

As mentioned earlier in this chapter, spinal injuries can cause irreversible paralysis. As a first responder, you must know how to properly handle a patient and provide prompt treatment. Errors may make the injury worse.

Mechanisms of Injury

If one or more vertebrae are injured, the spinal cord may also be injured. A displaced vertebra, swelling, or bleeding **Figure 14-32 ▶** may put pressure on the spinal cord and damage it. In severe cases, the cord may be severed. If all or part of the spinal cord is cut, nerve impulses (which are like signals in a telephone cable) cannot travel to and from the brain. Then the patient is paralyzed below the point of injury. Injury to the spinal cord high in the neck paralyzes the diaphragm and results in death. Gunshot wounds to the chest or abdomen may produce spinal cord injury at that level. Falls, motor vehicle collisions, and stabbings are other common causes of spinal injuries. Suspect spinal injury if the patient has suffered high-energy trauma.

Signs and Symptoms of Spinal Cord Injury

To determine if a patient has sustained an injury to the spinal cord, carefully examine and talk to the patient and attempt to determine the mechanism of injury. Gently conduct a hands-on examination, as described in Chapter 7, to detect

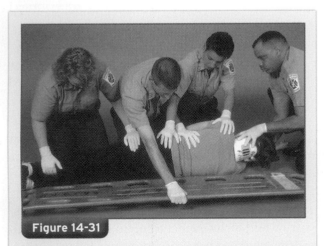

Figure 14-31

Keep the head and spine in alignment by using the log-roll technique.

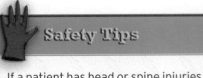
Safety Tips

If a patient has head or spine injuries, use a log roll to move the patient onto his or her side. Do not place these patients in the recovery position. Provide support for the head and neck.

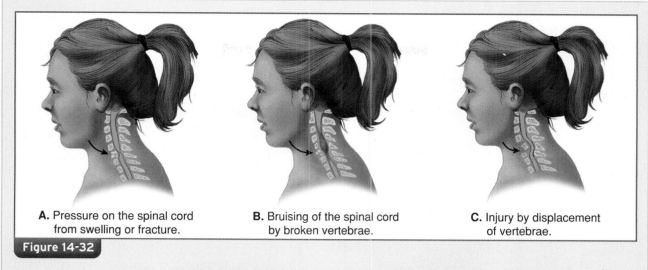

A. Pressure on the spinal cord from swelling or fracture.

B. Bruising of the spinal cord by broken vertebrae.

C. Injury by displacement of vertebrae.

Figure 14-32

Types of spinal injuries. **A.** Pressure on the spinal cord from swelling or fracture. **B.** Bruising of the spinal cord by broken vertebrae. **C.** Injury by displacement and fractured vertebrae.

paralysis or weakness. Ask the patient to describe any points of tenderness or pain. Do not move the patient during the examination. Further, do not allow the patient to move. The key signs and symptoms of a spinal injury are noted in the Signs and Symptoms box below. During your examination, be extremely careful. Take your time. Position yourself so that the patient will not need to move his or her head to communicate with you. Do not move patients unless they are in a hazardous area.

Treatment of Spinal Injuries

If any one sign or symptom of spinal injury is present, proceed as follows:

1. Place the head and neck in a neutral position. Avoid unnecessary movement of the head.

Signs and Symptoms

Spinal Injuries

- Laceration, bruise, or other sign of injury to the head, neck, or spine
- Tenderness over any point on the spine or neck
- Extremity weakness, paralysis, or loss of movement
- Loss of sensation or tingling/burning sensation in any part of the body below the neck

2. Stabilize the head and prevent movement of the neck.
3. Maintain an open airway. Use the jaw-thrust technique to open the airway to avoid movement of the head and neck. Clear any blood or vomitus from the mouth with your gloved fingers.
4. Support the patient's breathing. A spinal cord injury may paralyze some or all of the respiratory muscles, resulting in abnormal breathing patterns. In some cases, only the diaphragm may be working. Breathing using the diaphragm only is called **abdominal breathing**. The abdomen (not the lungs) swells and collapses with each breath. Help the patient breathe by administering oxygen (if available) and by keeping the airway open.
5. Monitor circulation.
6. Assess pulse, movement, and sensation in all extremities.
7. Examine and treat other serious injuries.
8. Do not move the patient unless it is necessary to perform CPR or to remove him or her from a dangerous environment.
9. Assist in immobilizing the patient using a long or short backboard. (The steps for applying long and short backboards are covered in Chapter 5.)
10. Arrange for **prompt transport** to an appropriate medical facility.

Skill DRILL 14-7

Stabilizing the Cervical Spine and Maintaining an Open Airway

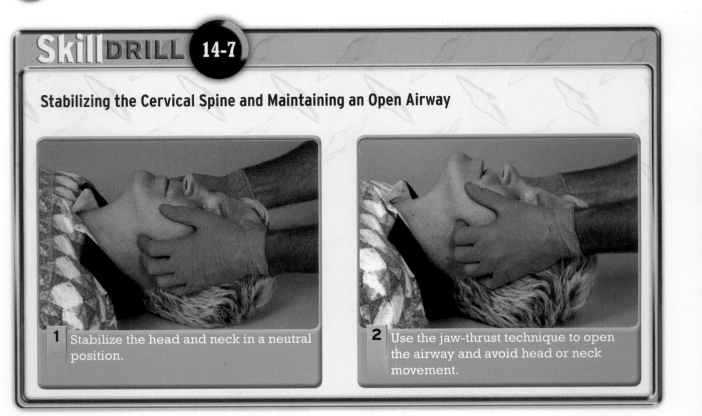

1 Stabilize the head and neck in a neutral position.

2 Use the jaw-thrust technique to open the airway and avoid head or neck movement.

Safety Tips

If you suspect the presence of a spinal injury, it is absolutely essential that the injury be splinted and protected until hospital tests rule out a spinal cord injury.

Stabilizing the Cervical Spine

Stabilization of the cervical spine is initially accomplished manually, as shown in **Skill Drill 14-7 ▲**:

Skill DRILL 14-7

1. Stabilize the head and prevent movement of the neck. Place the head and neck in a neutral position **Step 1**.
2. In this position, the rescuer can maintain an open airway with the jaw-thrust technique **Step 2**. Do not manipulate or twist the head and neck. After you have manually stabilized the head and neck, you must

maintain support until the entire spine is fully splinted. A rigid collar and a long or short backboard are used to splint the cervical spine. Review the steps for applying a cervical collar and a short backboard device, which are covered in Chapter 5.

Motorcycle and Football Helmets

Many patients with neck injuries are motorcyclists or football players who are wearing protective helmets. In almost all instances, helmets do not need to be removed. Indeed, they are frequently fitted so snugly to the head that they can be secured directly to the spinal immobilization device.

You should remove part or all of a helmet only under two circumstances:

1. When the face mask or visor interferes with adequate ventilation or with your ability to restore an adequate airway.
2. When the helmet is so loose that securing it to the spinal immobilization device will not provide adequate immobilization of the head.

Safety Tips

Do not move patients unless it is necessary to perform CPR or remove them from a dangerous environment.

When part of a motorcycle helmet interferes with ventilation, the visor should be lifted away from the face. In the case of a football helmet, the face guard should be removed. Some newer football helmets have a tough plastic strap fixing the face guard to the mask. Trainers and coaches should have a special tool readily available that can remove the face guard. The chin strap should also be loosened to facilitate the jaw-thrust technique. In most instances, exposing the face and jaw allows you access to the airway to secure adequate ventilation. Most football face guards are fastened to the helmet by four plastic clips, which can be cut with a sharp knife or unscrewed with a screwdriver to remove the face guard, as shown in **Skill Drill 14-8** :

SKILL DRILL 14-8

1. Stabilize the patient's head and helmet in a neutral, in-line position **Step 1**.
2. Then remove the mask in one of two ways.
   A. Unscrew the retaining clips for the face mask **Step 2**.
   B. Use a trainer's tool designed for cutting retaining clips **Step 3**.
3. Assess the patient's airway.

The second indication for helmet removal is a loose helmet that will not ensure adequate immobilization of the head when secured to the spinal immobilization device. A loose helmet can be removed easily while the head and neck are being stabilized manually. The procedure for helmet removal in this circumstance is shown in **Skill Drill 14-9** . Note that this procedure requires two experienced people.

SKILL DRILL 14-9

1. Kneel down at the patient's head, and open the face shield so that you can assess the airway and breathing. Remove the eyeglasses if the patient is wearing them **Step 1**.
2. Stabilize the helmet by placing your hands on either side of it, ensuring that your fingers are on the patient's lower jaw to prevent movement of the head. Your partner can then loosen the strap **Step 2**.
3. After the strap is loosened, your partner should place one hand on the patient's lower jaw and the other behind the head at the occiput **Step 3**.
4. Once your partner's hands are in position, gently slip the helmet off about halfway and then stop **Step 4**.
5. Have your partner slide his or her hand from the occiput to the back of the head to prevent the head from snapping back once the helmet is removed **Step 5**.
6. With your partner's hand in place, remove the helmet and stabilize the cervical spine. Apply a cervical collar and then secure the patient to a long backboard **Step 6**. Note: With large helmets or small patients, you may need to pad under the shoulders.

Injuries of the Chest

The chest cavity contains the lungs, the heart, and several major blood vessels. The cavity is surrounded and protected by the chest wall, which is made up of the ribs, cartilage, and associated chest muscles. The most common chest injuries are fractures of the ribs, flail chest, and penetrating wounds.

Fractures of the Ribs

Injury may produce fracture of one or more ribs. Even a simple fracture of one rib produces pain at the site of the fracture and difficulty breathing **Figure 14-33** . Multiple rib fractures result in significant breathing difficulty. The pain may be so intense that the patient cannot breathe deeply enough to take in adequate amounts of

Skill DRILL 14-8

Removing the Mask on a Sports Helmet

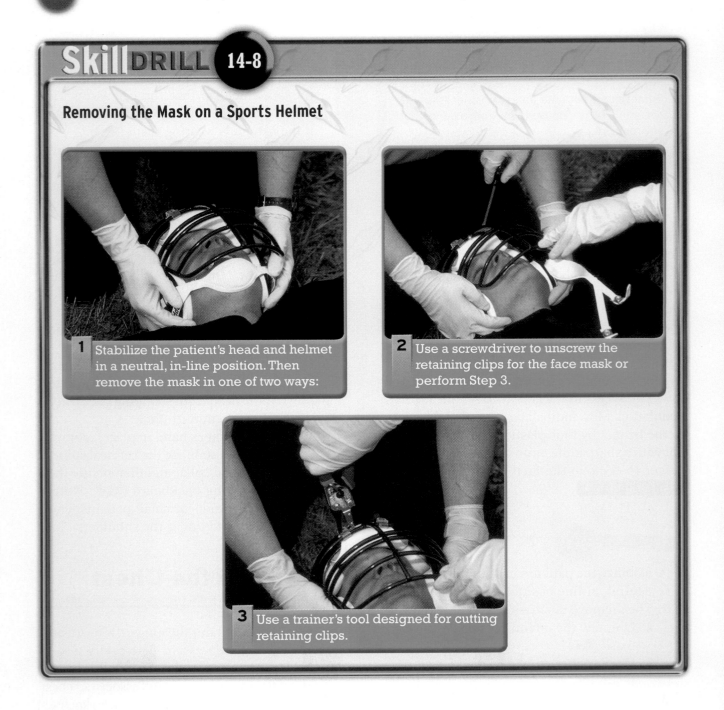

1 Stabilize the patient's head and helmet in a neutral, in-line position. Then remove the mask in one of two ways:

2 Use a screwdriver to unscrew the retaining clips for the face mask or perform Step 3.

3 Use a trainer's tool designed for cutting retaining clips.

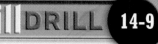

Removing a Helmet

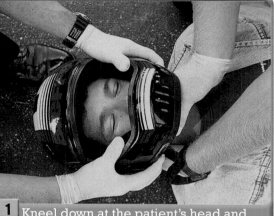

1 Kneel down at the patient's head and open the face shield to assess the airway and breathing.

2 Stabilize the helmet by placing your hands on either side of it, ensuring that your fingers are on the patient's lower jaw to prevent movement of the head. Your partner can then loosen the strap.

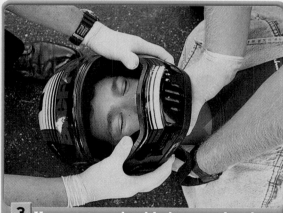

3 Your partner should place one hand on the patient's lower jaw and the other behind the head at the occiput.

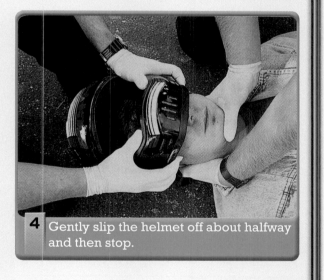

4 Gently slip the helmet off about halfway and then stop.

continued

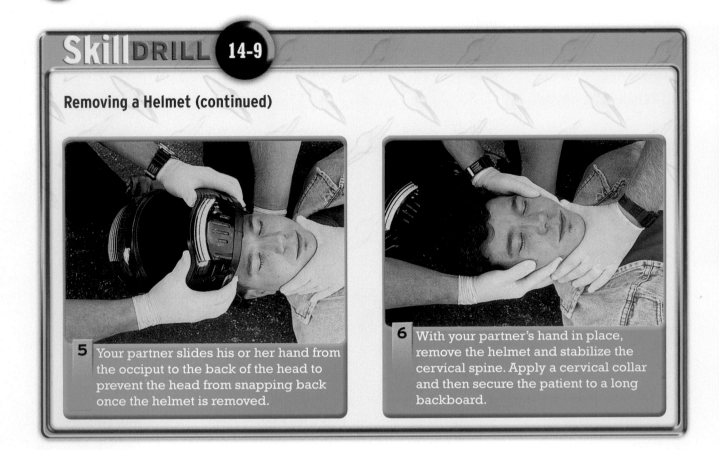

Skill DRILL 14-9

Removing a Helmet (continued)

5 Your partner slides his or her hand from the occiput to the back of the head to prevent the head from snapping back once the helmet is removed.

6 With your partner's hand in place, remove the helmet and stabilize the cervical spine. Apply a cervical collar and then secure the patient to a long backboard.

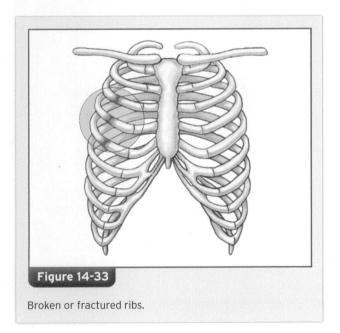

Figure 14-33

Broken or fractured ribs.

oxygen. Rib fractures may be associated with injury to the underlying organs.

To tell if a rib is bruised or broken, apply some pressure to another part of the rib. Pain in the injured area indicates a bruise, crack, or fracture.

If the injury is to the side of the chest, place one hand on the front of the chest and the other on the back and gently squeeze. To check an injury to the front or back of the rib cage, put your hands on either side of the chest and gently squeeze. If there is no pain, the rib is probably not broken. In cases of rib fractures, be alert for signs and symptoms of internal injury, particularly shock.

Treatment of Rib Fractures

Try to reassure and make a patient with rib fractures more comfortable by placing a pillow against the injured ribs to splint them. Prevent excessive movement of the patient as you prepare for **transport** to an appropriate medical facility. Administer oxygen if it is available and you are trained to use it.

Flail Chest

If three or more ribs are broken in at least two places, the injured portion of the chest wall does not move at the same time as the rest of the chest. The injured part bulges outward when the patient

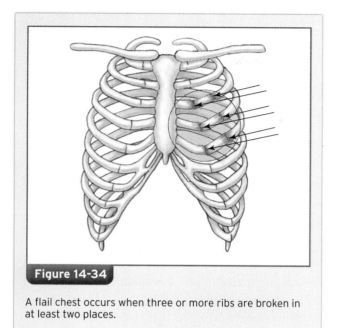

Figure 14-34

A flail chest occurs when three or more ribs are broken in at least two places.

exhales and moves inward when the patient inhales. This condition is called a flail chest **Figure 14-34 ▲**. A flail chest decreases the amount of oxygen and carbon dioxide exchanged in the lungs. It causes breathing problems that become progressively worse.

You can identify a flail chest by examining the chest wall and observing chest movements during breathing. If the injured portion of the chest moves inward as the rest of the chest moves outward (and vice versa), the patient has a flail chest **Figure 14-35 ▼**.

Treatment of Flail Chest

If the patient is having difficulty breathing, firmly place a pillow (or even your hand) on the flail section of the chest to stabilize it. In severe cases of flail chest, it may be necessary to support the patient's breathing. This can be done by EMTs or paramedics with mouth-to-mask or bag-mask resuscitation devices and by using supplemental oxygen. Monitor and support the patient's ABCs and arrange for **prompt transport** to an appropriate medical facility.

Penetrating Chest Wounds

If an object (usually a knife or bullet) penetrates the chest wall, air and blood escape into the space between the lungs and the chest wall **Figure 14-36 ▶**. The air and blood cause the lung

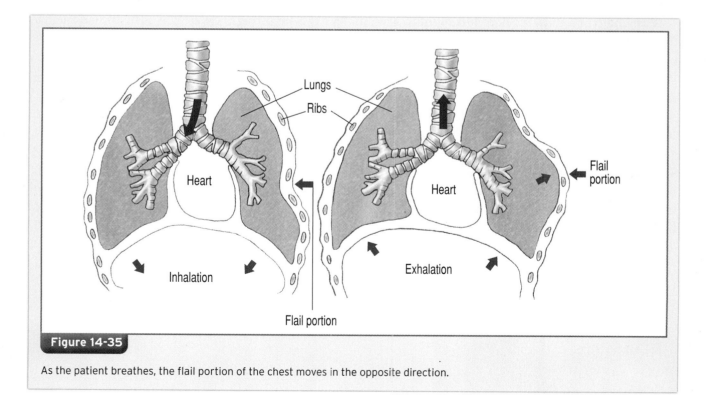

Figure 14-35

As the patient breathes, the flail portion of the chest moves in the opposite direction.

Voices of Experience

Life and Limb

The call came in at 4:35 PM on a Wednesday afternoon. An 18-year-old male had his arm pinned in a machine at a metal manufacturing company. I responded from home and arrived at the station with two other fire fighters. We had all recently finished a medical first responder class.

We arrived on the scene at 4:43 PM, and we were immediately directed to the machine shop. Upon entering the shop, I saw a scene that caused me to stop in order to gain my composure.

> **" I was surprised that there was not a lot of blood around us, because the patient was missing his arm and all of the vessels were severed. "**

Sitting on the floor was our patient, an 18-year-old-male, holding his left shoulder where his arm should have been. Along with another fire fighter, I immediately went to the patient and began to assess him. He was pale with a rapid pulse, dropping blood pressure, and an expression of complete disbelief. As my partner was taking his vitals, I held direct pressure on the shoulder and spoke to the patient, trying to reassure him. As I talked to the patient, I was sizing up the scene. I was surprised that there was not a lot of blood around us, because the patient was missing his arm and all of the vessels were severed. I was also wondering where the third fire fighter who had arrived with us had gone.

I looked away from the patient and saw that the third fire fighter was tearing the roller machine apart with the help of a shop worker. I thought to myself, "What is he doing?" I watched as he pulled the patient's left arm out of the machine. It had never dawned on me that they could reattach the patient's arm but in order to do so, they had to have a limb to work with!

We packaged the patient and his left arm for transportation to our local hospital. While en route, he received ALS care from the paramedics, who had arrived just before the ambulance was ready to leave. At the hospital, he was further stabilized, and then transferred by medical helicopter for treatment and surgery at the trauma center.

The surgery was a success and after many months of therapy and rehabilitation, the patient regained 85 percent use of the limb. The emergency department doctor attributed the successful outcome of this incident to the quick EMS response and our application of basic life support skills. Our first responder training helped us to react effectively to the situation and contribute to the EMS response that saved this patient's life and limb.

Alan E. Joos, Fire Fighter/EMT-I
Assistant Director—Training
Utah Fire and Rescue Academy
Provo, Utah

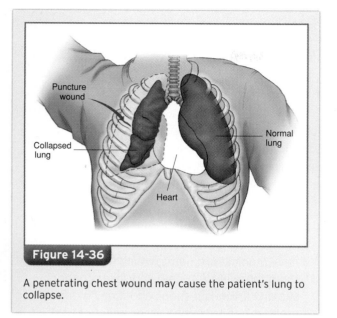

Figure 14-36

A penetrating chest wound may cause the patient's lung to collapse.

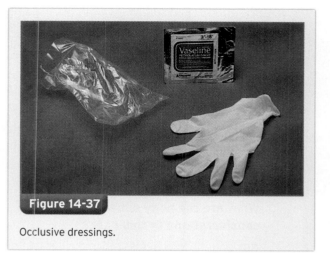

Figure 14-37

Occlusive dressings.

to collapse. Lung collapse greatly reduces the amount of oxygen and carbon dioxide that is exchanged and can result in shock and death. Blood loss into the chest cavity can produce hemorrhagic shock.

Treatment of Penetrating Chest Wounds

Quickly seal an open chest wound with something that will prevent more air from entering the chest cavity. (Occlusive dressings were discussed in Chapter 13 and are shown in **Figure 14-37 ▶**.) You can use petroleum jelly, gauze, aluminum foil, plastic wrap, or even cellophane. In rare cases, sealing the wound may increase the patient's breathing difficulty. If it is harder for a patient to breathe after you seal the wound, uncover one corner of the occlusive dressing to see if the breathing improves. Administer oxygen if it is available and

you are trained to use it. If a knife or other object is impaled in the chest, do not remove it. Seal the wound around the object with a dressing to prevent air from entering the chest. Stabilize the impaled object with bulky dressings.

Any chest injury that results in air leakage and bleeding requires prompt attention. For these reasons, patients with severe chest injuries require **rapid transport** to an appropriate medical facility.

A conscious patient with chest trauma may demand to be placed in a sitting position to ease breathing. Unless you must immobilize the spine or treat the patient for shock, help the patient assume whatever position eases breathing. If oxygen is available, administer it. If the patient's respirations are excessively slow or absent, perform mouth-to-mask breathing. A bag-mask device may also be used by trained personnel. If the patient's heart stops, begin chest compressions, regardless of whether there are chest injuries.

You are the Provider

SUMMARY

Review the *You are the Provider* case study provided at the beginning of the chapter.

It is a warm, sunny, spring day. You are dispatched to a residence for the report of a senior citizen who has fallen. When you arrive, you find a conscious and alert 74-year-old woman lying at the bottom of the four steps leading up to the front porch. The woman complains of pain in her right leg.

1. What are the body substance isolation considerations in this case?

Any patient with a possible musculoskeletal injury should be suspected of having open wounds. These may be simple abrasions from a fall or an open fracture. Take body substance isolation (BSI) precautions when examining and treating patients with musculoskeletal injuries. Wear approved gloves to protect yourself from any blood that is present.

2. What type of physical examination is needed for this patient?

Your patient examination should be systematic and complete. Older patients have decreased sensation to pain and may not be aware of their injuries. Brittle bones caused by osteoporosis may result in broken bones from a simple fall at home. Older patients are more likely to have medical problems, which make them more likely to fall. Your examination should include questions about any medical problems and a careful assessment of vital signs.

3. Under what conditions would you move this patient?

A patient who has possible bone or muscle injuries should not be moved unless the patient is in a position of danger and must be moved to safety. Whenever possible, it is better to leave the patient where they are found until more assistance arrives on the scene.

Prep Kit

Ready for Review

The Ready for Review thoroughly summarizes the chapter.

- Musculoskeletal injuries are caused by three types of mechanism of injury: direct force, indirect force, and twisting force.

- A fracture is a broken bone. Fractures can be closed (the bone is broken but there is no break in the skin) or open (the bone is broken and the overlying skin is lacerated).

- A dislocation is a disruption that tears the supporting ligaments of the joint.

- A sprain is a joint injury caused by excessive stretching of the supporting ligaments.

- The three steps in examining a patient with a limb injury include:
  - General assessment of the patient.
  - Examination of the injured part.
  - Evaluation of the circulation and sensation in the injured limb.

- Regardless of the extent or severity, all limb injuries are treated the same way in the field. For all open extremity wounds, first cover the entire wound with a dry, sterile dressing and then apply firm but gentle pressure to control bleeding, if necessary. The injured limb should then be splinted.

- The three basic types of splints are rigid, soft, and traction.

- It takes two people to adequately splint most limb injuries: one to stabilize and support the extremity and one to apply the splint.

- Severe head and spinal cord injuries can result from many different kinds of trauma. These injuries are common causes of death and can also lead to irreversible paralysis and permanent brain damage.

- Injuries of the head are classified as open or closed. In a closed head injury, bleeding and swelling within the skull may increase pressure on the brain, leading to irreversible brain damage. An open injury of the head usually bleeds profusely.

- When a sign or symptom of a head injury is present, immobilize the head and stabilize the patient's neck, maintain an open airway, support breathing, monitor circulation, check to see if cerebrospinal fluid or blood is seeping, control bleeding with dry, sterile dressings, treat other serious injuries, and arrange for prompt transport.

- Airway obstruction is the primary danger in severe facial injuries.

- When facial injuries are present, immobilize the head and stabilize the patient's head, maintain an open airway, support breathing, monitor circulation, control bleeding with dry, sterile dressing and apply direct pressure, treat other serious injuries, and arrange for prompt transport.

- When you suspect a spinal injury, do not move the patient during the examination. Further, do not allow the patient to move.

- When a sign or symptom of spinal injury is present, place the head and neck in a neutral position, stabilize the head and prevent movement of the neck, maintain an open airway, support breathing, monitor circulation, assess pulse, movement, and sensation, examine and treat other serious injuries, assist in immobilizing the patient using a long or short backboard, and arrange for prompt transport.

- The most common chest injuries are fractures of the ribs, flail chest, and penetrating wounds.

Technology

- Interactivities
- Vocabulary Explorer
- Anatomy Review
- Web Links
- Online Review Manual

www.FirstResponder.EMSzone.com

The Vital Vocabulary

The Vital Vocabulary are the key terms for this chapter.

abdominal breathing Breathing using only the diaphragm.

cerebrospinal fluid (CSF) A clear, watery, straw-colored fluid that fills the space between the brain and spinal cord and their protective coverings.

closed fracture A fracture in which the overlying skin has not been damaged.

closed head injury Injury where there is bleeding and/or swelling within the skull.

dislocation Disruption of a joint so that the bone ends are no longer in alignment.

forearm The lower portion of the upper extremity; from the elbow to the wrist.

joint The place where two bones come in contact with each other.

mechanism of injury The means by which a traumatic injury occurs.

open fracture Any fracture in which the overlying skin has been damaged.

osteoporosis Abnormal brittleness of the bones in older people caused by loss of calcium; affected bones fracture easily.

paralysis Inability of a conscious person to move voluntarily.

rigid splints Splints made from firm materials such as wood, aluminum, or plastic.

seizures Sudden episodes of uncontrolled electrical activity in the brain.

sling A bandage or material that helps to support the weight of an injured upper extremity.

soft splint A splint made from supple material that provides gentle support.

sprain A joint injury in which the joint is partially or temporarily dislocated and some of the supporting ligaments are either stretched or torn.

traction splint A splint that holds a lower extremity fracture (PSDE) in alignment by applying a constant, steady pull on the extremity.

trauma A wound or injury, either physical or psychological.

Assessment in Action

Assessment in Action presents a fictitious scenario to help you review what you learned in this chapter.

You are dispatched to a recreational bicycle trail for the report of an injured bicyclist. Upon arrival you find a 23-year-old female who lost control of her bicycle and was thrown to the pavement. She is complaining of pain in her right collarbone while cradling her right arm.

1. What kind of assessment should you perform on this patient?

   A. Examine only the areas that are painful.
   B. Examine only the upper extremities.
   C. Perform a head-to-toe examination.
   D. Complete all parts of the patient assessment sequence.

2. What parts of the body can be injured by this type of incident?

   A. Head and neck
   B. Upper extremities
   C. Trunk
   D. Any part of the body

3. If you identify pain and deformity of the collarbone, what type of splint would you apply?

   A. A sling
   B. A sling and swathe
   C. A rigid splint
   D. An air splint

4. Do you need to immobilize this patient's neck?

   A. Yes
   B. No

5. You discover swelling, deformity, and an open wound on the patient's leg. How should you treat this wound?

   A. Splint the leg and then apply a sterile dressing.
   B. Leave the wound exposed because it is associated with a possible fracture.
   C. Cover it with a sterile dressing.
   D. Elevate the leg to stop the bleeding.

6. The general rule for splinting is to

   A. Immobilize the fracture site.
   B. Immobilize the fracture site and the joint above it.
   C. Immobilize the fracture site and the joint below it.
   D. Immobilize the fracture site and the joints above and below it.

7. When is it appropriate to check circulation, sensation, and movement in a patient with a limb injury?

Childbirth, Pediatrics, and Geriatrics

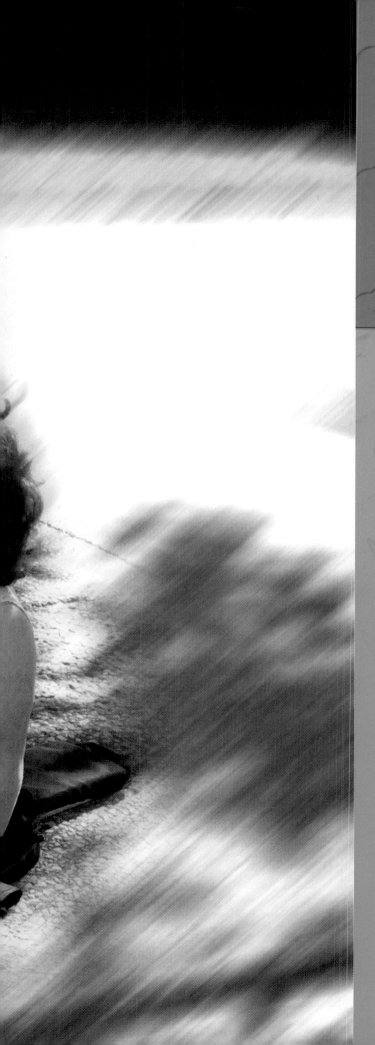

Childbirth

You are the Provider

As you are completing your morning check out of your vehicle and equipment, you and your partner Mary are dispatched for the report of a 24-year-old woman in labor. The address is about 8 minutes from your station and the closest EMS unit is transporting another patient to the hospital.

1. What information do you need to get from the patient?
2. What information is important to learn from your physical examination?
3. How do you determine whether to transport this patient or to prepare to assist with the delivery of the baby?

Introduction

As a first responder, you must sometimes assist in the birth of a child. A planned childbirth is an exciting, dramatic, and stressful event in itself. An unplanned childbirth, where you are called to assist, can be even more dramatic and stressful. However, if you remember some easy steps, you can effectively assist in the birth process and offer comfort and support to both mother and child.

Childbirth is a normal and natural part of life. If you are concerned about your ability to handle such a situation, just remember that thousands of deliveries occur each day and result in healthy babies. In many countries, medical assistance at childbirth is the exception, not the rule.

You may not have the time or necessary assistance to transport the expectant mother to the hospital. Therefore, you must be prepared to help the pregnant woman deliver the child wherever she is. In most cases, the pregnant woman is the one who delivers the child and you will only assist her as needed. During the birth process, the baby is literally pushed out of the pregnant woman. Your assistance involves "catching" the baby, helping it begin to breathe adequately, and keeping it warm.

Generally, pregnancy and the birth process are not a surprise for the mother and she may be quite knowledgeable and well-prepared. However, the call to you may come because the timing of the childbirth caught everyone by surprise or because a complication has developed. In reviewing this chapter, you will find that the birth process has several stages. The two key indicators of an impending birth that concern you are the frequency of <u>contractions</u> and <u>crowning</u>, or the appearance of the baby's head during a contraction.

The Anatomy and Function of the Female Reproductive System

The major female reproductive organs are the ovaries, which produce eggs, and the <u>uterus</u> (<u>womb</u>), which holds the fertilized egg as it develops during pregnancy. The egg released by the ovaries travels through the fallopian tube to the uterus. The external opening of the female reproductive system is called the <u>birth canal</u> or the <u>vagina</u>. The developing baby (<u>fetus</u>) is encased in an amniotic sac for support and floats in amniotic fluid. The <u>placenta</u>, or afterbirth, draws nutrients from the wall of the mother's uterus. These nutrients and oxygen are delivered to the fetus through the <u>umbilical cord</u>. **Figure 15-1 ▾** shows the anatomy of a pregnant female.

Technology

- Interactivities
- Vocabulary Explorer
- Anatomy Review
- Web Links
- Online Review Manual

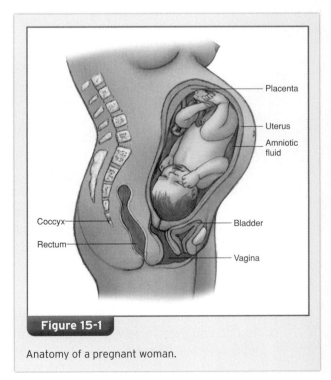

Figure 15-1

Anatomy of a pregnant woman.

Assessing the Birth Situation

Should you help deliver a baby away from the hospital or arrange to transport the mother to the hospital? To make this decision, you need to understand that normal **labor** (the process of delivering a baby) consists of three distinct stages.

Stages of Labor

Stage One is when the mother's body prepares for birth. This stage is characterized by the following conditions: initial contractions occur; the "water" breaks; the bloody show occurs, but the baby's head does not appear during the contractions. Carefully check the mother to determine whether the baby is crowning. Report your findings to the responding ambulance crew so that they can decide whether to transport the mother to the hospital during this stage of labor. Stage Two involves the actual birth of the baby. You will see the baby's head crowning during contractions, at which time you must prepare to assist the mother in the delivery of the baby **Figure 15-2 ▼**. No time for transport now! Stage Three, the final stage, involves delivery of the placenta (afterbirth). You must assist in stabilizing the mother and baby and delivering the placenta.

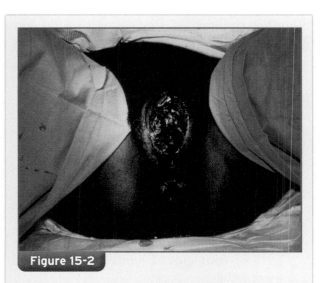

Figure 15-2

Crowning occurs when the infant's head appears at the vaginal opening.

Is There Time to Reach the Hospital?

The following questions will help you to determine how close the mother is to delivering her baby and whether there is time to transport the mother to the hospital or if you need to prepare for a delivery.

1. *Has the woman had a baby before?* The length of labor for a first-time mother is usually longer than for a woman who has had previous children. A woman who is experiencing her first labor will usually have more time to reach the hospital. It is also helpful to ask the woman when the baby is due, although labor can start before the baby's due date.

2. *Has the woman experienced a bloody show?* As the baby starts its descent toward the birth canal, a plug of mucus, often mixed with blood, called the **bloody show** is expelled from the cervix and discharged from the vagina. This occurs as the first stage of labor is about to begin.

3. *Has the bag of waters broken?* The **bag of waters** is the amniotic sac and fluid in which the baby floats. The bag of waters usually breaks toward the end of the first stage of labor and may give some idea of the progress of the birth process. In a few cases, the bag of water may not break until the birth is actually occurring (see the section on complications of delivery).

4. *How frequent are the contractions?* If the contractions are more than 5 minutes apart, you can usually transport the woman to the hospital. Contractions less than 2 minutes apart usually indicate that delivery will occur very soon and you need to prepare to deliver the baby. If the contractions are 3 to 4 minutes apart, you should take the other factors listed here into account to make your decision.

5. *Does the woman feel an urge to move her bowels?* When the baby's head is in the birth canal, it presses against the rectum and the mother may feel the urge to move her bowels. DO NOT allow her to go to the toilet. This is an indication that delivery is imminent.

6. *Is the baby's head crowning?* Crowning indicates that the baby will be born in the next few minutes and you need to be ready to receive the baby.

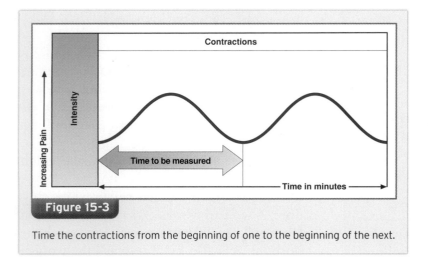

Figure 15-3

Time the contractions from the beginning of one to the beginning of the next.

7. *Is transportation available?* Find out not only if the ambulance is responding, but also how far it is to the hospital. Will bad weather, a natural disaster, or rush-hour traffic prevent prompt arrival of transportation?

Timing Contraction Cycles

Time the contraction cycles from the beginning of one contraction to the beginning of the next Figure 15-3 ▲ . Do not time the interval between contractions. If contractions are less than 3 minutes apart, delivery is close.

Detecting Crowning

To determine whether the baby's head is crowning, you must observe the vagina during a contraction. If you see the baby's head crowning during the contraction, prepare for the delivery (see Figure 15-2). Do not risk transporting the woman to the hospital.

Preparing for Delivery

As you prepare to assist in the delivery of a baby, keep these two things in mind:

1. Calm the woman. Delivery is a natural process.
2. Calm yourself. You are there to help.

Because you are not in a hospital, you will not be able to maintain sterile conditions. However, you must attempt to be as clean as possible. Wash your hands thoroughly. If you don't have a sterile delivery kit, use the gloves from your first re-

sponder life support kit (or even clean kitchen gloves, if they are available). If a shower curtain is available, place it on the bed for protection. Cover the shower curtain with clean newspapers, and then cover the newspapers with a clean sheet. Have plenty of clean towels ready to cover the baby and to clean the mother after delivery has occurred. Childbirth is bloody and messy. Your practical and mental preparations to deal with the messiness can keep it from affecting your performance.

As the woman's contractions become more forceful, they push the baby down the vagina. The woman should be in a comfortable position. This is often on her back with knees bent and legs drawn up and apart.

Body Substance Isolation and Childbirth

Because a woman in childbirth will expel both blood and body fluids, body substance isolation (BSI) techniques should be used during the delivery. Try not to get any more blood or fluids on you than is absolutely necessary. Use sterile gloves during any delivery whenever possible. Sterile gloves protect not only the woman and infant from infection, but also you from any bloodborne diseases the woman might have Skill Drill 15-1 ▶ .

SKILL DRILL 15-1

1. Carefully open the sterile glove package without touching the gloves Step 1 .
2. Pick up the first glove by grasping one edge Step 2 .
3. Pull on the first glove, being careful not to touch the outside Step 3 .
4. Grasp the second glove by sliding two fingers of your gloved hand into the rolled edge Step 4 .
5. Put on the second glove Step 5 .
6. Keep gloves as sterile as possible Step 6 .

Skill DRILL 15-1

Putting on Sterile Gloves

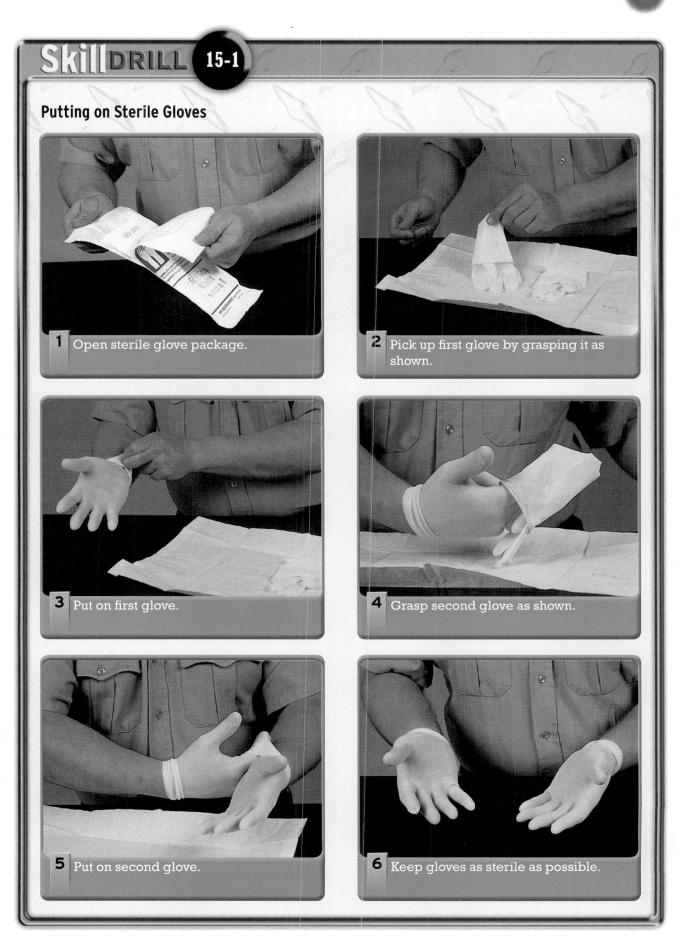

1 Open sterile glove package.

2 Pick up first glove by grasping it as shown.

3 Put on first glove.

4 Grasp second glove as shown.

5 Put on second glove.

6 Keep gloves as sterile as possible.

Because you could get splattered on the face during the delivery process, wear face and eye protection to keep possible splatter out of your eyes, nose, and mouth. Wearing a surgical gown can help keep fluids off your body. As a first responder, you will not have all the protective equipment that is available in a hospital. Do what you can to prevent unnecessary exposure to body fluids and report all direct exposures of blood or fluids to the emergency physician or to your medical director.

Equipment

You should have a prepackaged obstetrical (OB) delivery kit in your emergency care equipment Figure 15-4 ▼.

The delivery kit includes:
- Sterile gloves
- Umbilical cord clamp
- Sterile drapes and towels
- Sanitary pads
- 4-inch × 4-inch gauze pads
- A towel or blanket for the baby
- Bulb syringe

In addition, you will need:
- Sheets or towels for the mother
- Suction (if available)
- Oxygen (if available and if you are trained to use it)
- Infant mask

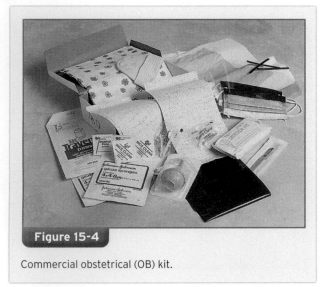

Figure 15-4

Commercial obstetrical (OB) kit.

If you do not have a delivery kit, look for appropriate substitute materials. You can probably find most of these items in your first responder life support kit or in most homes. Even if you do not have any equipment, remember that you can still assist in delivering a child with no more equipment than common sense and gloved hands.

Assisting With Delivery

Remember that your primary purpose is to assist in the delivery of the baby. The woman is going to feel pressure in the vaginal area, as if she has to move her bowels. This is a normal feeling during the delivery process. Do not let her go to the bathroom and do not hold her legs together.

Be as clean as possible during the entire delivery process. Follow the BSI techniques described. Do not touch the vaginal area except during the delivery. If you have a partner, have him or her stay with you during the delivery.

Have the woman lie on her back. If pillows or blankets are available, cover them with clean towels or sheets and place them under the mother's buttocks to elevate her hips slightly. Have the mother draw up her knees and spread her legs apart.

The baby's head should emerge slowly to prevent undue stress on the baby and tearing of the vagina. As the head emerges, support the baby's head and tell the mother to stop pushing. To help her stop, tell her to take quick, short breaths (advise her to blow like she is blowing out a candle). Some EMS systems advise their personnel to use the palm of the hand to provide slight counterpressure over the baby's head to slow down the birth process. Be sure to check with your local medical authority on your EMS protocols for this situation.

Do not attempt to pull the baby during delivery. In a normal birth, the baby will turn to its side by itself after the head emerges and the rest of the body will be delivered spontaneously Figure 15-5 ▶. Continue to support the baby's head and be ready to catch the baby in a clean towel. Remember, the baby will be wet and slippery. As the torso and the legs are delivered, support the infant with both hands. Grasp the baby's feet as they are delivered. Keep the infant's head at about the level of the woman's vagina. If the amniotic sac has not broken as the baby's head starts to deliver, tear it with your fingers and push it away from the infant's head and mouth. As the head emerges, check to make sure that the umbilical cord is not wrapped around the infant's neck. If it is, attempt to slip the cord over the baby's shoulder. If you cannot do this, attempt to reduce the pressure on the cord. Never pull on the umbilical cord; it is extremely fragile and you do not want to tear or cut it until it is safe to do so.

Caring for the Newborn

As soon as you are holding the newborn baby in a clean towel, lay him or her down between the mother's legs and immediately clear the baby's mouth and nose. Suction the mouth and the nostrils two to three times. Use a bulb syringe from the delivery kit if one is available Figure 15-6 ▶ . Be careful not to reach all the way to the back of the baby's mouth. If a bulb syringe is not available, wipe the baby's mouth and nose with a gauze pad.

You can place the infant on the mother's abdomen. This will help keep the baby from losing too much warmth. Wipe blood and mucus from the baby's mouth and nose with sterile gauze or with the cleanest object available. If the baby is not breathing, suction the baby's mouth and nose again. Rub the baby's back or flick the soles of the baby's feet to stimulate breathing Figure 15-7 ▶ . Use the towel to dry the infant and then wrap the child in a blanket to keep it warm. Place the infant on his or her side with the head slightly lower than the trunk. This will help to aid the drainage of secretions from the airway.

When the umbilical cord stops pulsating, tie it with gauze between the mother and the newborn. In a normal delivery, there is no need for you to cut the umbilical cord. Keep the infant warm and wait until more highly trained EMS personnel arrive. They will have the proper equipment to clamp and cut the umbilical cord in an approved manner.

Note the time of the delivery so it can be properly reported on the baby's birth certificate.

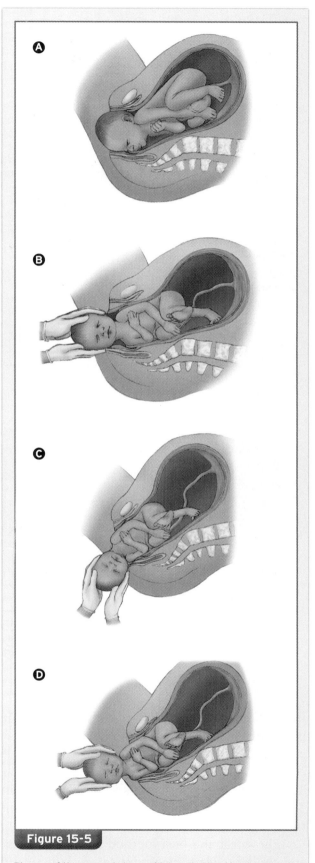

Figure 15-5

Phases of the second stage of labor. **A.** Head begins to deliver. **B.** Delivery of head. **C.** Delivery of upper shoulder. **D.** Delivery of lower shoulder.

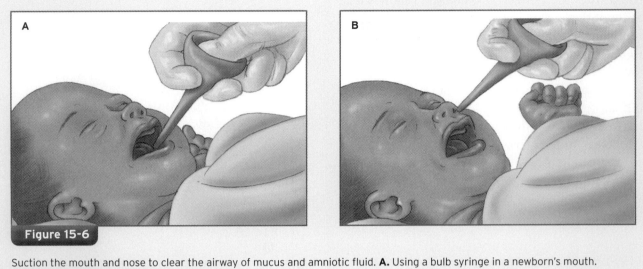

Suction the mouth and nose to clear the airway of mucus and amniotic fluid. **A.** Using a bulb syringe in a newborn's mouth. **B.** Using a bulb syringe in a newborn's nose.

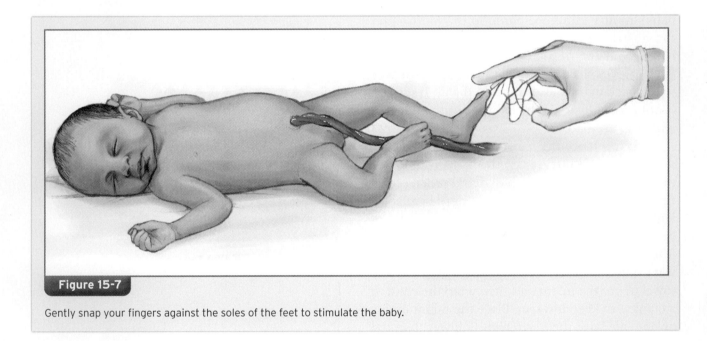

Gently snap your fingers against the soles of the feet to stimulate the baby.

In the rare event that there may be multiple births, prepare for the second delivery.

Delivery of the Placenta

The placenta will deliver on its own, usually within 30 minutes of the baby's delivery. Never pull on the umbilical cord to help deliver the placenta!

The safest and best method for both mother and child is to leave the umbilical cord uncut and attached to both the placenta and the baby—at least until the transporting EMS unit arrives. After the placenta is delivered, wrap it in a towel or newspaper with three quarters of the umbilical cord. Then, place it in a plastic bag and transport it to the hospital with the mother and child so it can be examined by a physician. Try to keep the placenta at the same level as the baby to help prevent any blood from the infant flowing back out into the placenta. This is especially important if you are unable to tie the umbilical cord

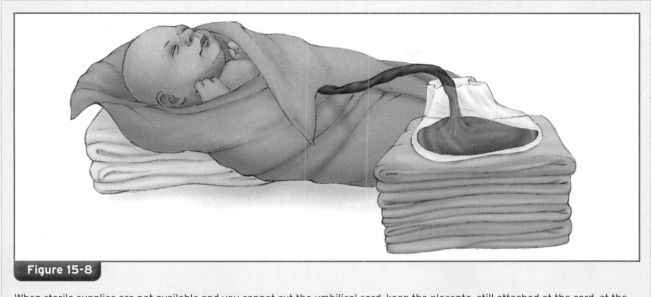

Figure 15-8

When sterile supplies are not available and you cannot cut the umbilical cord, keep the placenta, still attached at the cord, at the same level as the baby during transport to the hospital.

Figure 15-8 ▲. The mother can be transported to the hospital before the placenta is delivered, if necessary.

Bleeding usually stops after the placenta is delivered. You can massage the uterus to help stop the bleeding. To massage the uterus, place one hand with fingers fully extended just above the mother's pubic bone. Use your other hand to press down into the abdomen and gently massage the uterus until it becomes firm. This should take 3 to 5 minutes. As the uterus firms up, it should feel about the size of a softball or large grapefruit.

Aftercare of the Mother and Newborn

Continue to carefully observe both the mother and child and keep them both warm. Cover the baby's head and body to prevent loss of body heat. About every 3 to 5 minutes, recheck the uterus for firmness. Also recheck the vagina to see if there is any excessive bleeding. In a normal delivery, the mother will lose about 300 to 500 mL (1 to 2 cups) of blood. Continue to massage the uterus if it is not firm or if bleeding continues.

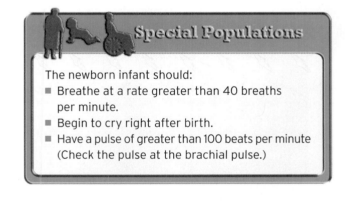

Special Populations

The newborn infant should:
- Breathe at a rate greater than 40 breaths per minute.
- Begin to cry right after birth.
- Have a pulse of greater than 100 beats per minute (Check the pulse at the brachial pulse.)

Clean the mother with clean, moist towels or cloths. Cover the vaginal opening with a clean sanitary pad or large dressing, but do NOT pack. Replace the sheets with clean ones, if possible. If the mother is thirsty, you can give her small amounts of water to drink.

FYI

Resuscitating the Newborn

If the infant does not breathe on its own within the first minute after birth, proceed with the following steps **Skill Drill 15-2** ▶ :

Skill DRILL 15-2

Resuscitating a Newborn Infant

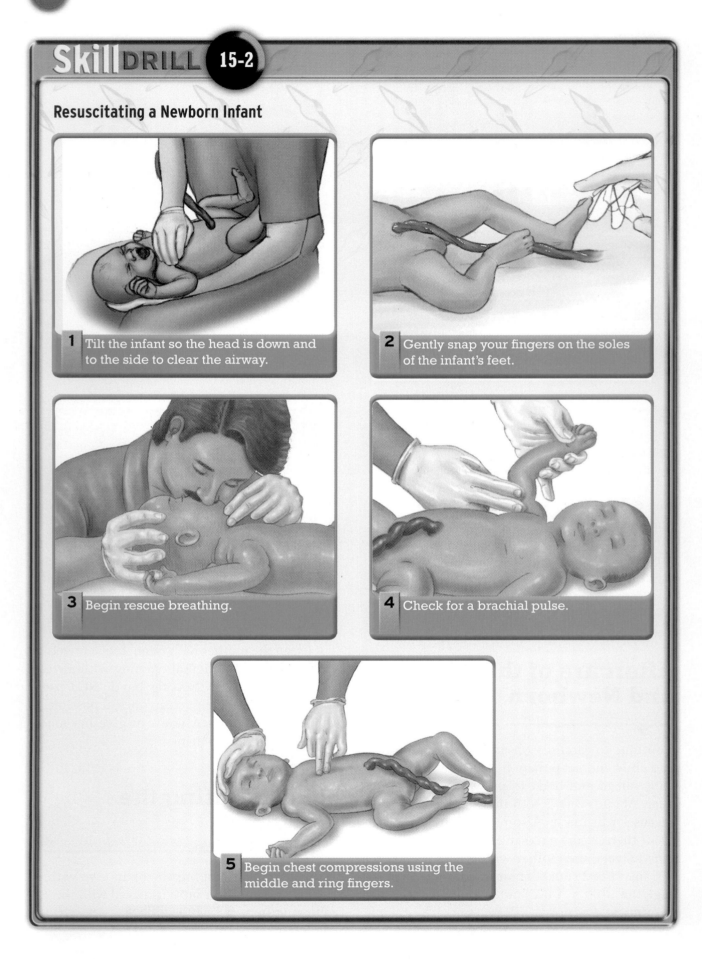

1 Tilt the infant so the head is down and to the side to clear the airway.

2 Gently snap your fingers on the soles of the infant's feet.

3 Begin rescue breathing.

4 Check for a brachial pulse.

5 Begin chest compressions using the middle and ring fingers.

SKILL DRILL 15-2

1. Tilt the infant's head down and to the side to encourage drainage of mucus **Step 1**.

2. Suction the mouth and nose with a bulb syringe (if available) after delivery of the shoulders. Drying and **suctioning** are usually enough stimulation to induce breathing. Other ways to stimulate breathing include gently snapping your fingers against the soles of the baby's feet and/or rubbing the infant's back. Rough handling is not needed. An infant responds best to simple, gentle techniques, but if the infant is still not breathing, proceed to the next step **Step 2**.

3. Begin mouth-to-mouth-and-nose or mouth-to-mask breathing by gently puffing twice into the infant's mouth and nose **Step 3**. If the infant begins breathing on its own, support and assist respirations and recheck the airway to be sure it remains clear (see Chapter 6).

4. If the infant is still not breathing, continue mouth-to-mouth-and-nose or mouth-to-mask breathing and check for a brachial pulse **Step 4**.

5. If you cannot feel a brachial pulse or if the heart rate is less than 60 beats per minute, begin closed-chest cardiac compressions. Use your middle and ring fingers to depress the infant's chest **Step 5** (see Chapter 9).

6. Continue CPR until the infant begins breathing or until it is pronounced dead by a physician. Provide **rapid transport** to the hospital. Do not give up!

Automobile Crashes and the Pregnant Woman

Any pregnant woman involved in an automobile crash or suffering other trauma should be examined by a physician. The forces involved in even minor crashes may be great enough to injure the mother or the unborn child, even though the child is usually well protected in the uterus.

Promptly assess and **transport** a pregnant woman who has been involved in an auto crash to the hospital. If the woman exhibits signs or symptoms of shock, monitor the airway, breathing, and circulation. Arrange for administration of high-flow oxygen. Have the mother lie on her left side rather than on her back. This will relieve pressure on the uterus and the abdominal organs and allow blood to return through the major veins in the abdomen.

In rare circumstances, a crash can be severe enough to kill the mother, yet the unborn child can still be saved. Provide CPR to the mother while transporting her to the closest medical facility.

Complications of Childbirth

Although the vast majority of births are normal, you should be aware of possible complications.

Unbroken Bag of Waters

In rare instances, the bag of amniotic fluid that surrounds the baby does not break. If the baby is born surrounded by the bag of waters, carefully break the bag and push it away from the baby's nose and mouth so he or she can breathe. Be careful not to injure the baby in the process. Then suction the baby's nose and mouth to help him or her begin to breathe.

Breech Birth

In a breech birth, some part of the baby other than the top of its head comes down the birth canal first. In this abnormal delivery, the first thing you see may be the baby's leg, arm, shoulder, or buttocks. This type of delivery can result in injury to both the baby and the mother.

If, instead of the normal crowning, you see a **breech presentation**, make every attempt to arrange for **prompt transport** to a medical facility. A breech birth slows the labor, so there will be more time for transport to the emergency department. If you are stranded and cannot transport the mother to the emergency room, you will have to assist with the breech birth.

Voices of Experience

Follow Your Protocols

I was the Chief of a suburban police department, when one of my officers was involved in a medical emergency that changed the entire department's thinking toward emergency childbirth. The shift had started slowly, when the radio announced his first call: "Report of a baby not responding. Caller is frantic." Luckily, he was within a block of the residence.

> **The real success of this call was in teaching our department to follow protocols in every emergency situation.**

When the officer arrived, the man who opened the door was visibly upset and pointed to a nearby bedroom. He told the officer that his wife was having a baby, and things were not going well.

When the officer entered the darkened room, he was presented with a situation that he hadn't expected or prepared for. The family had decided on a home delivery with a midwife. This baby was not the patient's first. The baby was stuck in the birth canal, and it was not breathing. The officer responded without hesitation and assisted the midwife and the mother in the delivery. The complications that he found were a prolapsed cord, which was around the baby's neck, and there were no signs of respirations. Upon delivery, he cleared the airway, suctioned the nose and mouth, and performed CPR on the newborn. Within seconds the sounds of a healthy baby filled the room.

Within 5 minutes the ALS unit arrived and took over the care of the infant and mother. The officer was excited and proud of the work he was able to do that truly saved the life of the newborn, and he was complimented for a job well done.

About 6 hours later, the department telephone rang. The caller requested to talk to the officer, and then urged him to come to the hospital, as they needed to talk to him. The child had tested positive for hepatitis.

All of his excitement over the events of the day was now disappearing as he remembered that in his hurry to help the child and mother, he had not used his personal protective equipment, and he hadn't been concerned with body substance isolation procedures.

This day's events made the officer and the entire department much more aware of the need for first responder training and the reasons that we all need to follow our protocols. For my department, this was an eye-opening event that woke all of us up to the reality of the dangers that we face in the field. As a result, we changed both our operations and training procedures, new equipment was purchased, strict protocols were put into place, and yearly training updates became required for all officers. These changes have truly made us more efficient and professional first responders.

This story has a happy ending, as the baby and the officer both came out of the situation without any serious side effects. But the real success of this call was in teaching our department to follow protocols in every emergency situation. No matter how rushed we feel or how good our intentions are, first responder and patient safety are the number one concerns of every call.

David M. Schwartz
Director of Public Safety, retired
Forest Lake Police Department
Forest Lake, Minnesota

FYI cont.

Support the baby's legs and body as they are delivered; the head usually follows on its own. If the head does not deliver within 3 minutes, arrange for **prompt transport** to a hospital. Insert a gloved hand into the vagina and use your fingers to keep the baby's airway open by forming a pocket over the infant's nose and mouth.

In very rare cases, the arm is the first part of the baby to appear in the birth canal. This circumstance is an extreme emergency that cannot be handled in the field. You must arrange for **rapid transport** to the hospital by ambulance.

Prolapse of the Umbilical Cord

On rare occasions, the umbilical cord comes out of the vagina before the baby is born. This is called **prolapse of the umbilical cord**. If this happens, the cord may be compressed between the baby and the mother's pelvis during contractions, cutting off the baby's blood supply. This is a serious emergency that requires immediate transport to a hospital.

Get the mother's hips up! Place the mother on her back and prop her hips and legs higher than the rest of her body with pillows, blankets, or articles of clothing. Keep the cord covered and moist and do not try to push it back into the vagina. Administer oxygen to the mother if it is available and you are trained to use it. Arrange for **rapid transport** to the hospital.

Some EMS systems recommend placing the mother in a kneeling position (knee-chest position) to take the pressure off the cord. Check with your medical director regarding local procedures.

Excessive Bleeding After Delivery

In addition to the early bloody show that precedes birth, about 1 or 2 cups of blood are lost during normal childbirth. If the mother is bleeding se-

FYI cont.

verely, place one or more clean sanitary pads at the opening of the vagina, elevate her legs and hips, treat her for shock, and arrange for **rapid transport** to the hospital by ambulance.

Encourage the baby to nurse at the mother's breast because nursing contracts the uterus and can often help stop the bleeding. Massage the uterus with your hand, as described earlier in this chapter.

If the area between the mother's vagina and **anus** is torn and bleeding, treat it as you would an open wound. Apply direct pressure, using sanitary pads or gauze dressings.

Miscarriage

A **miscarriage** (spontaneous abortion) is the delivery of an incomplete or underdeveloped fetus. If a miscarriage occurs, you should save the fetus and all the tissues that pass from the vagina. Control the mother's bleeding by placing a sanitary pad or other large dressing at the vaginal opening. You should also treat her for shock. Arrange for **prompt transport** to a hospital so that a physician can examine her and the fetal tissues and control any additional bleeding.

A mother who miscarries will be upset about losing the baby and will need your psychological support as well as your emergency medical care. Be sensitive to the needs and concerns of the mother and other members of the family.

Stillborn Delivery

Resuscitation should be started and continued on all newborns who are not breathing. However, sometimes a baby dies long before delivery. The baby will generally have an unpleasant odor and will not exhibit any signs of life. Such a life-

FYI
cont.

less fetus is referred to as a stillborn. In a case like this, you should turn your attention to the mother in order to provide physical care and psychological support. Carefully wrap the stillborn in a blanket.

Premature Birth

Any baby weighing less than $5\frac{1}{2}$ pounds or delivered before 37 weeks of pregnancy is called premature. Premature infants are smaller, thinner, and usually redder than full-term babies.

You must keep **premature babies** warm because they lose body heat rapidly. Wrap the infant in a clean towel or sheet and cover its head.

FYI
cont.

Wrapping the premature baby in an additional length of aluminum foil can also help maintain its temperature. Arrange for **prompt transport** to a medical facility.

Multiple Births

In the event of multiple births (such as twins), another set of labor contractions will begin shortly after the delivery of the first baby. A mother generally knows of a multiple birth in advance. However, occasionally everyone is surprised. Do not worry—just get ready to repeat the procedures you completed for the first baby!

You are the Provider   SUMMARY

Review the *You are the Provider* case study provided at the beginning of the chapter.

As you are completing your morning check out of your vehicle and equipment, you and your partner Mary are dispatched for the report of a 24-year-old woman in labor. The address is about 8 minutes from your station and the closest EMS unit is transporting another patient to the hospital.

1. What information do you need to get from the patient?

Your patient history should elicit whether the patient has had children before, whether there has been a bloody show, and whether the bag of waters has broken.

2. What information is important to learn from your physical examination?

Your examination of the patient should determine the frequency of contractions and whether the baby's head is crowning.

3. How do you determine whether to transport this patient or to prepare to assist with the delivery of the baby?

As you respond, it is important to assess the amount of time it will take for a transporting EMS unit to arrive on the scene and how much time it will take to transport the patient to the nearest appropriate medical facility. Assessing all these factors will give the data you need to determine whether to transport the woman to a hospital or to prepare for a home delivery.

Prep Kit

Ready for Review

The Ready for Review thoroughly summarizes the chapter.

- This chapter presents the skills and knowledge you need to assist in the birth of a child.

- The key indicators in estimating how soon a delivery will occur are crowning and the time between contractions. By using these two factors, you can determine whether a woman should be transported to a medical facility or whether the baby will be born outside the hospital.

- Normal labor consists of three distinct stages:

  - Stage One is characterized by the following conditions: initial contractions occur; the "water" breaks; the bloody show occurs, but the baby's head does not appear during the contractions.

  - Stage Two involves the actual birth of the baby. You will see the baby's head crowning during contractions, at which time you must prepare to assist the mother in the delivery of the baby.

  - Stage Three involves delivery of the placenta. You must assist in stabilizing the mother and baby and delivering the placenta.

- Exercise good body substance isolation techniques when assisting with a delivery.

- After the delivery, you have two patients to care for—the mother and the infant.

- If the infant does not breathe on its own within the first minute after birth, proceed with the steps to resuscitate a newborn infant.

- Although the vast majority of births are normal, you should be aware of possible complications including unbroken bags of water, breech birth, prolapse of the umbilical cord, excessive bleeding after delivery, miscarriage, stillborn delivery, premature birth, and multiple births.

- Keep in mind that childbirth is normally a happy event. You are there to assist in the delivery, which in most cases has a happy, healthy outcome.

Technology

- Interactivities
- Vocabulary Explorer
- Anatomy Review
- Web Links
- Online Review Manual

Vital Vocabulary

The Vital Vocabulary are the key terms for this chapter.

anus The distal or terminal ending of the gastro-intestinal tract.

bag of waters The amniotic fluid that surrounds the baby before birth.

birth canal The vagina and the lower part of the uterus.

bloody show The bloody mucus plug that is discharged from the vagina when labor begins.

breech presentation A delivery in which the baby's buttocks, arm, shoulder, or leg appears first rather than the head.

contractions Muscular movements of the uterus that push the baby out of the mother.

crowning Appearance of the baby's head during a contraction as it is pushed outward through the vagina.

fetus A developing baby in the uterus or womb.

labor The process of delivering a baby.

miscarriage Delivery of the fetus before it is mature enough to survive outside the womb (about 20 weeks), from either natural (spontaneous abortion) or induced causes.

placenta Life-support system of the baby during its time inside the mother (commonly called the after-birth).

premature babies Babies who deliver before 37 weeks of gestation or who weigh less than $5\frac{1}{2}$ pounds at birth.

prolapse of the umbilical cord A delivery in which the umbilical cord appears before the baby does; the baby's head may compress the cord and cut off all circulation to the baby.

suctioning Aspirating (sucking out) fluid by mechanical means.

umbilical cord Rope-like attachment between the mother and baby; nourishment and waste products pass to and from the baby and the mother through this cord.

uterus (womb) Muscular organ that holds and nourishes the developing baby.

vagina The opening through which the baby emerges.

Assessment in Action

Assessment in Action presents a fictitious scenario to help you review what you learned in this chapter.

While you are on patrol at the state campground, a young man comes running up to you and states that his wife is in labor. You radio your dispatcher to send an ambulance and follow the man to his campsite.

1. What are the signs and symptoms that a birth is imminent?

2. As soon as the head of the baby is delivered, you should:

   A. Look, listen, and feel for breathing.
   B. Apply high-flow oxygen via a nonrebreather mask.
   C. Check the neck to be sure the umbilical cord is not around it.
   D. Clamp the umbilical cord.

3. If the amniotic sac has not broken once the baby's head has delivered, you should:

   A. Tear it with your fingers and push it away from the baby's face.
   B. Suction the mouth and nose of the baby.
   C. Clamp the umbilical cord.
   D. Arrange for immediate transport.

4. The baby has just delivered but is not yet breathing on her own. What should you do?

   A. Begin ventilations at a rate of 40 times per minute.
   B. Suction the airway dry and stimulate the baby.
   C. Begin CPR.
   D. Administer oxygen via a nonrebreather and rapidly transport to the baby to the hospital.

5. CPR should be started on the newborn if:

   A. There is no brachial pulse or if the heart rate is less than 60 beats per minute.
   B. Only if there is no brachial pulse.
   C. The newborn is breathing on her own.
   D. CPR should not be done on any child under 3 months of age.

6. All of the following should be done to treat the mother who is bleeding severely after the delivery of the placenta, EXCEPT:

   A. Having the baby nurse
   B. Massaging the uterus
   C. Elevating her legs and hips and treating for shock
   D. Positioning her on her back with her head raised

7. In a breech delivery, you should:

   A. Clamp the umbilical cord before the head delivers.
   B. Pull gently on the legs to aid in the delivery of the head.
   C. Support the baby's legs and body as they are delivered.
   D. Massage the uterus to aid in the delivery.

Pediatric Emergencies

Skill Objectives

1. Determine a child's respiratory rate, pulse rate, and body temperature. (p 394)
2. Perform the following respiratory skills on a child:
   - Opening the airway (p 396)
   - Basic life support (p 397)
   - Suctioning (p 397-398)
   - Inserting an oral airway (p 398)
3. Treat the following conditions:
   - Partial (mild) airway obstruction in children and infants (p 398)
   - Complete (severe) airway obstruction in children and infants (p 399)
4. Cool a child with a high fever. (p 407-408)

*These are chapter learning objectives.

Pediatric Emergencies

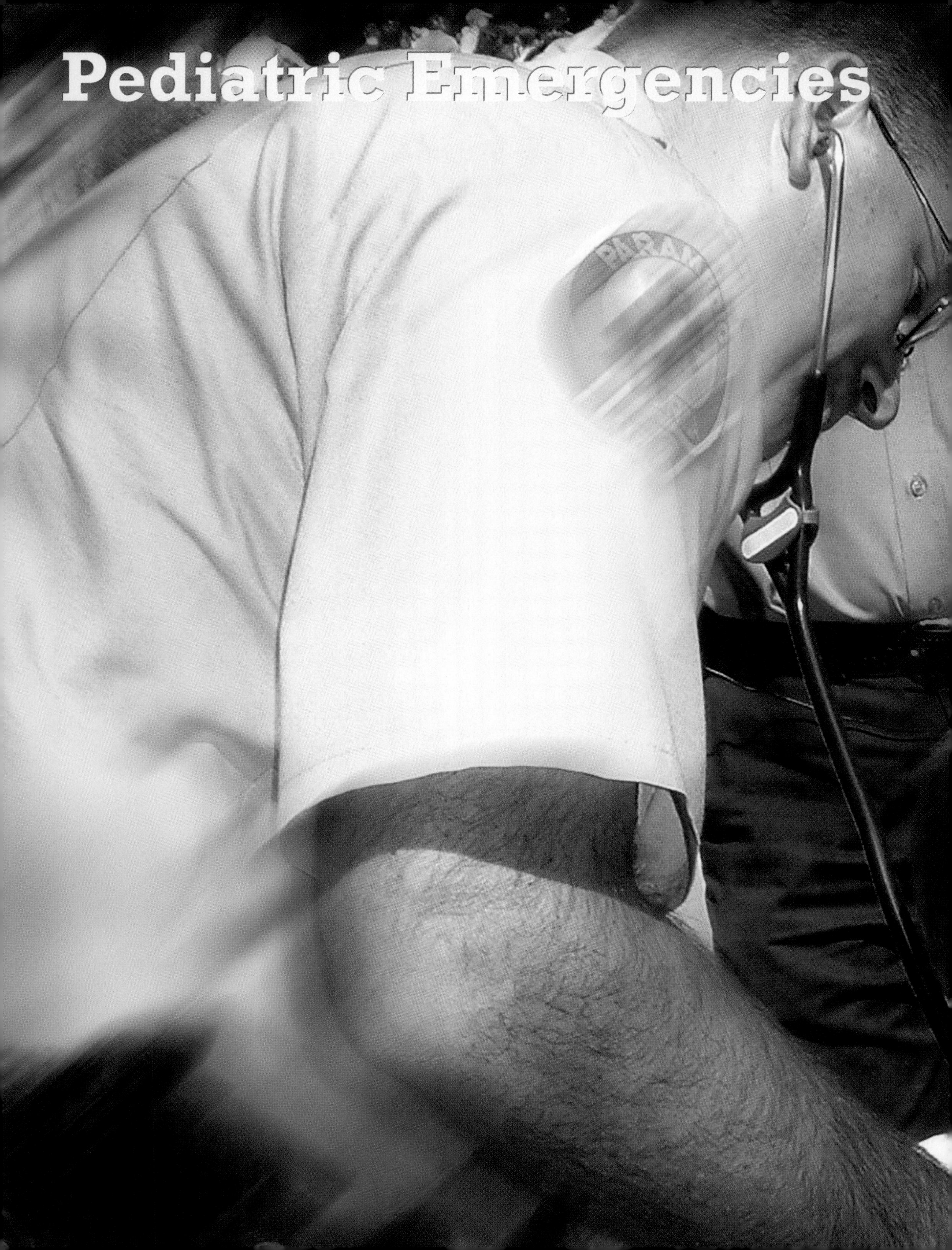

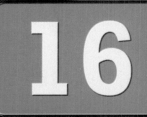

You are the Provider

Your unit is dispatched to a daycare center for the report of a sick child. After you and your partner arrive at the scene, you note a 3-year-old girl who is sitting in the lap of a daycare worker. She appears to have an increased rate of respirations and her breathing is noisy. Your partner examines the child while she remains in the caregiver's lap.

1. What are the differences between the airway of an adult and the airway of a child?
2. How can you quickly form an initial impression of the severity of this child's condition?
3. Why did your partner choose to examine this patient while the child remained in the lap of the caregiver?

Introduction

Sudden illnesses and medical emergencies are common in children and infants. This chapter covers the special knowledge and skills the first responder needs to assess and treat children and infants. This chapter covers the differences between the anatomy of an adult and a child and highlights the special considerations for examining pediatric patients. It describes how the pediatric assessment triangle is a valuable tool for determining the severity of a child's illness or injury.

Respiratory care for children is extremely important. This chapter reviews the following respiratory skills: opening the airway, basic life support, suctioning, and relieving airway obstructions. The signs of respiratory distress, respiratory failure, and circulatory failure in children and infants are explained.

It is important that you learn some basic information and treatment for the following conditions: altered mental status, asthma, croup, epiglottitis, drowning, heat illnesses, high fever, seizures, vomiting and diarrhea, abdominal pain, poisoning, and sudden infant death syndrome. Because trauma is the leading cause of death in children, this chapter covers patterns of injury and the signs of traumatic shock in children. Finally, you should be able to recognize some of the signs and symptoms of child abuse and sexual abuse of children so you can take the proper steps to get help.

Technology

- Interactivities
- Vocabulary Explorer
- Anatomy Review
- Web Links
- Online Review Manual

General Considerations

Managing a pediatric emergency can be one of the most stressful situations you face as a first responder. The child is frightened, anxious, and usually unable to communicate the problem to you clearly. The parents are anxious and frightened. In this atmosphere, where everyone else is tense, you must behave in a calm, controlled, and professional manner.

EMS personnel often have mixed feelings when treating a child. In some cases, the child reminds them of someone they know. Even the most experienced personnel respond emotionally to a seriously ill or injured child. Unless you are prepared, your anxiety and fear may interfere with your ability to deliver proper care.

The Parents

The child's parents or caregivers can be either allies or another problem. You must respond to them as much as to the child, although in a different way. Talk to both parents and to the child as much as possible. Parents are understandably concerned about their child's condition, especially if they don't clearly understand the situation or if they think the situation is more serious than it is. For instance, imagine a parent's reaction to a bleeding laceration of a child's forehead. You know that scalp wounds can bleed profusely, but that such bleeding can be easily controlled with direct pressure. However, most parents do not know that and may become emotional.

Children get many of their behavioral cues from their parents. Calm the parents, talk with them, and ask their assistance in calming the child. It is a good idea to allow a parent to hold the child if the illness or injury permits **Figure 16-1A ▶**. If the injury doesn't permit the parent to hold the child on a lap, let the parent hold the child's hand or keep the parents where the child can see them.

Quickly try to develop rapport with the child. Tell the child your first name, find out what the child's name is, and use the child's name as you explain what you are doing. Do not stand over the child. Squat, kneel, or sit down and establish

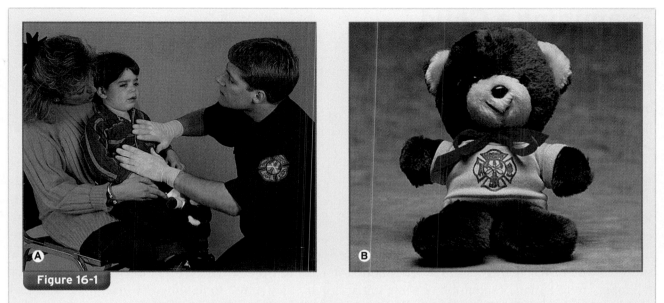

A. Allow the parent to hold the child if possible. **B.** The trauma teddy bear helps keep a child calm while being examined.

eye contact. Ask the child simple questions about the pain and ask the child to help you by pointing to (or touching) the painful area.

Be honest with the child. For instance, if you must move an arm or leg in order to splint it, tell the child what you are going to do and explain that the movement may hurt. Ask the child to help by being calm, lying still, or holding a bandage. The level of understanding and cooperation you can receive from an ill or injured child is often remarkable and may surprise you. Some emergency service agencies provide the child with a trauma teddy bear to hold while being examined Figure 16-1B ▲ .

Pediatric Anatomy and Function

Children and adults have the same body systems that perform the same functions, but there are certain differences, particularly in the airway, that you should know. A child's airway is smaller in relation to the rest of the body. Therefore, secretions or swelling from illnesses or trauma can more easily block the child's airway. Because a child's tongue is relatively larger than the tongue of an adult, a child's tongue can more easily block the airway if the child becomes unresponsive. Because a child's upper airway anatomy is more flexible than that of an adult,

you must remember to avoid hyperextending (overextending) the neck of an infant or child when attempting to open the airway. Position the head in a neutral or slight sniffing position, but do not hyperextend the neck. Hyperextension of a child's neck can occlude the airway. For at least the first 6 months of their lives, infants can breathe only through their noses. If an infant's nose becomes blocked by mucous secretions, the infant cannot breathe through the mouth. Therefore, it is important to clear the nose of an infant to enable breathing.

Children can quickly compensate as the demands on their respiratory system change. They can increase their breathing rate and their breathing efforts for a short period of time. However, they will "run out of steam" in a relatively short period of time. When this happens, the child may soon show signs of severe respiratory distress and rapidly progress into respiratory failure. Therefore, it is important to perform a complete and thorough patient assessment and to monitor the child's vital signs. Recheck the vital signs at least every 5 minutes when caring for seriously ill or injured pediatric patients.

Infants and children also have limited abilities to compensate for changes in temperature. Children have a greater surface area relative to the mass of their body. This means that they lose relatively more heat than adults do. Therefore, you need to keep the body temperature of children as close to normal as possible and warm them if they become chilled.

Examining a Child

Observe the child carefully when you first meet. Does the child appear to be ill or injured? Children often "look sick" or you may note an obvious injury Figure 16-2 ▾ . The child who is unresponsive, lackluster, and appears ill should be evaluated carefully because lack of activity and interest can signal serious illness or injury. Infants and young children normally cry in response to fear or pain; a child who is not crying may have a decreased level of consciousness, an upper airway infection, or swelling in the airway. If the child is crying, does the cry sound like a normal healthy cry or is it a subdued whimper? A systematic evaluation of these initial observations can be done using the pediatric assessment triangle, which is explained later.

After your initial assessment, carry out the routine patient examination described in Chapter 7, paying special attention to mental awareness, activity level, respirations, pulse rate, body temperature, and color of the skin.

Respirations

You can calculate the respiratory rate of a child by counting respirations for 30 seconds and multiplying by two. Counting for less than 30 seconds can cause inaccurate results because children often have irregular breathing patterns.

As you examine a child, look to see how much work the child is doing to breathe. This work of

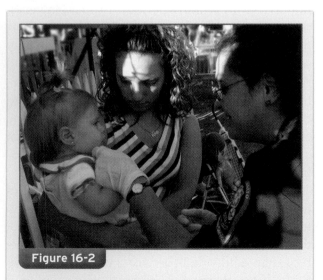

Figure 16-2

Observe the child carefully for signs of illness or injury.

breathing will help to determine if the child is in respiratory distress. Look for abnormal breath sounds such as noisy breathing, snoring, crowing, grunting, or wheezing. Look to determine if they are holding themselves in an abnormal position. Are they supporting themselves with their arms while leaning forward (known as the tripod position) or do they refuse to lie down? Check for retractions of the neck or chest. Look for flaring of the nostrils. The presence of any of these signs indicates that they are having some difficulty breathing and may be experiencing respiratory distress. Respiratory distress is discussed under respiratory emergencies.

Pulse Rate

The normal pulse rate of a child is faster than an adult's normal rate. For a child under 1 year of age, take the brachial pulse, which is halfway between the shoulder and the elbow on the inside of the upper arm or directly over the heart Figure 16-3 ▸ . Table 16-1 ▾ describes the usual, normal vital signs for children at various ages.

TABLE 16-1	Normal Vital Signs in Children at Rest	
Age	**Heart Rate**	**Respirations**
Newborn (0 to 1 month)	90–180	30–60
Infant (1 month to 1 year)	100–160	25–50
Toddler (1 to 3 years)	90–150	20–30
Preschool age (3 to 6 years)	80–140	20–25
School age (6 to 12 years)	70–120	15–20
Adolescent (12 to 18 years)	60–100	12–16

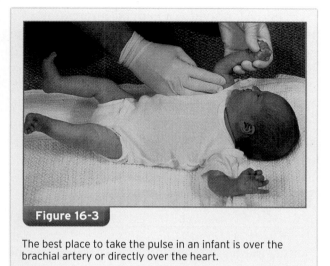

Figure 16-3

The best place to take the pulse in an infant is over the brachial artery or directly over the heart.

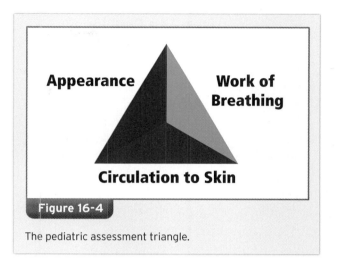

Appearance   Work of Breathing

Circulation to Skin

Figure 16-4

The pediatric assessment triangle.

High Body Temperature

High temperatures in children are often accompanied by flushed, red skin, sweating, and restlessness. You can often feel a high temperature just by touching the child's chest and head. A child's heart rate increases with each degree of temperature rise.

The Pediatric Assessment Triangle

It is important to form a general impression of a child's condition. The **pediatric assessment triangle (PAT)** is designed to give a quick general impression of the child using only your senses of sight and hearing. It is a valuable tool that can be used to assess a child from a distance and help you determine what steps need to be taken first. Three components of the PAT will help to determine the child's overall condition. These are: (1) the child's overall appearance, (2) the work of breathing, and (3) circulation to the skin **Figure 16-4 ▶**.

Appearance

The first leg of the pediatric assessment triangle is appearance. The child's general appearance is important in determining the severity of the child's illness or injury. The general appearance is an indicator of how well the heart and lungs are working. Appearance is also a good indication of how well the central nervous system is working. As you assess a child, compare his or her appearance and actions to what you would expect from a healthy child of the same age. Look at the child

to see if he or she has good muscle tone. Is the child crying or able to speak? Does the child have a blank, unfocused stare or does he or she look at others? Is the child able to interact in a manner that is age appropriate? If the child is conscious, it is better to start your assessment from across the room than to disturb the child by removing him or her from the caregiver's arms. A child with good eye contact, good muscle tone, and good color would seem to be normal. A child who makes poor eye contact and is pale and listless should be of concern to you. As you evaluate the initial appearance of a child, keep in mind that the child's appearance can change quickly. Therefore, you need to reassess the child's appearance regularly.

Work of Breathing

The second leg of the pediatric assessment triangle is the work of breathing. In children, assessing the work of breathing is a more accurate indicator of a child's condition than merely determining the rate of respirations. The work of breathing is determined by measuring four factors: (1) abnormal breath sounds, (2) abnormal positioning, (3) retractions of the neck or chest, and (4) flaring of the nostrils. Abnormal breath sounds include noisy breathing, snoring, crowing, grunting, or wheezing. Abnormal positioning includes leaning forward while supporting themselves with their arms and a refusal to lie down. Retractions can occur above the collarbone or between the ribs. Flaring of the nostrils occurs during inspiration. Assess

TABLE 16-2	Characteristics of Work of Breathing
Characteristic	**Features to Look for**
Abnormal breath sounds	Noisy breathing, snoring, crowing, grunting, or wheezing
Abnormal positioning	Leaning forward while using the arms for support
Retractions	Retractions above the collarbone or between the ribs
Flaring	Flaring of the nostrils

these four factors to determine the work of breathing Table 16-2 ▲ . This assessment can be made without touching the child and can be done across the room.

Circulation to the Skin

The third leg of the pediatric assessment triangle is circulation to the skin. The three characteristics for determining circulation to the skin are paleness, mottling, and cyanosis. Check the skin for paleness or pallor. White or pale skin indicates an inadequate blood flow to the skin. The second characteristic of circulation to the skin is mottling. **Mottling** is a patchy skin discoloration that is caused by too little or too much circulation to the skin. The third characteristic used in assessing the skin is cyanosis. Cyanosis is a bluish discoloration of the skin that is caused by low levels of oxygen in the blood Table 16-3 ▾ . You can establish the status of the circulation to the skin without touching the child.

TABLE 16-3	Characteristics of Circulation to the Skin
Characteristic	**Features to Look for**
Pallor	White or pale skin or mucous membranes
Mottling	Patchy skin discoloration caused by too much or too little blood flow to the skin
Cyanosis	Bluish discoloration of the skin and mucous membranes

The PAT provides a general impression of a pediatric patient and will help to determine the severity of the child's illness or injury. It should be used with the other parts of the patient assessment sequence that you learned in Chapter 7. It is a helpful tool because it allows you to quickly obtain valuable information without touching and agitating the child, and it helps set the priorities for further assessment and treatment.

Respiratory Care

Neither adults nor children can tolerate a lack of oxygen for more than a few minutes before permanent brain damage occurs.

It is important for the first responder to open and maintain the airway and to ventilate adequately any child with respiratory problems. Otherwise, the child may suffer respiratory arrest, followed by cardiac arrest because of the lack of oxygen to the heart. This is a different situation than adults, who usually suffer cardiopulmonary arrest as a result of a heart attack.

Some of the specific causes of cardiopulmonary arrest in children include suffocation caused by the aspiration of a foreign body, infections of the airway such as croup and acute epiglottitis, sudden infant death syndrome (SIDS), accidental poisonings, and injuries around the head and neck. This chapter covers each problem in detail.

Treating Respiratory Emergencies in Infants and Children

Opening the Airway

Use the same general techniques to open the airway of a child or an infant that you use for an adult patient. The head tilt–chin lift technique can be used for children who have not suffered an injury to the neck or head Figure 16-5 ▸ . When using the head tilt–chin lift technique on a child, be sure that you do not hyperextend the neck when you tilt the head back. Hyperextending a child's neck can occlude the airway. Use a neutral or slight sniffing position. You can place a folded towel under the child's shoulders to help maintain this position. If the possibility of injury

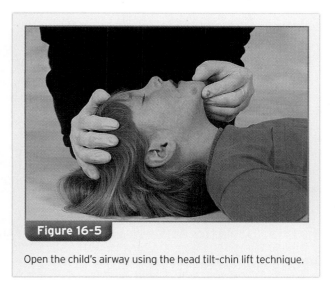

Figure 16-5

Open the child's airway using the head tilt–chin lift technique.

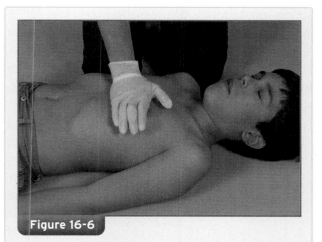

Figure 16-6

Place one or two hands in the middle of the chest, between the nipples.

to the head or neck exists, try the jaw-thrust technique to open the airway. If the jaw-thrust technique does not open the airway, you should use the head tilt–chin lift technique because opening the airway is a top priority for an unresponsive patient.

Basic Life Support

Because children are smaller than adults, you must use specific techniques when you perform CPR on children. There are special procedures for hand placement, compression pressure, and airway positioning.

CPR for children (1 year of age to the onset of puberty) is different from adult CPR in three ways:

1. If you are alone, without help, and EMS has not been called, you should perform five cycles or 2 minutes of CPR before activating the EMS system.

2. Use the heel of one hand or two hands to perform chest compressions, depending on the size of the child **Figure 16-6 ▲** .

3. Compress the sternum one half to one third the depth of the chest.

CPR for infants (less than 1 year of age) has six differences from adult CPR:

1. Check for responsiveness by tapping the foot or gently shaking the shoulder.

2. Give gentle rescue breaths, using mouth-to-mouth-and-nose ventilations.

3. Check the pulse by using the brachial pulse as shown in Figure 16-3.

4. Use your middle and ring fingers to compress the sternum just below the nipple line.

5. Compress the sternum to a depth of one half to one third the depth of the chest.

Suctioning

Airways that are blocked by secretions, vomitus, or blood should be cleared initially by turning the patient on the side and using gloved fingers to

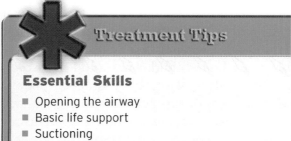

Treatment Tips

Essential Skills

- Opening the airway
- Basic life support
- Suctioning
- Using airway adjuncts

Treatment Tips

CPR for infants and children is described in detail in Chapters 6 and 9. To review these techniques, see these chapters.

scoop out as much of the substance as possible. You can use **suctioning** (aspirating or sucking out fluid by mechanical means) to remove the foreign substances that cannot be removed with your gloved fingers. Suctioning to open a blocked airway can be a lifesaving procedure.

The procedure used for suctioning infants and children is generally the same as for adults, with the following exceptions:

1. Use a tonsil tip or rigid tip to suction the mouth. Do not insert the tip any farther than you can see.
2. Use a flexible catheter to suction the nose of a child; set the suction on low or medium.
3. Use a bulb syringe to suction the nose of an infant. Remember that an infant can only breathe through the nose.
4. Never suction for more than 5 seconds at one time.
5. Try to ventilate and reoxygenate the patient before repeating the suctioning.

For a complete description of how to use suctioning, review the material presented in Chapters 6 and 15.

Airway Adjuncts

Oral airways can maintain an open airway after you have opened the patient's airway by manual means. Use the following steps to insert an oral airway in a child or an infant:

1. Select the proper size oral airway by measuring from the patient's earlobe to the corner of the mouth.
2. Open the patient's mouth with one hand using the jaw-thrust technique.

Treatment Tips

You must be careful not to overextend the neck. In infants and some small children, the overextension may actually obstruct the airway because of the flexibility of the child's neck. Smaller children may breathe easier if the neck is held in a neutral position rather than overextended. To maintain the neutral position, you can use a towel to support the shoulders.

3. Depress the patient's tongue with two or three stacked tongue blades. Press the tongue forward and away from the roof of the mouth.
4. Follow the anatomic curve of the roof of the patient's mouth to slide the airway into place.
5. Be gentle. The mouths of children and infants are fragile.

First responders usually do not use nasal airways for children. If you have questions about using nasal airways in pediatric patients, check with your medical director.

Partial or Mild Airway Obstruction

You can usually relieve a partial (mild) airway obstruction by placing the child on his or her back (supine), tilting the head, and lifting the chin in the usual manner (the head tilt–chin lift maneuver).

A blocked airway from an aspirated foreign object (small toy, piece of candy, or balloon) is a common problem in young children, particularly in children who are crawling. If the foreign object is only partially blocking the airway, the child will probably be able to pass some air around the object. You can remove the object if it is clearly visible in the mouth and can be removed easily. However, if you cannot see the object or if you do not think it can be removed easily, you should not attempt to remove it as long as the child can still breathe air around the object. Sometimes trying to remove an object that is partially blocking the airway can result in a severe airway blockage, which is an extremely serious situation.

Children with a partial (mild) airway obstruction should be transported to the hospital. You should talk constantly to a child with a partially obstructed airway about what you are doing. Talking also comforts the child and reduces the terror of having something "stuck in the throat."

The presence of a parent during transport can provide psychological support to both the parent and the child. The parent's presence can often reassure and calm the child. You should judge each situation carefully. Not all parents can remain calm themselves during such a serious situation. However, most of the time, when the parents realize the seriousness of the situation, they are able to redirect their emotions and work with you to reassure and calm the child.

If you have oxygen available and are trained in its use, administer it by carefully placing the oxygen mask over the child's mouth and nose. Do not try to get an airtight seal on the mask; hold it 1 or 2 inches away from the child's face. If you tell the child what you are doing with the oxygen and how it will make breathing easier, you may be able to calm and relax the child. Carefully monitor this critical situation to ensure that the mild obstruction does not become a severe obstruction!

Complete or Severe Airway Obstruction in Children

A complete or severe airway obstruction is a serious emergency. A severe airway obstruction exists when there is poor air exchange, increased breathing difficulty, a silent cough, the inability to speak, or no air movement because of an obstruction. You have only a few minutes to act before permanent brain damage occurs. Use the Heimlich maneuver (abdominal thrusts) **Figure 16-7 ▾** because it provides enough energy to expel most foreign objects that could completely block a child's airway.

Airway Obstruction in a Child

The steps for relieving an airway obstruction in a conscious child (1 year of age to the onset of puberty) are the same as for an adult patient. However, the anatomic differences between adults and children require that you make some adjustments in your technique. When opening the airway of

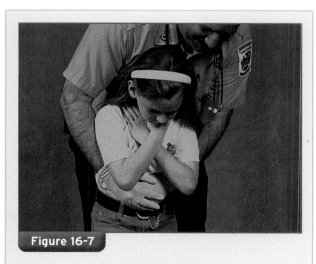

Figure 16-7

Performing abdominal thrusts on a child.

a child or infant, tilt the head back just past the neutral position. Tilting the head too far back (hyperextending the neck) can actually obstruct the airway of a child or infant. If you are by yourself and a child with an airway obstruction becomes unresponsive, perform CPR for five cycles (about 2 minutes) before activating the EMS system.

A skill performance sheet titled "Child: Foreign Body Airway Obstruction" is included for your review and practice **Figure 16-8 ▸**.

Complete or Severe Airway Obstruction in Infants

An infant (under 1 year of age) is very fragile. Infants' airway structures are very small and they are more easily injured than those of an adult. If you suspect an airway obstruction, first assess the baby to determine if there is any air exchange. If the baby is crying, the airway is not completely obstructed. If no air is moving in or out of the baby's mouth and nose, suspect an obstructed airway. Find out what was happening when the episode began. Someone may have seen the baby put a foreign body into the mouth. To relieve an airway obstruction in a conscious infant, use a combination of back slaps and the **chest-thrust maneuver**. Be sure you are holding the infant securely as you alternate the back slaps and the chest thrusts.

Airway Obstruction in an Infant

If there is no movement of air from the infant's mouth and nose, a sudden onset of severe breathing difficulty, a silent cough, or a silent cry, suspect a severe airway obstruction. To relieve an airway obstruction in an infant, use a combination of back slaps and chest thrusts. Review the following sequence until you can carry it out automatically. To assist a conscious infant with a severe airway obstruction, you must:

1. Assess the infant's airway and breathing status. Determine that there is no air exchange.
2. Place the infant in a face-down position over one arm so that you can deliver five back slaps. Support the infant's head and neck with one hand and place the infant face-down with the head lower than the trunk. Rest the infant on your forearm and support your forearm with

Child: Foreign Body Airway Obstruction

Steps	Adequately Performed
1. Ask "Are you choking?"	
2. Give abdominal thrusts.	
3. Repeat thrusts until foreign body is dislodged or until patient becomes unresponsive.	
If the patient becomes unresponsive:	
4. If a second rescuer is available, have him or her activate the EMS system.	
5. Begin CPR: ■ Open the airway by using the head tilt-chin lift technique. ■ Look into the mouth for any foreign object. Use finger sweeps only if you can see a foreign object. ■ Give two rescue breaths. ■ If first breath is unsuccessful, retilt the child's head and reattempt ventilation. ■ If both breaths are unsuccessful, administer 30 chest compressions. (This part of the CPR sequence is covered in Chapter 9).	
6. Continue CPR for five cycles (about 2 minutes) and then activate the EMS system if you are by yourself.	
7. Continue CPR until more advanced EMS personnel arrive.	

*If victim is unresponsive but breathing , place in recovery position.
Source: Based on the 2005 CPR and ECC guidelines.

Figure 16-8

Skill Performance Sheet.

your thigh. Use the heel of your hand and deliver five back slaps forcefully between the infant's shoulder blades **Figure 16-9A ▶** .

3. Support the head and turn the infant face-up by sandwiching the infant between your hands and arms. Rest the infant on his or her back with the head lower than the trunk.

4. Deliver five chest thrusts in the middle of the sternum. Use two fingers and deliver the thrusts firmly **Figure 16-9B ▶** .

5. Repeat the series of back slaps and chest thrusts until the foreign object is expelled or until the infant becomes unresponsive.

If the infant becomes unresponsive, continue with the steps below.

6. Ensure that EMS has been activated.

7. Begin CPR:
■ Open the airway by using the head tilt–chin lift maneuver.
■ Look into the mouth for any foreign object. Use the finger sweep only if you can see a foreign object.
■ Give two rescue breaths.
■ Administer 30 chest compressions. (This part of the CPR sequence is covered in Chapter 9.)

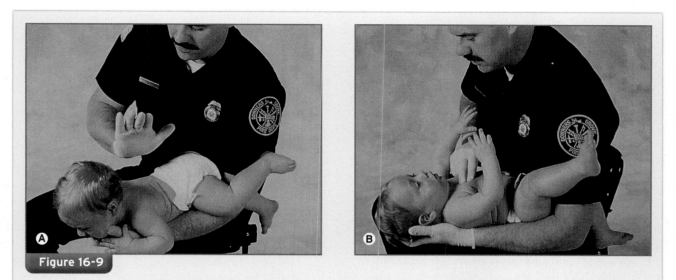

Figure 16-9

Administering back slaps and chest thrusts in an infant. **A.** Hold the infant face-down with the body resting on your forearm. Support the jaw and face with your hand without blocking the airway and keep the head lower than the rest of the body. Give the infant five back slaps between the shoulder blades, using the heel of your hand. **B.** Sandwich the infant between your hands, turn the infant over, and give the infant five quick chest thrusts, using two fingers placed on the lower half of the sternum (finger position should be the same as CPR for infants).

8. Continue these CPR steps until more advanced EMS personnel arrive.

Note: If you are alone, administer CPR for five cycles (about 2 minutes) and then activate EMS.

Recent studies have shown that administering chest compressions on an unresponsive patient increases the pressure in the chest similar to administering chest thrusts and may relieve an airway obstruction. Therefore, performing CPR on an infant who has become unresponsive has the same effect as administering chest thrusts on a conscious patient.

A skill performance sheet titled "Infant: Foreign Body Airway Obstruction" is included in **Figure 16-10 ▸** for your review and practice.

Swallowed Objects

Children often swallow small, round objects like marbles, beads, buttons, and coins. If they do not become airway obstructions, they usually pass uneventfully through the child and are eliminated in a bowel movement. However, sharp or straight objects such as open safety pins, bobby pins, and bones are dangerous if swallowed. Arrange for **prompt transport** to an appropriate medical facility because special instruments and techniques are required to locate and remove the object from the stomach and intestinal tract.

Respiratory Distress

Respiratory distress indicates that a child has a serious problem that requires immediate medical attention. Often respiratory distress quickly leads to respiratory failure.

You must be able to recognize the following signs of respiratory distress:

1. A breathing rate of more than 60 breaths per minute in infants
2. A breathing rate of more than 30 to 40 breaths per minute in children
3. Nasal flaring on each breath
4. Retraction of the skin between the ribs and around the neck muscles
5. Stridor (a high-pitched sound on inspiration)
6. Cyanosis of the skin
7. Altered mental status
8. Combativeness or restlessness

If any of the listed signs is present, try to determine the cause. Support the child's respirations by placing the child in a comfortable position, usually sitting. Keep the child as calm as possible by letting a parent hold the child if practical. Prepare to administer oxygen if it is available and you are trained in its use. Monitor the child's vital signs and arrange for **prompt transport** to an appropriate medical facility.

Infant: Foreign Body Airway Obstruction

Steps	Adequately Performed
1. Confirm severe airway obstruction. Check for sudden onset of serious breathing difficulty, ineffective cough, silent cough, or silent cry	
2. Give five back slaps and five chest thrusts.	
3. Repeat Step 2 until foreign body is dislodged or until infant becomes unresponsive.	
If the infant becomes unresponsive:	
4. If a second rescuer is available, have him or her activate EMS.	
5. Begin CPR: ■ Open the airway by using the head tilt-chin lift maneuver. ■ Look into the mouth for any foreign object. Use finger sweeps only if you can see a foreign object. ■ Give two rescue breaths. ■ If first breath is unsuccessful, retilt head and reattempt ventilation. ■ If both breaths are unsuccessful, administer chest compressions. (This part of the CPR sequence is covered in Chapter 9.)	
6. Continue these steps for five cycles (about 2 minutes) and then activate EMS if you are alone.	
7. Continue CPR until more advanced EMS personnel arrive.	

Source: Based on the 2005 CPR and ECC guidelines.

Figure 16-10

Skill Performance Sheet.

Respiratory Failure/Arrest

Respiratory failure often results as respiratory distress proceeds. It can be caused by many of the same factors that cause respiratory distress.

Respiratory failure is characterized by the following conditions:

1. A breathing rate of fewer than 20 breaths per minute in an infant
2. A breathing rate of fewer than 10 breaths per minute in a child
3. Limp muscle tone
4. Unresponsiveness
5. Decreased or absent heart rate
6. Weak or absent distal pulses

A child in respiratory failure is on the verge of respiratory and cardiac arrest. You must immediately assess the child and take whatever steps are appropriate to support the patient. Support respirations by performing mouth-to-mask ventilations. Administer oxygen if it is available and you have been trained to use it. Begin chest compressions if the heart rate is absent or below 60 beats per minute. Arrange for **prompt transport** to an appropriate medical facility. Continue to monitor the patient's vital signs and support the airway, breathing, and circulation functions as well as you can.

Circulatory Failure

The most common cause of circulatory failure in children is respiratory failure. Uncorrected respiratory failure in children can lead to circulatory failure and uncorrected circulatory failure can lead to cardiac arrest. That is why it is so important to correct respiratory failure before it progresses to circulatory failure. However, this is not always possible, so you should learn the signs of circulatory failure and its treatment. An increased heart rate, pale or bluish skin, and changes in mental status indicate circulatory failure. If the child or infant's heart rate is more than 60 beats per minute, your treatment consists of completing the patient assessment sequence, supporting ventilations, administering oxygen if available, and observing vital signs for any changes. If the heart rate of a child or infant is less than 60 beats per minute and there are signs of poor circulation such as cyanosis, you should begin chest compressions and rescue breathing.

Sudden Illness and Medical Emergencies

Not many illnesses occur suddenly in young children, but most of the medical calls for children will involve these sudden illnesses. It is important that you be able to recognize and treat these key pediatric illnesses.

Treating Altered Mental Status

Altered mental status in children can be caused by a variety of conditions, including low blood sugar, poisoning, postseizure state, infection, head trauma, and decreased oxygen levels. Sometimes you will be able to determine the cause of the altered mental status and take steps to correct the problem. For example, if the parent tells you that the child is diabetic and suffering from insulin shock, you can give sugar to in-

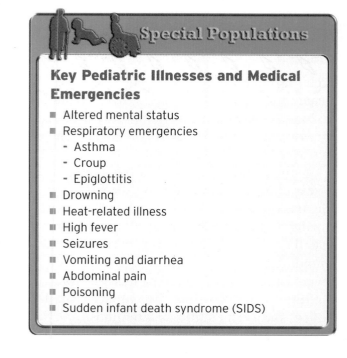

Special Populations

Key Pediatric Illnesses and Medical Emergencies

- Altered mental status
- Respiratory emergencies
  - Asthma
  - Croup
  - Epiglottitis
- Drowning
- Heat-related illness
- High fever
- Seizures
- Vomiting and diarrhea
- Abdominal pain
- Poisoning
- Sudden infant death syndrome (SIDS)

crease the patient's blood sugar. However, in many cases, you will not be able to determine the cause and will have to treat the patient's symptoms.

Complete your patient assessment, paying particular attention to any clues at the scene. Question any bystanders or family about the situation and try to get as much medical history as possible. Pay particular attention to the patient's initial vital signs. Recheck vital signs regularly to monitor any changes. Calm the patient and the patient's family. Be prepared to support the patient's airway, breathing, and circulation if needed. Place unconscious patients in the recovery position to help keep an open airway and to aid them in handling their secretions.

Treating Respiratory Emergencies

A respiratory problem in an infant or child can range from a minor cold to complete blockage of the airway. Because infants breathe primarily through their noses, even a minor cold can cause breathing difficulties. The excessive mucus in the nose resulting from a cold makes it more difficult for an infant to breathe than for an older child who can breathe through both the nose and mouth. Although most common respiratory problems in children are caused by colds, you should also be able to recognize and treat the three more serious conditions: asthma, croup, and epiglottitis.

Asthma

A child who has **asthma** is usually already being treated for the condition by a physician and is taking a prescribed medication. The parents call for assistance or transport only if the child experiences unusual breathing difficulty.

Asthma can occur in children greater than 1 year of age; it is rare during the first year of life. It is caused by a spasm or constriction (narrowing) of the smaller airways in the lungs that usually produces a characteristic wheezing sound. Asthma attacks can range from mild to severe and can be triggered by many factors, including feathers, animal fur, tobacco smoke, pollen, and even emotional situations.

A child who is having an asthma attack is in obvious respiratory distress. During a severe attack, you can often hear the characteristic wheezing on exhalation—even without a stethoscope. The child can inhale air without difficulty but must labor to exhale. The effort to exhale is both frightening and tiring for the child.

Your primary treatment consists of calming and reassuring both the parents and the child. Tell them everything possible is being done and encourage them to relax.

Place the child in a sitting position to make breathing more comfortable. Ask the child to purse his or her lips, as if blowing up a balloon. Tell the child to blow out with force while doing this. Pursed-lip breathing helps in two ways: Both parents and the child feel that "something is being done" and this type of breathing relieves some of the internal lung pressures that cause the asthma attack **Figure 16-11 ▶** .

If a child has asthma medication but has not yet taken it, help the parent administer the medication. The parents should contact the child's physician for further advice. If the child's physician is not available, arrange for **prompt transport** to a hospital emergency department.

Croup

Croup is an infection of the upper airway that usually occurs in children from 6 months to 4 years of age. The lower throat swells and

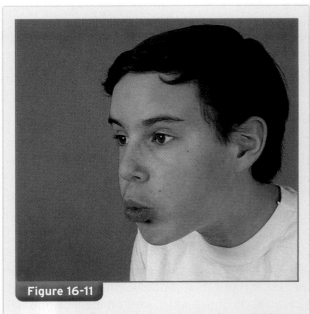

Figure 16-11

Pursed-lip breathing can help relieve an asthma attack.

compresses (narrows) the airway, resulting in a characteristic hoarse, whooping noise during inhalation and a seal-like barking cough.

Croup occurs often in colder climates (during fall and winter) and is frequently accompanied by a cold. The child usually has a moderate fever and a croupy noise that has developed over time. The worst attacks of croup usually occur in the middle of the night. Lack of fright or anxiety and a willingness to lie down are important because they help you distinguish croup from epiglottitis. Epiglottitis is a more serious condition discussed in the next section.

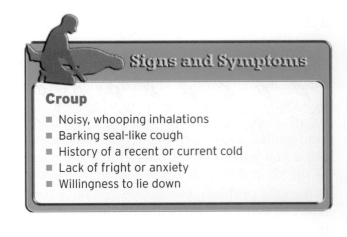

Signs and Symptoms

Croup

- Noisy, whooping inhalations
- Barking seal-like cough
- History of a recent or current cold
- Lack of fright or anxiety
- Willingness to lie down

Voices of Experience

Who Said Pediatric Calls Aren't "Basic" in Nature?

The unsettling call of a "baby not breathing" was the dispatch we received on that quiet Sunday afternoon. As we approached the house in the ambulance, a hysterical mother met us on the sidewalk. The baby was still inside the house with the grandmother. As I ran into the house with my airway bag, the mother was screaming the answers to my questions. I learned that the baby had been crawling and then appeared to collapse to the floor. I asked her one of the standard questions, "Does the baby have any allergies or past medical history that we need to know about?" The mother very audibly stated, "NO!" As we entered the house, I saw that the grandmother was on the floor with the lifeless baby. She was on the phone with dispatch, trying to administer CPR. The baby was unresponsive and very cyanotic in color. I began what we learned in CPR class: checking unresponsiveness, opening the airway, and giving two breaths, but then I noticed that the air was not going in. I repositioned the baby's head and tried again. The air still did not go in. I began looking on the floor, which was very clean, and only noticed a Winnie the Pooh pacifier on the floor. I was baffled. What is going on with this baby's airway? My plan was to get a secure airway prior to leaving; we could perform the other interventions en route to the hospital. I began the obstruction protocol for this baby with back slaps and chest compressions, and then visualizing for anything in the mouth. I decided to open the mouth a little wider to make sure there wasn't anything in the mouth before I began a more advanced procedure. Once I got past the tongue, I could see that there was a flesh-colored object sitting at the back of the throat. I thought, "What is that?" I grabbed my Magill forceps and pulled it out. Believe it or not, it was the tip of the pacifier. I grabbed the pacifier that was on the ground and sure enough, it was missing the end portion. You could see where the infant's teeth had bit down on it and severed it. My partner began BVM ventilations with good rise and fall of the chest. Within four respirations, the baby began coughing and crying and his color was returning. We transported the baby to the hospital for an exam and everything turned out to be just fine.

> **Knowing and understanding the basics can save you time, effort, and energy.**

The main lesson that I learned from this call is: In EMS, it is all about the basics. EMS providers love to get into the advancement of our profession, which is absolutely great and needed at times, but sometimes the basics are all we need to make wonderful things happen. It is great to learn as much as there is to learn about emergency medical services, but never forget the basics. Sometimes knowing and understanding the basics can save you time, effort, and energy. The knowledge of a first responder is used across all levels of emergency medicine and it is the foundation for any pediatric call.

Tammy Samarripa, AAS, EMT-LP
EMT/Paramedic Course Coordinator
Central Texas College
Killeen, Texas

Although croup is frightening for parents, it may not frighten children. As with many childhood emergencies, you must respond to the psychological needs and concerns of the parents as well as the medical needs of the child. Do not assume that noisy breathing is caused by croup! Look to see if the child is choking on a toy, food, or foreign object caught in the airway.

If the EMS unit is delayed, ask the parents to turn on the hot water in the shower and close the bathroom door. After the bathroom steams up, ask the parents to wait in there with the child until the EMS unit arrives. The moist, warm air relaxes the vocal cords and lessens the croupy noise. This effectively treats the child and reassures the parents. Have the parents contact the child's physician for further instructions or arrange for **transport** to an appropriate medical facility.

Epiglottitis

The third, and most severe, major respiratory problem is epiglottitis. __Epiglottitis__ is a severe inflammation of the epiglottis, the small flap that covers the trachea during swallowing. In this condition, the flap is so inflamed and swollen that air movement into the trachea is completely blocked. Epiglottitis usually occurs in children from 3 to 6 years of age.

At first examination, you may think the child has croup. However, because epiglottitis poses an immediate threat to life, you must be able to recognize the differences and know the signs and symptoms of epiglottitis; this is a serious respiratory emergency. Little can be done except to make the child comfortable with as little handling as possible, keep everyone calm, administer oxygen (if you have it available and have been trained

Treatment Tips

The child with epiglottitis must have medical attention to ensure an open airway.

Signs and Symptoms

Epiglottitis
- The child is usually sitting upright (he or she does not want to lie down).
- The child cannot swallow.
- The child is not coughing.
- The child is drooling Figure 16-12 ▾ .
- The child is anxious and frightened (he or she knows that something is seriously wrong).
- The child's chin is thrust forward.

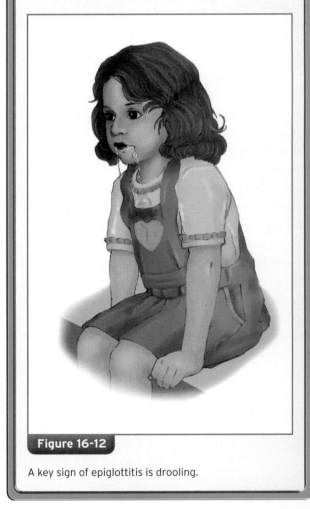

Figure 16-12

A key sign of epiglottitis is drooling.

Safety Tips

Do not examine a child's throat if you suspect epiglottitis! An examination can cause more swelling of the epiglottis, resulting in a complete airway blockage.

to use it), and arrange for **prompt transport** to an appropriate medical facility. You may consider letting a parent hold the child during transport if the emotional attitudes of the child and parent are appropriate.

FYI cont.
Drowning

Drowning is caused by submersion in water and initially causes respiratory arrest. It is the second most common cause of accidental death among children 5 years of age or younger in the United States. Although swimming pools, lakes, streams, and oceans present significant risks of drowning, ordinary water sources around the home increase the risk of drowning for young children. Children left unattended in washbowls or bathtubs—even a few minutes—can drown. Buckets of water and toilet bowls also pose threats to young children who put their heads down to look into the water, lose their balance, fall in, and are unable to get out.

The many sources of water around a home increase the chance that you, as a first responder, may encounter a drowning situation in responding to a medical emergency involving a child. If you respond to a drowning situation, make sure that you do not put yourself in danger as you attempt a rescue. (See Chapter 20 for more information on water rescues.) After the child is removed from the water, begin assessment and treatment. Signs and symptoms of drowning include lack of breathing and no pulse. Begin by assessing the airway, breathing, and circulation. Make sure the airway is clear of water. Turn the child to one side and allow the water to drain out. Use suction if it is available, start rescue breathing if necessary, and administer supplemental oxygen if it is available. If no pulse is present, start chest compressions. Because there is a chance that the cervical spine was injured, stabilize the neck. To reduce the risk of hypothermia, dry the child with towels and cover with dry blankets or jackets. Arrange for **prompt transport** of the patient to an appropriate medical facility. All patients who have experienced submersion need to be evaluated by a physician because they may develop serious respiratory problems several hours after submersion.

FYI
Heat-Related Illnesses

Heat-related illnesses may range from relatively minor muscle cramps to vomiting, heat exhaustion, and heatstroke. The most dangerous heat-related illness in children is heatstroke. Any child who is in a closed, parked car on a hot day or in a poorly ventilated room and who has hot, dry skin may be suffering from heatstroke. This is a serious and potentially fatal condition that requires rapid treatment from you to cool the child and reduce body temperature. Undress and sponge or immerse the child up to the shoulders with water and fan him or her to help lower body temperature quickly. You may wrap the child in wet sheets (if they are available) to speed up the evaporation and cooling process, but do not let the child become chilled. Finally, be sure that you have arranged for **rapid transport** to an appropriate medical facility. (See Chapter 10 for a more detailed description of heatstroke.)

Treating High Fevers

Fevers are quite common in children and can be caused by many different infections, especially ear and gastrointestinal infections. Because the temperature-regulating mechanism in young children has not fully developed, a very high temperature (104°F to 106°F or 40°C to 41°C) can develop quickly even with a relatively minor infection. Most children can tolerate temperatures as high as 104°F (40°C), but a high fever may require that the child be hospitalized so that the underlying cause can be discovered and treated.

Your first step in treating a child with a high fever is to uncover the child so that body heat can escape. Layers of clothing or blankets retain body heat and can increase body temperature high enough to cause convulsions. About 10% of children between 1 and 6 years of age are susceptible to seizures brought on by high fevers. Remember that in attempting to reduce high fever, you are only treating the symptom and not the source. The child must be seen by a physician as soon as possible to determine the cause of the fever.

If you encounter a child with a fever above 104°F (40°C), take these steps to treat the fever symptoms:

1. Make certain the child is not wrapped in too much clothing or too many blankets.

2. Attempt to reduce the high temperature by undressing the child.

3. Fan the child to cool him or her down.

4. Protect the child during any seizure (do not restrain the child's motion) and make certain that normal breathing resumes after each seizure.

Treating Seizures

Seizures (convulsions) can result from high fever or from disorders such as **epilepsy** (see Chapter 10). Seizures can vary in intensity from simple, momentary staring spells (without body movements) to generalized seizures in which the entire body stiffens and shakes severely.

Although seizures can be frightening to parents, bystanders, and rescuers, they are not usually dangerous. During a seizure, a child loses consciousness, the eyes roll back, the teeth become clenched, and the body shakes with severe jerking movements. Often, the child's skin becomes pale or turns blue. Sometimes the child loses bladder and bowel control and soils his or her clothing. Seizures caused by high fever usually last about 20 seconds.

If a seizure occurs, place the child on a soft surface (sofa, bed, or rug) to protect the child from injury during the seizure. Reassure the child's parents who may be frightened by the seizure. If they become too emotional, ask them to leave the room. Carefully monitor the child's airway during and after the seizure.

As a first responder, you can provide the following treatment for seizures:

1. Place the patient on the floor or a bed to prevent injury.

2. Maintain an adequate airway after the seizure ends.

3. Provide supplemental oxygen after the seizure if it is available and you are trained to use it.

4. Arrange for **prompt transport** to an appropriate medical facility.

5. Continue to monitor the patient's vital signs and support the ABCs if necessary.

6. After the seizure is over, cool the patient if the patient has a high fever.

FYI cont.

Vomiting and Diarrhea

Children are very susceptible to vomiting and diarrhea, which are usually caused by gastrointestinal infections. Prolonged vomiting and diarrhea may produce severe dehydration. The dehydrated child is lethargic and has very dry skin, which can be especially noticeable around the mouth and nose. Hospitalization may be required to replace fluids through the veins. If you suspect that a child may be dehydrated, arrange for **transport** to an appropriate medical facility.

Abdominal Pain

One of the most serious causes of abdominal pain in children is appendicitis. Although it can occur at any age, appendicitis is often seen in people who are between 10 and 25 years old. A cramping pain usually starts in the belly button area of the stomach. Within a matter of hours, the pain moves to the right lower quadrant of the abdomen, becoming steady and more severe. Usually the child is nauseated, has no appetite, and occasionally will vomit.

Because there are several potential causes of abdominal pain, including appendicitis, do not try to make a diagnosis in the field. Even physicians may find it difficult to diagnose the cause of abdominal pain. A good rule to follow is to treat every child with a sore or tender abdomen as an emergency and arrange for **transport** to an appropriate medical facility for an appropriate diagnosis.

Poisoning

Little children are curious and often like to sample the contents of brightly colored bottles or cans looking for something good to eat or drink. However, many common household items contain poisonous substances. The two most common types of poisonings in children are caused by ingestion and absorption.

Ingestion

An ingested poison is taken by mouth. A child who has ingested a poison may have chemical burns, odors, or stains around the mouth and be suffering from nausea, vomiting, abdominal pain, or diarrhea. Later symptoms may include abnormal or decreased respirations, unconsciousness, or seizures.

If you believe a child has ingested a poisonous substance, you should:

1. Try to identify what the child has swallowed, attempt to estimate the amount ingested, and send the bottle or container along with the child to the emergency department.
2. Gather any spilled tablets if the child swallowed tablets from a medicine bottle and replace them in the bottle so they can be counted. The emergency physician may then be able to determine how many tablets the child has taken.
3. Contact your local poison control center if transportation to an appropriate medical facility is delayed. The poison control center will need to know:
   - Age of the patient
   - Identification of the poison
   - Weight of the patient
   - Estimated quantity of the poison taken
4. Follow the directions provided by the poison control center. You may need to:
   - Dilute the poison by giving the child large amounts of water.
   - Administer activated charcoal if it is available and you have been trained in its use (the usual dose for pediatric patients is 12.5 to 25 grams).
5. Monitor the child's breathing and pulse closely. This is a critical step and you must be prepared to give emergency care, including rescue breathing and CPR.
6. Arrange for **transport** to an appropriate medical facility for examination by a physician.

> ### Treatment Tips
>
> Do not attempt to give liquids or induce vomiting in an unconscious or partially conscious child because of the danger of aspiration of the vomitus.

Absorption

Poisoning by absorption occurs when a poisonous substance enters the body through the skin. A child who has absorbed poison may have localized symptoms, such as skin irritation or burning, or may have systemic signs and symptoms of the poisoning, such as nausea, vomiting, dizziness, and shock.

If you believe a child has absorbed a poisonous substance, you should:

1. Ensure that the child is no longer in contact with the poisonous substance.
2. Protect yourself from exposure to the poison. Call for specially trained personnel if indicated.
3. Remove the child's clothing if you think it is contaminated.
4. Brush off any dry chemical. After you have removed all dry chemical, wash the child with water for at least 20 minutes.
5. Wash off any liquid poisons by flushing with water for at least 20 minutes.
6. Try to identify the poison and send any containers with the child to the emergency department.

> ### Safety Tips
>
> Be careful not to get any chemical onto your skin.

> ### Treatment Tips
>
> Chemical burns to the eyes cause extreme pain and injury. Gently flush the affected eye or eyes with water for at least 20 minutes. Hold the eye open to allow water to flow over its entire surface. Direct the water from the inner corner of the eye to the outward edge of the eye. After flushing the eyes for 20 minutes, loosely cover both eyes with gauze bandages and arrange for **prompt transport** to an appropriate medical facility.

7. Monitor the child for any changes in respiration and pulse. Be prepared to administer rescue breathing or CPR if needed.

8. Arrange **transport** to an appropriate medical facility for examination by a physician.

See Chapter 11 for additional information on emergency treatment of poisoning.

Sudden Infant Death Syndrome

A condition that is frequently mistaken for child abuse is sudden infant death syndrome (SIDS), also called crib death. It is the sudden and unexpected death of an apparently healthy infant. SIDS usually occurs in infants between the ages of 3 weeks and 7 months. The babies are usually found dead in their cribs.

Currently, no adequate scientific explanation exists for SIDS. These deaths are not the result of smothering, choking, or strangulation. SIDS deaths often remain unexplained, even after a complete and thorough autopsy.

You can imagine the shock and grief felt by parents who find their apparently healthy babies dead in bed. Your actions and words can help relieve their feelings of remorse and guilt.

If the infant is still warm, begin CPR and continue until help arrives (infant CPR is described in Chapters 6 and 9). In many cases, the infant has been dead several hours and the body is cold and lifeless. Do not mistake the large, bruise-like blotches on the baby's body for signs of child abuse. The blotches are caused by the pooling of the baby's blood after death. Sometimes you may find a small amount of bloody foam on the infant's lips. If the child is obviously dead, follow the protocol in your community for dealing with deceased patients.

Know your local guidelines for the management of SIDS. Remember that the parents could do nothing to prevent the death. Be compassionate and supportive during this tragic situation.

Pediatric Trauma

Trauma remains the number one killer of children. Each year, many young lives are lost because of accidental injury, particularly automobile crashes.

Treat an injured child as you would treat an injured adult, but remember the following differences:

1. A child cannot communicate symptoms as well as an adult.

2. A child may be shy and overwhelmed by adult rescuers (especially those in uniform), so it is important to develop a good relationship quickly to reduce the child's fear and anxiety.

3. You may have to adapt materials and equipment to the child's size.

4. A child does not show signs of shock as early as an adult but can progress into severe shock quickly.

Patterns of Injury

The patterns of injuries suffered by children will be related to the type of trauma they experience, the type of activity causing the injury, and the child's anatomy. Motor vehicle crashes produce different patterns of injuries depending on whether the patient was using a seat belt, whether the patient was strapped in a car seat, and whether an air bag inflated in the crash. Unrestrained patients tend to have more head and neck injuries. Restrained passengers often suffer head injuries, spinal injuries, and abdominal injuries. Children struck while riding a bicycle often have head injuries, spinal injuries, abdominal injuries, and extremity injuries. The use of bicycle helmets greatly reduces the number and severity of head injuries. Pedestrians who are struck by a vehicle often suffer chest and abdominal injuries with internal bleeding, injured thighs, and head injuries. Falls from a height or diving accidents tend to cause head and spinal injuries and extremity injuries. Burns are a major cause of injuries to children. Injuries from sports activities cause a wide variety of injuries depending on the type of sports activity. By learning some of the basic patterns of injury, you can anticipate the injuries you may find when carefully examining pediatric patients.

If the child has been hit by a car, look for the common types of injuries shown in **Figure 16-13 ▶**. Major trauma in children usually results in multiple system injuries. No matter what the cause of injury, your first priority is always to check the patient's ABCs. Stop severe bleeding, treat the patient for shock, and proceed with the head-to-toe examination described in Chapter 7 to determine the extent of any other injuries Figure 16-14 ▾ . The head-to-toe examination is a hands-on procedure. A complete examination is especially important because a child cannot always communicate symptoms. Involve the child in the physical examination as much as possible. Ask the child simple questions. Complete the head-to-toe examination even if the patient is too young to understand what is happening. Then stabilize all injuries you find. Splint suspected fractures, bandage wounds, and immobilize suspected spinal injuries.

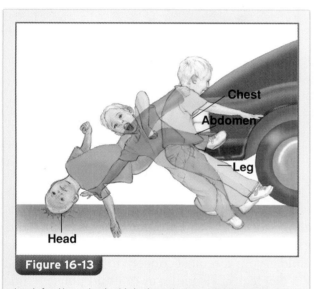

Figure 16-13

Look for these typical injuries when a child has been hit by a car.

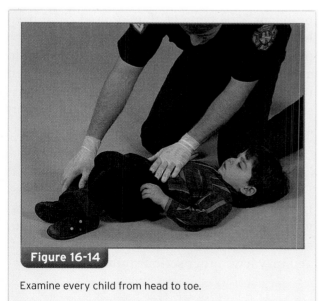

Figure 16-14

Examine every child from head to toe.

If you are dealing with head lacerations, remember that the generous blood supply to the scalp can result in severe bleeding. These wounds can be treated with direct pressure and appropriate bandaging techniques. See Chapter 13 for a review of effective bandaging techniques.

Traumatic Shock in Children

Children show shock symptoms much more slowly than adults, but they progress through the stages of shock quickly. An injured child displaying obvious shock symptoms such as cool, clammy skin; a rapid, weak pulse; or rapid or shallow respirations is already suffering from severe shock. It is vital that you learn to recognize and treat shock quickly. Review the signs and symptoms of shock in Chapter 13.

Immediate treatment for an injured child suffering from shock includes controlling external bleeding, elevating the feet and legs, keeping the child warm, and administering oxygen if it is available. Children who show signs of shock should be transported as soon as possible to an emergency department. Seizures are relatively common in children who have sustained a serious head injury. Be prepared to manage this problem by maintaining the airway and protecting the child from further injury.

The greatest dangers to any patient who has suffered trauma are airway obstruction and hemorrhage. The most important things you can do for the injured child are to:

- Open and maintain the airway.
- Control bleeding.
- Arrange for **prompt transport** to an appropriate medical facility.

 FYI

Car Seats and Children

The impact of mandatory child restraint laws means that first responders are finding more children still strapped into car seats after vehicle crashes. You should become familiar with child restraint seats and understand how to gain access to children restrained in them. If you find a child properly restrained in a car seat, leave the child in the car seat until the ambulance arrives Figure 16-15 ▸ . In many cases, a child can be secured in the seat, the seat removed from the vehicle, and both the seat and the child transported together Figure 16-16 ▸ to the hospital.

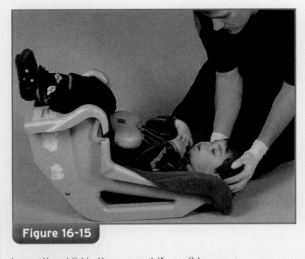

Figure 16-15

Leave the child in the car seat if possible.

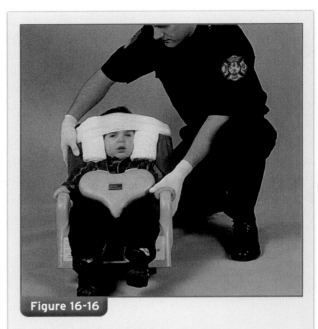

Figure 16-16

A child can be immobilized in the car seat.

Treatment Tips

Children under 9 years of age who are in seatbelts without a booster seat are at risk for sliding out of the lap belt during the crash. Rapid, jackknife bending increases the chances of intra-abdominal, spinal cord, and brain injuries.

Child Abuse

Child abuse is not limited to any ethnic, social, or economic group or to families with any particular level of education. Suspect child abuse if the child's injuries do not match the story you are told about how the injuries occurred. Child abuse is often masked as an accident. The abused or battered child may have many visible injuries—all at different stages of healing. The child may appear to be withdrawn, fearful, or even hostile. You should be concerned if the child refuses to discuss how an injury occurred. Occasionally, the child's parents or caretaker will reveal a history of several "accidents" in the past. Treat the child's injuries and, if you think you are dealing with a case of child abuse, ensure the safety of the child.

Make sure that the child receives **transport** to an appropriate medical facility. If the parents object to having the child examined by a physician, summon law enforcement personnel and explain your concerns to them. The safety of the child is your foremost concern in these situations.

Neglect is also a form of child abuse. Children who are neglected are often dirty or too thin or appear developmentally delayed because of lack of stimulation. You may observe such children when you are making calls for unrelated problems. The parents of an abused child need help and the child may need protection from the parents' future actions. Handle each situation in a nonjudgmental manner. Know whom you need to contact (usually the emergency department staff or law enforcement personnel) and report any instances of suspected child abuse.

Sexual Assault of Children

Sexual abuse occurs in children as well as adults. It may occur in both male and female infants, young children, and adolescents. In addition to sexual assault, the child may have been beaten and may have other serious injuries.

Signs and Symptoms

Child Abuse

- Multiple fractures
- Bruises in various stages of healing (especially those clustered on the torso and buttocks) **Figure 16-17A** ▾

- Human bites **Figure 16-17B** ▾
- Burns (particularly cigarette burns and scalds from hot water) **Figure 16-17C** ▾
- Reports of bizarre accidents that do not seem to have a logical explanation

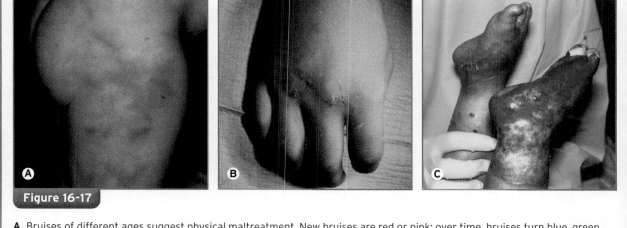

Figure 16-17

A. Bruises of different ages suggest physical maltreatment. New bruises are red or pink; over time, bruises turn blue, green, yellow-brown, and faded. **B.** A human bite wound has a characteristic appearance. **C.** Stocking/glove burns of the hands and feet in the infant or toddler are almost always inflicted injuries.

Signs and Symptoms

Neglect

- Lack of adult supervision
- Malnourished-appearing child
- Unsafe living environment
- Untreated chronic illness

If you suspect sexual assault has occurred, obtain as much information as possible from the child and any witnesses. Realize that the child may be hysterical or unwilling to talk, especially if the abuser is a brother or sister, parent, or family friend. A caring approach to these children is extremely important and they should be shielded from onlookers.

All victims of sexual assault should receive **transport** to an appropriate medical facility. Sexual assault is a crime and you should cooperate with law enforcement officials during their investigation.

First Responder Debriefing

As a first responder, you will respond to many calls that involve children. These calls tend to produce strong emotional reactions. At times you may experience a feeling of helplessness when an innocent child is seriously injured or gravely ill. You may be reminded of your own children when you see an ill or injured child. You may feel especially angry or helpless when you suspect the neglect or abuse of a child.

After you have completed your treatment and transferred the responsibility for care to other EMS personnel, you may need to talk about your frustrations with a counselor or with another member of your department. After a major incident or an especially emotional incident involving children, it may be helpful to set up a critical incident stress debriefing (CISD) session. Although you cannot change the types of traumatic events you see, you can use your department's resources to work through your feelings about these events. By debriefing, you can maintain a healthy approach to future calls.

You are the Provider SUMMARY

Review the *You are the Provider* case study provided at the beginning of the chapter.

Your unit is dispatched to a daycare center for the report of a sick child. After you and your partner arrive at the scene, you note a 3-year-old girl who is sitting in the lap of a daycare worker. She appears to have an increased rate of respirations and her breathing is noisy. Your partner examines the child while she remains in the caregiver's lap.

1. **What are the differences between the airway of an adult and the airway of a child?**

   There are several differences between a child's airway and an adult's airway. A child's airway is smaller in relation to his or her body than the airway of an adult. A child's tongue is relatively larger than the tongue of an adult. A child's airway is more flexible than the airway of an adult. These differences mean that a child's airway can be more easily closed by a foreign object or by swelling. It is important that you carefully assess, monitor, and correct airway problems in children.

2. **How can you quickly form an initial impression of the severity of this child's condition?**

   You can assess the overall condition of this patient by using the pediatric assessment triangle. Determine the overall appearance of the child, the work of breathing being done, and the quality of the circulation to the patient's skin. Using the PAT will give you a quick impression of the severity of this child's illness. Assessing a child using the PAT requires only your senses of sight and hearing.

3. **Why did your partner choose to examine this patient while the child remained in the lap of the caregiver?**

   Allowing the child to remain in the caregiver's lap helps to prevent the child from becoming upset. This makes your examination easier and your findings more accurate. Anything you can do to keep this child more comfortable and less frightened will help you to accomplish your patient-care goals.

Prep Kit

Ready for Review

The Ready for Review thoroughly summarizes the chapter.

- Sudden illnesses and medical emergencies are common in children and infants. Because the anatomy of children and infants differs from that of adults, special knowledge and skills are needed to assess and treat pediatric patients.

- Managing a pediatric emergency can be a stressful situation for first responders. Because both the child and the parents may be frightened and anxious, you must behave in a calm, controlled, and professional manner.

- A child's airway is smaller in relation to the rest of the body; therefore, secretions and swelling from illnesses or trauma can more easily block the child's airway. Because the tongue is relatively larger than the tongue of an adult, a child's tongue can more easily block the airway. Hyperextension of a child's neck can occlude the airway.

- The child who is unresponsive, lackluster, and appears ill should be evaluated carefully because lack of activity and interest signal serious illness or injury. After you conduct your initial assessment, you should carry out the routine patient examination, paying special attention to mental awareness, activity level, respirations, pulse rate, body temperature, and color of the skin.

- The pediatric assessment triangle (PAT) is designed to give you a quick general impression of the child using only your senses of sight and hearing. The three components of the PAT are overall appearance, work of breathing, and circulation to the skin.

- It is important to open and maintain the airway and to ventilate adequately any child with respiratory problems. Otherwise, the child may suffer respiratory arrest, followed by cardiac arrest.

- CPR for children and infants differs from adult CPR in several important ways. You should be certain that you understand these differences and are able to perform the appropriate steps confidently in the field.

- Suctioning removes foreign substances that you cannot remove with your gloved fingers from the airway of a child. Oral airways can be used to maintain an open airway after you have opened the child's airway by manual means.

- Young children often obstruct their upper and lower airway with foreign objects, such as small toys or candy. If the object is only partially blocking the airway, the child should be able to pass some air around it. You should attempt to remove the object only if it is clearly visible and you can remove it easily.

- In complete or severe airway obstruction in a conscious child, you should perform the Heimlich maneuver (abdominal thrusts). If the child becomes unresponsive, you should begin CPR.

- To relieve airway obstruction in an infant, use a combination of back slaps and chest thrusts.

- Children in respiratory distress require immediate medical attention. Signs of respiratory distress include a rapid or slow breathing rate, nasal flaring, retraction of the skin between the ribs and around the neck muscles, stridor, cyanosis, altered mental status, and combativeness. Respiratory distress can lead to respiratory failure, which in turn can lead to circulatory failure.

- Three serious respiratory problems are asthma, croup, and epiglottitis. A child who has asthma is usually already being treated for the condition by a physician; your primary treatment consists of calming and reassuring the parents and child. Croup is an upper airway infection that results in a barking cough. Although epiglottitis resembles croup, it is a serious respiratory emergency and you must arrange for prompt transport.

Technology

- Interactivities
- Vocabulary Explorer
- Anatomy Review
- Web Links
- Online Review Manual

Prep Kit

- Other pediatric medical emergencies include drowning, heat-related illnesses such as heatstroke, high fevers, seizures, vomiting and diarrhea, and abdominal pain.

- Children's natural curiosity may lead them to sample medications or household items that contain poisonous substances. The two most common types of poisonings in children are caused by ingestion (taken by mouth) and absorption (entering through the skin).

- Sudden infant death syndrome (SIDS), also called crib death, is the unexpected death of an apparently healthy infant. You should know your local guidelines for the management of SIDS. Remember that the parents could do nothing to prevent the death.

- When dealing with pediatric trauma patients, remember that you may have to adapt materials and equipment to the child's size and that children do not show signs of shock as early as adults, although they can progress into severe shock quickly.

- Major trauma in children usually results in multiple system injuries. Your first priority is always to check the ABCs and then stop severe bleeding, treat for shock, and proceed with the physical examination.

- If you suspect child abuse or sexual assault, you must transport the child to an appropriate medical facility.

Vital Vocabulary

The Vital Vocabulary are the key terms for this chapter.

asthma An acute spasm of the smaller air passages marked by labored breathing and wheezing.

chest-thrust maneuver A series of manual thrusts to the chest to relieve upper airway obstruction; used in the treatment of infants, pregnant women, or extremely obese people.

croup Inflammation and narrowing of the air passages in young children, causing a barking cough, hoarseness, and a harsh, high-pitched breathing sound.

drowning Submersion in water that results in suffocation or respiratory impairment.

epiglottitis Severe inflammation and swelling of the epiglottis; a life-threatening situation.

epilepsy A disease manifested by seizures, caused by an abnormal focus of electrical activity in the brain.

mottling Patchy skin discoloration caused by too little or too much circulation.

pediatric assessment triangle (PAT) An assessment tool that measures the severity of a child's illness or injury by evaluating the child's appearance, work of breathing, and circulation to the skin.

suctioning Aspirating (sucking out) fluid by mechanical means.

Technology

- Interactivities
- Vocabulary Explorer
- Anatomy Review
- Web Links
- Online Review Manual

Assessment in Action

Assessment in Action presents a fictitious scenario to help you review what you have learned in this chapter.

You are called to a home where a 3-year-old girl is sitting in her mother's lap. The mother tells you that her daughter seemed hot and did not eat or drink much all day. She says that the child vomited once. You notice that the girl's forehead seems hot.

1. In what order should you examine this child?
   1. Level of consciousness
   2. Head to toe
   3. Airway, breathing, and circulation
   4. Depends on the history of the illness
      A. 3, 4, 2, 1
      B. 3, 1, 4
      C. 1, 3, 2
      D. 4, 2, 3, 1

2. Based on the history and assessment of this child, which of the following conditions would be of concern to you?
   A. Possibility of seizures
   B. Possibility of gastrointestinal illness
   C. Dehydration
   D. All of the above

3. The best place to examine this child is:
   A. Lying on a table
   B. Lying on the floor
   C. In the mother's lap
   D. With the child on her back

4. If this child started to seize, you should do all of the following EXCEPT:
   A. Place the child on a soft surface.
   B. Monitor the airway after the seizure ends.
   C. Cool the patient after the seizure is over.
   D. Keep the child on her back.

5. Your first responder treatment in this case is to:
   A. Cancel any EMS units that have been dispatched to this address.
   B. Help arrange for transportation to an appropriate medical facility.
   C. Tell the mother to call her physician in the morning.
   D. Advise the mother that her child needs to drink some fluids.

Geriatric Emergencies

Chapter Objectives*

Knowledge and Attitude Objectives

1. Describe some of the physiological changes that occur with aging. (p 420)
2. Explain how to ensure more effective communication with elderly patients who have hearing or sight impairment. (p 421-422)
3. Describe why geriatric patients are at high risk for broken bones. (p 422)
4. Explain the types of cardiovascular and respiratory diseases that are prevalent among elderly patients. (p 423)
5. Describe how to approach the assessment and treatment of chronically ill patients. (p 424-425)
6. Explain your responsibility in dealing with patients who show signs of depression or dementia. (p 427)
7. Describe the purpose of hospice care. (p 428)
8. Explain the purpose of advance directives and living wills. (p 428)
9. Describe the signs and symptoms of elder abuse. (p 428-429)

Skills Objectives

There are no skills objectives for this chapter.

*These are chapter learning objectives.

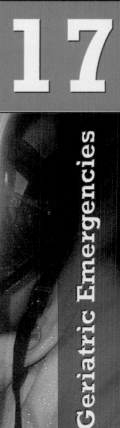

You are the Provider

At 2:09 AM, your dispatcher breaks the relative quiet of your radio: "Unit 429, respond to 592 West Buckeye Drive, Apartment 2B, for an 87-year-old man who has fallen. The patient is reported to be conscious." You remember that Buckeye Drive is located in a senior citizen's complex.

1. What medical conditions are more likely to be present with a patient this age?
2. Why should you be concerned about the increased possibility of broken bones with this patient?
3. How would your approach to this patient change if you learned that this patient had Alzheimer's disease?

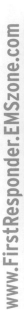

FYI

The material in this chapter is not required by the U.S. DOT National Standard Curriculum.

Introduction

A **geriatric patient** is commonly defined as a patient who is more than 65 years of age. The geriatric population of the United States is the fastest growing segment of society. The U.S. Census Bureau reports that there are 35 million people in the United States who are over 65 years of age. This chapter addresses concerns particular to geriatric patients, including sensory changes such as hearing loss and vision impairment, changes in mobility, and changes in medical conditions. Special considerations for the care of patients with chronic conditions are addressed. Mental conditions that commonly affect older patients such as depression and senility are covered. The chapter concludes with a discussion of end-of-life issues, hospice care, advance directives, and methods of recognizing signs of elder abuse.

The natural aging process results in a decline in the functioning of all body systems. This slow-down is gradual and begins shortly after the body reaches maturity. Heredity and lifestyle choices such as diet, stress level, and amount of exercise influence the speed with which this decline occurs.

It is important that first responders not pre-judge the physical or mental condition of older patients. Some people are vibrant and healthy at 80, while others suffer from chronic debilitating diseases at 50. The same is true of mental capacity: Although you may encounter middle-aged patients who have become senile, many elderly people retain their full mental capacity.

Because older patients experience health problems more frequently than younger people, most EMS systems respond to a great many calls involving geriatric patients. These calls will be much easier for you to handle if you understand some of the physical and mental changes involved in the aging process. These calls will also be less stressful for the patient and for you if you understand how to effectively communicate with older patients. You will achieve a greater rapport with older patients if you deal with each as an individual, rather than as a member of some arbitrary group defined by age **Figure 17-1 ▼**.

Elderly people often wear more clothing than younger people, even during warmer months. Do not use layers of clothing as an excuse to perform a less-than-complete physical examination: It is essential that you conduct a complete head-to-toe examination on all patients.

The loss of bowel and bladder control occurs frequently in the geriatric population. This situation can be distressing and embarrassing to both you and the patient. Do not let this problem interfere with appropriate patient care.

Technology

Interactivities

Vocabulary Explorer

Anatomy Review

Web Links

Online Review Manual

Figure 17-1

Deal with every patient as an individual.

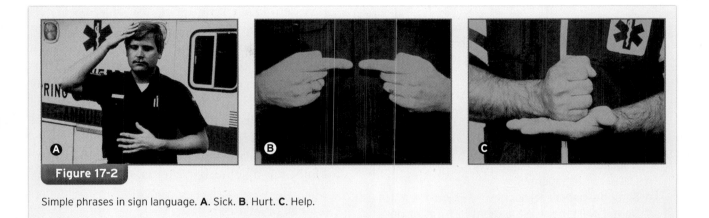

Figure 17-2

Simple phrases in sign language. **A.** Sick. **B.** Hurt. **C.** Help.

When responding to a call for an elderly patient, remember that the patient's spouse is probably apprehensive as well. Try to keep the spouse informed of what is happening to alleviate some of his or her anxiety.

Sensory Changes

Two of the most socializing senses are hearing and sight. Many people suffer some loss of hearing as they age and the ability to see often diminishes as well. For some older people, this means the need for reading glasses. Others develop conditions such as cataracts or macular degeneration, which may prevent them from driving or reading the newspaper.

Hearing-Impaired or Deaf Patients

Hearing loss is an invisible disability. Hearing loss may be related to repeated exposures to loud noises or to heredity. Often hearing losses are most pronounced in certain frequencies. This means that a person may be able to hear a person with a low-pitched voice but not hear a person with a higher pitched voice.

Be certain an elderly patient can hear and understand what you say. Make sure you identify yourself and speak slowly and clearly. If you think the patient has difficulty hearing you, do not shout. Ask the patient if he or she can hear you. Speak directly into the patient's ear or talk while facing the patient and maintaining eye contact. Many elderly patients read lips to help compensate for hearing loss. If this fails, write down your questions and offer paper and pencil to the patient to respond. Some emergency responders learn sign language so they can communicate with hearing-impaired people who know sign language Figure 17-2 ▲.

Visually Impaired or Blind Patients

During your initial assessment of the scene, look for signs indicating that the patient may be visually impaired. These signs may include the presence of eyeglasses, a white cane, or a service dog Figure 17-3 ▼. As you approach, introduce yourself to the patient. If you think the patient is blind, ask, "Can you see?"

A visually impaired patient may feel vulnerable, especially during the chaos of an emergency incident. The patient may have learned to use

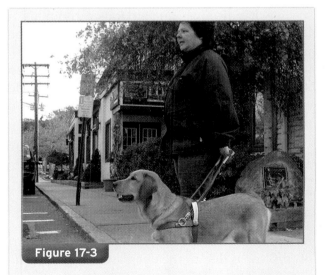

Figure 17-3

Blind patients may have a service dog.

Techniques for Communicating With Older Patients

- Identify yourself.
- Look directly at the patient.
- Speak slowly and distinctly.
- Explain what you are going to do in clear, simple language.
- Listen to the patient.
- Show the patient respect.
- Do not talk about the patient in front of the patient.
- Be patient.

other senses such as hearing, touch, and smell, to compensate for the loss of sight. The sounds and smells of an accident may be disorienting. The patient may have to rely on you to make sense of everything. Tell the patient what is happening, identify noises, and describe the situation and surroundings, particularly if you must move the patient. Find out what the patient's name is and use it throughout your examination and treatment, just as you would with a sighted patient. A reaffirming, supportive touch may provide psychological support.

If an older patient wears eyeglasses, keep them with the patient if at all possible. If the eyeglasses are lost during a medical emergency, search everywhere to try and find them! The patient may be severely handicapped and anxious without his or her glasses; knowing that the glasses are close and not lost will be a great relief. Imagine how you would feel if you were in an emergency situation and could not see; bring that understanding and empathy to your dealings with visually impaired patients.

Musculoskeletal and Mobility Issues

As a person ages, the muscles lose strength. Part of this loss is due to the decrease in physical activity, which can be offset by a good exercise program, and part is an inevitable part of the aging process. At the same time, the bones in the skeletal system lose strength because of a loss of calcium. This loss of bone strength is especially pronounced in postmenopausal women, who can develop a condition called <u>osteoporosis</u>. Osteoporosis is a decrease in the density of bone. Many older people also suffer some loss of balance due to a wide variety of reasons. Together the loss of muscular strength, weakened bones, and decreased balance result in an increased incidence of falls among elderly patients.

Slowed Movements

When you assist an older patient, remember that as a person ages, movements become slower. Lend a helping hand or supporting arm. Most elderly patients are afraid of falling and your support will help them overcome this fear. Allow enough time for patients to move safely rather than trying to rush them.

Fractures

Fractures occur often in the geriatric population because of the loss of bone density due to osteoporosis. Osteoporosis affects both women and men. Be aware that a simple fall at home can result in multiple severe fractures in an older patient who has weakened bones. Fractures of the wrist, spine, and hip are particularly common. Some of these fractures can occur with little trauma. Geriatric patients may also have a diminished awareness of pain. They may experience little pain even with a major fracture and they may not realize the seriousness of their injury.

Hip fractures are a common result of osteoporosis. They usually result from a fall and occur most frequently in elderly women. As you do your initial assessment, remember that other conditions may have contributed to the fall. Patients may have experienced a minor stroke, heart attack, or confusion before the fall or they may not have seen an obstacle.

In a hip fracture, the injured leg is usually (but not always) shortened as compared to the other leg. The toes of the injured leg are pointed outward (<u>externally rotated</u>) and there may be so much pain that the patient cannot move the leg. Every elderly patient who complains of pain after a fall must be X-rayed for possi-

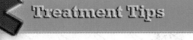

Treatment Tips

Carefully examine geriatric patients for signs and symptoms of fractures.

TABLE 17-1	Disabilities That May Occur With Age

- Hearing loss or impairment
- Sight loss or impairment
- Slowed movements
- Fractures
- Senility
- Loss of bowel or bladder control

ble fractures. Splint the patient as described in Chapter 14 and arrange for **prompt transport** to an appropriate medical facility.

The types of disabilities that occur with age are listed in Table 17-1 ▲.

Medical Considerations

With increasing age comes an increase in the incidence of many different medical conditions. Two types of medical conditions that cause the greatest number of deaths are cardiovascular diseases and respiratory diseases.

Cardiovascular Diseases

Cardiovascular diseases are conditions that affect the heart and blood vessels. Heart attacks, angina, and congestive heart failure are three common heart conditions that affect geriatric patients. Strokes and abdominal aortic aneurysms are two common conditions related to problems with blood vessels. Some patients may have suffered one of these conditions in the past. Their current medical emergency may be related to the ongoing results of a past stroke or heart attack. With other patients, the immediate cause of their medical emergency may be a heart attack or stroke that is occurring at that moment.

When dealing with geriatric patients, it is important to understand that the signs and symptoms of medical conditions may be different from the classic signs and symptoms you would expect. Often older patients have a decreased awareness or sensation to the pain of a medical or trauma condition. Older patients are more likely to have a silent heart attack where they do not suffer acute pain; hence they may not realize that they are suffering a heart attack. Some patients who are experiencing a stroke will not be aware of the signs and symptoms that are present. Treat older patients with a high degree of suspicion. It is better to err on the side of overtreating than it is to fail to treat and arrange for transport.

Respiratory Diseases

Respiratory diseases are another cause of sickness and death in elderly patients. There are two major types of respiratory diseases: chronic respiratory diseases and acute respiratory diseases.

Patients with chronic obstructive pulmonary disease (COPD) may live with this condition for many years. They call for emergency medical assistance when change in their life causes them to suffer shortness of breath. A cold or other respiratory infection can upset their normal equilibrium and result in a medical emergency.

Acute respiratory diseases can strike a patient quickly. Pneumonia is one infectious disease that is common in elderly patients. Because many elderly patients have a weakened immune system, they are especially susceptible to pneumonia. Pneumonia frequently kills older people. Minor symptoms can become a major illness in a short period of time. A physician should examine any elderly patient with congestion and a possible fever.

Your role in caring for elderly patients with a possible respiratory condition is to carefully examine them, secure an accurate medical history (past and present), treat their presenting symptoms, and arrange for **transport** to an appropriate medical facility when indicated.

Cancer

Cancer is a frequent cause of disability and death in elderly patients. Cancer can strike any part of the body. Patients do not call for emergency medical service because they have cancer. They call for help when complications from cancer result in acute pain, shortness of breath, or shock. These patients require prehospital support and then **transport** to a medical facility for stabilization. Patients with cancer and their families are experiencing a major family crisis. Your support and understanding will help them to get through this difficult time.

Altered Mental Status

Many of the medical conditions that commonly occur in elderly patients can result in altered mental status. Patients may be confused or unresponsive for a wide variety of reasons. Three common causes of decreased responsiveness in elderly patients are lack of adequate oxygen to the brain, low blood sugar, and hypothermia. These conditions can be caused by a variety of problems. Your treatment of patients with decreased responsiveness involves carefully assessing the patient and treating according to the signs and symptoms you note. Knowing some of the common causes of altered mental status may help you in treating these patients.

Medications

Because elderly patients suffer from a variety of chronic conditions, many of them take a large number of medications every day. They may be seeing several doctors for different conditions. If there is not good communication between these doctors, there is a chance that some medications may interfere with the action of other medications. Many medications have side effects, such as dizziness, when taken in excess quantities. Elderly patients may be taking many different types of medications so they may take the wrong dosage of a particular medication or miss doses altogether Figure 17-4 ▶ .

It is important for EMS personnel to determine what types of medication a patient takes. If the patient is being transported to a medical facility, gather up his or her medications and bring them to the hospital with the patient.

Chronic-Care Patients

Modern medical science has made great advances in treating patients with chronic conditions. In the past, most patients with serious chronic medical

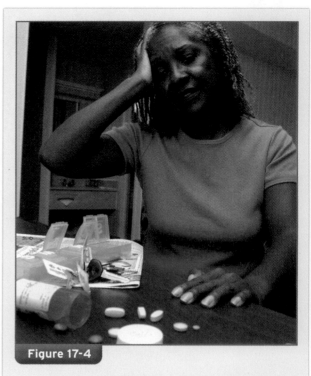

Figure 17-4

Elderly patients may take many different medications at the same time.

conditions were treated in hospitals or rehabilitation facilities; many died shortly after their conditions were diagnosed. Today, many patients are treated at home by nurses or family members and their lifespan has increased. Patients with chronic conditions may be of any age. Because the majority of patients with chronic problems are older, this topic is being addressed in this chapter. However, remember that young children with complex chronic-care conditions are often treated at home as well.

A variety of complex medical devices are used with chronic-care patients. Devices that help patients breathe include ventilators that push oxygen into the patients' lungs, oxygen-enrichment devices, surgically inserted breathing tubes, and monitors that sound an alarm if a patient stops breathing. Patients with certain heart conditions may have pacemakers and automatic defibrillators under their skin. Tubes inserted into a patient's arm, neck, or stomach may provide fluids or food. Catheters drain urine from the patient's bladder. To make matters even more complex, chronic-care patients must often take a wide variety of medications.

As a first responder, you may be called to assist with these patients for a variety of reasons, ranging from trauma or illness to mechanical failures or transport needs. What may be a minor illness for a healthy person can be life threatening for a patient with a chronic condition. Some patients fall and suffer musculoskeletal trauma, while others simply may need help getting back into bed. Medical equipment may stop working because the power or backup batteries failed. Patients may need transport to a hospital for assessment and treatment.

When you receive such a call, remember your role as a first responder. Your job is to assess the immediate problem and use your training to take the appropriate steps in caring for the patient. Do not get overwhelmed or distracted by the complex equipment **Figure 17-5 ▾**. You are not expected to understand how all these complex medical devices work. The people caring for the patient are familiar with the equipment they use each day. Do not be afraid to ask them about the equipment and condition of the patient. Do not hesitate to question the patient and the patient's caregivers about the problem. They can probably tell you what the problem is and how you can help. Keep in mind the principles of your training. These patients need open airways and adequate breathing and circulation. In most situations, you need to help stabilize the patient for only a few minutes until more highly trained EMS providers arrive to provide care.

Mental Considerations

Older people are not immune from mental problems. A wide variety of problems are experienced by this age group. Three types of mental problems seen frequently in older people are depression, suicide, and dementia or Alzheimer's disease. It is helpful for you to have some understanding of why these conditions are common in elderly people and what you can do when you encounter them.

Depression

Depression is the most common psychiatric condition experienced by older adults. It is estimated that there are 2 million older American adults who are suffering from depression. This condition is more common in women than in men. Depression is common among residents of nursing homes, assisted-living facilities, and with elderly

Special Populations

Do not overlook signs of mental health problems in elderly patients.

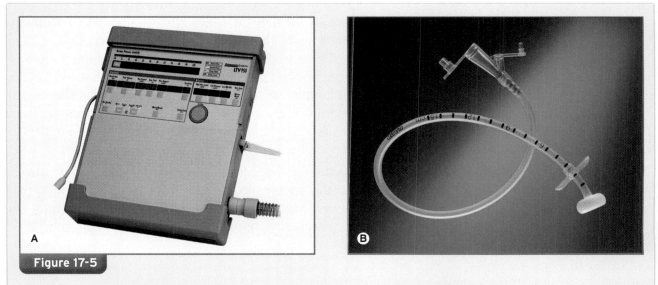

Figure 17-5

Complex medical devices may be used to treat chronic-care patients. **A.** Ventilator. **B.** Feeding tube.

Voices of Experience

Improving Lives by Caring

The most special person in my life was my grandmother. When I was a child, she taught me many things that still direct my life today. We used to have our heart-to-heart talks when I accompanied her on visits to some of her elderly friends who were in nursing homes. When I would question their confusion or need for assistance with simple tasks, my grandmother would point out how they had taken care of their children and family, now it was their time to be taken care of.

> **Some of the most important calls are the ones in which we help our patients in a more basic way.**

As EMS professionals, we all dream of helping with the large traumas and accidents that make the news. We enjoy the excitement, the infusion of adrenaline, and that powerful feeling of being needed. However, some of the most important calls are the ones in which we help our patients in a more basic way.

One day, while I was working in the yard, my husband drove into the driveway and said he thought that the woman living at the end of our road was in need of assistance. I asked if anyone had dialed 9-1-1, but he said "I think you had better check on her first." As I approached her house, I could see her inside an enclosed porch waving a white tissue. She was a frail elderly woman in her 80s with wispy grey hair in a neat twist. I opened the porch door and asked if she needed help. She had tears running down her cheek and was holding a portable phone. She held the phone out to me and said, "It doesn't work." I asked if she was hurt or needed any assistance. She just looked down and shook her head. The whole time I was talking, I was looking around at the house for hazards. All that training in assessment was working automatically. I was also looking at her, from head to toe, for apparent bleeding or injuries. As I took her arm and we walked back inside her house, she continued to cry and tell me how the phone was broken and she could not reach her son. I tried the phone and got a dial tone. I asked for her son's number and dialed it. It was ringing, but there was no answer. We sat on the couch while she explained how long she had lived in the house and how her kids use to play in the front yard. She was worried about her husband, who she said had not come home from work. I knew that she was confused because he had been dead for years. My EMS training and the wonderful lessons from my grandmother allowed me to really listen and ask the right questions. My neighbor was dehydrated and had not eaten properly for several days. Her son, who would normally check in on her daily, had been in the hospital. Her confusion and fear at not being able to reach anyone became overwhelming. I was able to comfort her and decrease her loneliness and uncertainty. As EMS providers, we learn what services are available and we can provide our patients and their families with a wealth of information that they might not have. I made a few calls and was able to get community services, Meals on Wheels, and visitation from the local church to assist in her care. For my dear elderly neighbor, those resources and my willingness to take the time improved her life and allowed her to continue living at home for a while longer.

As a first responder, it is important to treat older patients with respect and patience. It is important to understand that geriatric patients have different needs than other patients and that age-related factors can cause geriatric emergencies. In this case, the patient had not been involved in a trauma or physical emergency, but without assistance, her lack of care and her fear could easily have resulted in a true geriatric emergency.

Roxann Gabany, RN, BSBA EMT Instructor
EMS Educator
Peninsula Center for Life Support
Bena, Virginia

people living by themselves. The recent loss of a spouse or loss of a close friend can contribute to depression. People who are suffering from declining health, chronic health conditions, or terminal illnesses are especially likely to suffer from depression. Emergency medical providers should be aware of the high incidence of depression in elderly patients. You should be alert for signs and symptoms of persistent feelings of sadness or despair. If you observe signs or symptoms of depression, bring this to the attention of other EMS providers or other medical professionals.

Suicide

Older men have a high rate of <u>suicide</u> in the United States. When older people attempt suicide, they choose more lethal means than younger people do. This results in more deaths from suicide than in some other age groups. Many factors contribute to this. Physical illnesses, especially terminal ones, can lead to suicide. Loss of a loved one and alcohol abuse are also contributing factors. As a first responder, listen carefully to the patient. Be alert for indications of hopelessness, depression, or attempts at suicide. If you think a patient may be considering suicide, arrange for **transport** to an appropriate medical facility **Figure 17-6 ▸**. Be alert for your safety because weapons may be involved. Know the protocols in your department for handling this type of situation.

Dementia

As people get older, some of them experience a decrease in mental function. A pattern of decline in mental function is called <u>dementia</u>. Dementia is a progressive and usually irreversible decline in mental functions. It is marked by impairment in memory and may result in decreases in reasoning, judgment, comprehension, and ability to communicate verbally. It is estimated that 20% to 40% of people over the age of 85 have some degree of dementia. You may hear people refer to demented patients as suffering from <u>senile dementia</u>. Senile dementia is a general term used to describe abnormal decline in mental functioning seen in elderly patients. Dementia can be caused by many different conditions including small strokes, hardening of the arteries, and/or heredity.

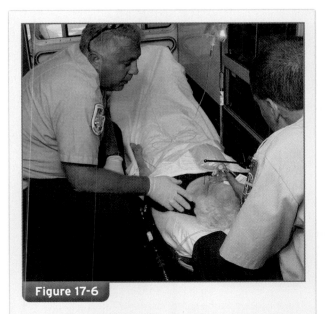

Figure 17-6

If you think a patient may be considering suicide, arrange for transport to an appropriate medical facility.

The most common type of dementia is <u>Alzheimer's disease</u>. Alzheimer's disease is a chronic degenerative disorder that attacks the brain and results in impaired memory, behavior, and thinking. It is estimated that Alzheimer's disease affects 4 million people in the United States. During the course of this illness, the patient may experience mood swings and feelings that people are plotting against them. Patients with Alzheimer's disease may wander at night and are at increased risk for falls. In the terminal stages of this disease, patients may be unable to walk, lose control of their bowels and bladder, and become unable to swallow.

When dealing with patients suffering from dementia, it is important to speak clearly to them using their name. Let the patient know what you are doing at each step of your assessment and treatment. You will need to rely on family members or caregivers for a medical history. Try to avoid asking the patient if it is OK to do something. It is better to inform the patient what you need to do. Realize that patients who are senile are confused and will pick up on your calm attitude and approach or they will pick up your apprehension and respond accordingly. A lot of nonverbal communication is possible with patients who are unable to communicate verbally. Your kind and caring approach will make the patient more comfortable and will make your job easier **Figure 17-7 ▸**.

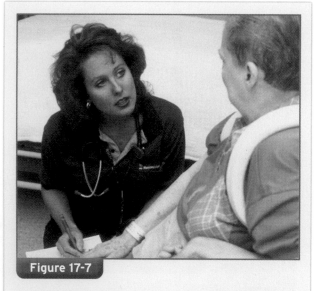

Figure 17-7

Use a kind and caring approach when dealing with patients who have dementia.

End-of-Life Issues

Hospice Care

A <u>hospice</u> is a health care program that brings together a variety of caregivers to provide physical, spiritual, social, and economic care for patients who have terminal illnesses and who are expected to die within the next 6 months. Hospice care is provided in the patient's home or in a special hospice facility.

The hospice's interdisciplinary programs are designed to provide pain relief and other supportive care when there is no hope that the patient can recover from the illness. One of the goals of a hospice is to provide pain relief without the use of needles or IVs. Pain relief is provided through oral medications, special pain-relieving patches, and medicine that is placed in the mouth between the gum and the cheek. Most hospice patients are suffering from some type of cancer.

When the hospice care is working well, EMS providers are usually not called. However, if the patient experiences unexpected problems such as shortness of breath, EMS may be requested by a family member or by a caregiver. In the event that you are called to care for someone who is under the care of hospice, it is helpful for you to know the purpose of the hospice and the types of care they give. Patients who are under the care

of hospice may have advance directives that request that they not be resuscitated. (See the following section for more on living wills and advance directives.) If there is any question about whether you should begin treatment, you should begin treatment and let the physician at the hospital make the decision about further treatment.

Advance Directives

Patients who have a terminal condition may have drawn up a document to give instructions to physicians and other medical caregivers regarding the care they want to receive if they are not able to speak to the caregivers. These documents are called advance directives, living wills, or do not resuscitate (DNR) orders. It is important for you to know the regulations concerning these documents in your state. Some states have systems, such as bracelets, to identify patients with advance directives. If you are not able to determine if a living will or advance directive is valid, you should begin appropriate medical care and leave the questions about living wills to physicians. You also should know your local protocols relating to advance directives.

Elder Abuse

Elderly people who are physically weak or mentally compromised are at high risk for abuse by a spouse, other family members, friends, or caregivers. <u>Elder abuse</u> is hard to detect because those who are at the highest risk of abuse are also isolated from public view if they are confined to their homes or to an assisted-care facility. As an EMS provider, you may be in a position to recognize physical or emotional abuse in geriatric patients. Elder abuse may be in the form of physical abuse, sexual abuse, emotional abuse, or neglect **Figure 17-8 ▶**. Patients with severe physical conditions or with senility may not be able to report abuse.

The signs and symptoms of abuse include bruises, especially on the buttocks, lower back, genitals, cheeks, neck, and earlobes. Look for pressure bruises caused by a human hand grabbing the patient. Look for multiple bruises in different states of healing. Burns are another means of abuse. These may be caused by cigarettes or hot fluids. Suspect

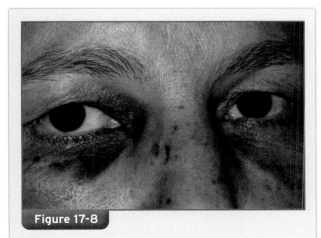

Figure 17-8

Physical abuse is one form of elder abuse.

sexual abuse if there is trauma in the genital area. Finally, look for signs of neglect. Does the patient appear to be malnourished? If you suspect abuse, you need to report it to the proper authorities. Learn the requirements for reporting elder abuse in your state and know how to follow the protocols for reporting within your department.

Many community-based programs assist in supporting geriatric patients who need physical assistance, nutritional support, or emotional help. It is only by reporting signs and symptoms of abuse to the proper authorities that the condition can be improved.

You are the Provider   SUMMARY

Review the *You are the Provider* case study provided at the beginning of this chapter.

At 2:09 AM, your dispatcher breaks the relative quiet of your radio: "Unit 429, respond to 592 West Buckeye Drive, Apartment 2B, for an 87-year-old man who has fallen. The patient is reported to be conscious." You remember that Buckeye Drive is located in a senior citizen's complex.

1. What medical conditions are more likely to be present with a patient this age?

Elderly patients are more likely to have some type of disease involving the heart, blood vessels, or lungs. Elderly patients may fall because they suffer from low blood pressure and black out when they get up suddenly. You should determine the patient's medical history and any past medical conditions. Try to determine the types of medications the patient is currently taking.

2. Why should you be concerned about the increased possibility of broken bones with this patient?

As people age, their bones become weaker due to the loss of calcium. Lack of physical activity contributes to this weakening. Often it is hard to determine if a patient fell because of poor balance or fainting, or

because he or she broke a bone. Elderly people often have a diminished perception of pain and may not realize that they have broken a bone. Therefore, it is important to thoroughly examine any elderly patient who has fallen for signs and symptoms of a possible broken bone.

3. How would your approach to this patient change if you learned that this patient had Alzheimer's disease?

If you were told that this patient has Alzheimer's disease, it is especially important to introduce yourself by name and use the patient's name when talking with the patient. You will probably need to get an account of what happened from a family member or caregiver. In addition, current medical conditions and medications often will have to be obtained from family members and caregivers.

Prep Kit

Ready for Review

The Ready for Review thoroughly summarizes the chapter.

- This chapter describes the special considerations and skills needed when working with geriatric patients.

- The natural aging process results in a decline in the functioning of all body systems, including sensory and musculoskeletal changes.

- Fractures occur often in older people because of the loss of bone density due to osteoporosis. A simple fall at home can result in multiple severe fractures in an older patient who has weakened bones. Fractures of the wrist, spine, and hip are particularly common.

- Common medical concerns for geriatric patients include cardiovascular and respiratory diseases.

- Many of the medical conditions that commonly occur in elderly patients can result in altered mental status, including lack of adequate oxygen to the brain, low blood sugar, and hypothermia.

- You may be called to assist with chronic-care patients for a variety of reasons, ranging from trauma or illness to mechanical failures or transport needs. What may be a minor illness for a healthy person can be life threatening for a patient with a chronic condition.

- Do not overlook signs of mental health problems in elderly patients. Three types of mental problems seen frequently in older people are depression, suicide, and dementia.

- Elderly people who are physically weak or mentally compromised are at high risk for abuse by a spouse, other family members, friends, or caregivers. As an EMS provider, you may be in a position to recognize abuse in geriatric patients. Elder abuse may be in the form of physical abuse, sexual abuse, emotional abuse, or neglect.

Vital Vocabulary

The Vital Vocabulary are the key terms for this chapter.

Alzheimer's disease A chronic progressive dementia that accounts for 60% of all dementia.

dementia A progressive irreversible decline in mental functioning; marked by memory impairment and decrease in reasoning.

depression A psychiatric disorder marked by persistent feelings of sadness, hopelessness, and decreased interest in daily activities. The person may have persistent thoughts of suicide.

elder abuse An action taken by a family member or caregiver that results in the physical, emotional, or sexual harm to a person over 65 years of age.

externally rotated Rotated outward, as a fractured hip.

geriatric patient A patient who is over 65 years of age.

hospice An interdisciplinary program designed to reduce or eliminate pain and address the physical, spiritual, social, and economic needs of terminally ill patients.

osteoporosis Abnormal brittleness of the bones caused by loss of calcium; affected bones fracture easily.

senile dementia General term for dementia that occurs in older people.

suicide Intentionally causing one's own death. Suicide is especially common in elderly and chronically ill persons.

Technology

- Interactivities
- Vocabulary Explorer
- Anatomy Review
- Web Links
- Online Review Manual

Assessment in Action

Assessment in Action presents a fictitious scenario to help you review what you learned in this chapter.

You are dispatched to a residence for the report of an elderly person with an unknown medical problem. Your dispatcher indicates that she does not have any further information because a neighbor made the call. When you arrive at the house, you are met by the neighbor, who states that Mrs. Jones "does not seem to be herself" today.

1. As you begin to talk to your patient, her neighbor states that she can't hear very well. Based on this information, you should:

   A. Not speak to her.
   B. Speak slowly and clearly while facing the patient.
   C. Shout so that the patient can hear you better.
   D. Have the neighbor talk to her.

2. During your examination of Mrs. Jones, you notice that she is dressed in several layers of clothing, even though it is about 80°F (26°C) outside. You should:

   A. Take her vital signs only.
   B. Remove her clothing only if she stays in a warm place.
   C. Remove as much of her clothing as you need to examine her properly.
   D. Do a less-than-complete physical exam.

3. There is an increased chance that Mrs. Jones may have a broken bone because of:

   A. Diabetes
   B. Senility
   C. Arthritis
   D. Osteoporosis

4. If it becomes necessary to transport Mrs. Jones to a medical facility, you should make sure that the EMS crew also takes along her:

   A. Medical insurance policy
   B. Coat
   C. Address book
   D. Medications

5. If this patient were blind, you should:

   A. Speak loudly so the patient knows where you are.
   B. Verbally explain everything you are doing during your assessment and treatment.
   C. Avoid touching the patient when not necessary because your unexpected touch may scare the patient.
   D. Secure the service dog in another area to prevent the dog from interfering with your assessment.

While returning to your station from the last call, you are dispatched to a nursing home for a patient who has fallen out of bed. When you arrive, a staff member takes you to the patient's room which has a couple of complex medical devices, one of which has an alarm sounding.

6. In regard to the medical equipment, you should:

   A. Unplug the equipment.
   B. Disconnect the patient from the equipment but leave it turned on.
   C. Disregard the equipment.
   D. Ask the staff member to explain the equipment.

EMS Operations

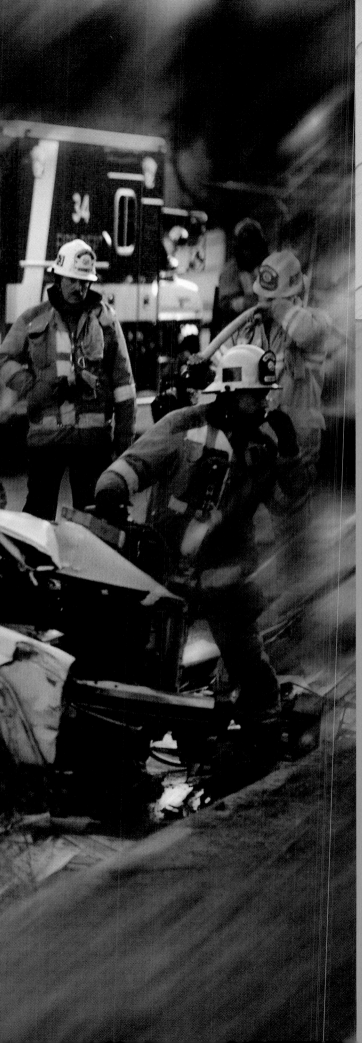

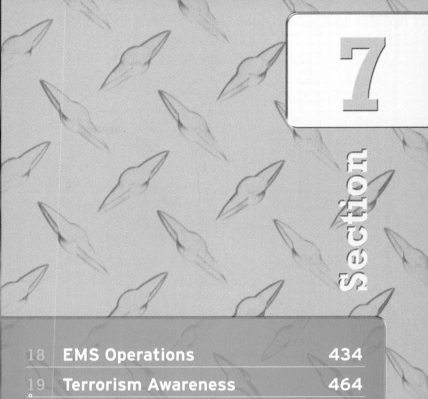

EMS Operations

National Standard Curriculum Objectives

Cognitive

7-1.1 Discuss the medical and nonmedical equipment needed to respond to a call. (p 436-437)

7-1.2 List the phases of an out-of-hospital call. (p 436-438)

7-1.3 Discuss the role of the First Responder in extrication. (p 439-440)

7-1.4 List various methods of gaining access to the patient. (p 445)

7-1.5 Distinguish between simple and complex access. (p 445)

7-1.6 Describe what the First Responder should do if there is reason to believe that there is a hazard at the scene. (p 440-441)

7-1.7 State the role the First Responder should perform until appropriately trained personnel arrive at the scene of a hazardous materials situation. (p 450)

7-1.8 Describe the criteria for a multiple-casualty situation. (p 450)

7-1.9 Discuss the role of the First Responder in the multiple-casualty situation. (p 453, 455-458)

7-1.10 Summarize the components of basic triage. (p 453-456)

Affective

7-1.11 Explain the rationale for having the unit prepared to respond. (p 436)

Psychomotor

7-1.12 Given a scenario of a mass-casualty incident, perform triage. (p 453-456)

Chapter Objectives*

Knowledge and Attitude Objectives

1. Explain the medical and nonmedical equipment needed to respond to a call. (p 436-437)
2. List the five phases of an emergency call for a first responder. (p 436-438)
3. Discuss the role of a first responder in extrication. (p 439-440)
4. List the seven steps in the extrication process. (p 440)
5. List the various methods of gaining access to a patient. (p 445-447)
6. Describe the simple extrication procedures that a first responder can perform. (p 445-447)
7. List the complex extrication procedures that require specially trained personnel. (p 448)
8. State the responsibilities of the first responder in incidents where hazardous materials are present. (p 450)
9. Describe the actions that a first responder should take in hazardous materials incidents before the arrival of specially trained personnel. (p 450)
10. Define a multiple-casualty incident. (p 450)
11. Describe the role of a first responder in a multiple-casualty incident. (p 453, 455-458)
12. Describe the purpose of the National Incident Management System. (p 458-460)
13. Describe the steps in the START triage system. (p 458-459)

Skill Objectives

1. Perform simple procedures for gaining access to a wrecked vehicle. (p 445-447)
2. Triage a simulated multiple-casualty incident using the START triage system. (p 455-458)

*These are chapter learning objectives.

You are the Provider

Just after your shift starts, you are dispatched for the report of a single vehicle collision with possible injuries. The vehicle is reported to be a package delivery truck that hit a tree on an interstate highway that runs through your community. There has been a light rain for the last half hour. Dispatch reports that the EMS has an estimated time of arrival of 8 to 9 minutes.

1. What are the actions you should take at this call?
2. What is your principal role in this incident if hazardous materials are present?
3. What are the initial actions you should take if this incident is a mass-casualty incident?

Introduction

As a first responder in an EMS operation, you must take several steps to render care to an ill or injured patient. Be prepared to respond when the call comes in. Respond in a safe and timely manner and have the proper equipment to render care. In addition, you must be able to perform simple extrication procedures and assist other responders with patient extrication. Because many first responders work with air medical EMS providers, this chapter covers basic information on that aspect of EMS operations as well. First responders should also be able to identify the signs of a hazardous materials incident and prevent injury to themselves and to others in the first minutes of a hazardous materials incident. Because you may be involved in a multiple-casualty incident, it is important for you to understand the purpose of an incident management system and the framework of the National Incident Management System. Your knowledge of basic triage and the ability to utilize the START triage system are also important.

Preparing for a Call

In your primary role as a law enforcement officer, a fire fighter, or other, you are also on call as a medical first responder. In preparing yourself

for a call, you must understand your role as a member of the emergency medical system. You may respond using a fire department vehicle, a law enforcement vehicle, your private vehicle, or on foot. Be prepared to respond promptly, using the most direct route available. Have the proper equipment to perform your job, including the medical equipment in your first responder life support kit, your personal safety equipment, and equipment to safeguard the accident scene. Suggested contents of a first responder life support kit are shown in **Figure 18-1 ▶** and listed in **Table 18-1 ▶**. This equipment must be stocked and maintained on a regular basis according to the schedule specified by your agency.

Response

Response to an emergency call involves five different phases. The sequence of actions in an emergency call was covered in Chapter 1; you may find it helpful to review this material.

Dispatch

The dispatch facility is a center that citizens can call to request emergency medical care. Most centers are part of a 9-1-1 system that is responsible for dispatching fire, police, and EMS. You should understand how the dispatch facility used by your department operates. Your job will be easier if the dispatcher obtains the proper information from the caller. Dispatchers should also be able to instruct callers on how to perform lifesaving techniques such as CPR until you arrive.

You may receive your dispatch information by telephone, radio, pager, computer terminal, or written printout. Regardless of the transmission method, the information should include the nature of the call, the name and location of the patient, the number of patients, and any special problems. The dispatcher should also obtain a call-back number in case you need more information from the caller. Without good dispatch information, you will not be able to respond properly.

Response to the Scene

Your first priority in responding to the scene is to get there quickly and safely. Consider traffic pat-

TABLE 18-1	Suggested Contents of a First Responder Life Support Kit		
Patient Examination Equipment	1 flashlight	Extrication Equipment	1 spring-loaded center punch 1 pair heavy leather gloves
Personal Safety Equipment	5 sets of gloves 5 face masks 1 bottle of hand sanitizer	Miscellaneous Equipment	2 blankets (disposable) 2 cold packs 1 pair of bandage scissors 1 obstetrical kit
Resuscitation Equipment	1 mouth-to-mask resuscitation device 1 portable hand-powered suction device 1 set oral airways 1 set nasal airways	Other Equipment	1 set personal protective clothing (helmet, eye protection, EMS jacket) 1 reflective vest 1 fire extinguisher (5 lb ABC dry chemical) 1 *Emergency Response Guidebook* 6 fusees 1 pair of binoculars
Bandaging and Dressing Equipment	10 gauze-adhesive strips 1″ 10 gauze pads 4″ × 4″ 5 gauze pads 5″ × 9″ 2 universal trauma dressings 10″ × 30″ 1 occlusive dressing for sealing chest wounds 4 conforming gauze rolls 3″ × 15′ 4 conforming gauze rolls 4½″ × 15′ 6 triangular bandages 1 adhesive tape 2″ 1 burn sheet		
Patient Immobilization Equipment	2 (each) cervical collars: small, medium, large, or 2 adjustable cervical collars 3 rigid conforming splints (SAM splints), or 1 set air splints for arm and leg, or 2 (each) cardboard splints 18″ and 24″		

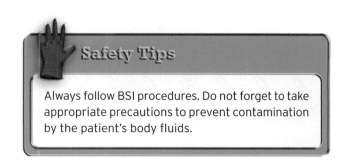

Figure 18-1 Suggested contents of a first responder life support kit.

terns and the time of day before you select the best route to the scene. Follow the safety procedures outlined by your department, including the use of safety belts and the proper use of vehicle-warning devices. Above all else, drive so you are not involved in an accident.

Arrival at the Scene

When you arrive at the scene, remember to place your vehicle in a safe location to minimize the chance of injury. Consider how best to use your vehicle warning lights. Remember to overview the scene as outlined in the patient assessment sequence (Chapter 7) and consider scene safety.

Take into account the number of patients and determine if you need additional resources. Follow the patient assessment sequence you learned in Chapter 7. Practice being as efficient and as organized as you can.

Safety Tips

Always follow BSI procedures. Do not forget to take appropriate precautions to prevent contamination by the patient's body fluids.

Transferring the Care of the Patient to Other EMS Personnel

As more highly trained EMS personnel arrive on the scene, you will have to transfer care of the patient to them. Give them a brief report of the situation as you initially observed it and tell them what care you have provided. Ask them if they have any questions for you. Finally, offer to assist them in caring for the patient.

Postrun Activities

You may think you are done with a call after you have cared for the patient and provided assistance to other EMS personnel—however, your job is not done until you have completed the paperwork. Documentation is important, as emphasized in Chapter 1 and Chapter 8. In addition to completing paperwork, you must also clean your equipment and replace needed supplies. Only after you have completed these activities should you resume regular duties or notify your dispatcher or supervisor that you are ready for another call.

Helicopter Operations

Helicopters are used by EMS systems to reach patients, transport patients to medical facilities, or remove patients from inaccessible areas **Figure 18-2 ▾**. If your EMS system uses a helicopter, obtain a copy of the ground operations procedures or schedule an orientation session with helicopter personnel. As a first responder, you may be responsible for making the initial call for helicopter assistance or for setting up and preparing a landing site in the field.

Helicopter Safety Guidelines

Helicopters can provide lifesaving transport for patients with serious injuries to an appropriate medical facility. However, helicopters are also dangerous to untrained personnel. The main rotor of the helicopter spins at more than 300 revolutions per minute (rpm) and may be just 4 feet above the ground. The tail rotor spins at more than 3,000 rpm, and may be invisible to an unwary person. Additionally, the rotors can generate a "wash" equivalent to winds of 60 to 80 miles per hour (mph). Because a rescuer who approaches without caution may be severely injured by walking upright or by raising an arm above the head, it is important to understand safe helicopter operations.

Setting Up Landing Zones

When choosing a landing site, remember that pilots usually land and take off into the wind. The size of a landing zone will vary and depends on the size of the helicopter. Most civilian helicopters need a landing zone of at least 100 feet × 100 feet (10,000 square feet). Military aircraft may need a larger area. The landing zone should be as flat as possible and free of debris that could become airborne in the 60-mph winds generated by the helicopter. Check carefully for any nearby wires. Wires that you

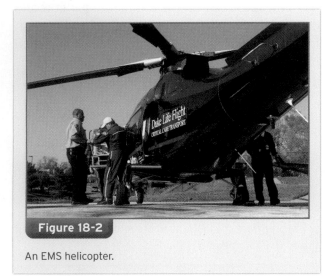

Figure 18-2

An EMS helicopter.

✋ Safety Tips

1. Be alert for electrical wires when identifying a landing zone for a helicopter.
2. Always approach helicopters from the front so the pilot can see you. Approaching a helicopter from the rear is dangerous because the tail rotor is nearly invisible when spinning.
3. Do not approach the helicopter until the pilot signals that it is safe to do so.
4. Helicopters are very noisy and you may not be able to hear a shouted warning. Maintain eye contact with the pilot.
5. Keep low when you approach the helicopter to avoid the spinning main rotor blades.
6. Follow the directions of the helicopter crew.

can see may be invisible to the pilot. If the site slopes or has any obstacles, notify the pilot.

Check with your helicopter service to see how you should secure and mark the perimeter of the site. Avoid using traffic cones, flags, or other objects that can be blown away by the force of the helicopter-rotor wash. <u>Fusees</u> (red signal flares) create a fire hazard and should not be used. Turn off unnecessary white lights and avoid flashing emergency lights because they interfere with the pilot's vision during landing and takeoff. Keep vehicles clear of the landing zone. Close the windows and doors of any nearby vehicles and remove any loose objects on the vehicles that could become airborne. Some helicopter services request that a charged hose line be available for fire emergencies.

Loading Patients Into Helicopters

Certain safety precautions must be followed during the loading of a helicopter patient. Secure all loose clothing, sheets, and instruments such as stethoscopes. Use eye protection to prevent debris from getting into your eyes. Approach a helicopter from the front and only after the pilot or a crew member signals that it is safe **Figure 18-3 ▼**.

The helicopter crew may need help carrying equipment to the patient. Follow their instructions. Give your patient report to the crew, away from the helicopter's noise, and offer your assistance. It is harder to load a helicopter stretcher than an ambulance stretcher. Because loose sheets

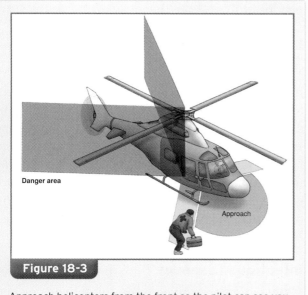

Figure 18-3

Approach helicopters from the front so the pilot can see you.

Safety Tips

Several "DO NOTs" are important. DO NOT approach the helicopter landing zone unless necessary. DO NOT approach a helicopter from the upside if it is on a slope. DO NOT run near a helicopter. DO NOT raise your hand when approaching a helicopter.

or blankets can blow off the stretcher, patients need to be packaged (prepared) properly and securely.

As a first responder, you can provide ground support and assistance during helicopter ambulance operations, provided that you take proper safety precautions. If you will be working with a helicopter ambulance, arrange an orientation with helicopter personnel so you will be prepared in an emergency.

Extrication

This section describes simple techniques you can use to access, treat, and extract patients who are trapped inside wrecked vehicles. The ability to think quickly and use the principles and guidelines that are presented here are essential for the first responder. You will also need several hours of practical exercises to become skilled in the process of <u>extrication</u>.

Your first responder course should include a demonstration of the entire extrication operation. You should be familiar with extrication equipment, its use, and the hazards involved in the extrication operation. You should know what equipment is available in your community and what to do to summon this equipment. First responders usually use extrication techniques for automobile accidents, but many of the same principles apply to other situations. Resourcefulness, common sense, and a knowledge gained through training are key attributes of the first responder, which underlie every act of patient care.

The safety of all rescuers and patients is an important consideration during the extrication process. Ideally, rescuers should wear protective equipment similar to a fire fighter's outfit: full bunker gear consisting of coat, pants, boots, helmet with face shield, and gloves. Minimally, a helmet with face shield or goggles and gloves should be worn.

A situation in which patients are trapped in an automobile can be complex enough to tax the skills and resources of even the most highly trained and well-equipped EMS system. To ensure the best care, many different agencies may need to cooperate: law enforcement personnel, the fire department, EMS personnel, and sometimes the utility company and a wrecker operator. Achieving the cooperation and mutual understanding that is needed for a safe, smooth extrication effort requires prior coordination and practice.

As you read this section, keep in mind these basic guidelines:

- Know the limitations of your training, equipment, and skill.
- Identify any hazards (gasoline, power lines or wires, or hazardous materials).
- Control those hazards for which you are trained and equipped.
- Gain access to the patients.
- Provide patient care and stabilization.
- Move the patients only if absolutely necessary.

As a first responder, you have two primary extrication goals: to obtain safe access to the patients and to ensure patient stabilization. To achieve these goals, your role in the extrication process can be divided into the seven steps listed in the box on this page. As a first responder, you will usually be responsible only for the first four steps of the extrication process. However, you will often have to assist other EMS personnel in completing the remaining steps. You cannot give this assistance unless you fully understand what must be done and how it is accomplished. Think safety so that you do not become injured. An injured rescuer becomes a second patient.

The actions you take as the first trained person on the scene can make the difference between an organized and a disorganized rescue effort, perhaps even the difference between life and death! You set the stage and you have an essential role in the extrication process. Remember this as you review the example of an automobile crash described in this section.

Step One: Overview of the Scene

As soon as the dispatcher tells you of the incident, begin to anticipate and plan for what you are likely to find upon arrival. You may, for instance, know

In the Field

Steps in the Extrication Process

1. Conduct an overview of the scene.
2. Stabilize the scene, control any hazards, and stabilize the vehicle.
3. Gain access to patients.
4. Provide initial emergency care.
5. Help disentangle patients.
6. Help prepare patients for removal.
7. Help remove patients.

that a certain type of accident frequently occurs at a particular intersection or along a specific stretch of highway. Do not, however, become complacent about responding to the "same old thing." Use your knowledge, but be flexible in planning.

If the dispatch information is complete, you will know the types of vehicles involved (for example, two cars, a car and motorcycle, a truck and car, or a train and truck) and whether there are injured or trapped people, burning vehicles, or hazardous materials present.

As you approach the accident scene and before you exit your vehicle, get an overview of the entire incident **Figure 18-4 ▶**. Remember that you must locate the patients before you can treat them! Rapidly determine the extent of the accident or incident, try to estimate the number of patients, and try to locate any hazards that may be present. Then call for whatever assistance you may need to manage the accident.

Step Two: Stabilization of the Scene and Any Hazards

It is especially important to keep a sharp lookout for hazards that can result in injury, disability, or death to a patient, yourself, other emergency personnel, or bystanders. Some of the most common hazards found at automobile crash scenes include infectious diseases, traffic, bystanders, spilled gasoline or other hazardous materials, automobile batteries, downed electrical wires, unstable vehicles, and vehicle fires **Figure 18-5 ▶**.

Infectious Diseases

Many patients involved in motor vehicle crashes will have soft-tissue injuries and active bleeding

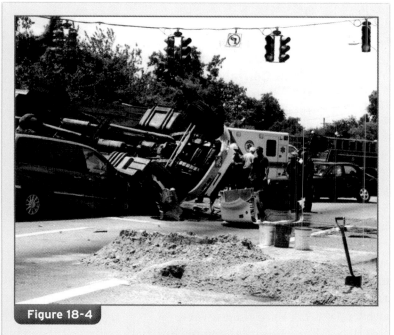

Figure 18-4

As you approach an accident, look over the entire scene.

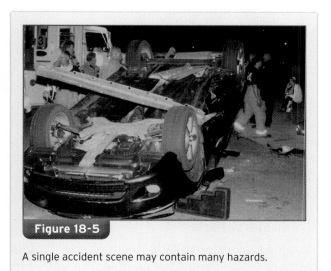

Figure 18-5

A single accident scene may contain many hazards.

situations, park in a location that does not obstruct open traffic lanes, but do not hesitate to use your vehicle to block traffic to protect you, your patients, and other rescuers. If other emergency personnel are already on the scene, ask them where you should park your vehicle. Consider the design of your vehicle's warning lights and park so you can use them to their best advantage. Do not leave your trunk lid open after removing your emergency equipment; the lid may block your warning lights!

Another way to protect the scene is to ignite fusees or warning flares as soon as possible. Place the flares or fusees up and down the road to warn oncoming traffic and give other drivers time to slow down safely. After you've taken these traffic-protective measures, survey the scene for other hazards.

Bystanders

Keep bystanders away from the crash scene to minimize the danger to themselves and patients. It is not usually enough to ask everyone to move back. You should give specific directions such as, "Move back to the other side of the road" or "Move back onto the sidewalk." You can also pick out one or two bystanders and ask them to assist you in keeping others away from the scene.

A rope or police/fire barrier tape is very effective if it is available. People respond appropriately to such "barriers" and usually will not cross them once they are set up.

Spilled Gasoline

Gasoline spills are common during automobile crashes. Expect to find a fuel spill if an automobile has been hit near the rear, is on its side, or is

from open wounds or from their mouth or nose. Follow standard BSI precautions at all motor vehicle crash scenes. If sharp glass or metal is present, you should wear heavy-duty rescue type gloves over your latex or vinyl gloves; otherwise, vinyl or latex gloves should be sufficient. If there is the danger of splattering blood, you should consider using face protection.

Traffic Hazards

First, park your vehicle and other emergency vehicles so that they protect the scene and warn oncoming traffic to avoid the crash site. In most

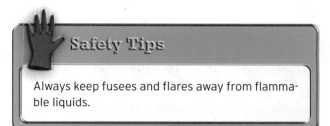

Safety Tips

Always keep fusees and flares away from flammable liquids.

upside down. If there are fuel spills (or if the car is in a position that suggests there will be), call the fire department to minimize the fire hazard and to clean up any spilled fuel.

If patients are in a car with a fuel spill and the fire department has not arrived, consider covering the fuel with dirt. This reduces the amount of vapor coming from the spill, which, in turn, reduces the danger of fire. Fuel vapors tend to stay close to the ground and will travel with the wind. In any event, be sure to call the fire department whenever you suspect a fuel spill.

Automobile Batteries

Automobile batteries are hazardous and you must avoid contact with them. In a front-end collision, the battery may already be broken open and acid will be leaking. Reduce the possibility of an electrical short circuit by turning off the automobile's ignition. Do not attempt to disconnect the battery because you could be injured by a short circuit, explosion, or contact with battery acid.

Downed Electrical Wires

Downed electrical wires may be caused by weather problems or by a vehicle hitting a utility pole. Sometimes, downed electrical wires explode in arcs of spectacular flashes and sparks; other times,

they simply lay across the vehicle, fully charged with electricity and capable of causing injury or death to the unwary.

Locate the wires but avoid contact! If a vehicle has a downed wire across it and passengers are trapped inside, immediately instruct them to stay inside the car. Then summon the utility company and fire department. Move bystanders back in all directions, to at least the distance between two power poles.

Do not forget that electrical hazards can come from other sources as well, including traffic-light control boxes and underground power feeds. Be sure to check everywhere, including under the vehicles, for electrical hazards. However, you should not attempt to deal with electrical hazards at accident scenes.

Unstable Vehicles

Assume that every vehicle involved in a crash is unstable, unless you have manually stabilized it. Vehicles on a hill, on their sides, upside down, or teetering over the edge of an embankment or bridge are obviously unstable **Figure 18-6 ▶**. However, no matter how stable the vehicle appears to be, it may suddenly roll away or topple

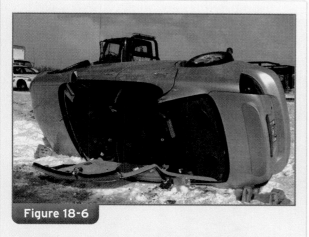

Figure 18-6

Vehicles on their sides are obviously unstable.

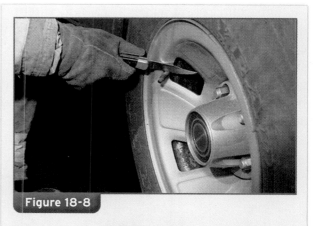

Figure 18-8

Deflating the tires will help to stabilize the vehicle.

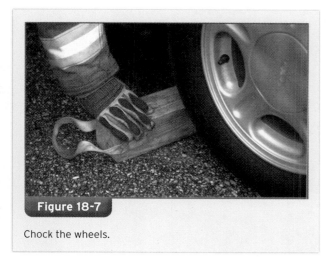

Figure 18-7

Chock the wheels.

Vehicles on Their Sides or Upside Down A vehicle on its side is extremely unstable. Fortunately, this position is fairly unusual. Stabilizing these vehicles is beyond the range of skills and equipment for many first responders and should be handled by rescue squads or fire departments. Many fire departments and rescue squads carry **wooden cribbing** and "step-chocks" to deal with this problem. If you must enter a vehicle on its side to respond to a life-threatening situation, do not climb on the vehicle. Carefully break the rear window glass and enter through the back of the vehicle. Bend over or crouch down to stay close to the ground. This will help prevent upsetting the car's center of gravity.

An upside-down vehicle is relatively stable. The primary hazard in this situation is spilled gasoline, which must be handled by the fire department.

Vehicle Fires

Even though fires happen infrequently at automobile crash sites, they are a cause of great concern among EMS personnel. There are two types of fires related to automobile crashes: impact fires and postimpact fires.

over. Be sure to check and ensure the stability of every vehicle before you attempt to enter it or treat the passengers inside.

Vehicles on Their Wheels If the car is upright and on its wheels, you can ensure stability by **chocking** the front or back of each wheel with hubcaps or pieces of wood Figure 18-7 ▲ . You can also deflate the tires by safely cutting or pulling the valve stems Figure 18-8 ▶ .

Safety Tips

If wooden blocks or hubcaps are not available, improvise by using materials found at the scene.

Safety Tips

Your purpose is to keep the vehicle in the position found. Do not move it. Any movement could cause the vehicle to move.

Impact fires occur when the gas tank ruptures during the collision. The vehicle is usually rapidly engulfed in flames, and it soon becomes impossible to approach it for a rescue attempt. Passengers rescued from this type of fire are usually saved by bystanders and witnesses to the accident who act immediately to remove them.

Postimpact fires are often caused by electrical short circuits and can be prevented by turning off the ignition. These fires usually do not develop into major fires if prompt action is taken. Should one occur, first turn off the ignition. Then extinguish the fire with a portable fire extinguisher. Remove the passengers from the vehicle as soon as possible.

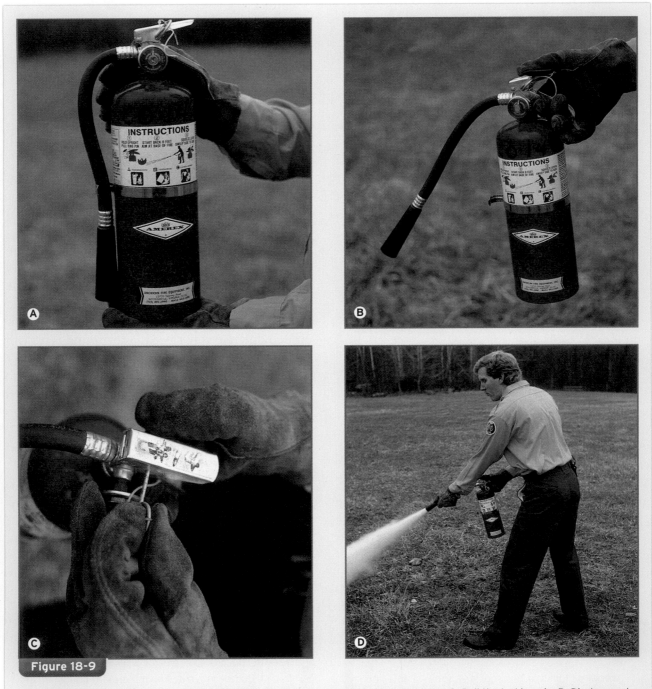

Figure 18-9

Use of a dry chemical fire extinguisher. **A.** Check the pressure gauge. **B.** Release the hose. **C.** Pull the locking pin. **D.** Discharge at the base of the fire.

Safety Tips

Do not mistake hot water vapor from a damaged radiator for smoke from an engine compartment fire. If the smoke disappears rapidly (10 feet to 15 feet away from the car), it is probably steam and not smoke.

Emergency Actions for Automobile Fires If you arrive at a crash scene and find a car on fire with people trapped inside, remember the following procedures:

- Use your dry chemical fire extinguisher **Figure 18-9 ◄** . Most dry chemical fire extinguishers can be used on ordinary combustibles, flammable liquids, or electrical fires. Be sure you know how to use the extinguisher in your vehicle.
- Use your extinguisher to keep flames out of the passenger compartment. Direct the extinguisher to the base of the fire—not at the passenger compartment.
- Do not be overly worried about discharging the extinguisher onto the passengers; the dry chemical powder is nontoxic. However, the dry chemical can be corrosive, so you should watch for respiratory problems.
- Immediately have someone else gather fire extinguishers from other vehicles on the scene. Do not wait until your extinguisher runs out!

- Remove patients as quickly as possible. Be careful because they may be injured.
- Move everyone at least 50 feet away from any vehicle that is on fire.

Step Three: Gain Access to Patients
Access Through Doors

Before you can provide patient care, you must gain access to the patient. Between 85% and 90% of all motor vehicle patients can be reached simply by stabilizing the vehicle and then opening a door or rolling down a window. Try all the doors first—even if they appear to be badly damaged. It is an embarrassing waste of time and energy to open a jammed door with heavy rescue equipment when another door can be opened easily and without any equipment. Attempt to unlock and open the least damaged door first. Make sure that the locking mechanism is released. Then try the outside and inside handles at the same time **Figure 18-10 ▼** .

Access Through Windows

If you believe that any passenger's condition is serious enough to require immediate care (for example, if the passengers are not sitting up and talking) and you cannot enter through a door, you should break a window.

Do not try to break and enter through the windshield because it is made of plastic-laminated glass **Figure 18-11 ▶** . The side and rear win-

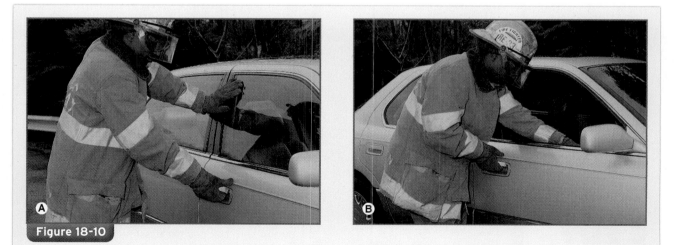

Figure 18-10

Access the vehicle through the doors, if possible. **A.** Try all doors first. **B.** Try inside and outside handles at the same time.

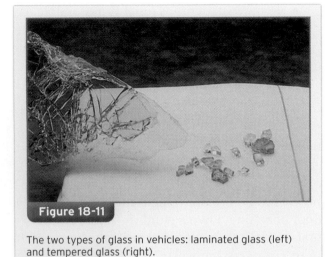

Figure 18-11

The two types of glass in vehicles: laminated glass (left) and tempered glass (right).

dows are made of **tempered glass** and will break easily into small pieces when hit with a sharp, pointed object such as a tire iron, spring-loaded center punch, or fire ax. Because these windows do not pose a safety threat, they should be your primary access route.

A spring-loaded center punch (available from many hardware stores) should be carried in your first responder's life support kit Figure 18-12 ▼ . It can be used rapidly, takes up little room in the kit, and is nearly always successful in breaking the side and rear windows on the first try.

If you must break a window to open a door or gain access, try to break one that is the farthest from the patient. However, if the patient's condition warrants your immediate entry, do not

hesitate to break the closest side or rear window, even if the glass will fall onto a patient.

Tempered pieces of glass do not usually pose a danger to people trapped in cars. Advise ambulance personnel if a passenger is covered with broken glass so they can notify the hospital emergency department. If there is glass on a passenger, pick it off—don't brush it off.

After breaking the window, use your gloved hands to pull the remaining glass out of the window frame so it does not fall onto any passengers or injure any rescuers.

If you are using something other than a spring-loaded center punch to break the window, always aim for a lower corner. That way, the window frame will help prevent the tool (such as a tire iron, fire ax, or large screwdriver) from sailing into the car and hitting the person inside.

Once you have broken the glass and removed the remaining pieces of glass from the frame, try to unlock the door again. Release the locking mechanism, and then use both inside and outside door handles at the same time. This will often enable you to force a jammed locking mechanism, even in a door that appears to be badly damaged.

To access a vehicle through the window, follow the steps in Skill Drill 18-1 ▶ :

Using the simple techniques described and illustrated in this section, you should be able to

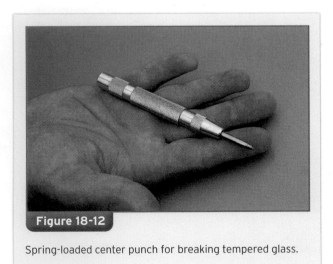

Figure 18-12

Spring-loaded center punch for breaking tempered glass.

SKILL DRILL 18-1

1. Place the spring-loaded center punch at the lower corner of the window Step 1 .
2. Press on the center punch to break the window Step 2 .
3. With gloved hands, remove the broken glass to the outside of the vehicle Step 3 .
4. Enter the vehicle through the window Step 4 .

Safety Tips

Always warn trapped car passengers that you are going to break the glass.

Skill DRILL 18-1

Accessing the Vehicle Through the Window

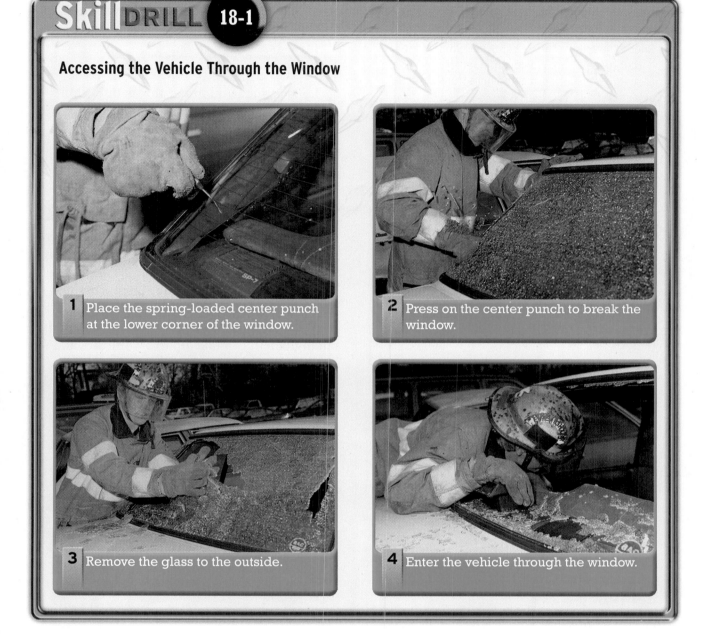

1 Place the spring-loaded center punch at the lower corner of the window.

2 Press on the center punch to break the window.

3 Remove the glass to the outside.

4 Enter the vehicle through the window.

gain access to nearly all automobile crash victims, even those in an upside-down car.

When you gain access to a wrecked vehicle, be alert for undeployed airbags. Airbags are mounted in the steering wheel on the driver's side and in the dashboard on the passenger's side. Many vehicles are also equipped with side-mounted airbags on the driver's side or passenger's side. If the airbags have not deployed in the crash, they represent a hazard to rescuers because

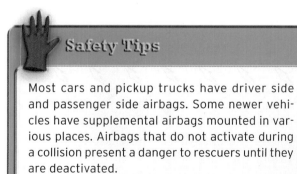

Safety Tips

Most cars and pickup trucks have driver side and passenger side airbags. Some newer vehicles have supplemental airbags mounted in various places. Airbags that do not activate during a collision present a danger to rescuers until they are deactivated.

Check the trunk. This is especially important in border areas where significant numbers of illegal aliens are transported in automobile trunks to avoid detection Figure 18-13 ▾ .

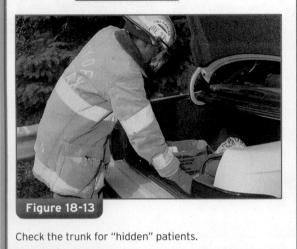

Figure 18-13

Check the trunk for "hidden" patients.

they may remain armed for some period of time. Avoid getting in front of an undeployed airbag until trained rescuers can assure you that it does not pose a hazard to you or to the patient.

If you cannot gain access, you must do what you can to assist the patients. This means stabilizing the vehicle and protecting the scene until the proper equipment arrives.

Step Four: Provide Initial Emergency Care

After you gain access to the passengers, immediately begin initial emergency medical care. Conduct a patient assessment on every patient. After you determine the status of each patient, you should monitor ABCs, control bleeding, treat for shock, stabilize the cervical spine, and provide psychological reassurance. Don't forget to maintain the patient's body temperature. If you have time, you can now perform a patient examination.

Leave the patients in the vehicle unless it is on fire or they are otherwise in immediate danger. Keep the patients stabilized and immobilized until they are properly packaged and can be removed from the vehicle by other rescuers.

Skill Drill 18-2 ▸ shows how to perform initial airway management when the patient is in a vehicle:

SKILL DRILL 18-2

1. Place one hand under the victim's chin and the other hand on the back of the victim's head Step 1 .
2. Raise the head to a neutral position to open the airway Step 2 .

Step Five: Help Disentangle Patients

Extrication operates on the principle of "removing the vehicle from around the patient." This process usually requires tools and specialized equipment, such as air chisels, manual or powered hydraulic rescue equipment, and air bags. In some serious extrication situations, disentanglement can take up to 30 minutes and requires advanced training Figure 18-14 ▾ .

Modern rescue crews use the concept of the **golden hour** when dealing with serious trauma situations. The golden-hour concept means that the

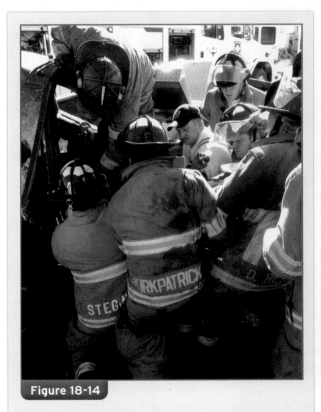

Figure 18-14

Significant entrapment requires teamwork from all responders.

Skill DRILL 18-2

Airway Management in a Vehicle

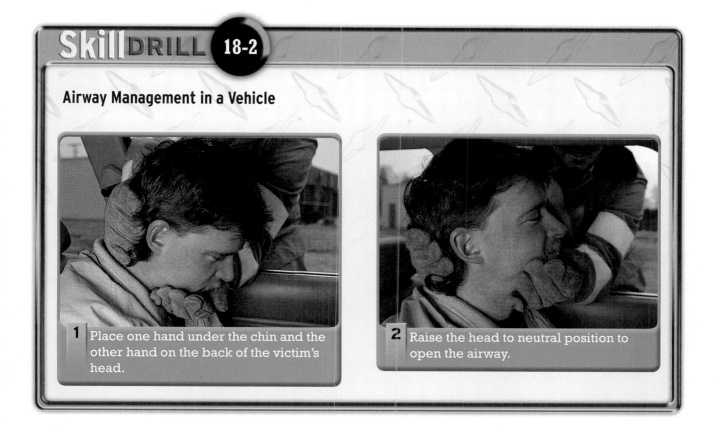

1 Place one hand under the chin and the other hand on the back of the victim's head.

2 Raise the head to neutral position to open the airway.

less time spent on the scene with a seriously injured patient, the better. The patient's chance for survival increases if rescuers can get the patient to a trauma center within 1 hour of the injury.

Your familiarity with the phases of the extrication effort may enable you to assist the rescue and extrication crews. You can do many things to help and you should take the time to find out about the rescue and extrication resources in your community. Ask the crews how you can assist them; they will probably be delighted to have your help and support.

Step Six: Help Prepare Patients for Removal

As disentanglement proceeds, the patient is prepared for removal. Dressings, bandages, and splints are applied and the head and spine are immobilized. If you are familiar with the procedures and equipment, you may be able to assist in this effort. For example, extra trained hands are useful to help move and secure the patient onto a long backboard for removal (see Chapter 5).

It is important to realize that the access route to the patient may not be adequate as an extrication route. The extrication route must be large enough to permit the safe removal of the packaged patient, whereas the access route may be a relatively small entry hole.

Step Seven: Help Remove Patients

Once packaged, the patient is removed from the vehicle and placed onto the stretcher of the transporting ambulance. Although a first responder is directly involved in only the first four of the seven extrication steps, you should be aware of the entire operation. Your actions or inaction can have a vital impact on the entire operation.

Review of the Extrication Process

Remember these steps when you arrive on the scene of a vehicle crash with trapped passengers:
- Call for extrication help.
- Specify the types of vehicles involved.
- Do not stand idly by while waiting for help:
  - Identify and contain hazards.
  - Park your vehicle so that its headlights and warning lights can be used to protect and light the scene.

- Clear a working area around the accident before you or rescue personnel attempt to stabilize the vehicle(s).
- Use your head! Think and use what tools you already have.
- Remember to try opening the doors first, rather than breaking windows.
- Once you gain access to the patients, assess and monitor their conditions.
- Above all, keep your cool!

Hazardous Materials Incidents

<u>Hazardous materials (HazMat)</u> are substances that are toxic, poisonous, radioactive, flammable, or explosive and can cause injury or death with exposure. During a HazMat incident, your top priority is to protect yourself and bystanders from exposure and contamination.

The single most important step when handling any HazMat incident is to identify the substance(s) involved. Federal law requires that all vehicles containing certain quantities of hazardous materials display a HazMat placard. When you see a HazMat placard, you know that a potential problem exists. You will have to find the proper response to the problem before beginning patient treatment **Figure 18-15 ▶** and **Figure 18-16 ▶**. The placard should also have a four-digit identification number, which can be used to identify the substance and to obtain emergency information.

The *Emergency Response Guidebook*, published by the U.S. Department of Transportation, lists the most common hazardous materials, their four-digit identification numbers, and the proper emergency actions to control the scene. It also describes the emergency care of patients who become ill or injured after exposure to these substances **Figure 18-17 ▶**. First responders should carry a copy of this guidebook in their vehicles.

Unless you have received training in handling hazardous materials and can take the necessary precautions to protect yourself, you should keep away from the contaminated area or <u>hot zone</u>.

Once the trained HazMat rescuers have been properly protected, the next step in HazMat inci-

dents is to identify victims who have sustained an acute injury as a result of exposure to hazardous materials. These patients should be removed from the contaminated area, decontaminated by trained personnel, given any necessary emergency care, and transported to a hospital.

There are very few specific antidotes or treatments for most HazMat injuries. Consequently, the emergency treatment of patients who have been exposed to hazardous materials is usually aimed at supportive care. Because most fatalities and serious injuries sustained in HazMat incidents result from breathing problems, you must constantly reevaluate the patient's vital signs, including breathing status, so that a patient whose condition worsens can be moved to a higher triage level.

Multiple-Casualty Incidents

As a first responder, you may face situations in which there is more than one sick or injured individual. These situations, known as <u>multiple-casualty incidents</u> (or <u>mass-casualty incidents</u>), may range from a serious automobile crash with three or four injured people to a building explosion with dozens of injured people. How do you determine which patient to treat first?

You must first be able to recognize the situation as a multiple-casualty incident. These incidents require a very different method of operation

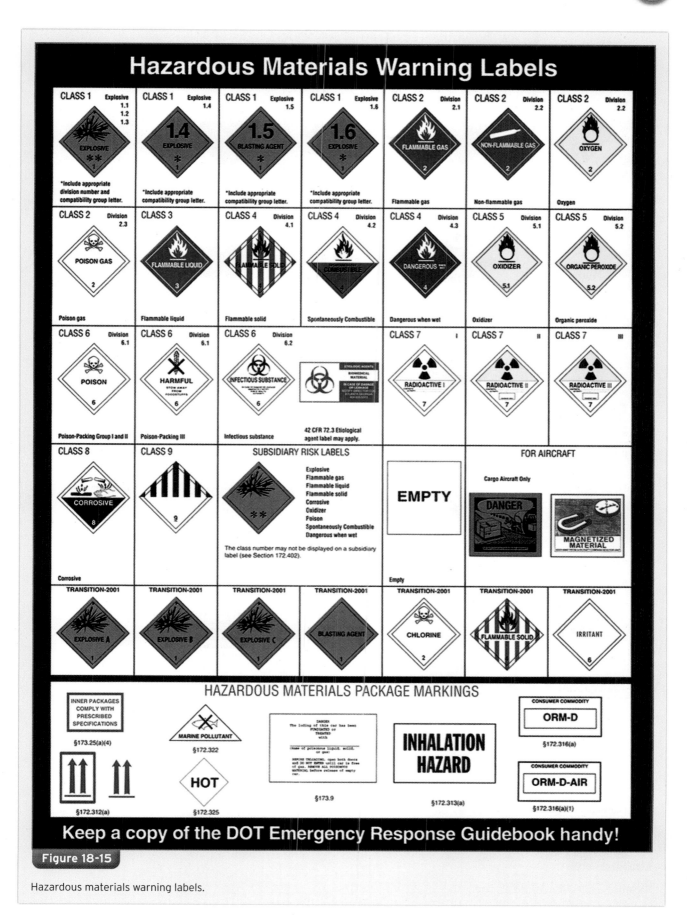

Figure 18-15

Hazardous materials warning labels.

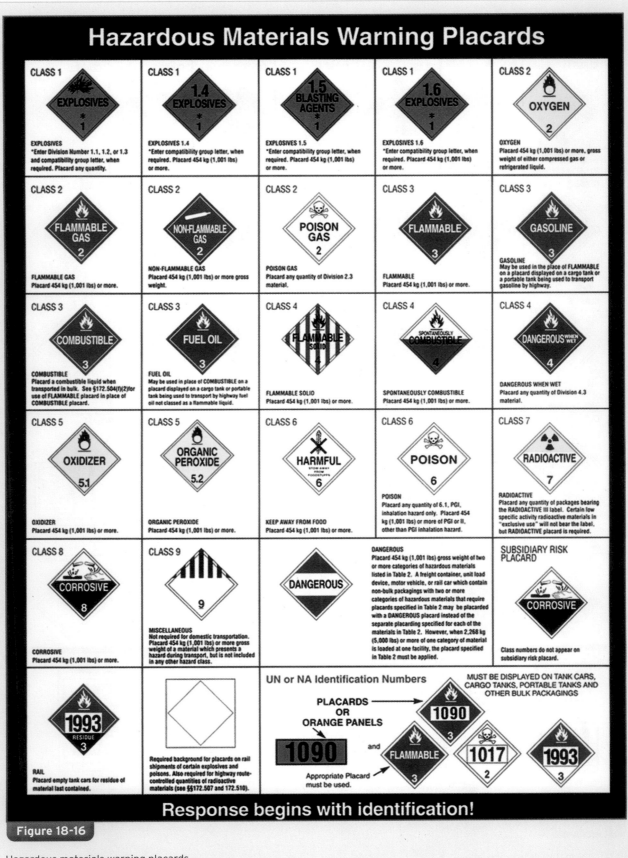

Figure 18-16

Hazardous materials warning placards.

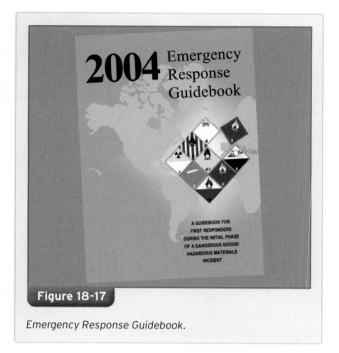

Figure 18-17

Emergency Response Guidebook.

from other emergency medical calls. During some multiple-casualty incidents, you (the first responder) may be on the scene 15 to 20 minutes before additional assistance arrives and it may be 45 to 60 minutes before enough rescue resources are available.

No easy formula exists for deciding when to shift from normal operations into the techniques of the multiple-casualty incident. Simulations provide realistic situations, but there are many variables, including the severity of the crash, access routes, available resources, response times, levels of emergency training, and overall experience of the EMS system.

The first responder's goal is to provide the greatest medical benefit for the greatest number of people and to match patients' medical needs with appropriate treatment and transportation. To accomplish this goal, you must be able to identify those most in need of treatment and those who can wait.

Casualty Sorting: Creating Order Out of Chaos

The sorting of patients into groups according to their need for treatment is called **triage**. Triage is a French word that has come to mean **casualty sorting** in the emergency care field. The purpose of casualty sorting is to determine the order in

which patients should be treated so that the most good can be done for the most people.

Ideally, your casualty-sorting system should be simple and fast, based on the skills and knowledge you already have. Do not worry about making a specific diagnosis before categorizing patients; a casualty-sorting system is meant to provide the basis for a system of rapid, lifesaving actions. A casualty-sorting system focuses your activities in the middle of a chaotic and confusing environment. You must identify and separate patients rapidly, according to the severity of their injuries and their need for treatment.

The Visual Survey: The Eye Sees It All

As you are on the way to the scene, you should be preparing yourself mentally for what you may find **Figure 18-18 ▶**. Perhaps you've responded to other accidents at the same location. Where will additional help come from? How long will it take for help to arrive?

When you arrive at the scene of a major incident, force yourself to stay as calm as possible. Make a visual assessment of the entire accident scene. This visual survey gives you an initial impression of the overall situation, including the potential number of patients involved and, possibly, the severity of their injuries. The visual survey should enable you to estimate how much and what kind of help you will need to handle the situation.

Your Initial Radio Report: Creating a Verbal Image

The initial radio report is often the most important radio message of a disaster because it sets the emotional and operational stage for everything that follows. As you key the microphone for that first vital report, use clear language, be concise, be calm, and do not shout into the microphone. Give the communications center a concise verbal picture of the scene.

The key points to communicate are:

- Location of the incident
- Type of incident
- Any hazards
- Approximate number of victims
- Type of assistance required

Voices of Experience

Provide the Best Possible Care

The initial call came in to 9-1-1 as "a car on fire." As a volunteer department, it was fortunate that we were already at the station. We were promptly en route to the car fire in the fire truck when additional reports came in that this was not a car fire, but rather a car wreck off a bridge. Other first responders were soon en route with the rescue truck. Upon arrival, we found that the car had gone off the bridge and landed upside down in the water. After descending the 20-foot embankment, we found the driver still strapped into the driver's seat by his seatbelt. The major problem was that he was unconscious from major trauma and the water level was rising rapidly in the car.

> **We were standing in thigh-deep water and the water level inside the car was up to the patient's eyes because he was hanging upside-down.**

The driver's door was undamaged in the wreck, so access to the patient was easy in that respect. However, we were standing in thigh-deep water and the water level inside the car was up to the patient's eyes because he was hanging upside-down. In addition, the car's motor was still running and leaking various fluids into the water. We had to make some quick decisions as to how to extricate this man.

Because of the victim's unconscious state, the rising water level, and the potentially dangerous environment from the leaking fluids, we elected to perform a rapid extrication. A long backboard was brought down, and with help from first responders, we unbuckled his seatbelt, and held him while turning him over to place him on the board. Due to the urgency of the situation, we had to suspend c-spine protection until after we removed him from the car. The patient was then transferred to the top of the upside-down car, where we climbed to make our initial assessment. Due to the steepness of the embankment, we had to wait until ropes could be set up to assist us in getting the patient up to the roadway. We decided that we would use a basket stretcher to carry the patient to the waiting medical helicopter. While the ropes were getting set up and we were waiting for the basket stretcher to be carried down to us, we began treatment. While the first responders assisted with c-spine immobilization by placing a cervical collar, immobilizing the head, and strapping the patient to the board, we inserted an endotracheal tube and started an IV for fluid resuscitation.

With the help of the ropes securing the basket and providing some traction, we were able to carry the patient to the top of the embankment. It was not easy since we didn't have all the proper equipment, but we worked as best as we could with the equipment that we had. It took several minutes to get him to the top of the embankment. Having to assist his ventilations made the climb even more difficult.

Even though the man died later as a result of the significant trauma, we provided him the best possible care under the extreme situation caused by his crash. We all used our training and tried very hard to save this man's life, but not every patient can be saved. The patient's family was thankful that we got him out of the car so quickly, and that he didn't drown.

Looking back on this difficult, challenging rescue operation, we realized that we were only able to accomplish this with everyone working as a team. The first responders were able to assist with the assessment, spinal immobilization, and extrication maneuvers. They applied all of the skills they learned in their first responder class.

John Reed, RN, EMT-P
Education Coordinator
Birmingham Regional Emergency Medical Services System (BREMSS)
Birmingham, Alabama

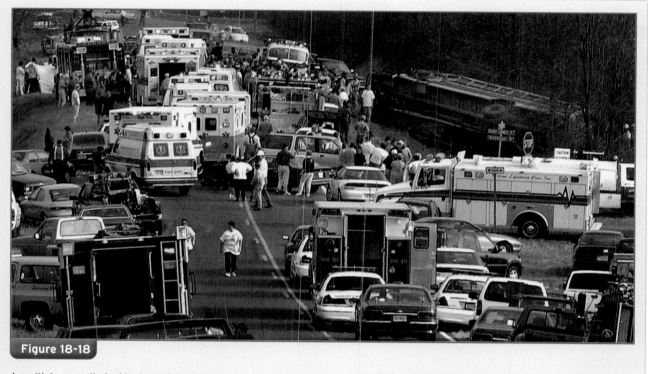

Figure 18-18

A multiple-casualty incident requiring triage.

Be as specific with your requests as possible. A good rule of thumb in mass-casualty situations is to request one ambulance for every five patients. For example, for 35 patients, request seven ambulances; for 23 patients, request five ambulances; and so forth. After taking several deep breaths (to give yourself time to absorb what you've seen and to try to calm your voice), you might give the following radio report about a commercial bus crash: "This is a major accident involving a truck and a commercial bus on Highway 233, about 2 miles west of Route 510. There are approximately 35 victims. There are people trapped. Repeat: This is a major crash. I am requesting the fire department, rescue squad, and seven ambulances at this time. Dispatch additional police units to assist."

In the Field

Recent studies show that the failure to provide adequate traffic control at the emergency scene is a common and often fatal error in multiple-casualty incidents. Immediately after radioing for help, establish a traffic control plan. This process should only take a couple of minutes.

1. Determine the perimeters for emergency vehicles only and exclude all other vehicles.
2. Establish a one-way route for emergency traffic to approach the scene and a separate one-way route for emergency traffic to exit the scene.
3. Allow adequate room for emergency vehicles that need to be close to the scene.
4. Keep vehicles and personnel that are not needed at a given time in a staging area.

Sorting the Patients

It is important not to become involved with treating the first or second patient you see. Remember that your job is to get to each patient as quickly as possible, conduct a rapid assessment, and assign patients to broad categories based on their need for treatment.

You cannot stop during this survey, except to correct airway and severe bleeding problems quickly. Your job is to sort (triage) the patients. Other rescuers will provide follow-up treatment.

The START System: It Really Works!

Different communities use many variations of triage systems, and you will need to learn the specific role that you have in your community's triage plan. Many EMS systems rely on the START system because it is simple and easy to remember and implement. The Simple Triage And Rapid Treatment (START) system lets first responders triage each patient in 60 seconds or less, based on three primary observations: breathing, circulation, and mental status (BCM).

The START system is designed to help rescuers find the most seriously injured patients. As more rescue personnel arrive, patients can be re-triaged for further evaluation, treatment, stabilization, and transportation. This system also allows first responders to open blocked airways and stop severe bleeding quickly.

Triage Tagging: Telling Others What You've Found

Patients are tagged so that other rescuers arriving on the scene can easily recognize their triage level. Tagging uses colored surveyor's tape or colored paper tags Figure 18-19 ▾ and Figure 18-20 ▸, and is based on the method determined by your local EMS system.

The Four Colors of Triage

The START system consists of four levels of triage, each with its own color code:

- Priority One (red tag): Immediate care/life threatening.
- Priority Two (yellow tag): Urgent care/can delay up to 1 hour.

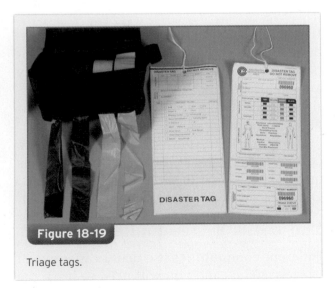

Figure 18-19

Triage tags.

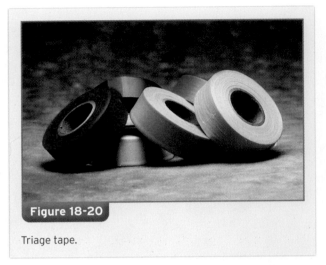

Figure 18-20

Triage tape.

- Priority Three (green tag): Delayed care (walking wounded)/can delay up to 3 hours.
- Priority Four (gray or black tag): Patient is dead/no care required.

The First Step in START: Get Up and Walk!

The first step in START is to tell all the people who can get up and walk to move to a specific area. If patients can get up and walk, they rarely have life-threatening injuries.

To make the situation more manageable, ask those victims who can walk to move away from the immediate rescue scene to a designated safe area. These patients are the "walking wounded" designated as Priority Three (green tag/delayed care). A patient who complains of pain when he or she attempts to walk or move should not be forced to move. Now you can concentrate on the patients who are left in the rescue scene.

The Second Step in START: Begin Where You Stand

Begin the second step of START by moving from where you stand. Move in an orderly and systematic manner through the remaining victims, stopping at each person for a quick assessment and tagging. The stop at each patient should never take more than 1 minute.

Your job is to find and tag the Priority One patients—those who require immediate attention. Examine these patients, correct life-threatening airway and breathing problems, tag the patients with a red tag, and move on!

How to Evaluate Patients Using BCM

The START system is based on the three observations: BCM. Each patient must be evaluated quickly, in a systematic manner, starting with breathing Figure 18-21 ▾ .

Breathing: It All Starts Here

If the patient is breathing, you need to determine the breathing rate. Patients with breathing rates greater than 30 breaths per minute are tagged Priority One (red tags). These patients are showing one of the primary signs of shock and need immediate care as soon as it is available.

If the patient is breathing at a rate less than 30 breaths per minute, move on to the circulation and mental status observations in order to complete your 60-second survey.

If the patient is not breathing, quickly clear the mouth of foreign matter. Use the head-tilt technique to open the airway. In a multiple- or mass-casualty situation, you may have to ignore the usual cervical spine guidelines when you are opening airways during the triage process. This is the only time in emergency care when you may not have time to properly stabilize every injured patient's spine. Open the airway, position the patient to maintain the airway, and—if the patient breathes—tag the patient Priority One (red tag). Patients who need help maintaining an open airway are Priority One (red tags). If you are in doubt as to the patient's ability to breathe, tag the patient as Priority One (red tag). If the patient is not breathing and does not start to breathe with simple airway maneuvers, tag the patient Priority Four (gray/black tag).

Circulation: Is Oxygen Getting Around?

The second BCM triage test is the patient's circulation. The best field method for checking circulation (to see if the heart is able to circulate blood adequately) is to check the carotid pulse. The carotid pulse is close to the heart. It is large and easily felt in the neck. To check the carotid pulse, place your index and middle fingers on the larynx and slide your fingers into the groove between the larynx and the muscles at the side of the neck. You must keep your fingers there for 5 to 10 seconds to find and measure the pulse rate (see Chapter 7). If the carotid pulse is weak or irregular, tag

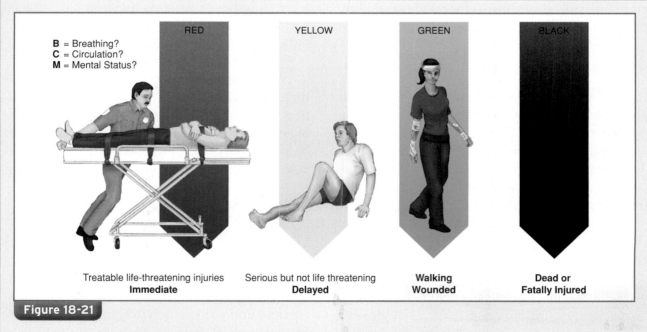

B = Breathing?
C = Circulation?
M = Mental Status?

RED   YELLOW   GREEN   BLACK

| Treatable life-threatening injuries | Serious but not life threatening | Walking | Dead or |
| **Immediate** | **Delayed** | **Wounded** | **Fatally Injured** |

Figure 18-21

Use START to sort patients into appropriate groups for treatment.

the patient Priority One (red tag). If the carotid pulse is strong, move on to the mental status observation, the third step of the BCM series.

Treat patients with a weak carotid pulse for shock by elevating the legs to return as much blood as possible to the brain, lungs, and heart. Then try to stop any severe bleeding. Do not spend time controlling the bleeding yourself. Get the patient to assist or ask one of the walking wounded Priority Three (green tag) patients to help. These patients are often eager to assist with emergency treatment. If the pulse is absent, tag the patient with a Priority Four (gray/black tag).

Mental Status: Open Your Eyes!

The last BCM triage test is the mental status of the patient. This observation is done on patients who have adequate breathing and adequate circulation. First determine whether the patient responds to verbal stimuli. Tell the patient to follow a simple command: "Open your eyes;" "Close your eyes;" "Squeeze my hand." Patients who can follow these simple commands and have adequate breathing and adequate circulation are tagged Priority Two (yellow tag). According to the AVPU scale, which is described in Chapter 7, such patients are considered to be "alert" and "responsive" to verbal stimuli. A patient who cannot follow this type of simple command is "unresponsive" to verbal stimuli, according to the AVPU scale. Tag these patients as Priority One (red tag).

START Is Just the Beginning

In every situation involving casualty sorting, the goal is to find, stabilize, and move Priority One patients first. The START system is designed to help rescuers find the most seriously injured patients. As more rescue personnel arrive on the scene, the patients will be retriaged for further evaluation, treatment, stabilization, and transportation.

Remember that injured patients do not stay in the same condition. The process of shock may continue and some conditions will become more serious as time goes by. As time and resources permit, go back and recheck the condition of Priority Two and Priority Three patients to catch changes in condition that may require upgrading to Priority One (red tag) attention **Figure 18-22**.

Working at a Multiple- or Mass-Casualty Incident

You may or may not be the first person to arrive on the scene of a multiple- or mass-casualty incident. If other rescuers are already at the scene when you arrive, be sure to report to the incident commander before going to work. Because many activities are going on at the same time, the incident commander will assign you to an area where your help and skills can best be used. The incident commander, based on training and local protocols, is in charge of the rescue operation. An effective incident command system (ICS) depends upon integrated, agreed-upon protocols and procedures involving fire department, law enforcement, and emergency medical services personnel. You should learn the ICS that is used in your community.

If you are the first on the scene, you will have to make the initial overview, clearly and accurately report the situation, and conduct the initial START triage. In addition, you will probably also be called on to participate in many other ways during multiple- and mass-casualty incidents.

As more highly trained rescue and emergency personnel arrive on the scene, accurately report your findings to the person in charge by using a format similar to that used in the initial arrival report. Note the following information:

- Approximate number of patients
- Number of patients that you have triaged into the four levels
- Additional assistance required
- Other important information

After you have reported this information, you may be assigned to provide emergency care to patients, to help move patients, or to assist with ambulance or helicopter transportation. You may also be asked to assist with traffic control or help provide fire protection depending on your training.

National Incident Management System

The **National Incident Management System (NIMS)** has been developed by the U.S. Department of Homeland Security to provide a consistent and unified approach to handling emergency incidents. NIMS is designed so that it can be used to effectively and efficiently handle the immedi-

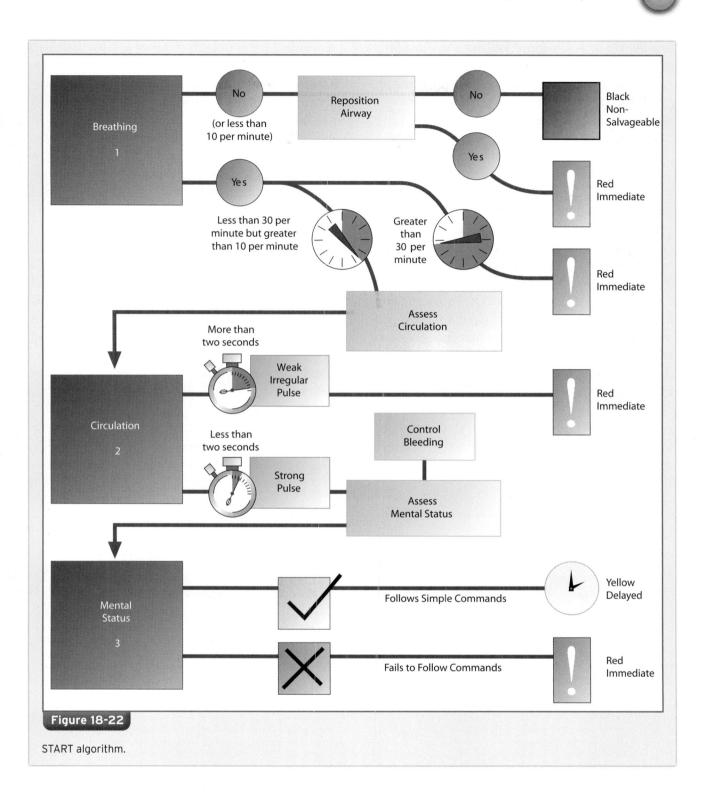

Figure 18-22

START algorithm.

ate response, mitigation, and long-term recovery of small and massive natural and man-made incidents. Effective implementation of NIMS helps local government agencies to work with regional, state, and federal agencies during all phases of a major emergency incident.

NIMS expands on the incident command system in your department, which may cover only one type of agency. NIMS is designed to address a unified command structure that includes all types of agencies responding to any type of man-made or natural disaster. In order to accomplish this, NIMS is flexible and yet contains standardized components.

Six major areas are addressed within the scope of NIMS. They are:

1. Command and Management
2. Preparedness
3. Resource Management
4. Communications and Information Management
5. Supporting Technologies
6. Ongoing Management and Maintenance

As a first responder, your role falls within the first box in the table, Command and Management. There are three major components within Command and Management: The Incident Command System, Multiagency Coordination Systems, and Public Information Systems. As a first responder, it is important for you to understand the function of the ICS and to understand your role within ICS. In large incidents, you may be working with people from other agencies, so you need to understand how the Multiagency Coordination Systems ensure unified operating procedures. It is important for you to understand the function of Public Information Systems in releasing information about an emergency incident. The other five components shown in Figure 18-23 ▾ are vital parts of NIMS, but your role as a first responder is not as directly related to these functions.

The federal government requires many agencies to utilize NIMS and you may be required to become trained in this system. Different levels of training are offered through Internet-based courses. Additional information on NIMS is available at the Federal Emergency Management Agency Web site. Taking advantage of training in incident management will help you to understand and work within the incident management system.

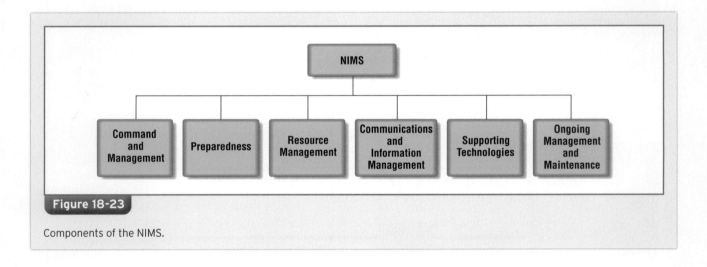

Figure 18-23

Components of the NIMS.

You are the Provider   SUMMARY

Review the *You are the Provider* case study provided at the beginning of this chapter.

Just after your shift starts, you are dispatched for the report of a single vehicle collision with possible injuries. The vehicle is reported to be a package delivery truck that hit a tree on an interstate highway that runs through your community. There has been a light rain for the last half hour. Dispatch reports that the EMS has an estimated time of arrival of 8 to 9 minutes.

1. What are the actions you should take at this call?

Your role as a first responder at the scene of a vehicle collision consists of the following tasks:

- Overview the scene.
- Identify and stabilize any hazards.
- Gain access to patients.
- Provide initial emergency care.
- Help disentangle patients.
- Help prepare patients for removal.
- Help remove patients.

2. What is your principal role in this incident if hazardous materials are present?

Your role in an incident that may involve hazardous materials is to look for and identify any hazardous materials involved while protecting yourself and keeping yourself and others away from the hazardous materials.

3. What are the initial actions you should take if this incident is a multiple-casualty incident?

Your role as a first responder in a multiple-casualty incident is to:

- Determine the approximate number of patients.
- Determine the number of patients that you have triaged.
- Report any additional assistance required.
- Report any other important information.

Prep Kit

Ready for Review

The Ready for Review thoroughly summarizes the chapter.

- In preparing yourself for a call, you must understand your role as a member of the emergency medical system and be prepared to respond promptly.

- As a first responder, you need the proper equipment on an emergency call, including the medical equipment in your life support kit, your personal safety equipment, and equipment to safeguard the accident scene.

- The five phases of an emergency call include dispatch, response to the scene, arrival at the scene, transferring care of the patient to other EMS personnel, and postrun activities.

- You should be able to perform the first four steps in the extrication process and assist other rescuers with steps five through seven.

- Because you may be the first trained person on the scene of an incident involving hazardous materials, you must be able to identify the potential problem and respond appropriately. During a HazMat incident, your top priority is to protect yourself and bystanders from exposure and contamination.

- You should understand the role of a first responder during the first few minutes of a multiple-casualty incident. The START system is a simple triage system that you can use at multiple-casualty incidents.

- The National Incident Management System (NIMS) is designed to provide a unified approach to emergency incidents of any size that involve multiple agencies anywhere in the United States.

- By learning these simple but important skills involving EMS operations, you can become an effective and lifesaving member of the EMS system in your community.

Vital Vocabulary

The Vital Vocabulary are the key terms for this chapter.

casualty sorting The sorting of patients for treatment and transportation.

chocking A piece of wood or metal placed in front of or behind a wheel to prevent vehicle movement.

extrication Removal from a difficult situation or position; removal of a patient from a wrecked car or other place of entrapment.

fusees Warning devices or flares that burn with a red color; usually used in scene protection at motor vehicle crash sites.

golden hour A concept of emergency patient care that attempts to place a trauma patient into definitive medical care within 1 hour of injury.

hazardous materials (HazMat) Substances that are toxic, poisonous, radioactive, flammable, or explosive and can cause injury or death with exposure.

hot zone A contaminated area.

multiple-casualty incidents (mass-casualty incidents) Accidents or situations involving more patients than you can handle with the initial resources available.

National Incident Management System (NIMS) The structure for managing an emergency incident, which may require a response of many different agencies; designed to provide efficient and effective management from initial response through recovery.

START system A system of casualty sorting using Simple Triage And Rapid Treatment.

tempered glass Safety glass that breaks into small pieces when hit with a sharp, pointed object.

triage The sorting of patients into groups according to the severity of their injuries; used to determine priorities for treatment and transport.

wooden cribbing Wooden 2- × 4-inch or 4- × 4-inch boards used for stabilization or bracing.

Technology

- Interactivities
- Vocabulary Explorer
- Anatomy Review
- Web Links
- Online Review Manual

Assessment in Action

Assessment in Action presents a fictitious scenario to help you review what you learned in this chapter.

You are dispatched to the intersection of Houghton and Broadway for a motor vehicle collision. Upon arrival, you find a small pickup truck that has struck a utility pole. The power line is resting on the roof of the truck. Two occupants are in the vehicle. Both appear to be conscious and alert.

1. What is your first step in this situation?

   A. Perform a scene size-up.
   B. Call for additional assistance.
   C. Assess the patient's ABCs.
   D. Begin removing the patients from the vehicle.

2. What additional resources would not be needed on this scene?

   A. Electric company
   B. HazMat team
   C. Fire department
   D. Additional ambulance

3. What hazards do you need to consider on this scene?

   A. Battery acid
   B. Transmission fluid
   C. Fuel leakage
   D. Live electric lines

4. The first step in the START system is to:

   A. Begin tagging patients.
   B. Walk among the injured patients.
   C. Instruct patients who can walk to move to a specified area.
   D. Ask each patient if he or she can walk to a different area.

5. Match each of the following colors with the appropriate level of triage in the START system.

   A. Green
   B. Black
   C. Red
   D. Yellow

   __ Immediate care/life threatening
   __ Urgent care can be delayed up to 1 hour
   __ Patient is dead; no care required
   __ Care can be delayed up to 3 hours

Terrorism Awareness

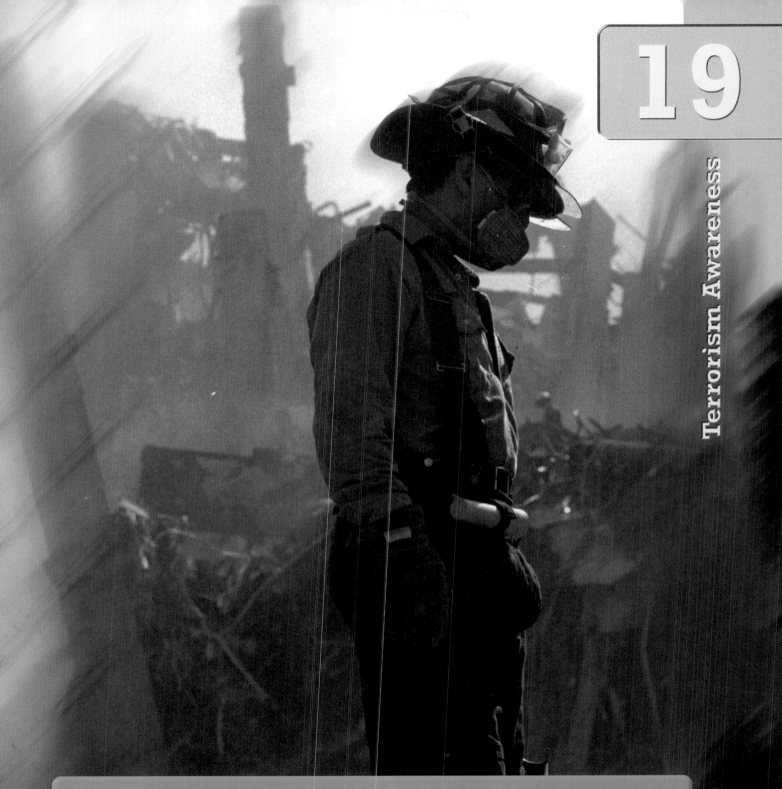

You are the Provider

You are enjoying a quiet afternoon when you hear the click of the intercom that signals an emergency call. "Unit 836 respond to assist EMS units at 116 City Mall Drive for the report of an explosion in a shopping mall. We are receiving reports of multiple injuries. Time out: 1543."

As you respond, you are directed to assist EMS units at a triage area in the parking lot on the south side of the mall.

1. What precautions should you take based on the information you received?
2. How would you determine if this might be a terrorist incident?

Introduction

The purpose of this chapter is to increase your awareness of terrorism. This chapter defines terrorism and describes the types of structures that might be targeted by terrorists. It describes how explosive, incendiary, chemical, biological, and radiological agents might be used by terrorists. It emphasizes the similarities between hazardous materials (HazMat) incidents and terrorist events. It explains the role of first responders at terrorist incidents; it stresses the importance of safety, preparedness, and the use of the incident command system to deal with these mass-casualty events. This chapter emphasizes that first responders should not rush into unsafe environments.

Because of the increase in both international and domestic terrorist activity, it is possible that you will be called to assist after a terrorist event at some point in your career. As a first responder, it is important that you be physically and mentally prepared to deal with the aftermath of such an attack.

What Is Terrorism?

Terrorism is the systematic use of violence by a group to intimidate a population or government in order to achieve a goal. Terrorism receives considerable public attention and is a high-profile crime. Terrorist acts may be instigated by a country's citizens or by people from other countries. The bombing of an abortion clinic by American citizens is considered a domestic terrorist event. The attacks on the World Trade Center and the Pentagon on September 11, 2001, were international terrorist events because the people who flew the planes into those buildings were citizens of other countries. A terrorist event may involve limited property damage with no injuries or it may involve the deaths of many people. Terrorists may use a wide variety of methods to incite terror, including the use of explosives, fire, chemicals, viruses, bacteria, and radiation. The success of terrorist events is measured by the intimidation produced, not just by the value of the property lost or the number of lives lost.

The agents used by terrorists are many of the same agents that produce hazards for first responders in everyday accidents and emergencies. A building collapse caused by a natural gas explosion and a building collapse caused by a terrorist attack are both collapsed buildings. They share many of the same hazards and require many of the same safety precautions for rescuers. The accidental release of a chemical causes a HazMat emergency; an intentional release of the same chemical by terrorists becomes a terrorist event. Still, the safety precautions for rescuers at both events are the same. A radiation leak from a nuclear power plant releases the same type of radiation that would be released by a terrorist. It is important to understand the agents and methods that are used by terrorists and to compare them with the agents that normally exist in communities. Many of the safety precautions used in accidental emergencies are the same precautions needed when dealing with terrorist events.

Weapons of Mass Destruction

A weapon of mass destruction (WMD) is any agent designed to bring about mass death, casualties, and/or massive damage to property and infrastructure (such as bridges, tunnels, airports, electrical power plants, and seaports). These instruments of death and destruction include explosive, chemical, biological, and nuclear weapons.

Technology

- Interactivities
- Vocabulary Explorer
- Anatomy Review
- Web Links
- Online Review Manual

To date, the preferred WMD for terrorists has been explosive devices. Terrorist groups have favored tactics that use truck or car bombs or pedestrian suicide bombers. Many previous terrorist attempts to use either chemical or biological weapons to their full capacity have been unsuccessful. Nonetheless, as a first responder, you should understand the destructive potential of these weapons.

Potential Targets and Risks

One step in understanding the threat that terrorists pose is to consider the places that terrorists might identify as targets for terrorist activities. Remember that terrorists strive to incite fear to achieve a political or ideological goal and their motives do not limit their choice of targets. Bridges, tunnels, pipelines, and harbors constitute infrastructure targets. The Washington Monument and the Statute of Liberty are examples of symbolic targets. Housing developments and automobile dealerships have been targeted by ecoterrorists. Computer networks and data systems might be targets for cyberterrorists. Farms and agricultural installations might be targets for terrorists trying to destroy or taint the nation's food sources. Civilian targets such as schools, government buildings, churches, and shopping centers represent high visibility targets for terrorists. Taken collectively, a wide variety of the places that represent most components in society might be considered as targets Figure 19-1 . In an open society in which people are largely free to

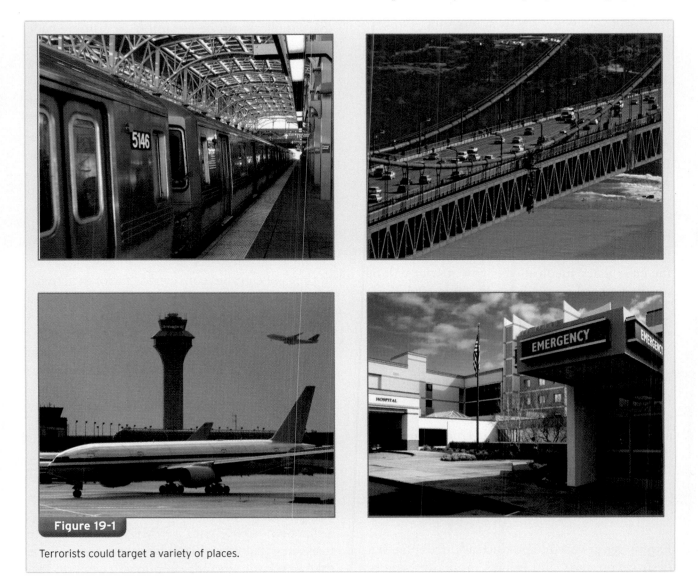

Figure 19-1

Terrorists could target a variety of places.

TABLE 19-1	Deaths in 2001
Cause of Death	**Number of Deaths**
Heart disease	700,142
Cancer	553,768
Accidents	101,537
Suicide	30,622
Murders	17,330
Terrorists	2,978

Source: Centers for Disease Control and Prevention.

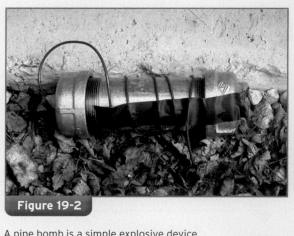

Figure 19-2

A pipe bomb is a simple explosive device.

move around as they wish, a person bent on committing a terrorist act can access most of the components of the infrastructure and turn any one of them into a target.

In spite of heightened security measures, a terrorist event could occur at any time. First responders should always be alert for hazards—those associated with a terrorist event as well as those connected to any other emergency. In any discussion of the risks of terrorist attacks, it is important to consider the number of terror-related deaths with other major causes of death. **Table 19-1 ▲** compares the number of deaths from terrorist events with deaths from other common causes. This comparison is not intended to minimize the tragedies of September 11, 2001; rather, it is intended to help you realize that terrorist events do not occur every day. Although you should be prepared for them, the majority of the emergency medical calls you answer will be for the types of events listed in Table 19-1.

Agents and Devices

A wide variety of agents and devices can be used to incite terror, including explosive devices, incendiary devices, chemical agents, biological agents, and radiological agents. Understand how these devices are used and the safety precautions to take as a first responder to ensure scene safety for rescuers and bystanders.

Explosives and Incendiary Devices

Explosives are used to produce a concussion that destroys property and inflicts injury and death. Some explosive devices, also known as incen-

diary devices, are designed to start fires. Incendiary devices can be as simple as a homemade firebomb or as complex as a highly technical device that may have been stolen from the military. An explosive device can be hand carried or transported in a heavy truck **Figure 19-2 ▲**. Often the first indication that an explosive or incendiary device is present is the explosion or fire that results from the deployment of the device. In some parts of the world, suicide terrorists carry explosive devices on their person and set them off to kill themselves and others.

Safety Considerations for First Responders

In times of elevated concern for terrorist activity, travelers are urged to be alert for bags or luggage left unattended. Be aware of suspicious vehicles and report them to the proper law enforcement officials. If you are called to respond to an explosion, be alert for safety hazards that may have been created by the explosion or by a terrorist. Do not enter any area that may be unsafe until properly trained personnel are able to assess the risks. Be alert for the possibility of a second explosive device that is timed to explode when rescuers are on the scene. Use the same safety skills you developed for other types of emergency situations to keep yourself safe.

When dealing with a WMD scene, it is safe to assume that you will not be able to enter where the event has occurred—nor do you want to. The best location for staging is upwind and uphill from the incident. Wait for assistance from those who are trained in assessing and managing WMD scenes.

Chemical Agents

Many different types of chemicals can be used as terrorist weapons. Industrial-process chemicals can be used to intentionally inflict harm on people. For example, chlorine is a gas that is used in many industrial processes and in water purification, but it was also used as a poisonous gas in World War I. Many of the **chemical agents** that could be used by terrorists are the same chemicals that create HazMat incidents when accidentally released.

Chemical agents can be divided into the following categories:

- Pulmonary (choking) agents
- Metabolic agents
- Insecticides
- Nerve agents
- Blister agents

Pulmonary Agents

Pulmonary agents are gases that cause immediate distress and injury. Their primary route of entry into the body is through the airway into the lungs. Once these chemicals are inhaled, they damage lung tissue, which causes fluid to escape into the lungs and leads to pulmonary edema. Pulmonary agents cause intense coughing, gasping, shortness of breath, and difficulty breathing. Two common pulmonary agents are chlorine and phosgene. Phosgene gas is produced by burning freon, which is found in most domestic air conditioners. The odor of this gas is similar to freshly mowed grass. The symptoms of phosgene gas exposure may be delayed for several hours after inhalation of the gas. Although pulmonary agents could be weapons of choice for terrorists, these chemicals are also present in a variety of domestic and industrial settings and might also be encountered following an accidental release. The safety precautions for an accidental release are the same as the precautions for an intentional release by terrorists: Keep a safe distance away until properly trained HazMat personnel can handle the situation.

Metabolic Agents

Metabolic agents affect the body's ability to use oxygen at the cellular level. The most common metabolic agents are cyanides. Cyanides are produced in large quantities and used in gold and silver mining, photography, and plastics processing. Cyanide is also produced by the combustion of plastics and textiles, so there is the potential for cyanide poisoning in any house fire. Contact with cyanides produces shortness of breath, flushed skin, rapid heartbeat, seizures, coma, and cardiac arrest. The safety precautions for an accidental release of cyanide are the same as the precautions for an intentional release by terrorists: Keep a safe distance away until properly trained HazMat personnel can handle the situation.

Insecticides

Insecticides are a class of poisonous chemicals that are inhaled or absorbed through the skin. Many insecticides belong to a class of chemicals that are called organophosphates. Absorption of these chemicals produces the following symptoms: salivation, sweating, lacrimation (excessive tearing), urination, diarrhea, gastric upset, and emesis (vomiting). The acronym for these symptoms is the word SLUDGE `Table 19-2 ▼`. Because insecticides are readily available, they could be used as agents by terrorists. It is important to realize that far more emergency providers have experienced accidental contact with insecticides than during terrorist-related events. If you encounter an incident involving an insecticide, keep bystanders far enough away to prevent additional contact with the chemical. If you encounter an emergency involving multi-

TABLE 19-2	Symptoms of Exposure to an Organophosphate Insecticide or Nerve Agent
S	Salivation, sweating
L	Lacrimation (excessive tearing)
U	Urination
D	Defecation, diarrhea
G	Gastric upset
E	Emesis (vomiting)

ple people with SLUDGE-like symptoms, assume you are dealing with poisoning from this type of chemical and call for help from a trained Haz-Mat team. Do not make contact with contaminated patients until they have been properly decontaminated by trained personnel.

Nerve Agents

Nerve agents are among the most deadly chemicals developed. These chemicals can kill large numbers of people with small quantities and cause cardiac arrest within seconds to minutes of exposure. Discovered by scientists in search of a superior pesticide, nerve agents are much stronger organophosphates than those found in insecticides. Nerve agents, like insecticides, block an essential enzyme in the nervous system and cause the SLUDGE-like symptoms listed in Table 19-2. Four of the most commonly mentioned nerve agents are sarin, soman, tabun, and V agent (VX).

In an emergency situation, your primary responsibility is to keep yourself, other rescuers, and bystanders from becoming contaminated. A well-trained HazMat team in special protective equipment is needed to remove and decontaminate people exposed to these agents. An antidote kit called a MARK 1 or a nerve agent antidote kit (NAAK) is available that contains drugs to counteract the effects of nerve agents.

Blister Agents

When blister agents come in contact with the skin, they produce burn-like blisters. If the vapors of these agents are inhaled, they cause burns of the respiratory system. Blister agents produce skin irritation, pain, eye irritation, severe shortness of breath, and severe coughing. Blister agents include sulfur mustard and Lewisite. As with other chemical agents, blister agents pose a threat to rescuers. Only well-trained and properly dressed rescuers with self-contained breathing apparatus should approach a scene that might contain these agents. Table 19-3 ▾ lists characteristics of some chemical agents.

TABLE 19-3   Chemical Agents

Name	Military Designations	Odor	Lethality	Onset of Symptoms	Primary Route of Exposure
Pulmonary agents	Chlorine (CL) Phosgene (CG)	Bleach (CL) Cut grass (CG)	Cause irritation choking (CL); severe pulmonary edema (CG)	Immediate (CL) Delayed (CG)	Vapor hazard
Metabolic agents	Hydrogen cyanide (AC) Cyanogen chloride (CK)	Almonds (AC) Irritating (CK)	Highly lethal chemical gases; can kill within minutes; effects are reversible with antidotes	Immediate	Vapor hazard
Nerve agents	Tabun (GA) Sarin (GB) Soman (GD) V agent (VX)	Fruity or none	Most lethal chemical agents; can kill within minutes; effects are reversible with antidotes	Immediate	Vapor hazard (GB) Contact hazard (VX) Both vapor and contact (GA, GD)
Blister agents	Mustard (H) Lewisite (L) Phosgene oxime (CX)	Garlic (H) Geranium (L)	Cause large blisters to form on victims; may severely damage upper airway if vapors are inhaled; severe, intense pain and grayish skin discoloration (L, CX)	Delayed (H) Immediate (L, CX)	Primarily contact with some vapor hazard

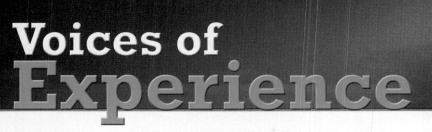

Voices of Experience

Voices of Experience

Create Order Out of Chaos

I had just finished my regular 8-hour paramedic shift in Lorain, Ohio. It was midnight, and I was about halfway through my 20-minute drive home, when I heard a distant thud to the south, toward Elyria. When I looked in the direction of the sound, I thought I saw a glow reflecting off the clouds in the distance. The EMS service I worked for covered both Lorain and Elyria, so I took the next right turn and headed toward the glow.

There had been an explosion at the Aztec Chemical Plant, which was inconveniently located in the middle of a city of about 50,000 residents. This occurred in the days before everyone had cell phones, and I didn't want to interfere with priority traffic by talking on the radio. One of the most important rules to remember as a first responder, and one of the most easily forgotten in the excitement of the moment is: Don't make things worse!

> **When the time comes, you must do what you have been trained to do.**

As I drove toward the scene, I looked for flags or smoke to check the wind direction. I was in luck, I was upwind. When I got into town, I could hear from the radio traffic that both fire and medical incident command were up and running. When there was a lull in radio traffic, I called dispatch and was directed to report to dispatch at the central station.

When I arrived at dispatch, I was told to wait for an assignment with several other off-duty personnel who were already there. After about an hour, we were sent to various schools where evacuation shelters were being set up by the Red Cross. Although the fire department had not been able to identify the chemicals released, there were reports of respiratory distress.

My partner and I took a squad and reported to one of the designated schools. What we saw on our arrival was amazing. Volunteers from the Red Cross were calmly and efficiently setting things up. They had already designated areas for decontamination, canteen, families, and intake. They had set up coolers, water, chairs, and cots, and they were bringing in food—and the explosion had occurred less than 2 hours before. Most of the volunteers were seniors, and they operated in a calm, friendly, and professional manner.

We were asked to set up a medical station to evaluate people who weren't feeling well. The chemical released was eventually reported to be a mild respiratory irritant, and the explosion was an accident caused by a worker, who was the only one to die in the blast. By morning, everyone was allowed to go back home.

It doesn't matter what the cause of a mass-casualty incident is—accident, terrorism, or criminal violence—the principles remain the same. First responders must respond quickly, but more importantly, they must respond wisely, calmly, and efficiently. The greatest service you can perform at a disorganized scene is to create order out of chaos, calm out of calamity. To do so, you must consciously work to control your emotions as well as your physiological response to stress. Slow down, breath slowly and deeply, and lower your voice. Tunnel vision is your worst enemy. Force yourself to look around, in all directions and dimensions, and use all of your senses. These skills do not come naturally—to be good in a crisis you must train and train and train, and when the time comes, you must do what you have been trained to do.

Guy H. Haskell, PhD, NREMT-P
Fire fighter, Benton Township Volunteer Fire Department, Unionville, Indiana
Paramedic, Brown Township Fire and Rescue, Mooresville, Indiana
Director, Emergency Medical and Safety Services Consultants, Bloomington, Indiana

Safety Considerations for First Responders

This brief summary about chemical agents does not make any first responder an expert. It is intended to give enough information to help you realize that the chemicals that might be used by terrorists, while deadly, are in the same classes as many of the chemicals encountered by HazMat teams. It is important to remember that any time there are multiple people suffering from unexplained symptoms, the first responder should suspect a common agent as the cause. Your primary role is to recognize that a problem exists and to avoid contaminating yourself, other rescuers, and bystanders. Stay upwind from any potential source and call for assistance from a properly trained HazMat team.

Biological Agents

Biological agents are naturally occurring substances that produce diseases. They may be bacteria such as anthrax or the plague or viruses such as smallpox or hemorrhagic fever. Many biological agents caused epidemics of disease in the past. Some of these agents, such as smallpox, have been wiped out; the last natural case of smallpox was seen in 1977. However, the smallpox organism has been maintained in laboratories and could be used intentionally to infect people. Although biological agents are hard to disperse to large numbers of people, there is some concern that they could be used as a deadly weapon by terrorists.

If terrorists intentionally dispersed a biological agent, the organism would have to come in contact with people in sufficient quantities to produce an illness. These diseases have an **incubation period**, which is the time from exposure to a disease organism to the time the person begins to show symptoms of the disease. This means that if people were exposed to an infectious organism today, it might be several days before they would show signs of the disease. The first awareness of a biological terrorist incident would probably come from hospital emergency departments and public health departments. The role of first responders in biological incidents is to report unusual patterns of illness and keep up-to-date with current information from your medical director and public health department.

Safety Considerations for First Responders

Safety considerations for first responders include being alert for unusual patterns of diseases with flu-like symptoms. Make every effort to review current information about disease trends from your medical director and public health department. Practice appropriate BSI precautions for the signs and symptoms exhibited by every patient. If you have any indications that a call might involve a biological agent, call for specially trained assistance and wait in a safe location.

First responders need to be aware of when they should suspect the use of biological agents. If the agent is in the form of a powder, such as in the October 2001 attacks involving anthrax mailed in letters, the incident must be handled by HazMat specialists. Patients who have come into direct contact with the agent need to be decontaminated before any EMS contact or treatment is initiated.

Radiological Agents

Ionizing radiation is a form of energy that is formed by the decay of a naturally occurring or manmade radioactive source. <u>Radiation</u> is used in hospitals, research facilities, and nuclear power plants, and for military weapons. Exposure to excess amounts of radiation can cause delayed illnesses, such as increase in the rate of certain cancers. Exposure to large amounts of radiation can cause people to become violently ill within a few hours of exposure and may produce death with hours or days. Table 19-4 ▼ lists some signs and symptoms of radiation sickness.

Radiation is a hidden hazard that is similar to electricity. You cannot see, feel, or detect radiation with any of your normal body senses. Special instruments are needed to detect and measure the amount of radiation that is present Figure 19-3 ▼ .

TABLE 19-4	Common Signs of Acute Radiation Sickness
Low exposure	Nausea, vomiting, diarrhea
Moderate exposure	First-degree burns, hair loss, depletion of the immune system (death of white blood cells), cancer
Severe exposure	Second- and third-degree burns, cancer, death

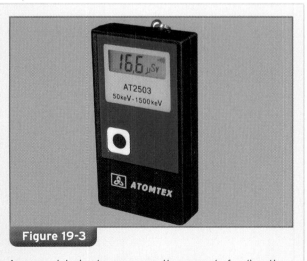

Figure 19-3

A personal dosimeter measures the amount of radioactive exposure received by an individual.

There is some concern that terrorists could detonate an explosive device containing a small amount of radioactive material (known as a dirty bomb). Such an explosion would spread radioactive material over the area of the explosion, and thereby contaminate anyone in the vicinity. In a case such as this, rescuers would have no means of determining if radioactivity was present unless special radiological monitors were used to check for radiation. Unless there was a warning issued about such an event, rescuers might not know about the presence of radiation.

Safety Considerations for First Responders

As a first responder, be alert to warnings about incidents involving radiation. If the presence of radiation is suspected, first responders should stay away from a blast or suspicious site until specially trained teams check for the presence of radiation with special monitoring devices. Know who in your community is equipped to handle such an event.

Your Response to Terrorist Events

The threat of terrorist activity is frightening to most people. It is important that all emergency responders have some awareness and knowledge of the various tactics and agents terrorists might use. Emergency response personnel need to develop an all-hazards approach to dealing with emergencies. Keep in mind that agents used by terrorists could be the same agents that first responders are already trained to deal with: explosions, fires, toxic chemicals, hazardous materials, infectious diseases, and radiation. Although you may feel apprehensive about dealing with a terrorist event, remember that in all emergencies, the same safety rules apply: good scene safety and vigilant BSI.

To prepare for a terrorist event, master the skills that enable you to be a good first responder. Be prepared and know the limits of your training. Many types of terrorist events require you to stay a certain distance away to avoid contaminating additional people. Teams with special training are required for incidents involving special hazards. Be alert for secondary devices placed by a terrorist and set to detonate after emergency responders arrive on the scene.

Terrorist events can affect large numbers of people. Establish an incident command system as soon as possible Figure 19-4 ▶ . Know your role in working within the incident command system. Treat these incidents as mass-casualty situations. Establish good working relationships with appropriate local, state, and federal agencies.

First responders have a vital role in working at terrorist events. You can do the most good by following your training and not exceeding the skills you have. Always be alert for your safety, the safety of other rescuers, and the safety of patients. Remember that you cannot be an effective rescuer if you become a victim yourself.

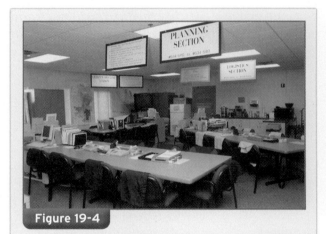

Figure 19-4

An incident command system needs to be set up for large-scale terrorist and mass-casualty events.

You are the Provider

SUMMARY

Review the *You are the Provider* case study provided at the beginning of the chapter.

You are enjoying a quiet afternoon when you hear the click of the intercom that signals an emergency call. "Unit 836 respond to assist EMS units at 116 City Mall Drive for the report of an explosion in a shopping mall. We are receiving reports of multiple injuries. Time out: 1543."

As you respond, you are directed to assist EMS units at a triage area in the parking lot on the south side of the mall.

1. What precautions should you take based on the information you received?

The steps you learned in the patient assessment sequence are appropriate in this situation. It is important to perform a scene size-up by reviewing dispatch information, observing BSI, ensuring scene safety, determining the mechanism of injury, and determining the need for additional resources. Some of these steps may have been taken care of by rescuers who arrived before you.

2. How would you determine if this might be a terrorist incident?

Suspect that this incident might be a terrorist event if you receive information from your dispatcher, from bystanders, or from officials on the scene. In most cases, you will have to exercise good safety procedures to ensure your safety, the safety of other rescuers, and the safety of bystanders. By exercising prudent safety precautions and by being alert for hazards, you stand the best chance of protecting yourself and others from injury or death.

Prep Kit

Ready for Review

The Ready for Review thoroughly summarizes the chapter.

- Terrorist attacks, although rare, are a concern for emergency providers. As a first responder, it is important that you be physically and mentally prepared to deal with the aftermath of such an attack.

- The goal of terrorists is to intimidate a population or government in order to achieve a goal. Terrorists may use a wide variety of methods to incite terror, including the use of explosives, fire, chemicals, viruses, bacteria, and radiation.

- Chemical agents are manmade substances that can have devastating effects on living organisms. These agents consist of pulmonary, metabolic, insecticides, nerve, and blister agents.

- Biological agents are organisms that cause disease. They are generally found in nature and can be weaponized to maximize the number of people exposed to the germ.

- Radiological weapons can create a massive amount of destruction. This type of weapon includes radiological dispersal devices, also know as dirty bombs.

- First responders need to consider their safety, the safety of other rescuers, and the safety of bystanders whenever dealing with a terrorist-related event. Identifying potential threats, ensuring safety, and calling for specially trained personnel to deal with these threats comprise the first responder's responsibilities in many of these situations.

Vital Vocabulary

The Vital Vocabulary are the key terms for this chapter.

biological agents Disease-causing bacteria or viruses that might be used by terrorists to intentionally cause epidemics of disease.

blister agents Chemicals that cause the skin to blister.

chemical agents Compounds that can be used by terrorists to inflict harm.

explosives Substances that release energy in a sudden and uncontrolled manner when detonated.

incubation period The time from exposure to a disease organism to the time the person begins to show symptoms of the disease.

insecticides Chemicals that are formulated to kill insects, but can intentionally or accidentally cause injury or death to humans.

metabolic agents Substances that are intended to produce injury or death by disrupting chemical reactions at the cellular level.

nerve agents Toxic substances that attack the central nervous system.

pulmonary agents Substances that produce respiratory distress or illness.

radiation The electromagnetic energy that is released from a radioactive material or a dirty bomb.

terrorism A systematic use of violence to intimidate or to achieve a goal.

weapon of mass destruction (WMD) Any agent designed to bring about mass death, casualties, and/or massive damage to property and infrastructure (bridges, tunnels, airports, electrical power plants, and seaports).

Technology

- Interactivities
- Vocabulary Explorer
- Anatomy Review
- Web Links
- Online Review Manual

Assessment in Action

Assessment in Action presents a fictitious scenario to help you review what you learned in this chapter.

You are dispatched for the report of several students who are short of breath and coughing at a local high school. As you arrive at the school, you find several students in the parking lot who are experiencing difficulty breathing.

1. Which of the following should not be one of your first actions?

   A. Park upwind of the school.
   B. Call for additional assistance.
   C. Enter the school building to investigate.
   D. Transmit an initial report to the dispatcher.

2. What type of assistance would you request?

   A. Fire department support
   B. HazMat team
   C. Law enforcement personnel
   D. Highway department

3. What type of substance(s) would you suspect might be involved in this incident?

   A. Blister agent
   B. Pulmonary agent
   C. Insecticide
   D. Chemical agent

4. Why would you suspect this or these types of agents?

   A. Because multiple people have the same symptoms at the same time
   B. Because high schools could be a terrorist target
   C. Because the students are coughing
   D. Because the students are short of breath

5. When would it be safe for you to treat these patients?

   A. As soon as you can
   B. As soon as they are triaged
   C. After the HazMat team has cleared them
   D. As soon as you put on gloves

6. Your role in an incident like this might be to:

   A. Treat patients as they exit the school.
   B. Prevent rescuers and bystanders from becoming contaminated.
   C. Assist with decontamination of these patients.
   D. Find the source of the problem.

7. In order for an incident such as this to be handled effectively, you need:

   A. A triage trailer
   B. Medical directors on the scene
   C. A certified emergency manager
   D. A strong incident command system

8. If this were a terrorist incident caused by a biological agent, what differences would you expect to see?

   A. There would be more patients with these symptoms.
   B. The patients should have cool, pale skin.
   C. The patients would be more likely to vomit.
   D. The symptoms would not occur as quickly because of the incubation period needed.

9. Responding to a terrorist event requires many of the same safety considerations as responding to a mass-casualty incident.

   A. True
   B. False

Enrichment

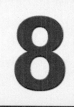

Section

8

Special Rescue

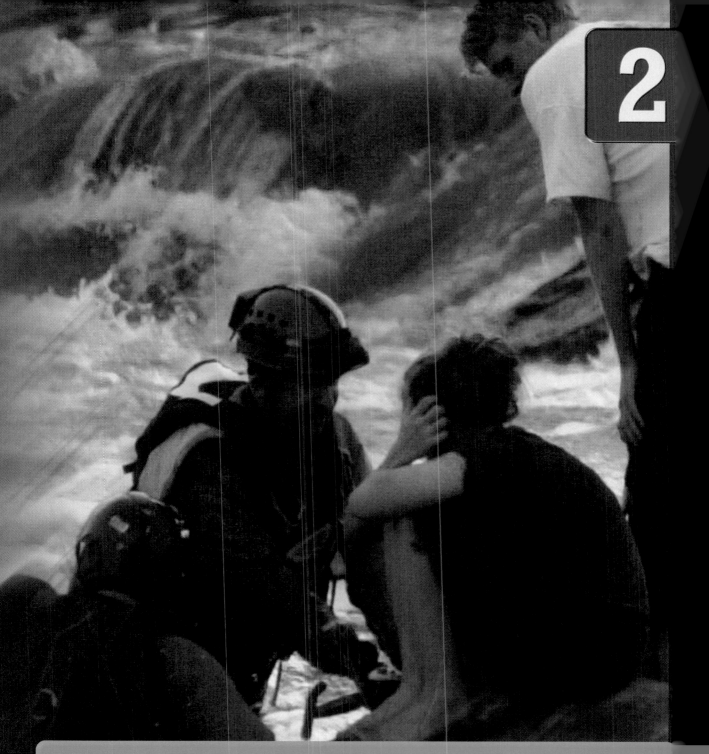

You are the Provider

At 5:37 AM, you are startled by your dispatcher. She announces, "Unit 433, respond to an unknown rescue situation at 10711 Lee Highway. This was a third-party call; no other information is available."

   You are concerned because you do not have enough information to begin to mentally prepare for this call.

1. If you are the first emergency provider to arrive on the scene, what is your role in handling a rescue situation?
2. What are the common safety principles that you need to follow during rescue operations?
3. What are the steps you should follow at any rescue situation?

Introduction

This chapter covers special rescue situations that can be life threatening to both the rescuer and the victim. These situations include water rescue, ice rescue, and confined space rescue. This chapter provides you with guidelines for dealing with these situations. It also covers guidelines for dealing with emergencies on farms and with bus collisions. In each situation, your first objective is to maintain your personal safety. In addition, there are basic rescue procedures you can perform without endangering yourself or the victim.

Water and Ice Rescue

You may encounter situations in which a person needs to be rescued from the water. The person may be fatigued, may have suffered a diving injury, or may have fallen through the ice in the winter. A book of this scope cannot teach you the skills of a certified lifesaver. It does describe some simple techniques you can use to perform a water or ice rescue without endangering your own safety.

Water Rescue

When you see a person struggling in the water, your first impulse may be to jump in to assist. However, that action may not result in a successful rescue and can endanger your own life. If you are faced with a water rescue situation, remember the steps listed and illustrated in **Figure 20-1 ▶**: **Reach-throw-row-go**. If you follow these steps, you may be able to perform a successful water rescue without ever entering the water. It may even be possible for someone who cannot swim to rescue a struggling person.

Reach

Use any readily available object to reach the threatened person. If the victim is close to shore, a branch, pole, oar, or paddle may be long enough. If you are at a swimming pool, there may be a specially designed pole available for this purpose. Use it.

Throw

If you cannot reach the person, throw something. At a swimming pool, dock, or supervised beach, a **flotation device** (such as a ring buoy) may be available. If a life buoy is available, throw it to the person in distress. If no buoy is handy, then improvise. Throw a rope, plastic milk jug, or sealed Styrofoam cooler. Even a car's spare tire can support several people in the water. Think before you act!

Row

If you cannot reach the person by throwing something that floats, you may be able to row out to the drowning person if a small boat or canoe is available. Consider this only if you know how to operate or propel the craft properly. Protect yourself by wearing an approved personal flotation device.

Go

As a last resort, you may have to go into the water to save the victim. Enter the water only if you are a capable swimmer trained in lifesaving techniques. Remove encumbering clothing before en-

Technology

- Interactivities
- Vocabulary Explorer
- Anatomy Review
- Web Links
- Online Review Manual

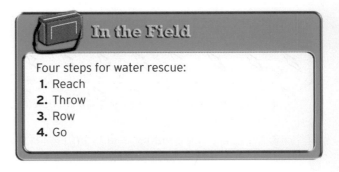

In the Field

Four steps for water rescue:
1. Reach
2. Throw
3. Row
4. Go

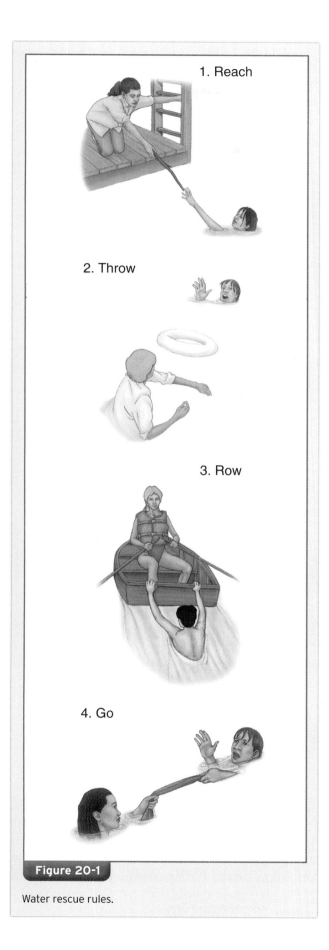

1. Reach

2. Throw

3. Row

4. Go

Figure 20-1

Water rescue rules.

tering the water. Take a flotation device with you if one is available.

Initial Treatment of a Person in the Water

If you are in a water rescue situation, your primary concerns must be to open an airway, establish breathing and circulation, and stabilize spinal cord injuries. Turn patients who are face down in the water face up **Skill Drill 20-1 ▶**:

SKILL DRILL 20-1

1. Support the back and head with one hand and place the other hand on the front of the patient to keep the head and neck stabilized **Step 1**.
2. Keep the head in the neutral position and carefully turn the patient as a unit **Step 2**.
3. Stabilize the patient's head and neck **Step 3**.

Use the jaw-thrust technique to open the airway. Do not hyperextend the neck because of the high risk of associated spinal cord injuries. Look, listen, and feel for signs of breathing. If the patient is not breathing, start rescue breathing while the

> **In the Field**
>
> If you are using something like a plastic milk jug or picnic jug, fill the container with about 1 inch of water to add weight before you seal it and throw it to the victim.

> **Safety Tips**
>
> Currents in streams or strong currents (**riptides**) at ocean beaches can pull both victim and rescuer rapidly away from shore. In an area below a dam, rapids, or waterfall, deadly currents may be present. An untrained rescuer should never attempt to enter the water under these conditions. If you do, both you and the victim will probably need to be rescued.

Skill DRILL 20-1

Turning a Patient in the Water

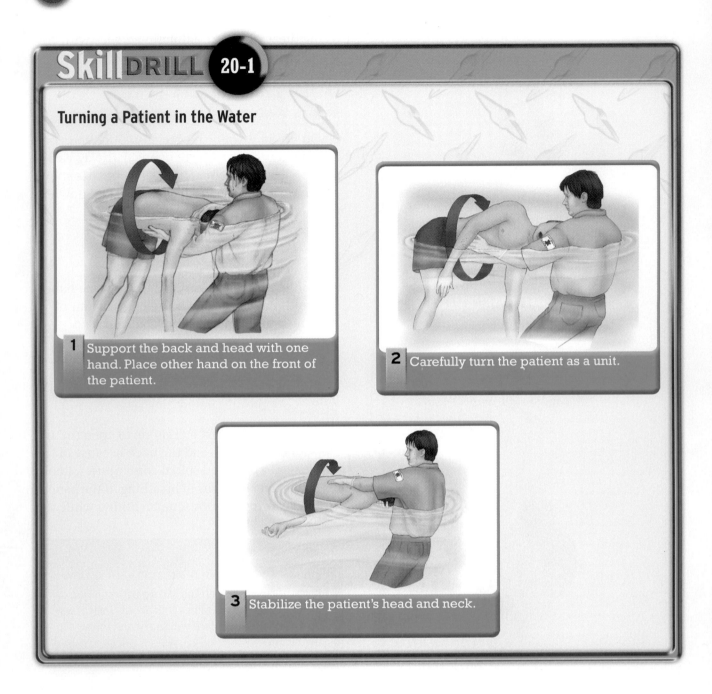

1 Support the back and head with one hand. Place other hand on the front of the patient.

2 Carefully turn the patient as a unit.

3 Stabilize the patient's head and neck.

patient is still in the water **Figure 20-2 ▶** . Ventilation will be much easier if you can stand on the bottom.

If the patient has suffered cardiac arrest, quickly stabilize the head and neck and remove the patient from the water. Place the patient on a hard surface before you begin CPR (see Chapter 9).

Treat a patient who is unconscious in the water as if a spinal cord injury were present. Also assume the presence of a spinal cord injury if a conscious patient in the water com-

plains of numbness or tingling in the arms or legs, inability to move the extremities, or neck pain. Support the patient by floating a backboard in the water under the patient **Figure 20-3 ▶** . Strap the patient to the backboard, stabilize the head and neck, and remove the patient from the water. If no rigid device is available and the patient must be removed from the water before EMS personnel arrive, six people, using their hands, can lift and support the patient **Figure 20-4 ▶** .

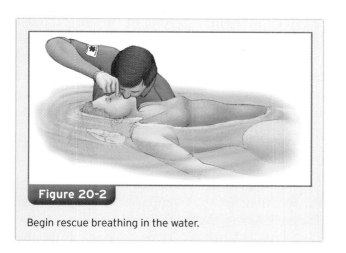

Figure 20-2

Begin rescue breathing in the water.

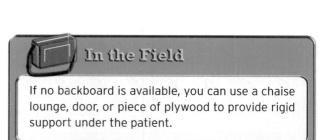

Figure 20-3

Apply the backboard while the patient is still in the water.

Diving Problems

First responders may be called to care for people involved in diving accidents. Most recreational divers use self-contained underwater breathing apparatus (scuba). Scuba gear consists of an air tank, a regulator, a mouthpiece, and a face mask. Commercial divers use either scuba gear or equipment that supplies air through a hose.

Most underwater diving accidents occur in coastal regions or in areas with large lakes. Diving accidents can cause trauma, near drowning, or specialized injuries. In cases involving trauma or drowning, remove the patient from the water and treat the patient using information and skills you have already learned.

Two specialized injuries are associated with diving: __air embolism__ and __decompression sickness (the bends)__. Usually it will not be possible for you to differentiate between these two conditions. Both are caused by air bubbles being released in the body as a result of the changes in pressure while diving. If an air bubble affects the brain or spinal cord, the signs and symptoms may be similar to those of a stroke. These include dizziness, difficulty speaking, difficulty seeing, and decreased level of consciousness. Pa-

In the Field

If no backboard is available, you can use a chaise lounge, door, or piece of plywood to provide rigid support under the patient.

tients may have difficulty in maintaining an open airway. If the air bubble causes a collapsed lung, the signs and symptoms will include chest pain, shortness of breath, and pink or bloody froth coming from the mouth or nose. If the air bubble obstructs

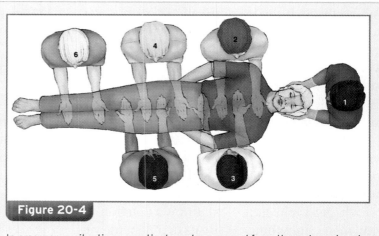

Figure 20-4

In emergency situations, a patient can be removed from the water using six people.

blood flow to the abdomen, the patient will experience severe abdominal pain and may be bent over. If the air bubble involves a joint, there will be severe pain in that joint.

To treat a patient with a suspected air embolism or decompression sickness, you must maintain the patient's airway, breathing, circulation, and normal body temperature. Oxygen should be administered as soon as it is available. Some physicians recommend placing the patient on their left side with the head of the patient slightly lowered. This may help to prevent further damage if there is an air bubble in the central nervous system. Patients with diving injuries may need to be transported to a hospital that is equipped with a hyperbaric (recompression) chamber. If you live in an area where diving injuries occur, you should receive specialized training and be familiar with the protocols of your local EMS system.

Ice Rescue

Ice rescue is extremely hazardous because no ice is safe ice! Ice is changeable and should always be considered unsafe. Think safety first; do not exceed the limits of your training and do not put yourself at undue risk. You cannot save anyone if you go through the ice yourself. As soon as you arrive at the scene of an ice rescue, visually mark the location where the person was last seen. This will enable other rescuers to concentrate their efforts on a limited area. You should know who is responsible for ice rescue in your community and call this team as soon as possible.

The basic rules of ice rescue are the same as water rescue: reach-throw-row-go. Reach for the victim using anything that will extend your natural stretch, such as a ladder, a pike pole, a tree branch, or a backboard. Next, throw a flotation device, rope, or anything that floats to pull in the victim. Third, row or propel a small boat to the victim, if you can break through the ice or use a tobog-

gan to get across the ice. Using a toboggan will spread your weight over a wider area and reduce your chances of falling through the ice. Be sure that you have a rope and that the boat or toboggan is secured to the shore as well. Finally, if you must go, secure yourself to shore with a rope around your waist, lie on your stomach, and proceed across the ice. Spreading your weight over a wider area reduces your chances of falling through the ice **Figure 20-5 ▶**. Be sure you have good communication with other rescuers.

A car on the ice presents a risky situation. Instruct the car's occupants to avoid unnecessary movement. If the car has not gone through the ice, instruct the occupants to open the car doors. This may help to slow the sinking of the car if the ice breaks. If the doors cannot be opened, instruct the occupants to roll down the windows so they have a better escape route. If you must approach the car, remember that the added weight of rescuers can cause movement of the car. Do not place your head inside the car. If the car sinks, you may be unable to get out.

During ice rescues, both victims and rescuers are at risk for hypothermia. Keep all rescuers as warm as possible. Rescue personnel who are not directly involved in the rescue operation should remain in a warm vehicle until they are needed. Victims should be dried and warmed as soon as they are removed from the water. Remember that people can survive for an extended period of time in cold water. If the patient has no pulse, start CPR and continue until the patient has been transported to a hospital and warmed. See Chapter 10 for more information on treating hypothermia.

Confined Space Rescue

Confined spaces are structures designed to keep something in or out. Confined spaces may be below ground, ground level, or elevated structures. Below-ground confined spaces include manholes, below-ground utility vaults or storage tanks, old mines, cisterns, and wells. Ground-level confined spaces include industrial tanks and farm storage silos. Elevated confined spaces include water towers and storage tanks.

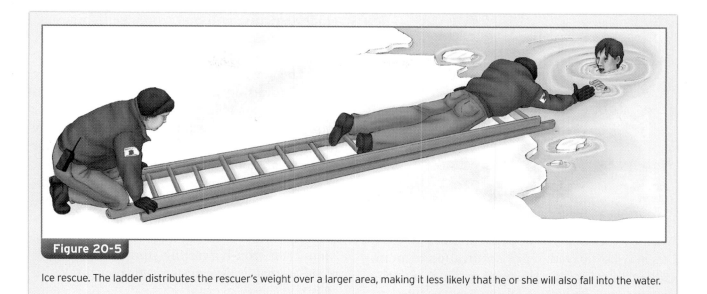

Figure 20-5

Ice rescue. The ladder distributes the rescuer's weight over a larger area, making it less likely that he or she will also fall into the water.

Rescue situations involving confined spaces have two deadly hazards. The first hazard is respiratory. There may be insufficient oxygen to support life or a poisonous gas may be present **Figure 20-6 ▼**. Rescuers must never enter a confined space without the proper respiratory protection. Anyone entering a confined space without proper respiratory protection stands a good chance of becoming a second victim.

The second hazard is the danger of collapse. In a mine, for example, rescuers may need to shore up the confined space before they can safely enter. Confined space rescue requires a specially trained team. As soon as you determine there is a confined space situation, call for additional assistance and do not enter the space until help arrives.

Farm Rescue

Farms are located in most parts of the country. They range from a few acres of land with limited machinery and a small number of animals to large complexes that contain many acres of land, complex machines, large animals, and many hazards. Farm accidents pose a wide variety of challenges for rescuers. Because many farmers

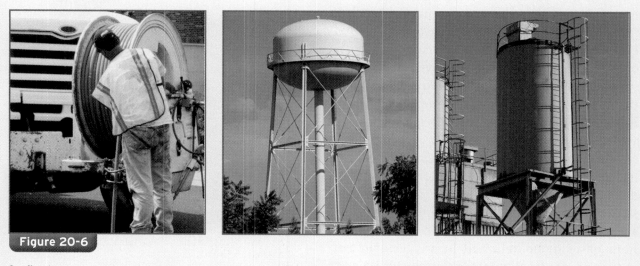

Figure 20-6

Confined spaces may have insufficient oxygen to support life without a self-contained breathing apparatus.

work by themselves, the reporting of emergencies may be delayed. Once notification of an incident is received, there may be a lengthy response in getting to a farm. Once rescuers arrive at a farm, it may be hard to pinpoint the exact location of the emergency. Poor roads, nonexistent roads, and muddy soil may require you to leave your vehicle some distance from the patient. All of these factors can delay your response in getting to the patient.

Farms contain a wide variety of hazards. Animals can seriously injure farmers and pose a serious risk to rescuers. Be alert for the dangers posed by animals. Also, farms contain a wide range of chemicals that can be hazardous. These include pesticides, herbicides, and fertilizers such as anhydrous ammonia. Any of these chemicals, if improperly handled, can create a dangerous situation for farmers and rescuers. Hazardous materials incidents are not always on highways! In addition, farms use a large number of electrically powered machinery. Be alert for the shock hazard posed by the presence of electrical lines and electrical devices on any part of a farm. Some accidents involve tall barns or silos. These accidents often require rescuers trained in high-angle rescue techniques Figure 20-7 ▶ . Some farm silos are sealed and are designed to operate in an oxygen-deficient atmosphere. Silos should always be treated as a hazardous confined space. Under certain conditions, these silos can explode. In addition, some farms contain below-grade manure storage pits. These pits may be filled with poisonous gases or be deficient in oxygen. Do not enter any confined space or enclosed below-grade structure without proper self-contained breathing apparatus and proper training.

Farms also contain a wide variety of machinery. Machinery is used in every step of growing crops and raising animals. Accidents with farm machinery usually involve rollovers of farm tractors, entrapment in machinery, or severing of body tissue by sharp objects Figure 20-8 ▶ . Tractor rollovers are more common with older tractors, which do not have roll bars or reinforced cabs. Rollovers most commonly occur on steep slopes and often result in the operator being pinned beneath the tractor. Entrapments can occur with a number of crop-harvesting equipment, mechanized animal feeding systems, or power take-off (PTO) systems.

As a first responder, your role in farm rescues consists of stabilizing the scene and providing initial medical care for the patient. Follow the seven steps of extrication that you learned in Chapter 18 Table 20-1 ▶ . Carefully overview

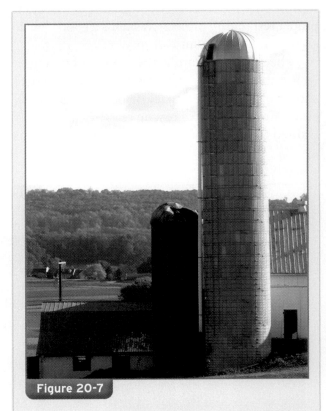

Figure 20-7

Farm silos represent high-angle hazards, confined space hazards, and explosive hazards.

the scene to determine the scope of the problem. Call for adequate assistance from fire, rescue, and EMS organizations. In some communities, rescue personnel utilize farm implement mechanics for assistance with complex farm rescues. Helicopter transport of patients may be beneficial. Remember, it is better to call for help and not need it than it is to delay adequate help from arriving on the scene. Stabilize any hazards that you can while keeping yourself and the patient safe. Shut off any electric power and turn off any machinery that is still operating. Realize that you do not have the training and equipment to stabilize all rescue scenes. If possible, gain access to the patient. Provide initial emergency care to the patient. Initial care consists of establishing responsiveness, supporting the patient's ABCs, controlling bleeding, and maintaining the patient's body temperature. It is important to talk with the patient and provide psychological support. As other rescuers arrive on the scene, help them to disentangle the patient, prepare the patient for removal, and remove the patient.

Your actions at a farm rescue incident can make a difference to the patient. Farm rescues can be challenging, but they require you to follow the same steps of patient care and extrication that you would use for other types of emergencies.

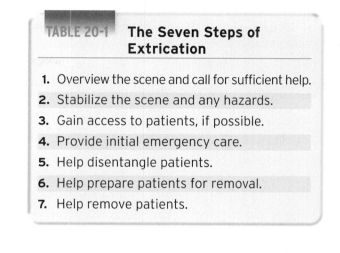

TABLE 20-1	The Seven Steps of Extrication

1. Overview the scene and call for sufficient help.
2. Stabilize the scene and any hazards.
3. Gain access to patients, if possible.
4. Provide initial emergency care.
5. Help disentangle patients.
6. Help prepare patients for removal.
7. Help remove patients.

Above all, remember your safety and the safety of the patient.

Bus Rescue

Buses operate in most communities. School buses transport students to school and to school-sponsored events. Cities operate fleets of municipal buses over established routes. Charter buses transport people of all ages to special events and on vacation trips. Specially equipped buses transport people with limited mobility. Interstate buses transport people all over the country.

Because of the large numbers of people being transported by buses, there is significant potential for bus collisions to occur in any community. Buses are multiple-casualty events waiting to happen! Therefore, you need to understand some guidelines for providing care to patients involved in bus crashes.

Bus collisions range from minor incidents with no injuries to multiple-casualty incidents. If you are a first responder at a bus collision, perform an overview of the scene and call for adequate police, fire, and EMS resources. Establish an incident command system if there are multiple casualties. Set up a one-way traffic pattern for responding vehicles to avoid congestion and gridlock at the emergency scene. For example, you might direct all responding emergency vehicles to approach the scene from the east and depart the scene traveling toward the west. When multiple patients must be removed from a bus, pass equipment into the bus through

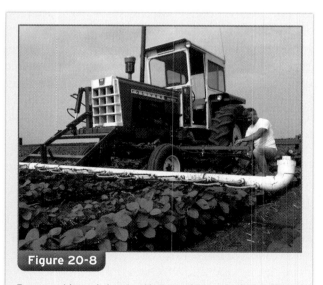

Figure 20-8

Farm machinery is involved in many farm rescue situations.

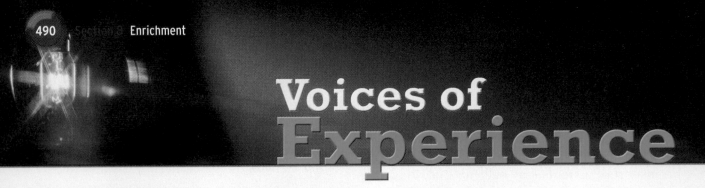

Voices of Experience

Thinking Positively in the Trenches

Throughout my 21-plus years with the New York City Fire Department, with 18 of those years spent in special operations, there has been only one time that I truly believed we would not be able to rescue a victim.

It was a cold, rainy, and windy day at 1500 hours, and I was returning from a multiple-alarm fire in Manhattan, when the dispatcher contacted me to respond to a man buried in a trench in Queens. The preliminary report indicated that the victim was a male worker who had been installing a new sewer main adjacent to a major expressway. The significant rainfall in conjunction with a disregard of trench and excavation safety regulations led to the victim becoming buried.

> ❝ Overcoming my negative thoughts at this incident raised my confidence in my ability to perform successful rescue operations. ❞

I arrived on the scene and immediately assumed the position of the operations chief. The first thing that I did was conduct my scene size-up. I started gathering information from two of the officers of the special units that were already operating on the scene. I observed one male victim entombed in a 10 foot-deep trench. He was buried up to his neck and pinned under a 24-inch sewer main pipe. Most victims who are trapped in trenches are buried in a vertical position, but this victim was in a supine position. The victim stated that he had been digging underneath and along the side of the pipe when he got trapped.

The first order of business was to shore the trench and get a paramedic into the trench to assess the victim's injuries and mental status. The victim had a compound fracture of his right leg, had difficulty breathing, and hypothermia was starting to set in. The medic assessed all of the victim's vital signs and injuries, and then administered an IV to address the issue of crush syndrome. We stopped the rescue operation, which lasted close to five hours, every fifteen minutes to reassess the victim.

Some of the issues I had to address during the operation were the horrendous weather conditions, the water that was escaping from the sewer pipe, and a 27 KV electric line that was located in a concrete junction box 6 inches below the sewer main pipe. These conditions created a dangerous work area for the rescuers as well as for the victim.

As the operation continued into the night, we had to set up lighting, which I had already requested since I had anticipated a prolonged operation. At a special rescue, you must always be proactive and think about the equipment you may need for long duration operations. The victim was in a tremendous amount of pain; hypothermia had set in, and he was becoming very edgy. Several times we came close to removing the victim, but each time some soil seeped back in. Despite all of the obstacles, I was trying to keep negative thoughts out of my head and remain hopeful that the operation would come to a successful conclusion. There is no doubt in my mind that the actions of the operating members, along with the medical expertise, contributed to the survival of the victim. The victim was freed, the medic stabilized his leg, and he was placed into a Stokes stretcher for transport to the hospital.

This was a long-duration operation under arduous conditions that was successfully completed due to the teamwork of all the responders on the scene. It is not uncommon in these types of incidents for even a seasoned, competent officer to start to doubt his or her training and experience. In this particular rescue, I started to think negatively, and I knew that I would have to dissolve those negative thoughts rapidly because they could inhibit my ability to control and supervise rescue operations. Overcoming my negative thoughts at this incident raised my confidence in my ability to perform successful rescue operations.

Fred P. LaFemina
Battalion Chief, Rescue Operations, and Special Operations Command
New York City Fire Department
New York, New York

one door or window and remove the patients through a second door or window. This will improve the efficiency of the extrication process. When confronted with a large number of patients, triage the patients using the START triage system.

You are not expected to handle the command functions at a bus collision involving multiple casualties. However, knowing some of the basic elements of handling this type of incident will help to improve the efficiency and effectiveness of the care given to the patients **Figure 20-9 ▶**.

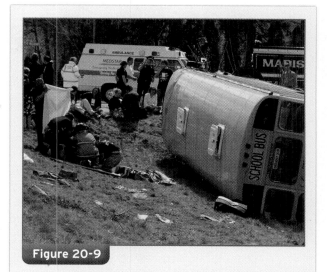

Figure 20-9

A bus collision requires a good incident command system.

You are the Provider

SUMMARY

Review the *You are the Provider* case study provided at the beginning of this chapter.

At 5:37 AM, you are startled by your dispatcher. She announces, "Unit 433, respond to an unknown rescue situation at 10711 Lee Highway. This was a third-party call; no other information is available." You are concerned because you do not have enough information to begin to mentally prepare for this call.

1. If you are the first emergency provider to arrive on the scene, what is your role in handling a rescue situation?

Your initial role at a rescue scene is to perform an overview of the scene, call for needed help, and ensure the safety of rescuers, patients, and bystanders. The actions you take to complete these tasks may vary from one situation to another, but the principles remain the same in different types of rescue.

2 What are the common safety principles that you need to follow during rescue operations?

Keep in mind the overriding safety principle of constantly assessing your safety, the safety of other rescuers, the safety of the patient, and the safety of bystanders. From the moment you begin to respond until you depart from the scene, keep safety in mind. Remember, in some situations, it will not be safe to approach the patient or attempt a rescue. Do not become a dead rescuer who has tried to save an already dead patient.

3. What are the steps you should follow at any rescue situation?

Regardless of the type of rescue situation, the same rescue and extrication steps apply. These are:

- Overview the scene and call for sufficient help.
- Stabilize the scene and any hazards.
- Gain access to patients if possible.
- Provide initial emergency care.
- Help disentangle patients.
- Help prepare patients for removal.
- Help remove patients.

You will need to determine what steps you can undertake safely and how much you can do in each rescue situation, yet the same general principles apply.

Prep Kit

Ready for Review

The Ready for Review thoroughly summarizes the chapter.

- Ice rescue, water rescue, underwater diving accidents, confined space rescue, farm rescue, and bus collisions are situations that require extensive skills and special training. It is important to help the victims, but not at the expense of your own safety.

- In water and ice rescue situations, there are some simple steps you can take to help the victim without endangering yourself, including reaching out to the victim with an object, throwing a flotation device to the victim, or rowing to the victim in a boat.

- You may not be able to distinguish between the two major medical emergencies created by underwater diving incidents, but you can provide basic care and summon appropriate assistance.

- In confined space rescue, your primary goals are to call for additional assistance and prevent other people, including yourself, from becoming victims.

- Farm emergencies and bus collisions are complex rescue situations, yet if you follow simple steps you can often stabilize these situations and provide initial aid to patients.

Technology

- Interactivities
- Vocabulary Explorer
- Anatomy Review
- Web Links
- Online Review Manual

Vital Vocabulary

The Vital Vocabulary are the key terms for this chapter.

air embolism A bubble of air obstructing a blood vessel.

decompression sickness (the bends) A condition seen in divers in which gas, especially nitrogen, forms bubbles in blood vessels obstructing them.

flotation device A life ring, life buoy, or other floating device used in water rescue.

reach-throw-row-go A four-step reminder of the sequence of actions that should be taken in water rescue situations.

riptides Unusually strong surface currents flowing outward from a seashore that can carry swimmers "out to sea."

Assessment in Action

Assessment in Action presents a fictitious scenario to help you review what you learned in this chapter.

You and your family are at the local swimming pool enjoying a break from the summer heat when you notice two boys rough housing near the shallow end of the pool. A few minutes later, you hear a boy screaming "Scott fell into the pool and hit his head on the bottom step! Help!" As you approach the side of the pool, you see a young boy floating face down in the pool.

1. What is the number one priority in the treatment of this patient?

   A. Remove the patient from the water.
   B. Establish an airway.
   C. Turn the patient over.
   D. Begin chest compressions.

2. It is impossible to put this patient on a backboard while still in the water.

   A. True
   B. False

3. When opening your patient's airway, what maneuver should you use?

   A. Head tilt–chin lift
   B. Head tilt–jaw thrust
   C. Jaw thrust

4. Opening the airway and maintaining stabilization of the neck can be accomplished at the same time.

   A. True
   B. False

5. If the patient must be removed from the water before EMS personnel arrive, how many people should assist in removing the patient?

   A. Two
   B. Four
   C. Six
   D. Eight

Supplemental Skills

Chapter Objectives*

Knowledge and Attitude Objectives

1. Describe how to measure blood pressure by palpation. (p 498-499)
2. Describe how to measure blood pressure by auscultation. (p 499-500)
3. Describe the indications for using supplemental oxygen. (p 500)
4. Describe the equipment used to administer oxygen. (p 500-501)
5. Describe the safety considerations and hazards of oxygen administration. (p 501, 502)
6. Describe the indications and use of a bag-mask device. (p 503)
7. Describe the function and operation of a pulse oximeter. (p 505-506)

Skill Objectives

1. Measure blood pressure by palpation. (p 498-499)
2. Measure blood pressure by auscultation. (p 499-500)
3. Assemble the equipment used to administer oxygen. (p 500-501)
4. Administer supplemental oxygen using a nasal cannula and a nonrebreathing mask. (p 501)
5. Perform bag-mask ventilation. (p 503-505)
6. Perform pulse oximetry. (p 506)

*These are chapter learning objectives.

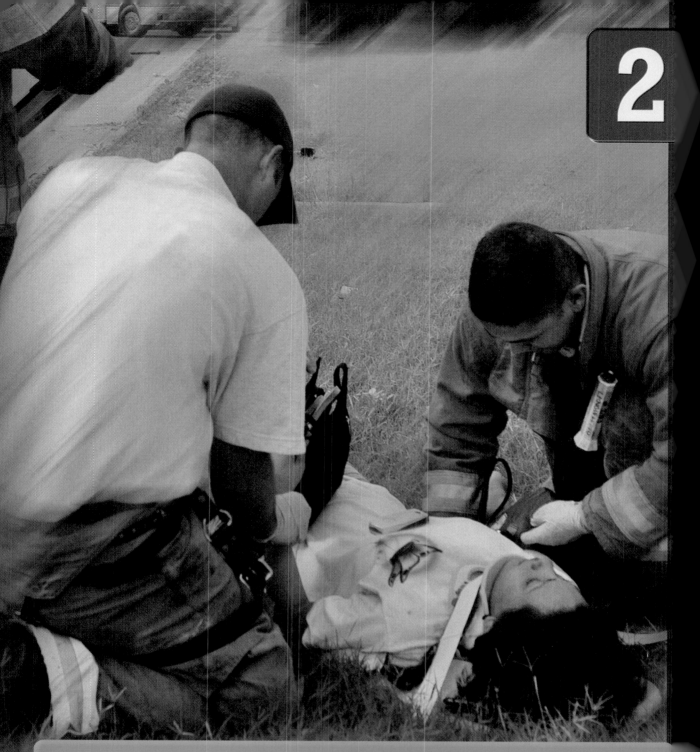

You are the Provider

As part of your training program, you are assigned to ride on one of the ambulances in your department. As you wait for the assigned crew to complete their shift change meeting, you think about the supplemental skills you just learned and how they might assist the on-duty crew in assessing and treating patients.

As the meeting ends, the crew leader, Markie, introduces herself and her partner, Jim. She welcomes you aboard and asks the following questions:

1. What supplemental assessment skills have you learned?
2. What methods of oxygen administration have you learned?
3. How would you care for a nonbreathing patient who has a pulse?

Introduction

In some EMS systems, first responders use supplemental skills to enhance the care they give their patients. These skills include taking blood pressure, administering supplemental oxygen, and assessing the level of oxygen in the blood. The topics covered in this chapter are not required by the national curriculum, but they may be adopted by some states or first responder systems. Even if these skills are not used by your system, the information contained in this chapter will help you to assist other EMS personnel in providing care for patients.

Blood Pressure

Blood pressure is one way to measure the condition of a patient's circulatory system. High blood pressure may indicate that the patient is susceptible to a stroke. Low blood pressure generally indicates one of various types of shock (see Chapter 13).

The blood pressure measurement consists of a reading of two numbers (for example, 120 over 80, or 120/80). These numbers represent the pressures found in the arteries as the heart contracts and relaxes. The numbers are determined by the

pressure exerted in millimeters of mercury (mm Hg), as shown on the dial. The higher number (120 in the example of 120 over 80) is called the **systolic pressure**. This measures the force exerted on the walls of the arteries as the heart contracts. The lower number (80 in the example of 120 over 80) is known as the **diastolic pressure**. It represents the arterial pressure during the relaxation phase of the heart.

Normal Blood Pressure

Blood pressure ranges may vary greatly. Excitement or stress may raise a person's blood pressure. **Hypertension** (high blood pressure) exists when the blood pressure remains greater than 140/90 after repeated examinations over several weeks. Hypertension is a serious medical condition that requires treatment by a physician.

Hypotension (low blood pressure) exists when the systolic pressure (the higher number) falls to 90 or below. A patient with this condition is usually in serious trouble. Treatment of shock should be started immediately if the patient is also experiencing other signs of shock (for example, cold, clammy, pale skin or dizziness).

Taking Blood Pressure by Palpation

To take a patient's blood pressure by **palpation** (by feeling it), apply the blood pressure cuff on the uninjured (or less injured) arm. Wrap the cuff around the upper arm. The bottom of the cuff should be 1 inch to 2 inches above the crease of the elbow. The arrow should point to the brachial artery, which is located on the medial side of the arm at the crease of the elbow.

Blood pressure cuffs come in different sizes for adults, children, and infants. Be sure to use the appropriate size for your patient, such as a narrow cuff for a child and an extra-large cuff for an obese adult. Cuffs that are too small may give falsely high readings, and cuffs that are too large may give falsely low readings. Place the indicator dial in a position where you can easily see the movement of the indicator needle. Turn the control knob on the blood pressure inflator bulb clockwise to close the valve. Do not tighten it too much. With the fingers of your other hand, locate the

Technology

- Interactivities
- Vocabulary Explorer
- Anatomy Review
- Web Links
- Online Review Manual

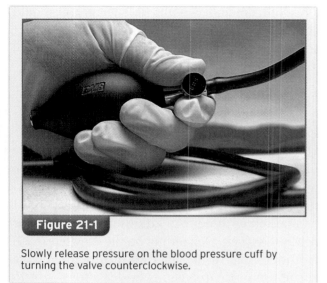

Figure 21-1

Slowly release pressure on the blood pressure cuff by turning the valve counterclockwise.

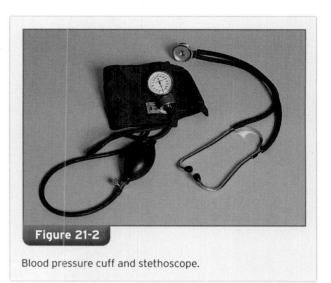

Figure 21-2

Blood pressure cuff and stethoscope.

radial pulse at the patient's wrist. Slowly pump up the blood pressure cuff until you can no longer feel the radial pulse. Continue to pump up the cuff for another 30 mm (millimeters) beyond the disappearing point of the radial pulse. Slowly release the pressure in the cuff by turning the valve counterclockwise **Figure 21-1 ▲**. Continue to feel for the radial pulse and when you first feel the pulse return, carefully note the position of the indicator needle on the dial. This number is the systolic pressure.

The palpation method of taking blood pressure does not give you a diastolic pressure. You will have only one number, the systolic pressure, instead of the two numbers. Report the results as "the blood pressure by palpation is 90."

Taking Blood Pressure by Auscultation

To take blood pressure by **auscultation** (by hearing it), you need both a blood pressure cuff and a stethoscope **Figure 21-2 ▶**. Apply the blood pressure cuff in the same manner and position as in the palpation method. After you apply the cuff, locate the brachial artery pulse on the medial side of the arm at the crease of the elbow.

Put the earpieces of the stethoscope in your ears with the earpieces pointing forward. Place the diaphragm of the stethoscope over the site of the brachial pulse. Using your index and mid-dle fingers, hold the diaphragm snugly against the patient's arm. Do not use your thumb! If you use your thumb, you may hear your own heartbeat in the stethoscope. Listen as you inflate the blood pressure cuff. When you can no longer hear the sound of the brachial pulse, note the pressure on the dial. Continue to inflate the cuff for another 30 mm over the pressure at which the brachial pulse disappeared. Then slowly and smoothly release air from the cuff by opening the control valve at a rate of 2 to 4 mm per second. Carefully watch the indicator needle, listen for the pulse to return, and note the pressure reading when you first hear the pulse return. This is the systolic pressure. As the cuff pressure continues to fall (at 2 to 4 mm per second), listen for the moment when the pulse disappears. Note the number when you can no longer hear the pulse; this is the diastolic pressure.

Blood pressure taken by auscultation **Figure 21-3 ▶** is reported as systolic pressure over diastolic pressure (the larger number over the smaller number) and is always given in even numbers (for example, 120/84, 90/40, or 186/98).

It takes practice to become skilled in taking blood pressures. Take every opportunity to practice on as many healthy, uninjured people as possible. Practice on children and older people as well as your friends and coworkers. This will help prepare you to measure the blood pressure of a seriously ill or injured patient.

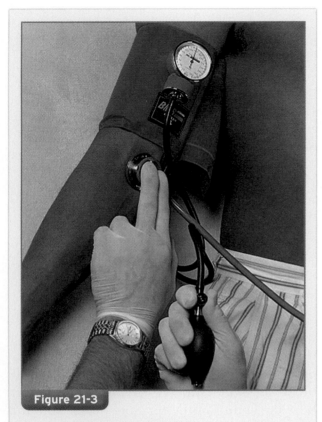

Figure 21-3

Taking blood pressure by auscultation.

Oxygen Administration

Under normal conditions, your body can operate efficiently using the oxygen that is contained in the air, even though air only contains 21% oxygen. The amount of blood lost after a traumatic injury could mean that insufficient oxygen is delivered to the cells of the body. This results in shock. Administering supplemental oxygen to patients showing signs and symptoms of shock increases the amount of oxygen delivered to the cells of the body and often makes a positive difference in the patient's outcome.

Patients who have suffered a heart attack or stroke or patients who have a chronic heart or lung disease may be unable to get sufficient oxygen from room air. These patients will also benefit from receiving supplemental oxygen.

Not all first responders know how to administer oxygen; however, knowing this skill can be helpful in areas where EMS response may be delayed. By learning this skill, you will be able to assist other members of the EMS team. You should administer oxygen only after receiving proper training and with the approval of your medical director.

Oxygen Equipment

Oxygen Cylinders

Oxygen is compressed to 2,000 pounds per square inch (psi) and stored in portable cylinders. The portable oxygen cylinders used by most EMS systems are either D or E size. Oxygen cylinders must be marked with a green color and be labeled as medical oxygen. Depending on the flow rate, each cylinder lasts for at least 20 minutes. A valve at the top of the oxygen cylinder allows you to control the flow of oxygen from the cylinder. Oxygen administration equipment is shown in **Figure 21-4 ▼**.

Pressure Regulator/Flowmeter

Oxygen in the cylinder is stored at 2,000 psi, but it can only be used when that pressure is regulated down to about 50 psi. This is done by the use of a pressure regulator. The regulator and the **flowmeter** are a single unit attached to the outlet of the oxygen cylinder **Figure 21-5 ▶**. Once the pressure has been reduced, you can adjust the flowmeter to deliver oxygen at a rate of 2 to 15 liters per minute. Because patients with different medical conditions require different amounts of oxygen, the flowmeter lets you select the proper amount of

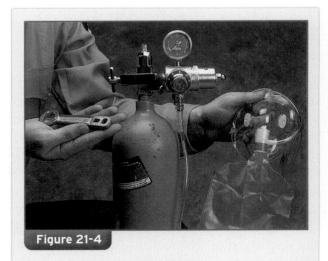

Figure 21-4

Oxygen administration equipment.

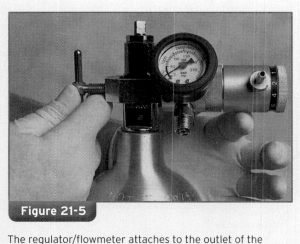

Figure 21-5

The regulator/flowmeter attaches to the outlet of the oxygen cylinder.

oxygen to administer. A gasket between the cylinder and the pressure regulator/flowmeter ensures a tight seal and maintains the high pressure inside the cylinder. Always check for this gasket before attaching the regulator.

Nasal Cannulas and Face Masks

The third part of an oxygen-delivery system is a device that ensures the oxygen is delivered to the patient and is not lost in the air. A **nasal cannula** has two small holes, which fit into the patient's nostrils. Nasal cannulas are used to deliver medium concentrations of oxygen (35% to 50%). A **face mask** is placed over the patient's nose and mouth to deliver oxygen through the patient's mouth and nostrils. Nonrebreathing masks are most commonly used by first responders. They deliver high concentrations of oxygen (up to 90%). These two oxygen-delivery devices are discussed more fully in the section on administering supplemental oxygen.

Safety Considerations

Oxygen does not burn or explode by itself. However, it actively supports combustion and can quickly turn a small spark or flame into a serious fire. Therefore, all sparks, heat, flames, and oily substances must be kept away from oxygen equipment. Smoking should never be permitted around oxygen equipment.

The pressurized cylinders are also hazardous because the high pressure in an oxygen cylinder can cause an explosion if the cylinder is damaged. Be sure the oxygen cylinder will not fall. If the shut-off valve at the top of the cylinder is damaged, the cylinder can take off like a rocket. Oxygen cylinders should be kept inside sturdy carrying cases that protect the cylinder and regulator/flowmeter. Handle the cylinder carefully to guard against damage.

Administering Supplemental Oxygen

To administer supplemental oxygen, place the regulator/flowmeter over the stem of the oxygen cylinder, and line up the pins on the pin-indexing system correctly **Figure 21-6 ▾**. Be sure to check for the mandatory gasket. Tighten the securing screw firmly by hand. With the special key or wrench provided, turn the cylinder valve two turns counterclockwise to allow oxygen from the cylinder to enter the regulator/flowmeter.

Check the gauge on the pressure regulator/flowmeter to see how much oxygen pressure remains in the cylinder. If the cylinder contains less than 500 psi, the amount of oxygen in the cylinder is too low for emergency use and should be replaced with a full (2,000 psi) cylinder.

To administer oxygen, you will need to adjust the flowmeter to deliver the desired liter-per-minute flow of oxygen. The patient's condition and the type of oxygen delivery device you use (a mask or a nasal cannula) dictates the proper

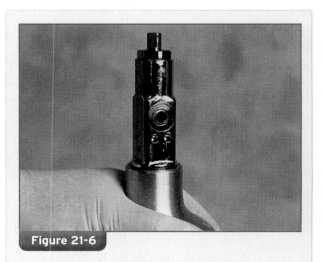

Figure 21-6

A valve stem with pin-index holes.

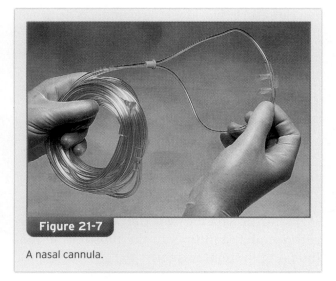

Figure 21-7

A nasal cannula.

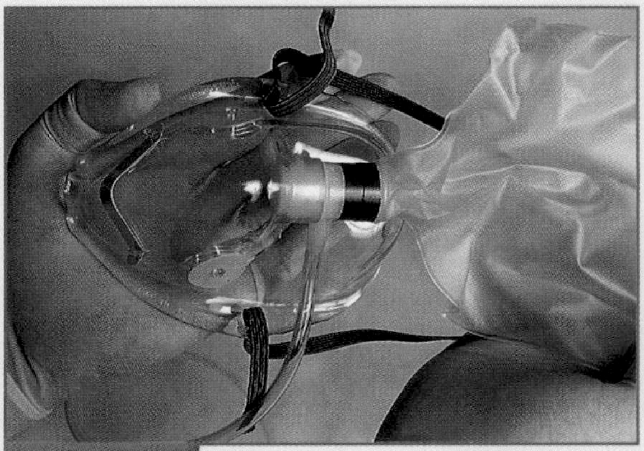

Figure 21-8

A nonrebreathing oxygen mask.

flow. When the oxygen flow begins, place the face mask or nasal cannula onto the patient's head.

Nasal Cannula

A nasal cannula is a simple oxygen-delivery device. It consists of two small prongs that fit into the patient's nostrils and a strap that holds the cannula on the patient's face **Figure 21-7 ▲**. A cannula delivers low-flow oxygen at 2 to 6 liters per minute and in concentrations of 35% to 50% oxygen. Low-flow oxygen can be used for fairly stable patients such as those with slight chest pain or mild shortness of breath.

To use a nasal cannula, first adjust the liter flow to 2 to 6 liters per minute and then apply the cannula to the patient. The cannula should fit snugly but should not be tight.

Nonrebreathing Mask

A nonrebreathing mask consists of connecting tubing, a reservoir bag, one-way valves, and a face piece **Figure 21-8 ▶**. It is used to deliver high flows of oxygen at 8 to 15 liters per minute. A nonrebreathing face mask can deliver concentrations of oxygen as high as 90%. This mask works by storing oxygen in the reservoir bag. When the patient inhales, oxygen is drawn from the reservoir bag. When the patient exhales, the air is exhausted through the one-way valves on the side of the mask.

Nonrebreathing face masks should be used for patients who require higher flows of oxy-

gen. These include patients experiencing serious shortness of breath, severe chest pain, carbon monoxide poisoning, and congestive heart failure (CHF). Patients who are showing signs and symptoms of shock should also be treated with high-flow oxygen from a nonrebreathing face mask.

To use a nonrebreathing mask, first adjust the oxygen flow to 8 to 15 liters per minute to inflate the reservoir bag before putting it on the patient. After the bag inflates, place the mask over the patient's face. Adjust the straps to secure a snug fit. Adjust the liter flow to keep the bag at least partially inflated while the patient inhales.

Hazards of Supplemental Oxygen

Supplemental oxygen can be lifesaving, but it must be used carefully in order to be safe. Although this gives you a basic outline on setting up oxygen equipment, you will need additional class work and practical training before you administer oxygen in emergency situations.

Safety Tips

Avoid using oxygen around fire or flames. Keep oxygen cylinders secured to minimize the danger of explosion.

Bag-Mask Device

The **bag-mask device** has three parts: a self-inflating bag, one-way valves, and a face mask Figure 21-9 ▾ . To use this device, a rescuer places the mask over the face of the patient and makes a tight seal. Squeezing the bag pushes air through a one-way valve, through the mask, and into the patient's mouth and nose. As the patient passively exhales, a second one-way valve near the mask releases the air.

The self-inflating bag refills when the rescuer releases the pressure on it. Without supplemental oxygen, the bag-mask device delivers 21% oxygen, the percentage of oxygen in room air. Supplemental oxygen is usually added to the bag-mask device. A bag-mask device can deliver up to 90% oxygen to a patient, if 10 to 15 liters per minute of oxygen is supplied into the reservoir bag. Many bag-mask devices are designed to be discarded after a single use.

The bag-mask device is used for the same purpose as a mouth-to-mask device—to ventilate a nonbreathing patient. Although the bag-mask device can administer up to 90% oxygen when used with supplemental oxygen, there are two disadvantages to its use. A single rescuer may find it difficult to maintain a seal between the face and mask with one hand. Additionally, the bag-mask device may be hard for people with small hands to use, because they may not be able to squeeze the bag hard enough to get an adequate volume of air into the patient.

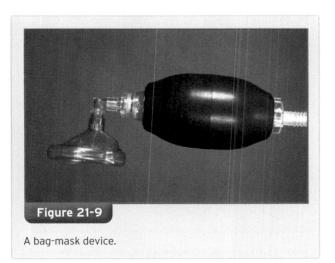

Figure 21-9

A bag-mask device.

Technique

The beginning steps for using a bag-mask device are the same steps you use for performing rescue breathing. Check to determine if the patient is unresponsive. Open the patient's airway using the head tilt–chin lift technique or the jaw-thrust technique for patients with suspected neck or spinal injuries. See if the patient is breathing: Look at the patient's chest, listen for the sound of air movement, and feel for the movement of air on the side of your face and ear. If the patient is not breathing, consider using an oral or nasal airway. The specific steps for using a bag-mask device are shown in Skill Drill 21-1 ▸ :

SKILL DRILL 21-1

1. Kneel above the patient's head. This position will enable you to keep the airway open, make a tight seal on the mask, and squeeze the bag. Maintain the patient's neck in an extended position. The bag-mask device does not maintain the patient's airway in an open position. You must continue to stabilize the head and maintain the head either in an extended position for the head tilt–chin lift or in a neutral position for the jaw-thrust technique.
2. Open the patient's mouth and check for fluids, foreign bodies, or dentures Step 1 . Suction if needed. Consider the use of an oral or nasal airway.
3. Select the proper mask size Step 2 . The mask should be big enough to seal over the bridge of the patient's nose and fit in the groove between the lower lip and the chin. A mask that is too small or too large may make it impossible to maintain a seal.
4. Place the mask over the patient's face. Start by putting the angled or grooved end of the mask over the bridge of the nose. Then bring the bottom of the mask against the groove between the lower lip and the chin Step 3 .
5. Seal the mask. Place the middle, ring, and little fingers of one hand under the angle of the jaw. Lift up on the jaw. Make a "C"

Skill DRILL 21-1

Using a Bag-Mask Device With One Rescuer

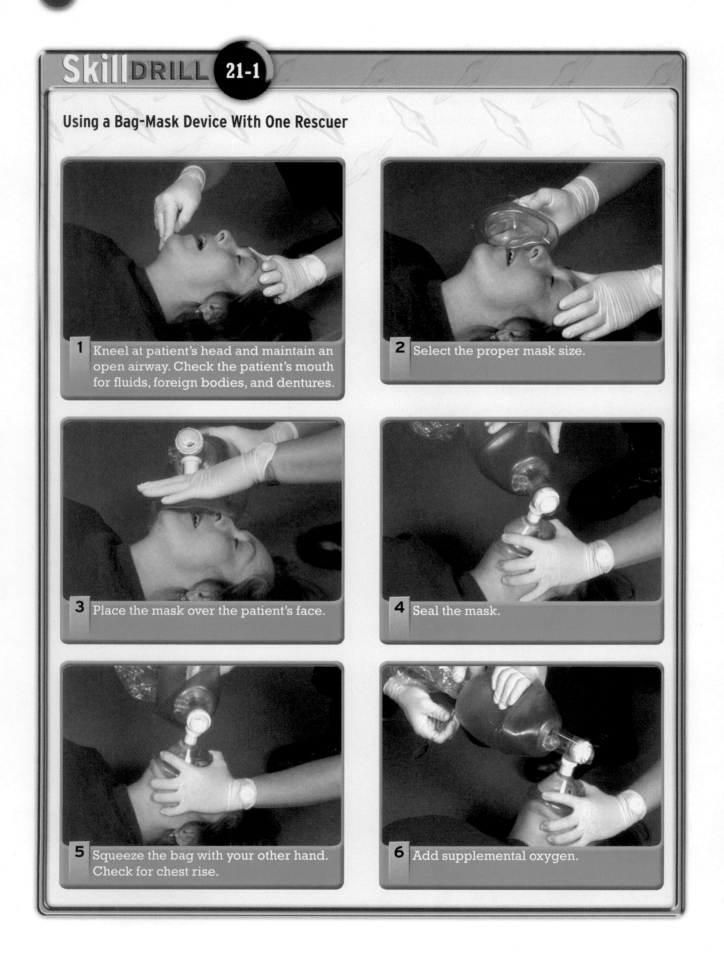

1 Kneel at patient's head and maintain an open airway. Check the patient's mouth for fluids, foreign bodies, and dentures.

2 Select the proper mask size.

3 Place the mask over the patient's face.

4 Seal the mask.

5 Squeeze the bag with your other hand. Check for chest rise.

6 Add supplemental oxygen.

with the index finger and thumb of the same hand, and place them over the mask. Clamp the mask by lifting the jaw and bringing the mask in contact with the jaw. Continue to hold the mask in position Step 4 .

6. Squeeze the bag. Using your other hand, squeeze the bag once every 5 seconds. Try to squeeze a large volume of air. Squeeze every 3 seconds for infants and children.

7. Check for chest rise Step 5 . As you squeeze the bag, watch for a rise in the chest. If you do not see the chest rise, air is probably leaking around the mask or there is an obstruction in the airway. If air is leaking around the mask, try to make a better seal between the mask and the patient's jaw. If you suspect an airway obstruction, follow the steps learned in Chapter 6.

8. Add supplemental oxygen Step 6 . Using a bag-mask device without supplemental oxygen supplies the patient with 21% oxygen. By adding 10 to 15 liters per minute of oxygen to the bag-mask device, you can increase the oxygen concentration to 90%. Adjust the liter flow on the pressure regulator/flowmeter to deliver between 10 and 15 liters per minute and connect the oxygen tubing from the flowmeter outlet to the inlet nipple on the bag-mask device. This higher percentage of oxygen is beneficial for a nonbreathing patient.

With sufficient training and practice, one person can ventilate a patient using a bag-mask device. However, it is difficult to maintain a good seal and squeeze the bag with only two hands. A bag-mask device should be done as a two-person operation if additional rescuers are present **Figure 21-10 ▶** . With two rescuers, one person squeezes the bag and the other person uses both hands to seal the mask to the patient. Use the middle, ring, and little fingers of both hands under the angles of the jaw, and use the index fingers and thumbs of both hands to form two "Cs" around the face mask. Most people can seal the mask much more easily using both hands.

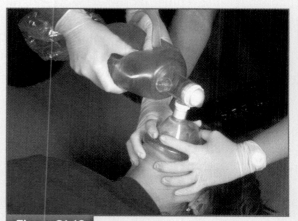

Figure 21-10

Using a bag-mask device with two rescuers.

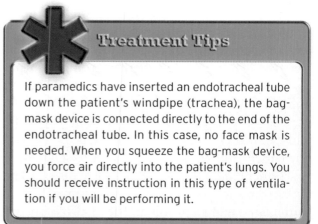

Treatment Tips

If paramedics have inserted an endotracheal tube down the patient's windpipe (trachea), the bag-mask device is connected directly to the end of the endotracheal tube. In this case, no face mask is needed. When you squeeze the bag-mask device, you force air directly into the patient's lungs. You should receive instruction in this type of ventilation if you will be performing it.

Using the bag-mask device requires proper training and practice. The bag-mask device can be a lifesaving tool. Your EMS service may use bag-mask devices for nonbreathing patients—or you may be asked to assist EMT-Bs or paramedics in ventilating nonbreathing patients so they can perform other needed skills. Check with your supervisor or medical director to learn the protocols for your service.

Pulse Oximetry

<u>Pulse oximetry</u> is used to assess the amount of oxygen saturated in the red blood cells. It does this through the use of a photoelectric cell that measures the light that passes through a fingertip or an earlobe. The machine that performs this

function is called a **pulse oximeter**. A pulse oximeter consists of a sensing probe and a monitor. The sensing probe attaches to the patient's fingertip or earlobe by means of a spring-loaded clip. The sensing probe contains a light source and a receiving chamber. The sensing probe attaches to the monitor of the pulse oximeter by means of a cable. The pulse oximeter monitor contains an on-and-off switch and a screen for displaying the percent of oxygen saturation **Figure 21-11 ▾**.

To operate the pulse oximeter, turn on the monitor. Most pulse oximeters perform a self-check to assure the operator that the machine is operating correctly. This self-check will vary from one brand of oximeter to another. Once you know that the monitor is operating correctly, place the sensing probe over the patient's fingertip or earlobe. The monitor should then display the percent of saturation of the patient's blood. In a healthy patient, the oxygen saturation should be between 95% and 100% when breathing room air.

If a patient has difficulty breathing due to an injury or a disease process, the percent of oxygen saturation may be much lower than 95%. The pulse oximeter cannot tell you what is wrong with the patient. You must perform a thorough patient assessment including a good medical history. The pulse oximeter can help you to recognize that the patient is having a problem. It can also help you to determine if your treatment is helping the patient. If the steps you are taking to treat the patient coincide with an increased percentage of oxygen saturation, that is a positive sign.

Like any other device, a pulse oximeter has certain limitations. It will not give an accurate reading if the patient is wearing nail polish or if the fingers are very dirty. Also, if the patient is cold and the blood vessels in their fingertips or earlobes are constricted, the pulse oximeter reading will not be accurate. Patients who have lost a lot of blood will also have an inaccurate pulse oximetry reading. Patients who are suffering from carbon monoxide poisoning will produce a false reading because their red blood cells are saturated with carbon monoxide instead of with oxygen. It is important to understand that the pulse oximeter is a valuable tool to help you assess a patient's condition. However, like any tool, it has certain limitations that you must consider. Remember, there is no machine that replaces the need for a careful patient assessment including a good medical history.

Assisting Other EMS Providers

Some first responders work closely with EMT-Bs and paramedics and may ride on ambulances with more advanced EMS providers. In these cases, it is helpful to know the types of equipment carried on the ambulance, where each piece of equipment is located, and how that equipment works. For example, it is helpful to know how to load and unload the ambulance cot and how to operate the controls that raise and lower the cot. In some EMS systems, you may be permitted to set up certain types of devices such as oxygen administration equipment or cardiac monitors. Being able to assist other EMS providers can improve the efficiency of patient care. You are encouraged to master additional skills as long as these skills are permitted by your local protocols, your medical director, and by your state regulations. Because the equipment varies widely from one system to another and because protocols and regulations vary, it is not possible to address all of these skills. You are encouraged to work within your local EMS system to assist other EMS providers.

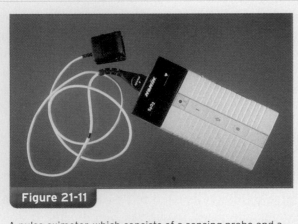

Figure 21-11

A pulse oximeter, which consists of a sensing probe and a monitor, is used to measure the percentage of oxygen saturation in the blood.

You are the Provider

SUMMARY

Review the *You are the Provider* case study provided at the beginning of this chapter.

As part of your training program, you are assigned to ride on one of the ambulances in your department. As you wait for the assigned crew to complete their shift change meeting, you think about the supplemental skills you just learned and how they might assist the on-duty crew in assessing and treating patients.

As the meeting ends, the crew leader, Markie, introduces herself and her partner, Jim. She welcomes you aboard and asks the following questions:

1. What supplemental assessment skills have you learned?

Supplemental assessment skills that contribute to patient assessment include blood pressure taken by palpation and by auscultation and pulse oximetry.

2. What methods of oxygen administration have you learned?

Oxygen can be administered by nasal cannula, nonrebreathing face mask, and by using a bag-mask device.

3. How would you care for a nonbreathing patient who has a pulse?

A patient who is not breathing can be ventilated with a bag-mask device with supplemental oxygen.

Participating in a ride along with other EMS providers can help you to learn about other parts of the EMS system. A ride along can also give you a chance to practice some of your first responder skills while working under the direction of an experienced EMS provider.

Prep Kit

Ready for Review

The Ready for Review thoroughly summarizes the chapter.

- In some EMS systems, first responders use supplemental skills to enhance the care they give their patients. These skills include taking blood pressure, administering supplemental oxygen, and assessing the level of oxygen in the blood.

- Blood pressure is one way to measure the condition of a patient's circulatory system. High blood pressure may indicate that the patient is susceptible to a stroke. Low blood pressure generally indicates one of various types of shock. You can take blood pressure by palpation (by feeling it) or auscultation (by hearing it).

- Administering supplemental oxygen to patients showing signs and symptoms of shock increases the amount of oxygen delivered to the cells of the body and often makes a positive difference in the patient's outcome. Patients who have suffered a heart attack or stroke or patients who have a chronic heart or lung disease may also benefit from receiving supplemental oxygen.

- Pulse oximetry is used to assess the amount of oxygen saturated in the red blood cells.

- Some first responders work closely with EMT-Bs and paramedics and may ride on ambulances with more advanced EMS providers. In these cases, it is helpful to know the types of equipment carried on the ambulance, where each piece of equipment is located, and how that equipment works.

Vital Vocabulary

The Vital Vocabulary are the key terms for this chapter.

auscultation Listening to sounds with a stethoscope.

bag-mask device A patient ventilation device that consists of a bag, one-way valves, and a face mask.

diastolic pressure The measurement of pressure exerted against the walls of the arteries while the left ventricle of the heart is at rest.

face mask A clear plastic mask used for oxygen administration that covers the mouth and nose.

flowmeter A device on oxygen cylinders used to control and measure the flow of oxygen.

hypertension High blood pressure.

hypotension Lowered blood pressure.

nasal cannula A clear plastic tube used to deliver oxygen that fits onto the patient's nose.

palpation To examine by touch.

pulse oximeter A machine that consists of a monitor and a sensor probe that measures the oxygen saturation in the capillary beds.

pulse oximetry An assessment tool that measures oxygen saturation in the capillary beds.

systolic pressure The measurement of blood pressure exerted against the walls of the arteries during contraction of the heart.

Technology

- Interactivities
- Vocabulary Explorer
- Anatomy Review
- Web Links
- Online Review Manual

Assessment in Action

Assessment in Action presents a fictitious scenario to help you review what you learned in this chapter.

You are dispatched to a residence for a report of a sick person. As you arrive at the residence, you find a 78-year-old man who is complaining of discomfort in his chest.

1. Which of the following will give you the most information about this patient's condition?

   A. Taking blood pressure by palpation
   B. Taking blood pressure by auscultation

2. You determine that the patient's blood pressure is 154/98 Hg mm by auscultation. This is:

   A. A normal blood pressure
   B. A high blood pressure
   C. A low blood pressure

3. An EMT-B who has also been dispatched on this call asks you to check the patient's pulse oximetry. You get a reading of 89% while the patient is breathing room air. This reading is:

   A. Low for a patient of this age
   B. In the normal range for this patient
   C. High for this patient

4. You need to administer oxygen by nasal cannula to this patient because he is slightly short of breath. How much oxygen should you give?

   A. 1 liter per minute
   B. 2-6 liters per minute
   C. 8-10 liters per minute
   D. 8-15 liters per minute

Glossary

abandonment Failure of the first responder to continue emergency medical treatment until relieved by someone with the same or higher level of training.

abdomen The body cavity between the thorax and the pelvis that contains the major organs of digestion and excretion.

abdominal aortic aneurysm (AAA) A condition in which the layers of the aorta in the abdomen weaken. This causes blood to leak between the layers of the artery, causing it to bulge and sometimes rupture.

abdominal breathing Breathing using only the diaphragm.

abrasion Loss of skin as a result of a body part being rubbed or scraped across a rough or hard surface.

absence seizure A seizure that is characterized by a brief lapse of attention. The patient may stare and not respond. Also known as a petit mal seizure.

acceptance The fifth stage of the grief process; when the person experiencing grief recognizes the finality of the grief-causing event.

acid A chemical substance with a pH of less than 7.0 that can cause severe burns.

acute abdomen The sudden onset of abdominal pain caused by disease or trauma which irritates the lining of the abdominal cavity and requires immediate medical or surgical treatment.

advance directive A legal document with specific instructions that the patient does not want to be resuscitated or kept alive by mechanical support systems. Also called a living will.

advanced life support (ALS) The use of specialized equipment such as cardiac monitors, defibrillators, intravenous fluids, drug infusion, and endotracheal intubation to stabilize the patient.

air embolism A bubble of air obstructing a blood vessel.

airway The passages from the openings of the mouth and nose to the air sacs in the lungs through which air enters and leaves the lungs.

airway obstruction Partial (mild) or complete (severe) obstruction of the respiratory passages resulting from blockage by food, small objects, or vomitus.

alveoli The air sacs of the lungs where the exchange of oxygen and carbon dioxide takes place.

Alzheimer's disease A chronic progressive dementia that accounts for 60% of all dementia.

amphetamines Stimulants that produce a general mood elevation, improve task performance, suppress appetite, or prevent sleepiness.

anaphylactic shock Severe shock caused by an allergic reaction to food, medicine, or insect stings.

anger The second stage of the grief reaction; when the person suffering grief becomes upset at the grief-causing event or other situation.

angina pectoris Chest pain with squeezing or tightness in the chest caused by an inadequate flow of blood to the heart muscle.

anterior The front surface of the body.

anus The distal or terminal ending of the gastrointestinal tract.

appropriate medical facility A hospital with adequate medical resources to provide continuing care to sick or injured patients who are transported after field treatment by first responders.

arm Part of the upper extremity that extends from the shoulder to the elbow.

arm-to-arm drag An emergency-patient move that consists of the rescuer grasping the patient's arms from behind; used to remove a patient from a hazardous place.

arterial bleeding Serious bleeding from an artery in which blood frequently pulses or spurts from an open wound.

aspiration Breathing in foreign matter such as food, drink, or vomitus into the airway or lungs.

aspirator A suction device.

assessment-based care A system of patient evaluation in which the chief complaint of the patient and other signs and symptoms are gathered. The care given is based on this information rather than on a formal diagnosis.

asthma An acute spasm of the smaller air passages marked by labored breathing and wheezing.

atherosclerosis A disease characterized by a thickening and destruction of the arterial walls and caused by fatty deposits within them; the arteries lose the ability to dilate and carry blood.

atrium Either of the two upper chambers of the heart.

auscultation Listening to sounds with a stethoscope.

automated external defibrillators (AEDs) Portable battery-powered devices that recognize ventricular fibrillation and advise when a countershock is indicated. The AED delivers an electric shock to patients with ventricular fibrillation.

AVPU scale A scale to measure a patient's level of consciousness. The letters stand for Alert, Verbal, Pain, and Unresponsive.

avulsion An injury in which a piece of skin is either torn completely loose from all of its attachments or is left hanging as a flap.

backboard A straight board used for splinting, extricating, and transporting patients with suspected spinal injuries.

bag of waters The amniotic fluid that surrounds the baby before birth.

bag-mask device A patient ventilation device that consists of a bag, one-way valves, and a face mask.

barbiturates Drugs that depress the nervous system; they can alter the state of consciousness so that the individual may appear drowsy or peaceful.

bargaining The third stage of the grief reaction; when the person experiencing grief barters to change the grief-causing event.

base station A powerful two-way radio that is permanently mounted in a communications center.

basic life support (BLS) Emergency lifesaving procedures performed without advanced emergency procedures to stabilize patients who have experienced sudden illness or injury.

behavioral emergencies Situations in which a person exhibits abnormal behavior that is unacceptable or cannot be tolerated by the patients themselves or by family, friends, or the community.

biological agents Disease-causing bacteria or viruses that might be used by terrorists to intentionally cause epidemics of disease.

birth canal The vagina and the lower part of the uterus.

blanket drag An emergency-patient move in which a rescuer encloses a patient in a blanket and drags the patient to safety.

blister agents Chemicals that cause the skin to blister.

blood pressure The pressure of the circulating blood against the walls of the arteries.

bloody show The bloody mucus plug that is discharged from the vagina when labor begins.

body substance isolation (BSI) An infection control concept that treats all bodily fluids as potentially infectious.

bounding pulse A strong pulse (similar to the pulse that follows physical exertion like running or lifting heavy objects).

brachial artery pressure point Pressure point located in the arm between the elbow and the shoulder; also used in taking blood pressure and for checking the pulse in infants.

brachial pulse Pulse located in the arm between the elbow and shoulder; used for checking pulse in infants.

breech presentation A delivery in which the baby's buttocks, arm, shoulder, or leg appears first rather than the head.

bronchi The two main branches of the windpipe that lead into the right and left lungs. Within the lungs, they branch into smaller airways.

bronchitis Inflammation of the airways in the lungs.

bruise Injury caused by a blunt object striking the body and crushing the tissue beneath the skin. Also called a contusion.

capillaries The smallest blood vessels that connect small arteries and small veins. Capillary walls serve as the membrane to exchange oxygen and carbon dioxide.

capillary bleeding Bleeding from the capillaries in which blood oozes from the open wound.

capillary refill The ability of the circulatory system to restore blood to the capillary blood vessels after it has been squeezed out by the examiner.

carbon dioxide (CO_2) The gas formed in respiration and exhaled in breathing.

carbon monoxide (CO) A colorless, odorless, poisonous gas formed by incomplete combustion, such as in a fire.

cardiac arrest Sudden cessation of heart function.

cardiogenic shock Shock resulting from inadequate functioning of the heart.

cardiopulmonary resuscitation (CPR) The artificial circulation of the blood and movement of air into and out of the lungs in a pulseless, nonbreathing patient.

carotid artery The principal arteries of the neck. They supply blood to the face, head, and brain.

carotid pulse A pulse that can be felt on each side of the neck where the carotid artery is close to the skin.

cartilage A tough, elastic form of connective tissue that covers the ends of most bones to form joints; also found in some specific areas such as the nose and the ears.

casualty sorting The sorting of patients for treatment and transportation.

central nervous system (CNS) The brain and spinal cord.

cerebrospinal fluid (CSF) A clear, watery, straw-colored fluid that fills the space between the brain and spinal cord and their protective coverings.

cervical collar A neck brace that partially stabilizes the neck following injury.

cervical spine That portion of the spinal column consisting of the seven vertebrae located in the neck.

chemical agents Compounds that can be used by terrorists to inflict harm.

chemical burns Burns that occur when any toxic substance comes in contact with the skin. Most chemical burns are caused by strong acids or alkalis.

chest compression Manual chest-pressing method that mimics the squeezing and relaxation cycles a normal heart goes through; administered to a person in cardiac arrest; also called external chest compression and closed-chest cardiac massage.

chest-thrust maneuver A series of manual thrusts to the chest to relieve upper airway obstruction; used in the treatment of infants, pregnant women, or extremely obese people.

chief complaint The patient's response to questions such as "What happened?" or "What's wrong?".

child Anyone between 1 year of age and the onset of puberty (12 to 14 years of age).

chocking A piece of wood or metal placed in front of or behind a wheel to prevent vehicle movement.

chronic obstructive pulmonary disease (COPD) A slow process of destruction of the airways, alveoli, and pulmonary blood vessels caused by chronic bronchial obstruction (emphysema).

circulatory system The heart and blood vessels, which together are responsible for the continuous flow of blood throughout the body.

clavicle The collarbone.

closed fracture A fracture in which the overlying skin has not been damaged.

closed head injury Injury where there is bleeding and/or swelling within the skull.

closed wound Injury in which soft-tissue damage occurs beneath the skin but there is no break in the surface of the skin.

clothes drag An emergency-patient move used to remove a patient from a hazardous environment; performed by grasping the patient's clothes and moving the patient head first from the unsafe area.

cocaine A powerful stimulant that induces an extreme state of euphoria. Legitimately, it is a potent local anesthetic. On the street, it is commonly known as coke. Synthetic cocaine is known as crack.

coccyx The tailbone; the small bone below the sacrum formed by the final four vertebrae.

coma A state of unconsciousness from which the patient cannot be aroused.

competent Able to make rational decisions about personal well-being.

congestive heart failure (CHF) Heart disease characterized by breathlessness, fluid retention in the lungs, and generalized swelling of the body.

contractions Muscular movements of the uterus that push the baby out of the mother.

cradle-in-arms carry A one-rescuer patient movement technique used primarily for children; the patient is cradled in the hollow formed by the rescuer's arms and chest.

cravat A triangular swathe of cloth that is used to hold a body part splinted against the body.

critical incident stress debriefing (CISD) A system of psychological support designed to reduce stress on emergency personnel after a major stress-producing incident.

croup Inflammation and narrowing of the air passages in young children, causing a barking cough, hoarseness, and a harsh, high-pitched breathing sound.

crowning Appearance of the baby's head during a contraction as it is pushed outward through the vagina.

cyanosis Bluish coloration of the skin resulting from poor oxygenation of the circulating blood.

decompression sickness (the bends) A condition seen in divers in which gas, especially nitrogen, forms bubbles in blood vessels obstructing them.

defibrillation Delivery of an electric current through a person's chest wall and heart for the purpose of ending lethal heart rhythms such as ventricular fibrillation.

delirium tremens (DTs) A severe, often fatal, complication of alcohol withdrawal that can occur from 1 to 7 days after withdrawal. It is characterized by restlessness, fever, sweating, confusion, disorientation, agitation, hallucinations, and convulsions.

dementia A progressive irreversible decline in mental functioning; marked by memory impairment and decrease in reasoning.

denial The first stage of a grief reaction; when the person suffering grief rejects the grief-causing event.

depression A psychiatric disorder marked by persistent feelings of sadness, hopelessness, and decreased interest in daily activities. The person may have persistent thoughts of suicide. Also, the fourth stage of the grief reaction; when the person expresses despair—an absence of cheerfulness and hope—as a result of the grief-causing event.

diabetes A disease in which the body is unable to use sugar normally because of a deficiency or total lack of insulin.

diabetic coma A state of unconsciousness that occurs when the body has too much sugar and not enough insulin.

diaphragm A muscular dome that separates the chest from the abdominal cavity. Contraction of the diaphragm and the chest wall muscles brings air into the lungs; relaxation expels air from the lungs.

diastolic pressure The measurement of pressure exerted against the walls of the arteries while the left ventricle of the heart is at rest.

digestive system The gastrointestinal tract (stomach and intestines), mouth, salivary glands, pharynx, esophagus, liver, gallbladder, pancreas, rectum, and anus, which together are responsible for the absorption of food and the elimination of solid waste from the body.

dislocation Disruption of a joint so that the bone ends are no longer in alignment.

distal Describing structures that are nearer to the free end of an extremity; any location that is farther from the midline than the point of reference named.

downers Depressants; barbiturates.

dressing A bandage.

drowning Submersion in water that results in suffocation or respiratory impairment.

duty to act A first responder's legal responsibility to respond promptly to an emergency scene and provide medical care (within the limits of training and available equipment).

dyspnea Difficulty or pain with breathing.

elder abuse An action taken by a family member or caregiver that results in the physical, emotional, or sexual harm to a person over 65 years of age.

electrical burns Burns caused by contact with high- or low-voltage electricity. Electrical wounds have an entrance and an exit wound.

emergency medical technician-basic (EMT-B) A person who is trained and certified to provide basic life support and certain other noninvasive prehospital medical procedures.

emergency services dispatch center A fire, police, or emergency medical services (EMS) agency; a 9-1-1 center; or a seven-digit telephone number used by one or all of the emergency agencies to receive and dispatch requests for emergency care.

emotional shock A state of shock caused by sudden illness, accident, or death of a loved one.

empathy The ability to participate in another person's feelings or ideas.

entrance wound Point where an injurious object such as a bullet enters the body.

epiglottis The valve located at the upper end of the voice box that prevents food from entering the larynx.

epiglottitis Severe inflammation and swelling of the epiglottis; a life-threatening situation.

epilepsy A disease manifested by seizures, caused by an abnormal focus of electrical activity in the brain.

esophagus The tube through which food passes. It starts at the throat and ends at the stomach.

exhalation Breathing out.

exit wound Point where an injurious object such as a bullet passes out of the body.

explosives Substances that release energy in a sudden and uncontrolled manner when detonated.

expressed consent Consent actually given by a person authorizing the first responder to provide care or transportation.

external cardiac compressions A means of applying artificial circulation by applying rhythmic pressure and relaxation on the lower half of the sternum.

externally rotated Rotated outward, as a fractured hip.

extremities The arms and legs.

extrication Removal from a difficult situation or position; removal of a patient from a wrecked car or other place of entrapment.

face mask A clear plastic mask used for oxygen administration that covers the mouth and nose.

fax machine A device used to send or receive printed text documents or images over a telephone or radio system.

femoral artery pressure point Pressure point located in the groin, where the femoral artery is close to the skin.

fetus A developing baby in the uterus or womb.

fire fighter drag A method of moving a patient without lifting or carrying him or her; used when the patient is heavier than the rescuer.

flail chest A condition that occurs when three or more ribs are each broken in two places, and the chest wall lying between the fractures becomes a free-floating segment.

floating ribs The eleventh and twelfth ribs, which do not connect to the sternum.

flotation device A life ring, life buoy, or other floating device used in water rescue.

flowmeter A device on oxygen cylinders used to control and measure the flow of oxygen.

forearm The lower portion of the upper extremity; from the elbow to the wrist.

fractures Breaks in a bone.

frostbite Partial or complete freezing of the skin and deeper tissues caused by exposure to the cold.

full-thickness burns Burns that extend through the skin and into or beyond the underlying tissues; the most serious class of burn.

fusees Warning devices or flares that burn with a red color; usually used in scene protection at motor vehicle crash sites.

gag reflex A strong involuntary effort to vomit caused by something being placed or caught in the throat.

gastric distention Inflation of the stomach caused when excessive pressures are used during artificial ventilation and air is directed into the stomach rather than the lungs.

generalized seizure A seizure characterized by contraction of all the body's muscle groups. May last for several minutes. Also known as a grand mal seizure.

genitourinary system The organs of reproduction, together with the organs involved in the production and excretion of urine.

geriatric patient A patient who is over 65 years of age.

golden hour A concept of emergency patient care that attempts to place a trauma patient into definitive medical care within 1 hour of injury.

Good Samaritan laws Laws that encourage individuals to voluntarily help an injured or suddenly ill person by minimizing the liability for any errors or omissions in rendering good-faith emergency care.

gunshot wound A puncture wound caused by a bullet or shotgun pellet.

hallucinogens Chemicals that cause a person to see visions or hear sounds that are not real.

hazardous materials (HazMat) Substances that are toxic, poisonous, radioactive, flammable, or explosive and can cause injury or death with exposure.

head tilt–chin lift technique Opening the airway by tilting the patient's head backward and lifting the chin forward, bringing the entire lower jaw with it.

heat exhaustion A form of shock that occurs when the body loses too much water and too many electrolytes through very heavy sweating after exposure to heat.

heatstroke A condition of rapidly rising internal body temperature that occurs when the body's mechanisms for the release of heat are overwhelmed. Untreated heatstroke can result in death.

Heimlich maneuver A series of manual thrusts to the abdomen to relieve an upper airway obstruction.

hemorrhage Excessive bleeding.

hives An allergic skin disorder marked by patches of swelling, redness, and intense itching.

hospice An interdisciplinary program designed to reduce or eliminate pain and address the physical, spiritual, social, and economic needs of terminally ill patients.

hot zone A contaminated area.

humerus The upper arm bone.

hypertension High blood pressure.

hypotension Lowered blood pressure.

hypothermia A condition in which the internal body temperature falls below 95°F after prolonged exposure to cool or freezing temperatures.

immobilize To reduce or prevent movement of a limb, usually by splinting.

impaled object An object such as a knife, splinter of wood, or glass that penetrates the skin and remains in the body.

implied consent Consent to receive emergency care that is assumed because the individual is unconscious, underage, or so badly injured or ill that he or she cannot respond.

incubation period The time from exposure to a disease organism to the time the person begins to show symptoms of the disease.

infant Anyone under 1 year of age.

inferior That portion of the body or body part that lies nearer the feet than the head.

inhalation Breathing in.

initial patient assessment The first actions taken to form an impression of the patient's condition; to determine the patient's responsiveness and introduce yourself to the patient; to check the patient's airway, breathing, and circulation; and to acknowledge the patient's chief complaint.

insecticides Chemicals that are formulated to kill insects, but can intentionally or accidentally cause injury or death to humans.

insulin A hormone produced by the pancreas that enables sugar in the blood to be used by the cells of the body; supplementary insulin is used in the treatment and control of diabetes mellitus.

insulin shock Condition that occurs in a diabetic who has taken too much insulin or has not eaten enough food.

intravenous (IV) fluids Fluids other than blood or blood products infused into the vascular system to maintain an adequate circulatory blood volume.

jaw-thrust technique Opening the airway by bringing the patient's jaw forward without extending the neck.

joint The place where two bones come in contact with each other.

labor The process of delivering a baby.

laceration An irregular cut or tear through the skin.

larynx A structure composed of cartilage in the neck that guards the entrance to the windpipe and functions as the organ of voice; also called the voicebox.

lateral Away from the midline of the body.

leg The lower extremity; specifically, the lower portion, from the knee to the ankle.

ligaments Fibrous bands that connect bones to bones and support and strengthen joints.

log rolling A technique used to move a patient onto a long backboard.

lumbar spine The lower part of the back formed by the lowest five nonfused vertebrae.

lungs The organs that supply the body with oxygen and eliminate carbon dioxide from the blood.

mandible The lower jaw.

manual suction devices Hand-powered devices used for clearing the upper airway of mucus, blood, or vomitus.

mechanical suction device An electrically or battery-powered device used for clearing the upper airway of mucus, blood, or vomitus.

mechanism of injury The means by which a traumatic injury occurs.

medial Toward the midline of the body.

metabolic agents Substances that are intended to produce injury or death by disrupting chemical reactions at the cellular level.

midline An imaginary vertical line drawn from the mid-forehead through the nose and the navel to the floor.

miscarriage Delivery of the fetus before it is mature enough to survive outside the womb (about 20 weeks), from either natural (spontaneous abortion) or induced causes.

mobile data terminal (MDT) A computer terminal mounted in a vehicle that sends and receives data through a radio communication system.

mobile radio A two-way radio that is permanently mounted in a vehicle such as a police car or fire truck.

mottling Patchy skin discoloration caused by too little or too much circulation.

mouth-to-mask ventilation device A piece of equipment that consists of a mask, a one-way valve, and a mouthpiece. Rescue breathing is performed by breathing into the mouthpiece after placing the mask over the patient's mouth and nose.

mouth-to-stoma breathing Rescue breathing for patients who, because of surgical removal of the larynx, have a stoma.

multiple-casualty incidents (mass-casualty incidents) Accidents or situations involving more patients than you can handle with the initial resources available.

nasal airway An airway adjunct that is inserted into the nostril of a patient who is not able to maintain a natural airway. It is also called a nasopharyngeal airway.

nasal cannula A clear plastic tube used to deliver oxygen that fits onto the patient's nose.

nasopharynx The posterior part of the nose.

National Incident Management System (NIMS) The structure for managing an emergency incident, which may require a response of many different agencies; designed to provide efficient and effective management from initial response through recovery.

negligence Deviation from the accepted standard of care resulting in further injury to the patient.

nerve agents Toxic substances that attack the central nervous system.

nerves Fiber tracts or pathways that carry messages from the spinal cord and brain to all body parts and back; sensory, motor, or a combination of both.

nervous system The brain, spinal cord, and nerves.

nitroglycerin A medication used to treat angina pectoris; it increases blood flow and oxygen supply to the heart muscle and reduces or eliminates the pain of angina pectoris.

occlusive dressing An airtight dressing or bandage for a wound.

one-person walking assist A method used if the patient is able to bear his or her own weight.

one-rescuer CPR Cardiopulmonary resuscitation performed by one rescuer.

on-scene peer support Stress counselors at the scene of stressful incidents to deal with stress reduction.

open fracture Any fracture in which the overlying skin has been damaged.

open wound Injury that breaks the skin or mucous membrane.

oral airway An airway adjunct that is inserted into the mouth to keep the tongue from blocking the upper airway. It is also called an oropharyngeal or nasopharyngeal airway.

oropharynx The posterior part of the mouth.

osteoporosis Abnormal brittleness of the bones in older people caused by loss of calcium; affected bones fracture easily.

oxygen (O_2) A colorless, odorless gas that is essential for life.

pack-strap carry A one-person carry that allows the rescuer to carry a patient while keeping one hand free.

paging systems Communications systems used to send voice or text messages over a radio system to specially designed radio receivers.

palpation To examine by touch.

paralysis Inability of a conscious person to move voluntarily.

paramedics Emergency medical technicians who have completed an extensive course of 800 or more hours, successfully passed a national or state certification, and who can perform advanced life support skills.

partial-thickness burns Burns in which the outer layers of skin are burned; these burns are characterized by blister formation.

pathogens Microorganisms that are capable of causing disease.

pediatric assessment triangle (PAT) An assessment tool that measures the severity of a child's illness or injury by evaluating the child's appearance, work of breathing, and circulation to the skin.

pelvis The closed bony ring, consisting of the sacrum and the pelvic bones, that connects the trunk to the lower extremities.

physical examination The step in the patient assessment sequence in which the first responder carefully examines the patient from head to toe, looking for additional injuries and other problems.

placenta Life-support system of the baby during its time inside the mother (commonly called the afterbirth).

plasma The fluid part of the blood that carries blood cells, transports nutrients, and removes cellular waste materials.

platelets Microscopic disk-shaped elements in the blood that are essential to the process of blood clot formation; the mechanism that stops bleeding.

pneumatic antishock garments (PASGs) Trouser-like devices placed around a shock victim's legs and abdomen and inflated with air.

pocket mask A mechanical breathing device used to administer mouth-to-mask rescue breathing.

poison Any substance that may cause injury or death if relatively small amounts are ingested, inhaled, or absorbed, or applied to, or injected into the body.

portable radio A hand-held, battery-operated, two-way radio.

portable stretcher A lightweight nonwheeled device for transporting a patient; used in small spaces where the wheeled ambulance stretcher cannot be used.

posterior The back surface of the body.

posterior tibial pulse Ankle pulse.

preincident stress education Training about stress and stress reactions conducted for public safety providers before they are exposed to stressful situations.

premature babies Babies who deliver before 37 weeks of gestation or who weigh less than 5½ pounds at birth.

pressure points Points where a blood vessel lies near a bone; pressure can be applied to these points to help control bleeding.

prolapse of the umbilical cord A delivery in which the umbilical cord appears before the baby does; the baby's head may compress the cord and cut off all circulation to the baby.

proximal Describing structures that are closer to the trunk.

psychogenic shock Commonly known as fainting; caused by a temporary reduction in blood supply to the brain.

psychotic behavior Mental disturbance characterized by defective or lost contact with reality.

pulmonary agent Substances that produce respiratory distress or illness.

pulse oximeter A machine that consists of a monitor and a sensor probe that measures the oxygen saturation in the capillary beds.

pulse oximetry An assessment tool that measures oxygen saturation in the capillary beds.

pulse The wave of pressure that is created by the heart as it contracts and forces blood out of the heart and into the major arteries.

puncture A wound resulting from a bullet, knife, ice pick, splinter, or any other pointed object.

pupils The circular openings in the middle of the eyes.

rabies An acute viral infection of the central nervous system transmitted by the bite of an infected animal.

radial pulse Wrist pulse.

radiation The electromagnetic energy that is released from a radioactive material or a dirty bomb.

radius The bone on the thumb side of the forearm.

reach-throw-row-go A four-step reminder of the sequence of actions that should be taken in water rescue situations.

recovery position A sidelying position that helps an unconscious patient maintain an open airway.

redirection A means of focusing the patient's attention on the immediate situation or crisis.

repeater A radio system that automatically retransmits a radio signal on a different frequency.

rescue breathing Artificial means of breathing for a patient.

respiratory arrest Sudden stoppage of breathing.

respiratory burn Burn to the respiratory system resulting from inhaling superheated air.

respiratory rate The speed at which a person is breathing (measured in breaths per minute).

respiratory system All body structures that contribute to normal breathing.

restatement Rephrasing a patient's own statement to show that he or she is being heard and understood by the rescuer.

ribs The paired arches of bone, 12 on either side, that extend from the thoracic vertebrae toward the anterior midline of the trunk.

rigid splints Splints made from firm materials such as wood, aluminum, or plastic.

riptides Unusually strong surface currents flowing outward from a seashore that can carry swimmers "out to sea."

road rash An abrasion caused by sliding on pavement. Usually seen after motorcycle or bicycle accidents.

Rule of Nines A way to calculate the amount of body surface burned; the body is divided into sections, each of which constitutes approximately 9% or 18% of the total body surface area.

sacrum One of three bones (sacrum and two pelvic bones) that make up the pelvic ring; forms the base of the spine.

saline Salt water.

SAMPLE history A patient's medical history. The letters stand for Signs/symptoms, Allergies, Medications, Pertinent past history, Last oral intake, Events associated with the illness or injury.

scoop stretcher A firm patient-carrying device that can be split into halves and applied to the patient from both sides.

seizures Sudden episodes of uncontrolled electrical activity in the brain.

self-contained breathing apparatus (SCBA) A complete unit for delivery of air to a rescuer who enters a contaminated area; contains a mask, regulator, and air supply.

senile dementia General term for dementia that occurs in older people.

shock A state of collapse of the cardiovascular system; the state of inadequate delivery of blood to the organs of the body.

shoulder girdles The proximal portions of the upper extremity; each is made up of the clavicle, the scapula, and the humerus.

sign A condition that you observe in a patient, such as bleeding or the temperature of a patient's skin.

situational crisis A state of emotional upset or turmoil caused by a sudden and disruptive event.

skull The bones of the head, collectively; serves as the protective structure for the brain.

sling A bandage or material that helps to support the weight of an injured upper extremity.

soft splint A splint made from supple material that provides gentle support.

splint A means of immobilizing an injured part by using a rigid or soft support.

spontaneous nosebleed A nosebleed with no apparent cause.

sprain A joint injury in which the joint is partially or temporarily dislocated and some of the supporting ligaments are either stretched or torn.

stair chair A small portable device used for transporting patients in a sitting position.

standard of care The manner in which an individual must act or behave when giving care.

START system A system of casualty sorting using Simple Triage And Rapid Treatment.

sternum The breastbone.

stoma An opening in the neck that connects the windpipe (trachea) to the skin.

straddle lift A method used to place a patient on a backboard if there is not enough space to perform a log roll.

straddle slide A method of placing a patient on a long backboard by straddling both the board and patient and sliding the patient onto the board.

suctioning Aspirating (sucking out) fluid by mechanical means.

suicide Intentionally causing one's own death. Suicide is especially common in elderly and chronically ill persons.

superficial burns Burns in which only the superficial part of the skin has been injured; an example is a sunburn.

superior Toward the head; lying higher in the body.

symptom A condition the patient tells you, such as "I feel dizzy."

systolic pressure The measurement of blood pressure exerted against the walls of the arteries during contraction of the heart.

telemetry A process in which electronic signals are transmitted and received by radio or telephone; commonly used for sending EKG tracings.

tempered glass Safety glass that breaks into small pieces when hit with a sharp, pointed object.

tendons Tough, rope-like cords of fibrous tissue that attach muscles to bones.

terrorism A systematic use of violence to intimidate or to achieve a goal.

thermal burns Burns caused by heat; the most common type of burn.

thoracic spine The 12 vertebrae that attach to the 12 ribs; the upper part of the back.

thready pulse A weak pulse.

topographic anatomy The superficial landmarks on the body that serve as location guides to the structures that lie beneath them.

toxic Poisonous.

trachea The windpipe.

traction splint A splint that holds a lower extremity fracture (PSDE) in alignment by applying a constant, steady pull on the extremity.

trauma A wound or injury, either physical or psychological.

triage The sorting of patients into groups according to the severity of their injuries; used to determine priorities for treatment and transport.

two-person chair carry Two rescuers use a chair to support the weight of the patient.

two-person extremity carry A method of carrying a patient out of tight quarters using two rescuers and no equipment.

two-person seat carry A method of carrying a patient in which two rescuers link arms behind the patient's back and under the patient's knees; requires no equipment.

two-person walking assist Used when a patient cannot bear his or her own weight; two rescuers completely support the patient.

two-rescuer CPR Cardiopulmonary resuscitation performed by two rescuers.

ulna The bone on the little-finger side of the forearm.

umbilical cord Rope-like attachment between the mother and baby; nourishment and waste products pass to and from the baby and the mother through this cord.

universal precautions Procedures for infection control that treat blood and certain bodily fluids as capable of transmitting bloodborne diseases.

uppers Drugs that stimulate the central nervous system. These include amphetamines and cocaine.

uterus (womb) Muscular organ that holds and nourishes the developing baby.

vagina The opening through which the baby emerges.

venous bleeding External bleeding from a vein, characterized by steady flow; the bleeding may be profuse and life threatening.

ventilations The movement of air in and out of the lungs.

ventricles The two lower chambers of the heart.

ventricular fibrillation An uncoordinated muscular quivering of the heart; the most common abnormal rhythm causing cardiac arrest.

vertebrae The 33 bones of the spinal column: 7 cervical, 12 thoracic, 5 lumbar, 5 sacral, and 4 coccygeal vertebrae.

vital signs Signs of life, specifically pulse, respiration, blood pressure, and temperature.

weapon of mass destruction (WMD) Any agent designed to bring about mass death, casualties, and/or massive damage to property and infrastructure (bridges, tunnels, airports, electrical power plants, and seaports).

wooden cribbing Wooden 2- × 4-inch or 4- × 4-inch boards used for stabilization or bracing.

xiphoid process The flexible cartilage at the lower tip of the sternum.

Index

NOTE: Page numbers followed by *f* or *t* indicate figures and tables respectively.

Photo Credits

Section 1

Opener © Glen E. Ellman

Chapter 1

Opener © Mark C. Ide; 1-1 © Keith Muratori/
ShutterStock, Inc.; 1-6B © Alfred Wekelo/ShutterStock,
Inc.; 1-8 © Jacqueline Shaw/Shutterstock, Inc.

Chapter 2

Opener © Steven Townsend/Code 3 Images; 2-2, 2-3
Courtesy of USDA; 2-7 Courtesy of Kimberly Smith/CDC;
2-9A © NDP/Alamy Images; 2-9B © Fancy
Photography/Veer

Chapter 3

Opener © Jim Ruymen/Reuters/Landov; 3-3 © Damian
Dovarganes/AP Photos; 3-4 © Bob Child/AP Photos

Chapter 4

Opener © Comstock Images/Jupiterimages

Chapter 5

Opener © Mark C. Ide

Chapter 6

Opener © Keith Srakocic/AP Photos

Section 3

Opener © Glen E. Ellman

Chapter 7

Opener © Glen E. Ellman; 7-2 © Dale A. Stork/
ShutterStock, Inc.; 7-17 Courtesy of the MedicAlert
Foundation®. © 2006, All Rights Reserved. MedicAlert® is
a federally registered trademark and service mark.

Chapter 8

Opener © Photodisc/Getty Images; 8-4 © Mark C. Ide;
8-8 Photographed by Kimberly Potvin

Chapter 9

Opener © Eddie Sperling; 9-4 Source: American Heart
Association

Section 5

Opener © Seth Gottfried/On Scene Photography

Chapter 11

Opener © Stockbyte Platinum/Getty Images; 11-5
Courtesy of Lynn Betts/NRCS; 11-6 Courtesy of Scott
Health & Safety; 11-7 © Michael Ledray/ShutterStock,
Inc.; 11-8 © Photos.com

Chapter 12

12-1 © LiquidLibrary; 12-5 © DigitalVues/Alamy Images

Chapter 13

Opener © Glen E. Ellman; 13-17A © Kiryay/
ShutterStock, Inc.; 13-39 © Suzanne Tucker/
ShutterStock, Inc.

Chapter 14

Opener © Glen E. Ellman; 14-6B © Charles Stewart and
Associates; 14-20 © E.M. Singletary, MD. Used with
permission.

Chapter 16

Opener © Eddie Sperling; 16-2 © Craig Jackson/
IntheDarkPhotography.com; 16-17C Courtesy of Ronald
Dieckman, MD

Chapter 17

Opener © Glen E. Ellman; 17-1 © Photodisc; 17-3
Courtesy of Guide Dog Foundation of the Blind, Inc.
(www.guidedog.org); 17-5A Courtesy of Pulmonetic
Systems; 17-5B Courtesy of Bard Access Systems; 17-8
© Ian Scott/ShutterStock, Inc.

Section 7

Opener © Corbis

Chapter 18

Opener © Glen E. Ellman; 18-2 Courtesy of Duke Life
Flight; 18-4 Courtesy of District Chief Chris E.
Mickal/New Orleans Fire Department, Photo Unit; 18-5
© Jack Dagley/ShutterStock, Inc.; 18-6 Courtesy of
Captain David Jackson, Saginaw Township Fire
Department; 18-14 © Glen E. Ellman; 18-15, 18-16, 18-
17 © U.S. Department of Transportation; 18-18 © David
Crigger, *Bristol Herald Courier*/AP Photos

Chapter 19

Opener Courtesy of Andrea Booher/FEMA; 19-1A
© Susan Tansil/ShutterStock, Inc.; 19-1B © Steve
Allen/Brand X Pictures/Alamy Images; 19-1C
© phdpsx/ShutterStock, Inc.; 19-1D © Galina Barskaya/
ShutterStock, Inc.; 19-2 Courtesy of Captain David
Jackson, Saginaw Township Fire Department; 19-3
Courtesy of Atomtex Scientific and Production Enterprise
(www.atomtex.com)

Section 8

Opener © Jeff Greenberg/PhotoEdit

Chapter 20

Opener © Robert Lahser, *The Charlotte Observer*/AP
Photos; 20-6A © Lynne Furrer/ShutterStock, Inc.; 20-6B
© Harris Shiffman/ShutterStock, Inc.; 20-6C © Joe
Gough/ShutterStock, Inc.; 20-7 © Nancy Hixson/
ShutterStock, Inc.; 20-8 Courtesy of Lynn Betts/NRCS
USDA; 20-9 © Dena Libner, *The Conway Daily Sun*/AP
Photos

Chapter 21

Opener © Glen E. Ellman

Unless otherwise indicated, photographs are under copyright
of Jones and Bartlett Publishers, courtesy of Maryland
Institute of Emergency Medical Services Systems, or the
Academy of Orthopaedic Surgeons.